PATIENT-BASED APPROACHES
TO COGNITIVE NEUROSCIENCE

ISSUES IN CLINICAL AND COGNITIVE NEUROPSYCHOLOGY

Jordan Grafman, series editor

Patient-Based Approaches to Cognitive Neuroscience
Martha J. Farah and Todd E. Feinberg, editors

Gateway to Memory: An Introduction to Neural Network Modeling of the Hippocampus and Learning
Mark A. Gluck and Catherine E. Myers

Neurological Foundations of Cognitive Neuroscience
Mark D'Esposito, editor

The Parallel Brain: The Cognitive Neuroscience of the Corpus Callosum
Eran Zaidel and Marco Iacoboni, editors

Fatigue as a Window to the Brain
John DeLuca, editor

Patient-Based Approaches to Cognitive Neuroscience
second edition
Martha J. Farah and Todd E. Feinberg, editors

PATIENT-BASED APPROACHES TO COGNITIVE NEUROSCIENCE

Second Edition

edited by
Martha J. Farah
Todd E. Feinberg

The MIT Press
Cambridge, Massachusetts
London, England

An abridged version of *Behavioral Neurology and Neuropsychology, Second Edition,* published by McGraw-Hill, New York, in 2003.

MIT Press books may be purchased at special quantity discounts for business or sales promotional use. For information, please email special_sales@mitpress.mit.edu or write to Special Sales Department, The MIT Press, 55 Hayward Street, Cambridge, MA 02142.

This book was set in Helvetica and Times. *10 0673374 2*
Printed and bound in the United States of America.

Library of Congress Cataloging-in-Publication Data

Patient-based approaches to cognitive neuroscience /edited by Martha J. Farah and Todd
E. Feinberg.—2nd ed.
    p. cm.—(Issues in clinical and cognitive neuropsychology)
Includes bibliographical references and index.
ISBN 0-262-56213-8 (alk. paper)
1. Clinical neuropsychology. 2. Cognitive neuroscience. I. Farah, Martha J. II. Feinberg, Todd E. III. Series.

RC341.B4242   2005
616.8—dc22
                                                2005045102

10 9 8 7 6 5 4 3 2 1

CONTENTS

PREFACE

Twenty years ago, a behavioral neurology fellow in Gainesville called a cognitive science postdoc in Boston to discuss mental imagery in neurology patients. The conversation lasted well over an hour—or perhaps we should say it has lasted 20 years, with the parties on each end of the line moving from Gainesville to New York and from Boston to Pittsburgh to Philadelphia.

In addition to whopping phone bills, several collaborative projects resulted from this relationship. Among them was the McGraw-Hill textbook *Behavioral Neurology and Neuropsychology,* edited by Todd and Martha, now in its second edition and weighing in at a hefty 69 chapters. Some of these chapters focus on clinical concerns (when should you shunt for normal pressure hydrocephalus in the elderly?), while others address basic questions of cognitive neuroscience with evidence from neurological patients. Although scientifically minded clinicians appreciate the combination of approaches, there are many other readers out there with an interest in patient-based approaches to cognitive neuroscience who have never pondered when to shunt. For these readers, we reedited the book to produce *Patient-Based Approaches to Cognitive Neuroscience.*

The first edition of *Patient-Based Approaches to Cognitive Neuroscience* was published in 2000 with the following inscribed on its back cover: "Although cognitive neuroscience is sometimes equated with cognitive neuroimaging, the patient-based approach to cognitive neuroscience is responsible for most of what we now know about the brain systems underlying perception, attention, memory, language, and higher order forms of thought including consciousness." While imaging continues to attract the attention of scientists and the public, the intervening years have seen renewed interest in complementary approaches to studying the brain, including transcranial magnetic stimulation (TMS), genetic analyses, and patient-based approaches. The integration of these different approaches is our best bet for continued progress in cognitive neuroscience.

The trend toward a broader methodological base for cognitive neuroscience is apparent in the second edition of *Patient-Based Approaches.* In addition to the updated coverage of perception, attention, memory, language, executive function, and development, the new edition includes expanded material on functional neuroimaging of normal subjects and of neurological patients, electrophysiological methods including TMS, and the genetics of neurocognitive disorders.

In closing, we want to thank the many different people who contributed to making the second edition of *Patient-Based Approaches* even better than the first: the chapter authors, the editorial staff at McGraw-Hill and MIT Press, and in particular Barbara Murphy of MIT Press.

Part I

HISTORY AND METHODS

Chapter 1

A HISTORICAL PERSPECTIVE ON COGNITIVE NEUROSCIENCE

Todd E. Feinberg
Martha J. Farah

ANTIQUITY THROUGH THE EIGHTEENTH CENTURY

The most fundamental fact of cognitive neuroscience was established in ancient times, when the Greeks first determined that the brain was the physical seat of the mind. Alcamaeon of Croton, who may have been a student of Pythagoras, is credited with making this basic advance in the fifth century B.C. on the basis of his observations of human patients with brain damage. The alternative hypothesis held the heart to be the organ responsible for sensation and thought. This was the accepted view among Egyptian writers and continued to attract adherents in ancient Greece centuries after Alcamaeon. Although Hippocrates and Plato held a cerebrocentric view of the mind, no less a thinker than Aristotle remained in the cardiocentric camp.

Among the ancient cerebrocentrists, the nature of the mind-brain relation was poorly understood. The brain itself was considered by many to be a mere package for the real substance of thought, the cerebrospinal fluid, and the most important anatomical features of the brain were therefore the ventricles. Although brain tissue itself was considered important by some writers, including Galen, for many centuries the mind was predominantly identified with cerebrospinal fluid. The present-day use of the word *spirit* to refer both to certain fluids and to the soul is vestige of this idea.

For the entire period of the middle ages in Europe (approximately the fourth to fourteenth centuries), the ventricles continued to be the focus of theories relating mind and brain.[1] For example, according to fourth-century church fathers, the anterior ventricles were associated with perception (later to be known as the *sensorium commune*), the middle with reason, and the posterior with memory.[2] It has been suggested that this focus on the ventricles accorded better with the dualism of Christian theology, as the hollow cavities could be said to contain the soul without hypothesizing an identity between mind and the physical substrate of brain tissue.[1] Figure 1-1 shows an early illustration of the ventricular system.

During the Renaissance, the ventricular doctrine and the role of the *rete mirabile* began to lose their influence on theories of mind-brain relations.[2,3,4] The seventeenth-century writings of René Descartes mark a transitional phase, in which the interaction between fluid in the ventricles and brain tissue itself was hypothesized to explain intelligent action, as shown in Fig. 1-2. For reflexive action, Descartes proposed a simple loop, in which stimulated nerves caused the release of animal spirits in the ventricles, which, in turn, caused efferent nerves and muscles to act. For intelligent human action, this loop was modulated by the soul via its effects on the pineal gland. The pineal gland was chosen in part because it is unpaired and centrally located and also because it is surrounded by cerebrospinal fluid. It was also mistakenly thought to be uniquely human. Of course, the pineal gland was just the vehicle for the mind's influence on the body; Descartes' theory still denied any form of identity between the mind and neural tissue.[3,5-8]

Descartes' theory was formulated at a time when neuroanatomic knowledge was quite primitive. This situation began to change with the work of such figures as Thomas Willis later in the seventeenth century[3,10] and Malpighi Pacchioni and Albrecht von Haller in the eighteenth.[11,12] For example, Von Haller stimulated the nerves of live animals in an effort to discover the pathways for perception and motor action, thus establishing the experimental method in neurophysiology. This work set the stage for the explosion of experimental and clinical research of the nineteenth century, in which the brain organization underlying perception, action, language, and many other cognitive functions was revealed.

THE LOCALISM/HOLISM DEBATE OF THE NINETEENTH CENTURY

One of the more notorious figures in the history of behavioral neurology is Franz Josef Gall, shown in Fig. 1-3. In the late eighteenth and early nineteenth centuries, he and his collaborator Johann Spurzheim made a number of important contributions to functional neuroanatomy, including proving by dissection the crossing of the pyramids and establishing the distinction between gray and white matter.[13-15] Gall is also credited with one of the earliest descriptions of aphasia linked to a lesion of the frontal lobes.[16] He is most famous, however, for his general theory of cerebral localization, known today as phrenology. At the age of 9, Gall had noted that his schoolmates who excelled at rote memory tasks had quite prominent eyes, *"les yeux à fleur de tête"* (cow's eyes). He reasoned that this was the result of the overdevelopment of the subjacent regions of the brain, and speculated that these regions of the brain might be particularly involved in language functions and especially verbal memory.

Gall identified 27 basic human faculties and associated them with particular brain centers that could affect the shape of the skull, as shown in Fig.

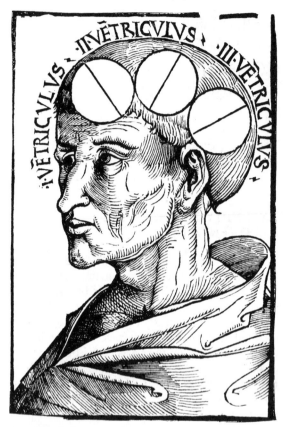

Figure 1-1
The ventricular system according to Albertus Magnus from his Philosophia naturalis (1506).[2]

1–4. These included memory of things and facts, sense of spatial relations, vanity, God and religion, and love for one's offspring.[15] His theory was based on hundreds of skulls and casts of humans and beasts. For instance, the disposition to murder and cruelty was based on a bump above the ear possessed by carnivorous animals. He located the same feature in sadistic persons whom he had examined personally,[3] skulls of famous criminals, and the busts and paintings of famous murderers.[12] Gall taught and practiced medicine in Vienna from 1781 to around 1802, until Emperor Francis I banned Gall's public lectures because they were materialistic and thus opposed to morality and religion.[12] Gall then took to the road,

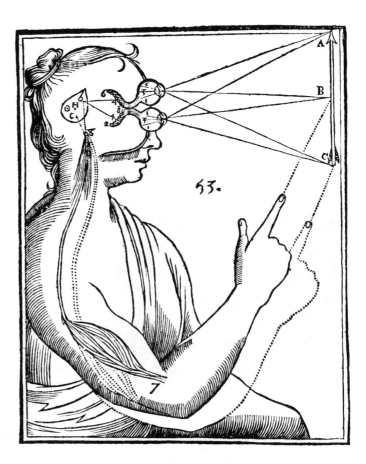

Figure 1-2
Descartes' conception of sensation and action as conceived in his De homine *(1662). Light was transferred from the retina to the ventricles, causing the release of animal spirits. The pineal gland modulated this mechanism for voluntary action.*[9]

lecturing across Europe to enthusiastic popular audiences. By the time he settled in Paris in 1807, he was hugely popular and internationally known. However, phrenology continued to create controversy in scientific circles.

The best-known critic of Gall was Marie-Jean-Pierre Flourens. Flourens mounted a scientific research program to disprove Gall's theory, but it appears to have been motivated at least as much by religious discomfort with the implications of Gall's straightforward mind-brain equivalences as by scientific considerations. Flourens viewed Gall's theory as tantamount to denying the existence of the soul, because it divided the mind and brain into functionally distinct parts and Flourens believed the soul to be unitary.[12,17–19] He carried out extensive lesion experiments on a variety of animal species to demonstrate the equipotentiality of cortex.

Gall's status as a popularizer, and Flourens's empirical attacks, helped to push localism out of the mainstream of contemporary scientific thought in the early nineteenth century. When, in 1825, Jean-Baptiste Bouillaud, shown in Fig. 1-5, presented a large series of clinical cases of loss of speech following frontal lesions,[12,18,19] his work was largely ignored. This landmark work, in which speech per se was distinguished from nonspeech movements of the mouth and tongue, is still relatively unknown.

Bouillaud was not the only one to suggest a frontal location for language functions. During this period and lasting up to the 1860s, numerous clinical reports of patients with frontal lobe

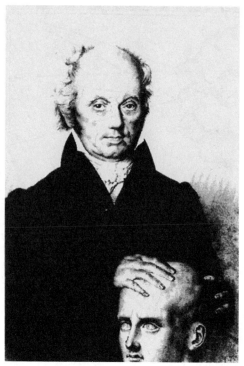

Figure 1-3
Franz Josef Gall (1758–1828).

reported his clinical observations of a patient whose frontal bone was removed following a suicide attempt. He reported that when the blade of a spatula was applied to the "anterior lobes," there was complete cessation of speech without loss of consciousness.[3,12,25] Aubertin went on to describe a patient of Bouillaud's who had a speech disturbance and was near death. Aubertin boldly vowed if this patient lacked a frontal lesion he would renounce his views.[12,24–27]

The 1861 debate is best known not for the presentations of Gratiolet and Aubertin but for the eventual participation of the society's founder and secretary, Paul Broca, shown in Fig. 1-7. Although Broca did not initially take a strong position, his observations of a patient then under his care led him to play a pivotal role in the debate. His patient, Leborgne, suffered from epilepsy,

Figure 1-4
An example of a porcelain phrenology bust with demarcations that demonstrate the reflection of the human faculties on the skull. (Photograph courtesy of Joseph A. Hefta.)

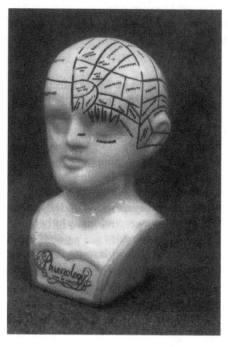

damage and loss of speech were recorded in Europe and America. Indeed, this idea had considerable historical precedence throughout antiquity.[20–22] However, intense interest in localization of brain functions, particularly language, was now developing. It was during this time that Marc Dax noted the association between left-hemispheric damage, right hemiplegia, and aphasia, based upon his examination of 40 patients over a 20-year period. This paper was handwritten in 1836 and not published at the time,[23] but copies may have been distributed to friends and colleagues.[3]

It was not until 1861 that the field reconsidered localism with a more open mind. That year the Société d'Anthropologie in Paris held a series of debates between Pierre Gratiolet, arguing in favor of holism or equipotentiality, and Ernest Aubertin, the son-in-law of Bouillaud, arguing in favor of localism.[12,24,25] Aubertin, shown in Fig. 1-6,

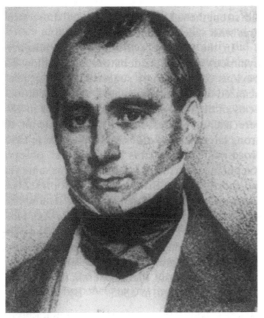

Figure 1-5
Jean-Baptiste Bouillaud (1796–1881).

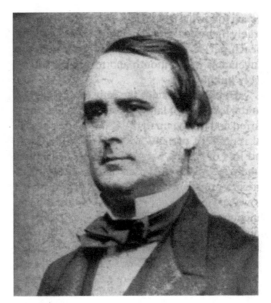

Figure 1-6
Ernest Aubertin (1825–1865).

Figure 1-7
Paul Broca (1824–1880).

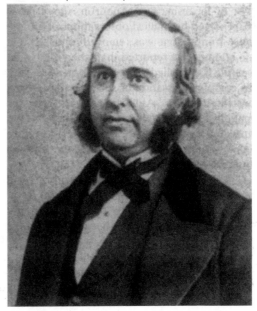

right hemiplegia, and loss of speech, the last for a period of over 20 years. Leborgne had been institutionalized for some 31 years and throughout the hospital was known by the name "Tan," as this was his only utterance along with a few obscenities.[3,9] In light of Aubertin's declaration, Broca invited him to examine Tan, which Aubertin did and afterward concluded that indeed the patient met the critieria of his prior challenge. Six days later Leborgne died; the following day, April 18, 1961, Broca presented the brain to the society along with a brief statement but without firm conclusions.[25] Figure 1-8 shows the brain of Leborgne.

Four months later, at a meeting of the Société Anatomique de Paris in August, Broca made a more extensive report. The brain of Leborgne had demonstrated an egg-sized fluid-filled cavity located in the posterior second and third frontal convolutions, with involvement of adjacent structures as well, including the corpus striatum.[36] In this report, Broca claimed that his findings would "support the ideas of M. Bouillaud on the seat of

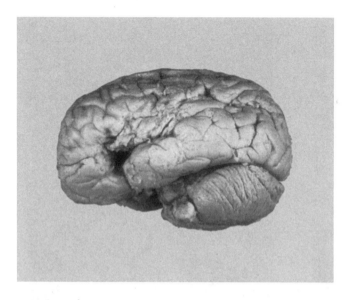

Figure 1-8
Photograph of the brain of Broca's first patient, Leborgne ("Tan"). It is now housed in the Musée Dupuytren.

the faculty for language";[25,28] he later suggested a possible localization of speech functions to the second or more probably third frontal convolution. Later the same year, Broca presented another patient with speech disturbance, an 84-year-old laborer whose lesion also involved the left second and third frontal convolutions. The lesion was more circumscribed than that found in Leborgne and strengthened the association of those structures with speech localization.

In the mid-1860s the issue of hemispheric asymmetry entered the debate on localization. The previous cases strongly suggested that speech is localized to the left hemisphere, and an additional series of eight cases published by Broca in 1863 were exclusively left-sided.[3,23,29] In spite of the strong lateralization of lesion locus in these cases, Broca made note of this "remarkable" observation but made no further claims.[23] In this same year and shortly before Broca's paper was presented,[3] Gustave Dax, son of Marc Dax, sent a handwritten copy of his father's manuscript to the Académie de Médecine in Paris. In this document, Marc Dax had previously described his view on the relation between speech and the left hemisphere. The paper was read before the Académie in December 1864 and published in 1865.[30,31] By

1865, Broca clearly expressed the opinion that the left hemisphere played a dominant role in speech production.[32,33] As far as the issue of priority of discovery is concerned (a matter of controversy among historians), most writers agree that the Dax paper in its original form in 1836 had no influence on Broca or the scientific community when first written. This paper did, however, make clear the association of language functions and the left hemisphere. While Broca alone clarified the role of the second and third frontal convolutions, he apparently did not take a firm position on the specific role of the left hemisphere until after the Dax paper was read before the Académie de Médecine in Paris in December 1964.[3] It appears that the reemergence of the Dax manuscript and Broca's discovery were nearly simultaneous events.

THE AFTERMATH OF 1861: THE EMERGENCE OF MODERN NEUROPSYCHOLOGY

The events in Paris in the 1860s constituted a turning point in the history of ideas regarding brain function. The concepts and methods developed in the course of debating the localization of speech were extended to a variety of different higher functions, experimental work on animals also developed apace. From this period onward, it is impossible to trace a single line of scientific development. Here we simply present a summary of some of the major advances seen in the behavioral neurology and neuropsychology of the late nineteenth and early twentieth centuries.

In the decade following Broca's contributions, two important developments took place in Germany. First, Edward Hitzig and Gustav Fritsch performed a series of experiments in which the cortex of a dog was stimulated while the dog lay on a dressing table in Hitzig's Berlin home.[4,9,34,42] These experiments established that motor functions are localized to anterior cortex and demonstrated experimentally the somatotopic organization of motor cortex inferred indirectly from previous clinical-anatomic correlations in humans. In their report, the investigators specifically noted that their results refuted the holism of Flourens. Following their work, Sir David Ferrier in England confirmed the findings of Hitzig and Fritsch and improved upon their method of stimulation to discover more detailed structure-function relationships.[11]

About the same time, the German neurologist Carl Wernicke began to investigate language functions other than speech. Wernicke, shown in Fig. 1-9, documented a form of aphasia different from the nonfluent variety that followed frontal damage. In what he called sensory aphasia, a posterior lesion in the region of the first temporal gyrus caused a disturbance in auditory comprehension, inappropriate word selection in spontaneous speech, and impaired naming and writing. In his landmark monograph *Der aphasische Symptomen-complex,* Wernicke reasoned that Broca's area was the center for the motor representation of speech, and the posterior first temporal gyrus was the center for "sound images." Wernicke also described global aphasia and explained it as a result of destruction of both anterior and posterior language areas. He also made a prediction that a disturbance of the pathways between these two areas would produce another variety of

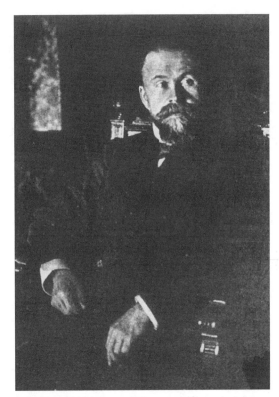

Figure 1-9
Carl Wernicke (1848–1904).

aphasia he called "conduction aphasia," in which comprehension would be preserved but output would be as impaired as in sensory aphasia.[35-38] Wernicke had, in effect, proposed a model that could explain a number of different aphasic syndromes by lesions to different combination of centers and connections between centers. This type of theorizing came to be known as "associationism," because language use was viewed in terms of associating representations in different brain centers, or as "connectionism," because of the emphasis that view put on the connections between centers, as shown in Fig. 1-10.

The connectionist paradigm was quickly extended to explain other disorders. Ludwig Lichtheim placed pure word deafness in this framework, predicting the critical lesion site as well as noting that, given the connectionist explanation

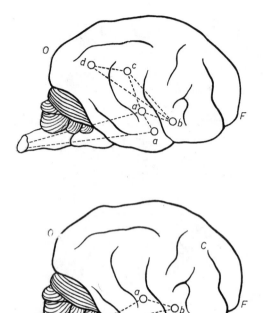

Figure 1-10
Wernicke's model of the speech mechanism.[36] *The auditory areas (a) project to centers subserving vocal output (b) and areas which contain tactile (c) and visual (d) images.*

for this syndrome, a disturbance in repetition should accompany conduction aphasia.[38,39] Hugo Liepmann described the apraxias, including ideomotor apraxia,[40] and, with Maas, callosal apraxia,[41] explaining them in terms of connectionist principles. Joseph Jules Déjerine, shown in Fig. 1-11, also used the framework of centers and connections in his explanation of alexia without agraphia.[42]

The nineteenth-century connectionist framework proved to have both parsimony and explanatory power. Rather than hypothesizing a new center for every ability or every observed deficit, after the fashion of Gall, a relatively small number of basic centers (vision, sound images, motor outputs) could be combined through connections to explain a wide variety of higher functions and

their deficits. Connectionist explanations of aphasia, apraxia, alexia, and other disorders survived well into the twentieth century; indeed, Norman Geschwind, one of the most influential behavioral neurologists of our time, championed them throughout his career.[43] Despite the current proliferation of theories and approaches in our field, the theories of Déjerine, Liepmann, Lichtheim, and Wernicke are still held to be correct by many.

Nevertheless, as successful as the connectionist framework was in late nineteenth century in explaining a variety of disorders, skeptics continued to reject the localism implicit in it. One of the most influential of these was the English neurologist John Hughlings Jackson, shown in Fig. 1-12. He viewed the nervous system not as a series of centers connected by pathways but rather as a hierarchically organized and highly interactive whole that could not be understood piecemeal.[24] Figure 1-13 shows Pierre Marie, a Parisian student of Broca and Charcot, who also took issue with the connectionist theorizing of the late nineteenth

Figure 1-11
Joseph Jules Déjerine (1849–1917).

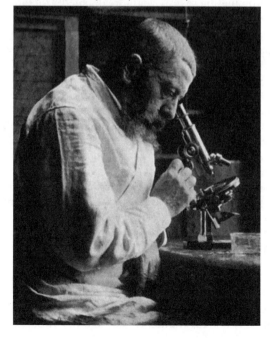

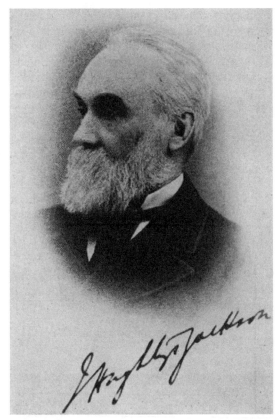

Figure 1-12
John Hughlings Jackson (1835–1911).

toward holism continued into the early twentieth century, with Jackson and Marie followed by a number of influential neurologists and psychologists, including Henry Head in England,[24] shown in Fig. 1-14, Kurt Goldstein in Germany,[45–47] shown in Fig. 1-15, and Karl Lashley in the United States.[48–51] This swing of the pendulum back toward holism has been explained by the waning of German influence following World War I[60] and the growing influence of Gestalt psychology.[61]

While these workers emphasized the brain's unity, other researchers had pointed out the difference between brain regions in cellular morphology, cell densities, and lamination and produced the first cytoarchitectonic maps. Oskar and Cécile Vogt[62,63] and Alfred W. Campbell[64,65] produced some of the earliest examples of these

Figure 1-13
Pierre Marie (1853–1940).

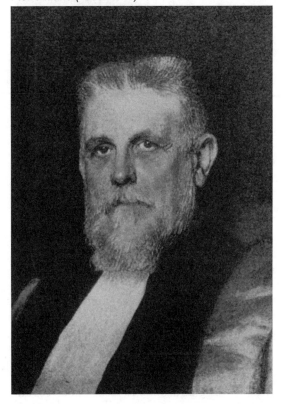

century. His style was direct, to say the least. One of his articles was so offensive to Déjerine that it provoked the latter to challenge Marie to a duel. His article questioning the empirical basis of the early claims concerning speech localization was entitled *"La troisiéme circonvolution frontale gauche ne joue aucun rôle spécial dans la fonction du langage"* ("The third frontal convolution plays no special role at all in the function of language").[44] Marie believed that there was just one basic form of aphasia, a posterior aphasia, which was a type of general intellectual loss not specific to language per se. He held that the speech problems of anterior aphasics were motoric in nature. When aphasia is viewed this way, a network of specialized centers is superfluous. A movement

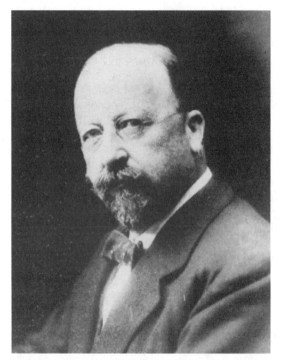

Figure 1-14
Henry Head (1861–1940).

architectonic maps, followed by many others, including those of Korbinian Brodmann,[58] whose cortical maps of the human brain have had the most widespread application. While these workers did not agree on the number and location of cortical areas (the Vogts counted over 200, Brodmann only 52[3]) it could not be contested that there were clear regional neuroanatomic differences.

The late nineteenth century also saw the beginnings of the modern study of memory and vision. Theodule Ribot introduced the distinction between anterograde and retrograde memory impairments and observed what is now known as "Ribot's law," that the most recently laid down memories were the most vulnerable to brain damage.[59–61] Ribot can also be credited with describing preserved learning in amnesia, thus anticipating the distinction between declarative and nondeclarative forms of memory that has been so intensively investigated in our own recent times. An ad-

ditional contribution to memory research in the latter nineteenth century was the description by Wernicke and Korsakoff (shown in Fig. 1-16) of the syndrome that bears their names, including Korsakoff's observations of what he called "pseudo-reminiscence," now known as confabulation.[70,71]

In 1881, Hermann Munk reported that when he ablated the occipital lobes of dogs, they seemed unable to recognize objects despite seeing well enough to navigate the visual environment.[72] Shortly thereafter, Lissauer presented one of the earliest clinical descriptions of visual recognition impairment in a human and suggested the distinction between apperceptive and associative impairment—a clinical dichotomy still in use today.[73] Freud would later introduce the term *agnosia* to describe these conditions.[74] In the decades that followed, the visuospatial functions of the right hemisphere finally attracted the attention of neu-

Figure 1-15
Kurt Goldstein (1878–1965).

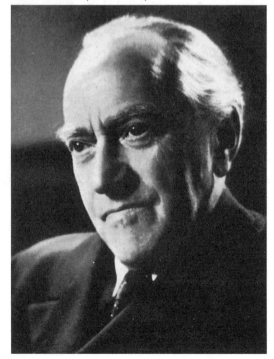

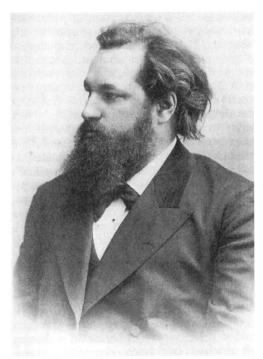

Figure 1-16
Sergei S. Korsakoff (1853–1900).

rologists and neuropsychologists.[67–69] The relatively delayed entry of this realm of functioning into the research arena is probably a result of the field's original focus on language and the left hemisphere, reflected in the nineteenth-century terminology of *major* and *minor hemisphere*.

THE RISE OF EXPERIMENTAL NEUROPSYCHOLOGY

Most of the advances described so far in this chapter were made by studying individual patients, or at most a small series of patients with similar disorders. In many instances, particularly before the middle of this century, patients' behavior was studied relatively naturalistically, without planned protocols or quantitative measurements. In the nineteen sixties and seventies, a different approach to the study of brain-behavior relations

took hold. Neurologists and neuropsychologists began to design experiments patterned on research methods in experimental psychology.

Typical research designs in experimental psychology involved groups of normal subjects given different experimental treatments (for example, different training or different stimulus materials), and the effects of the treatments were measured in standardized protocols and compared using statistical methods such as analysis of variance. In neuropsychology, the "treatments" were, as a rule, naturally occurring brain lesions. Groups of patients with different lesion sites or behavioral syndromes were tested with standard protocols, yielding quantitative measures of performance, and these performances were compared across patient groups and with non-brain-damaged control groups. Unlike the impairments studied previously in single-case designs, which were so striking that control subjects would generally have been superfluous, experimental neuropsychology often focused on group differences of a rather subtle nature, which required statistical analysis to substantiate.

The most common question addressed by these studies concerned localization of function. Often the localization sought was no more precise than left versus right hemisphere or one quadrant of the brain (which, in the days before computed tomography, often amounted to left versus right hemisphere with presence or absence of visual field defects and/or hemiplegia). Given the huge amount of research done during this period on language, memory, perception, attention, emotion, praxis, and so-called executive functions, it would be hopeless even to attempt a summary. For those interested in some examples of this approach, we cite here some classic papers from a variety of the active laboratories of the period, addressing the question "Is the right hemisphere specialized for spatial perception of properties such as location,[70–72] orientation,[73,74] and large-scale topography?[75,76]

The influential research program of the Montreal Neurological Institute also began during this period. In the wake of William Scoville's discovery that the bilateral medial temporal resection he performed on epileptic patient H. M. resulted in permanent and dense amnesia, Brenda Milner and her colleagues investigated this patient and groups of other operated epileptic patients. This enabled them to address questions of functional localization with the anatomic precision of known surgical lesions (e.g., see Refs. 77 and 78 for reviews of research from that period on frontal lobe function and temporal lobe function, respectively). At the same time, another surgical intervention for epilepsy, callosotomy, also spawned a productive and influential research program. Roger Sperry and his students and collaborators were able to address a wide variety of questions about hemispheric specialization by studying the isolated functioning of the human cerebral hemispheres.[79]

In addition to answering questions about localization, the experimental neuropsychology of the sixties and seventies also uncovered aspects of the functional organization of behavior. By examining patterns of association and dissociation among abilities over groups of subjects, researchers tried to determine which abilities depend on the same underlying functional systems and which are functionally independent. For example, the frequent association of aphasia and apraxia had been taken by some to support the notion that aphasia was not language-specific but was just one manifestation of a more pervasive loss of the ability to symbolize or represent ("asymbolia"). A classic group study by Goodglass and Kaplan[80] undermined this position by showing that severity of apraxia and aphasia were uncorrelated in a large sample of left-hemisphere-damaged subjects. A second example of the use of dissociations between groups of patients from this period is the demonstration of the functional distinction, by Newcombe and Russell, within vision between pattern recognition and spatial orientation.[81]

By the end of the seventies, experimental neuropsychology had matured to the point where many perceptual, cognitive, and motor abilities had been associated with particular brain regions, and certain features of the functional organization of these abilities had been delineated. Accord-

ingly, it was at this time that first editions of some of the best-known neuropsychology texts appeared, such as those by Hécaen and Albert,[82] Heilman and Valenstein,[83] Kolb and Whishaw,[84] Springer and Deutsch,[85] and Walsh.[86]

Despite the tremendous progress of this period, experimental neuropsychology remained distinct from and relatively unknown within academic psychology. Particularly in the United States, but also to a large extent in Canada and Europe (the three largest contributors to the world's psychology literature), experimental neuropsychologists tended to work in medical centers rather than university psychology departments and to publish their work in journals separate from mainstream experimental psychology. An important turning point in the histories of both neuropsychology and the psychology of normal human function came when researchers in each area became aware of the other.

THE BIRTH OF COGNITIVE NEUROSCIENCE

Patient-based cognitive neuroscience was born when the theories and methods of cognitive psychology and neuropsychology were finally combined. Both fields had strong incentives to overcome their isolation. Let us begin by reviewing the state of cognitive psychology prior to the birth of cognitive neuroscience.

The central tenet of cognitive psychology is that cognition is information processing. Although the effects of damage to an information-processing mechanism might seem to be a good source of clues as to its normal operation, cognitive psychologists of the seventies were generally quite ignorant of contemporary neuropsychology.

The reason that most cognitive psychologists of the 1970s ignored neuropsychology stemmed from an overly narrow conception of information processing, based on the digital computer. A basic tenet of cognitive psychology was the computer analogy for the mind: the mind is to the brain as software is to hardware in a computer. Given that the same computer can run different programs and the same program can be run on different computers, this analogy suggests that hardware and software are independent and that the brain is therefore irrelevant to cognitive psychology. If you want to understand the nature of the program that is the human mind, studying neuropsychology is as pointless as trying to understand how a computer is programmed by looking at the circuit boards.

The problem with the computer analogy is that hardware and software are independent only for very special types of computational systems: those systems that have been engineered, through great effort and ingenuity, to make the hardware and software independent, enabling one computer to run many programs and enabling those programs to be portable to other computers. The brain was "designed" by very different pressures, and there is no reason to believe that, in general, information-processing functions and the physical substrate of those functions will be independent. In fact, as cognitive psychologists finally began to learn about neuropsychology, it became apparent that cognitive functions break down in characteristic and highly informative ways after brain damage. By the early 1980s, cognitive psychology and neuropsychology were finally in communication with one another. Since then, we have seen an explosion of meetings, books, and new journals devoted to so-called cognitive neuropsychology. Perhaps more important, existing cognitive psychology journals have begun to publish neuropsychological studies, and articles in existing neuropsychology and neurology journals frequently include discussions of the cognitive psychology literature.

Let us take a closer look at the scientific forces that drove this change in disciplinary boundaries. By 1980, both cognitive psychology and neuropsychology had reached states of development that were, if not exactly impasses, points of diminishing returns for the concepts and methods of their own isolated disciplines. In cognitive psychology, the problem concerned methodologic limitations. By varying stimuli and instructions

and measuring responses and response latencies, cognitive psychologists made inferences about the information processing that intervened between stimulus and responses. But such inferences were indirect, and in some cases they were incapable of distinguishing between rival theories. In 1978 the cognitive psychologist John Anderson published an influential paper[87] in which he called this the "identifiability" problem and took as his example the debate over whether mental images were more like perceptual representations or linguistic representations. He argued that the field's inability to resolve this issue, despite many years of research, was due to the impossibility of uniquely identifying internal cognitive processes from stimulus-response relations. He suggested that the direct study of brain function could, in principle, make a unique identification possible, but he indicated that such a solution probably lay in the distant future.

That distant future came to pass within the next 10 years, as cognitive psychologists working on a variety of different topics found that the study of neurologic patients provided a powerful new source of evidence for testing their theories. In the case of mental imagery, taken by Anderson to be emblematic of the identifiability problem, the finding that perceptual impairments after brain damage were frequently accompanied by parallel imagery impairments strongly favored the perceptual hypothesis.[88] The study of learning and memory within cognitive psychology was revolutionized by the influx of ideas and findings on preserved learning in amnesia, leading to the hypothesis of multiple memory systems.[89–91] In the study of attention, cognitive psychologists had for years focused on the issue of early versus late attentional selection without achieving a resolution, and here too neurologic disorders were crucial in moving the field forward. The phenomena of neglect provided dramatic evidence of selection from spatially formatted perceptual representations, and the variability in neglect's manifestations from case to case helped to establish the possibility of multiple loci for attentional selection as opposed to a single early or late locus. The idea of separate visual feature maps, supported by cases of acquired color, motion, and depth blindness, provided the inspiration for the most novel development in recent cognitive theories of attention—namely, feature integration theory.[92]

What did neuroscience gain from the rapprochement with cognitive psychology? The main benefits were theoretical rather than methodologic. Traditionally, neuropsychologists studied the localization and functional organization of *abilities*, such as speech, reading, memory, object recognition, and so forth. But few would doubt that each of these abilities depends upon an orchestrated set of *component cognitive processes*, and it seems far more likely that the underlying cognitive components, rather than the task-defined abilities, are what is implemented in localized neural tissue. The theories of cognitive psychology therefore allowed neuropsychologists to pose questions about the localization and functional organization of the components of the cognitive architecture, a level of theoretical analysis that was more likely to yield clear and generalizable findings.

Among patients with reading disorders, for example, some are impaired at reading nonwords (e.g., *plif*) while others are impaired at reading irregular words (e.g., *yacht*). Rather than attempt to localize nonword reading or irregular word reading per se and delineate them as independent abilities, neuropsychologists have been able to use a theory of reading developed in cognitive psychology to interpret these disorders in terms of damage to a whole-word recognition system and a grapheme-to-phoneme translation system, respectively.[93] This interpretation has the advantage of correctly predicting additional features of patient behavior, such as the tendency to misread nonwords as words of overall similar appearance when operating with only the whole-word system.

In recent years the neuroscience of every major cognitive system has adopted the theoretical framework of cognitive psychology in a general way, and in some cases specific theories have been incorporated. This is reflected in the content and organization of the present book. For the most intensively studied areas of behavioral neu-

rology and neuropsychology—namely, visual attention, memory, language, frontal lobe function, and Alzheimer's disease—integrated pairs of chapters review the clinical and anatomic aspects of the relevant disorders and their cognitive theoretical interpretations. Chapters on other topics will cover both the clinical and theoretical aspects together.

COMPLEMENTARY METHODS IN COGNITIVE NEUROSCIENCE: PATIENT STUDIES AND FUNCTIONAL IMAGING

Following its introduction in the 1970s, positron emission tomography (PET) was quickly embraced by researchers interested in brain-behavior relations. This technique provides images of regional glucose utilization, blood flow, oxygen consumption, or receptor density in the brains of live humans. Resting studies, in which subjects are scanned while resting passively, have provided a window on differences between normal and pathologic brain function in a number of neurologic and psychiatric conditions. With the use of radioactive ligands, abnormalities can be localized to specific neurotransmitter systems as well as specific anatomic regions. Activation studies, in which separate images are collected while normal subjects perform different tasks (typically one or more active tasks and one resting baseline) yielded new insights on the localization of cognitive processes. These localizations were not studied region by region, as necessitated by the lesion technique, but could be apprehended simultaneously in a whole intact brain.

Positron emission tomography was soon joined by other techniques for measuring regional brain activity, each of which has its own strengths and weaknesses. Single photon emission computed tomography (SPECT) was quickly adapted for some of the same applications as PET, providing a less expensive but also less quantifiable and spatially less accurate method for obtaining images of regional cerebral blood flow. With new developments in the measurement and analysis of electromagnetic signals, the relatively old techniques of electroencephalography (EEG) and event-related potentials (ERPs), as well as magnetoencephalography (MEG), joined the ranks of functional imaging techniques allowing some degree of anatomic localization of brain activity, with temporal resolution that is superior to the blood flow and metabolic techniques. Most recently, functional magnetic resonance imaging (fMRI) has provided a particularly attractive package of reasonably good anatomic and temporal resolution, using techniques that are noninvasive and can be implemented with equipment available for clinical purposes in many hospitals.

Much of the early work with functional neuroimaging could be considered a form of "calibration," in that researchers sought to confirm well-established principles of functional neuroanatomy using the new techniques—for example, demonstrating that visual stimulation activates visual cortex. As functional neuroimaging matured, researchers began to address new questions, to which the answers were not already known in advance. An important development in this second wave of research was the introduction of theories and methods from cognitive psychology, which specified the component cognitive processes involved in performing complex tasks and provided a means of isolating them experimentally. In neuroimaging studies of normal subjects, as with the purely behavioral studies of patients, the entities most likely to yield clear and consistent localizations are these component cognitive processes and not the tasks themselves. Starting in the mid-1980s, a collaboration between cognitive psychologist Michael Posner and neurologist Marcus Raichle at Washington University led to a series of pioneering studies in which the neural circuits underlying language, reading, and attention were studied by PET (see Ref. 94 for a review). Since then, researchers at Washington University and a growing number of other centers around the world have adapted neuroimaging techniques to all manner of topics in cognitive neuroscience.

To many psychologists and neuroscientists, cognitive neuroscience is equivalent to cognitive neuroimaging. At the very least, we hope this book shows this idea to be mistaken. Although neuroimaging has had a huge and salutary effect on cognitive neuroscience, significantly expanding the range of questions that can be addressed, it has not replaced research with neurological patients. A full discussion of the complementary strengths and weaknesses of the two approaches could easily fill a chapter by itself, but a few of the most consequential differences can be summarized briefly here.

Lumping the different functional neuroimaging modalities together, they generally offer better spatial resolution than can be obtained in inferences from a few patients with focal brain lesions. Imaging also allows us to study normal brains, which lesion studies by definition do not. Furthermore, for some neurological conditions more than others there may be reason to suspect a degree of reorganization of remaining brain systems in response to damage. These are probably the greatest benefits of functional neuroimaging, although by no means the only ones.

The greatest weakness of neuroimaging is its inability to settle any issue concerning what might be called *mechanism*. An important goal of cognitive neuroscience is to identify the causal chain of neural events, or the mechanisms, underlying cognition. The data of functional neuroimaging are correlational: a certain area is activated when a certain cognitive process is occurring. Neuroimaging can never disentangle correlation from causation; in other words, it can never tell us which brain areas are causally involved in enabling a cognitive process. Activated regions could play a causal role or could be activated in an optional or even an epiphenomenal way. For this we must turn to studying the effects of brain damage, the "experiments of nature" that provide a direct test of the causal role of different brain areas by showing us how the system works in their absence. Given the complementary strengths of neuroimaging and patient studies, we predict that the most successful cognitive neuroscience research programs of the twenty-first century will be those that combine the two approaches.

REFERENCES

1. Pagel W: Medieval and Renaissance contributions to knowledge of the brain and its functions, in Poynter FNL (ed): *The Brain and Its Functions,* Oxford, England: Blackwell, 1958, pp. 95–114.
2. Clarke E. Dewhurst K: *An Illustrated History of Brain Function.* Berkeley, CA: University of California Press, 1972.
3. Finger S: *Origins of Neuroscience. A History of Explorations into Brain Function.* New York: Oxford University Press, 1994
4. Bakay L: *An Early History of Craniotomy.* Springfield, IL: Charles C Thomas, 1985.
5. Wozniak RH: *Mind and Body: René Descartes to William James.* National Library of Medicine, Bethesda, MD, and the American Psychological Association, Washington, DC, 1992.
6. Riese W: Descartes' ideas of brain function, in Poynter FNL (ed): *The Brain and Its Function.* Oxford, England: Blackwell, 1958, pp. 115–134.
7. Descartes R: *De homine figuris et latinitate donatus a Florentio Schuyl.* Leyden: Franciscum Moyardum and Petrum Leffen, 1662.
8. Descartes R: *Les passions de l'âme. Paris:* Henry Le Gras, 1649.
9. Clarke E, O'Malley CE: *The Human Brain and Spinal Cord.* Berkeley, CA: University California Press, 1968.
10. Willis T: *Cerebri anatome: Cui accessit nervorum descriptio et usus.* London: Martyn and Allestry, 1664.
11. Mazzolini RG: Schemes and models of the thinking machine. In Corsi P (ed): *The Enchanted Loom: Chapters in the History of Neuroscience.* New York: Oxford University Press, 1991, pp. 68–143.
12. Young RM: *Mind, Brain and Adaptation in the Nineteenth Century.* New York: Oxford University Press, 1990.
13. Stookey B: A note on the early history of cerebral localization. *Bull NY Acad Med* 30:559–578, 1954.
14. Ackerknecht EH: Contribution of Gall and the phrenologist to knowledge of brain function, in Poynter FNL (ed): *The Brain and Its Functions.* Oxford: Blackwell, 1958, pp. 149–153.
15. Pogliano C: Between form and function: A new science of man, in Corsi P (ed): *The Enchanted Loom: Chapters in the History of Neurosciences.* New York: Oxford University Press, 1991, pp. 144–203.
16. Brown JW, Chobor KL: Phrenological studies of aphasia before Broca: Broca's aphasia or Gall's aphasia? *Brain Lang* 43:475–486, 1992.
17. Flourens P: *Phrenology Examined* (Charles De Lucena Meigs, trans). Philadelphia: Hogan and Thompson, 1846.
18. Flourens P: *Recherches Expérimentales sur les Propriétés et les Fonctions du Système Nerveux dans les Animaux Vertèbras* (1824), 2d ed. Paris: Baillière, 1842.
19. Harrington A: Beyond phrenology: Localization theory in the modern era, in Corsi P (ed): *The Enchanted Loom. Chapters in the History of Neuroscience.* New York: Oxford University Press, 1991, pp. 207–239.
20. Bouillaud JB: *Traité clinique et physiologique de l'encephalite ou inflammation du cerveau.* Paris: Baillière, 1825.
21. Benton AL, Joynt RJ: Early descriptions of aphasia. *Arch Neurol* 3:205–221, 1960.
22. Benton AL, Joynt RJ: Three pioneers in the study of aphasia. *J His Med Sci* 18:381–383, 1963.
23. Joynt RJ, Benton AL: The memoir of Marc Dax on aphasia. *Neurology* 14:851–854, 1964.
24. Head H: *Aphasia and Kindred Disorders of Speech.* New York: Macmillan, 1926.
25. Stookey BL: Jean-Baptiste Bouillaud and Ernest Aubertin: Early studies on cerebral localization and the speech center. *JAMA* 184:1024–1029, 1963.
26. Critchley M: The Broca-Dax controversy, in Critchley M (ed): *The Divine Banquet of the Brain and Other Essays.* New York: Raven Press, 1979.
27. Joynt RJ: Centenary of patient "Tan": His contribution to the problem of aphasia. *Arch Intern Med* 108:953–956, 1961.
28. Broca P: Remarques sur le siège de la faculté du langage articulé: Suivies d'une observation d'aphemie. *Bull Soc Anat (Paris)* 6:330–357, 1861.
29. Broca P: Localisation des fonctions cérébrales: Sièe du langage articulé. *Bull Soc Anthropol (Paris)* 4:200–203, 1863.
30. Dax M: Lesions de la moitié gauche de l'encéphale coincident avec l'oublie des signes de la pensée. *Gaz hbd Méd Chir (Paris)* 2:259–262, 1865.
31. Dax G: Notes sur la mème sujet. *Gaz hbd Méd Chir (Paris)* 2:262, 1865.
32. Broca P: Sur le siège de la faculté du langage articulé. *Bull Soc Anthropol* 6:337–393, 1865.
33. Berker EA, Berker AH, Smith A: Translation of Broca's 1865 report: Localization of speech in the third left frontal convolution. *Arch Neurol* 43:1065–1072, 1986.
34. Fritsch G, Hitzig E: On the electrical excitability of the cerebrum (1870), in von Bonin G (ed): *Some*

Papers on the Cerebral Cortex. Springfield, IL: Charles C Thomas, 1960, pp. 73–96.

35. Geschwind N: Wernicke's contribution to the study of aphasia. *Cortex* 3:449–463, 1967.

36. Wernicke C: *Der aphasische Symptomemkomplex: Eine psychologische Studie auf anatomischer Basis.* Breslau: Cohn und Weigert, 1874.

37. Lecours AR, Lhermitte F: From Franz Gall to Pierre Marie, in Lecours AR, Lhermitte F, Bryans B (eds): *Aphasiology.* London: Baillière Tindall, 1983.

38. Geschwind N: Carl Wernicke, the Breslau School and the history of aphasia, in Carterette EC (ed): *Brain Function:* Vol. III. *Speech, Language, and Communication.* Berkeley, CA: University of California Press, 1963, pp. 1–16.

39. Lichtheim L: On aphasia. *Brain* 7:433–484, 1885.

40. Liepmann H: Das Krankheitsbild der Apraxie ("motorische Asymbolie") auf Grund eines Falles von einseitiger Apraxie, *Monatschr Psychiatr Neurol* 8:15–44, 102–132, 182–197, 1900.

41. Liepmann H, Maas O: Fall von linksseitiger Agraphie und Apraxie bei rechtsseitiger Lähmung. *J Psychol Neurol* 10:214–227, 1907.

42. Déjerine J: Contribution à l'étude anatomopathologique et clinique des différentes variétés de cécité verbale. *CRH Séances Mem Soc Biol* 44:61–90, 1892.

43. Geschwind N: Disconnexion syndromes in animals and man. *Brain* 88:237–294, 585–644, 1965.

44. Brais B: The third left frontal convolution plays no role in language: Pierre Marie and the Paris debate on aphasia (1906–1908). *Neurology* 42:690–695, 1992.

45. Goldstein K: *The Organism.* New York: American Book, 1939.

46. Goldstein K: *Language and Language Disturbances.* New York: Grune & Stratton, 1948.

47. Lecours AR, Cronk C. Sébahoun-Balsamo M: From Pierre Marie to Norman Geschwind, in Lecours AR, Lhermitte F, Bryans B (eds): *Aphasiology.* London: Baillière Tindall, 1983.

48. Franz SI, Lashley KS: The retention of habits by the rat after destruction of the frontal portion of the cerebrum. *Psychobiology* 1:3–18, 1917.

49. Lashley KS, Franz SI: The effects of cerebral destruction upon habit-formation and retention in the albino rat. *Psychobiology* 1:71–139, 1917.

50. Lashley KS: *Brain Mechanisms and Intelligence: A Quantitative Study of Injuries to the Brain.* Chicago: University of Chicago Press, 1929.

51. Lashley KS: In search of the engram. *Symp Soc Exp Biol* 4:454–482, 1950.

52. Geschwind N: The paradoxical position of Kurt Goldstein in the history of aphasia. *Cortex* 1:214–224, 1964.

53. Harrington A: A feeling for the "whole": the holistic reaction in neurology from the fin de siècle to the interwar years, in Teich M. Porter R (eds): *Fin de Siècle and Its Legacy.* Cambridge, England: Cambridge University Press, 1990.

54. Vogt O, Vogt C: Zur anatomischen Gliederung des cortex cerebri. *J Psychol Neurol* 2:160–180, 1903.

55. Haymaker WE: Cecile and Oskar Vogt, on the occasion of her 75th and his 80th birthday. *Neurology* 1:179–204, 1951.

56. Campbell AW: Histological studies on cerebral localization. *Proc R Soc* 72:488–492, 1903.

57. Campbell AW: *Histological Studies on the Localization of Cerebral Function.* Cambridge, England: Cambridge University Press, 1905.

58. Brodmann K: *Vergleichende Lokalisationslehre der Grosshirnrinde in ihren Prinzipien dargestellt auf Grund des Zellenbaues.* Leipzig: Barth, 1909.

59. Levin HS, Peters BH, Hulkonen DA: Early concepts of anterograde and retrograde amnesia. *Cortex* 19:427–440, 1983.

60. Ribot T: *Diseases of Memory.* London: Kegan Paul, Trench, 1882.

61. Squire LR, Slater PC: Anterograde and retrograde memory impairment in chronic amnesia. *Neuropsychologia* 16:313–322, 1978.

62. Victor M, Adams RD, Collins GH: *The Wernicke-Korsakoff Syndrome and Related Neurologic Disorders due to Alcoholism and Malnutrition,* 2d ed. Philadelphia: Davis, 1989.

63. Victor M, Yakovlev PI: SS Korsakoff's psychic disorder in conjunction with peripheral neuritis: A translation of Korsakoff's original article with brief comments on the author and his contribution to clinical medicine. *Neurology* 5:394–406, 1955.

64. Munk H: Über die Functionen der Grosshirnrinde: Gesammelte Mitteilungen aus den Jahren. Berlin: Hirschwald, 1877–1880.

65. Lissauer H: Ein fall von seelenblindheit nebst einem Beitrage zur Theori derselben. *Arch Psychiatr Nervenkrankh* 21–222-270, 1980.

66. Freud S: Zur Auffassung der Aphasien. Leipzig and Vienna: Deuticke, 1891.

67. Paterson A, Zangwill OL: Disorders of visual space perception associated with lesions of the right cerebral hemisphere. *Brain* 40:122–179, 1944.

68. Hécaen H, Ajuriaguerra J, Massonet J: Les troubles visuoconstructives par lésion pariéto-occipitale droite. *Encéphale* 40:122–179, 1951.

69. Benton A: Neuropsychology: Past, present and future, in Boller F. Grafman J (eds): *Handbook of Neuropsychology.* New York: Elsevier, 1988, vol. 1, pp. 3–27.

70. Hannay HJ, Varney NR, Benton AL: Visual localization in patients with unilateral brain disease. *J Neurol Neurosurg Psychiatry* 39:307–313, 1976.

71. Ratcliff G, Davies-Jones GAB: Defective visual localization in focal brain wounds. *Brain* 95:46–60, 1972.

72. Warrington EK, Rabin P: Perceptual matching in patients with cerebral lesions. *Neuropsychologia* 8:475–487, 1970.

73. De Renzi E, Faglioni P, Scotti G: Judgement of spatial orientation in patients with focal brain damage. *J Neurol Neurosurg Psychiatry* 34:489–495, 1971.

74. Carmon A, Benton AL: Tactile perception of direction and number in patients with unilateral cerebral disease. *Neurology* 19:525–532, 1969.

75. Hécaen H, Tzortzis C, Masure MC: Troubles de l'orientation spatiale dans une épreuve de recherche d'itinéraire lors des lesions corticales unilaterales. *Perception* 1:325–330, 1972.

76. Semmes J, Weinstein S, Ghent L, Teuber HL: Correlates of impaired orientation in personal and extrapersonal space. *Brain* 86:747–772, 1963.

77. Milner B: Some effects of frontal lobectomy in man, in Warren JM, Akert K (eds): *The Frontal Granular Cortex and Behavior.* New York: McGraw-Hill, 1964.

78. Milner B: Memory and the medical temporal regions of the brain, in Pribram KH, Broadbent DE (eds): *Biological Bases of Memory.* New York: Academic Press, 1970.

79. Trevarthen C, Roger W: Sperry's lifework and our tribute, in Trevarthen C (ed): *Brain Circuits and Functions of the Mind: Essays in Honor of Roger W. Sperry.* Cambridge, England: Cambridge University Press, 1990.

80. Goodglass H, Kaplan E: Disturbance of gesture and patomime in aphasia. *Brain* 86:703–720, 1963.

81. Newcombe F, Russell W: Dissociated visual perceptual and spatial deficits in focal lesions of the right hemisphere. *J Neurol Neurosurg Psychiatry* 32:73–81, 1969.

82 Hécaen H, Albert ML: *Human Neuropsychology.* New York: Wiley, 1978.

83. Heilman KM, Valenstein E: *Clinical Neuropsychology.* New York: Oxford University Press, 1979.

84. Kolb B, Whishaw I: *Fundamentals of Human Neuropsychology.* New York: Freeman, 1980.

85. Springer SP, Deutsch G: *Left Brain/Right Brain.* San Francisco: Freeman, 1981.

86. Walsh KW: *Neuropsychology: A Clinical Approach.* New York: Churchill Livingstone, 1978.

87. Anderson JR: Arguments concerning representation for mental imagery. *Psychol Rev* 85:249–277, 1978.

88. Farah MJ: Is visual imagery really visual? Overlooked evidence from neuropsychology. *Psychol Rev* 95:307–317, 1988.

89. Schacter DL: Implicit memory: History and current status. *J Exp Psychol Learn Mem Cog* 13:501–518, 1987.

90. Squire L: *Memory and Brain.* New York: Oxford University Press, 1987.

91. Weiskrantz L: On issues and theories of the human amnesic syndrome, in Weinberger N, McGaugh JL, Lynch G (eds): *Memory Systems of the Brain.* New York: Guilford Press, 1985.

92. Treisman A: Features and objects: The fourteenth Bartlett lecture. *Q J Exp Psychol* 40A:201–237, 1988.

93. Coltheart M: Cognitive neuropsychology and the study of reading, in Marin IP, Marin OSM (eds): *Attention and Performance XI.* London: Erlbaum, 1985.

94. Posner MI, Raichle ME: *Images of Mind.* New York: Scientific American Library, 1994.

Chapter 2

STRUCTURAL IMAGING OF PATIENTS IN COGNITIVE NEUROSCIENCE

Hanna Damasio
Antonio R. Damasio

The lesion method aims at establishing a correlation between a circumscribed region of brain damage, a lesion and a pattern of alteration in some aspect of an experimentally controlled cognitive or behavioral performance. The brain-damaged region is conceptualized as part of a large-scale network of cortical and subcortical sites that operate in concert, by virtue of their interlocking connectivity, to produce a particular function. Given a theoretical framework for how such networks are constituted and carry out that particular function, a lesion is thus a *probe* to test a specific hypothesis. A lesion probe allows the investigator to decide whether damage to a component of the putative network, responsible for function X, alters the network behavior according to the predictions made for it. In other words, given a theory about the operations of a normal brain, lesions are a means to support or falsify the theory.

The subjects for the lesion method may be humans or animals. The lesions may have been produced by neurologic disease alone or incurred in the process of treating it (e.g., a surgical procedure). They may be small or large and may be studied in vivo or at postmortem. The indispensable requirements are that lesions be stable, well demarcated, and referable to a neuroanatomic unit. In this chapter we focus on human lesions, produced by neurologic disease or surgical ablation and studied in vivo with modern neuroimaging techniques.

The lesion approach provided the first method in what was to become neuroscience. In the very least, it dates to Morgagni's demonstration of an association between unilateral brain disease and contralateral sensory and motor disabilities. Bouillaud's and Broca's finding of a correlation between speech and focal damage to the frontal lobe are reasonable signposts to mark the modern era of lesion studies.

In the latter decades of the nineteenth century, the lesion method led to pathbreaking discoveries. But although most of the findings have stood the test of time and gained wide acceptance, the theories that were associated with them did not. The pioneering neurologists conceived of the existence of brain centers capable of performing complex psychological functions with relative independence. What little interaction there was among those few and noncontiguous centers was achieved by unidirectional pathways. These concepts were subject to deserved criticism, the best known of which came from Sigmund Freud and Hughlings Jackson. As the theoretical account lost influence, the lesion method, which was closely interwoven with the theory, lost favor as a means of valid scientific inquiry.

The lesion method began to regain some prominence in the 1960s, perhaps as a reaction to the impasses of "equipotential" antilocalizationism and "black-box" behaviorism. The revival was spearheaded by Geschwind's reflections on the work of Wernicke, Lichtheim, Liepmann, and Déjerine and by the work of notable neuropsychologists, among whom were A. R. Luria, Henri Hécaen, Brenda Milner, Arthur Benton, Hans-Lukas Teuber, and Oliver Zangwill. The full value of the lesion method, however, only began to be appreciated after the development of new neuroimaging technologies—computed tomography (CT), which had its inception in 1973, and magnetic resonance imaging (MRI), which emerged a decade later.

It has gradually become evident that the lesion method should be separated from the theoretical accounts historically connected with it. As with any other approach, this method has limitations and misapplications. Nonetheless, it is one entity, with its virtues and pitfalls, and the theoretical constructs that make use of it represent another. Nothing prevents practitioners of the lesion method from proposing the richest and most dynamic accounts of brain function.

In short, the classically discovered links between certain brain regions of the cerebral cortex and signs of neuropsychological dysfunction have been validated, remain a staple of clinical neurology, and allow for relatively accurate predictions of *localization of damage* from neurologic signs. That is, more often than not, the presence of certain neuropsychological defects indicates to the clinical expert that there is dysfunction in a specific brain area. These valid links, however, should not be taken to mean that the functions disturbed by the lesion were inscribed in the tissue that the lesion destroyed. The complex psychological functions, which usually constitute the target of neuropsychological studies in humans, are not localizable at that level.

The neural architectures revealed by neuroanatomy and neurophysiology and the cognitive architectures revealed by experimental neuropsychology suggest that single-center functions, single-purpose pathways, and unidirectional cascades of information process are unrealistic. Moreover, the residual performance that follows focal brain insults, and the ensuing patterns of recovery, suggest that knowledge must be widely distributed, at multiple neural levels, and complex psychological functions must emerge from the cooperation of multiple components of integrated networks (see Chap. 7).

Two key developments made human lesion studies rewarding again. First, lesion studies in nonhuman primates brought major advances to the understanding of the neural basis of vision and memory, as demonstrated, among others, by Mishkin and colleagues. Second, the advent of CT and MRI began to permit human lesion studies in vivo. It is apparent now that the lesion method is indispensable to cognitive neuroscience, especially when it comes to human studies. The *new* lesion method is not concerned with "localizing functions," nor is it a contest for "localizing lesions." It is a means to test, at systems level, hypotheses regarding *both* neural structure *and* cognitive processes. What investigators from Déjerine to Geschwind gleaned from single cases can now be replicated systematically in a suitable group of subjects. Hypotheses old and new, including some advanced by the pioneer neuropsychologists, can be tested experimentally.

Beyond their intrinsic value, the results from the new lesion method in humans provide a welcome complement to results from neuroanatomic and neurophysiologic experiments in animals. Lesion work in humans has revealed characteristics of neural systems that could not have been investigated in experimental animals. The example of linguistic processes is the most obvious. Lesion results have also been the source of hypotheses that were further investigated in animals and in humans. Ungerleider and Mishkin's study of ventral and dorsal visual pathways in nonhuman primates[1] was inspired by Newcombe's work in humans.[2] Conversely, Ungerleider and Mishkin's work was followed up in humans, and the inferotemporal system has now been anatomically and functionally fractionated.[3–5] Moreover, the lesion method offers the possibility of conducting indepth experiments on some cognitive operations whose temporal characteristics are not suitable for other approaches (for instance, experiments requiring the monitoring of psychophysiologic variables).

We also see the lesion method as joining forces with two other approaches to the investigation of human brain function: electrophysiologic studies and functional imaging. The first includes the use of event-related potentials, the study of cognitive and behavioral changes induced by electrical stimulation of exposed cerebral cortex, and the direct recording of activity from cerebral cortex. The second involves the imaging of brain activity inferred from the differential emission of radio signals. It encompasses positron emission tomography (PET), single photon emission computed tomography (SPECT), and functional magnetic resonance imaging (fMRI). The combination of results from the lesion method with those from the other approaches will strengthen our conceptualization of the human brain and bring to light discrepancies that require new theorizing and experimentation. Many well-established facts from the lesion method remain the benchmark against which some results of the new dynamic methods must be measured. Moreover, the actual combination of procedures is likely to generate more powerful tools. This will become reality, for instance, with the performance of PET and fMRI studies in patients with focal lesions causing specific cognitive disorders.

The lesion method does have its limitations. Not every anatomic region of the human nervous system can be properly sampled by natural lesions, and the size of the lesions provides a natural limit to the structures the method can probe with confidence. And yet, in its modern incarnation, the approach provides data currently unavailable through other means.

Only a concerted set of approaches from the molecular to the systems levels, in both humans and experimental animals, can eventually provide answers to the questions currently posed in cognitive neuroscience. The lesion method is a key partner in systems-level studies.

THE MODERN PRACTICE OF
THE LESION METHOD IN HUMANS

There are at least five prerequisites for the modern practice of the lesion method: first, the availability of fine-grained structural imaging of the living human brain; second, the availability of a reliable method for the anatomic study of lesion probes; third, access to a large pool of subjects with lesions in varied brain sites, so that hypotheses regarding the operation of different systems can be experimentally tested in comparable target subjects and in appropriate controls; fourth, the availability of reliable techniques for various cognitive measurements; and fifth, the guidance of testable hypotheses concerning the neural basis of specific cognitive processes at systems level. In the following pages, we discuss some of these requisites.

Neuroanatomy from Neuroimaging

For many years, we have conceptualized the systematic neuroimaging studies pursued in our laboratory as a means to practice *human neuroanatomy from imaging data,* i.e., a means for detection and description of a lesion and consideration of its placement in the context of the anatomic systems to which it belongs. This purpose, which requires detailed knowledge of human neuroanatomy, is distinguishable from the traditional role of neuroimaging in *clinical neurologic diagnosis,* i.e., the detection of structural alterations and the prediction of its possible neuropathologic basis. The original tool for these studies was the template

technique,[6] but we have since developed a new technique for individualized lesion analysis based on the three-dimensional (3D) reconstruction of the human brain from high-resolution MRI.[7] This new technique is known as BRAINVOX. It permits us to identify reliably, in vivo, every major gyrus and sulcus of the human brain; to slice and reslice the human brain in whatever incidence is necessary for anatomic analysis; and to define and measure volumes or surfaces of interest in single cases and across groups. The technique dispenses with charting onto brain templates and permits instead a customized definition of each subject. We will comment on this technique first and complete this section with a review of the template technique.

BRAINVOX

BRAINVOX is a 3D volumetric imaging and analysis system. The software was originally developed to facilitate the 3D display and mapping of acquired human brain lesions using a volume-rendering approach, but it has grown to support a wide range of advanced multimodality neuroanatomic visualization and analysis techniques. Although BRAINVOX was designed for the analysis of high-resolution volumetric MRI, it can be used with CT and PET.

BRAINVOX consists of several interconnected software components: (1) a slice/contour–based tracing module, (2) a multivolume 3D rendering system, (3) a set of general-purpose volume-manipulation tools, (4) a basic volume–data-handling system, (5) a palette editor, and (6) a volumetric object-measurement system.

BRAINVOX allows for explicit definition of volumes bounded by tracings that can be separated from the full MRI volume. The software allows users to define many such volumes simultaneously, slice by slice, taking advantage of common borders, edge tracking, and flexible trace-editing tools. Volume and intersection volume statistics can be computed for all objects defined in this manner. Histograms of volumes and individual slices can be computed.

Lesion Analysis with BRAINVOX

Using the 3D reconstructed brain to determine which anatomic sectors of each hemisphere are damaged obviates the need to adjust the angle in which the MRI sections are obtained to the angle of available template systems. The accuracy of interpretation no longer depends on the "reading" of a template with the transferred lesion but rather on the direct reading from the identified landmarks in the unique brain in question.

The new technique permits a direct identification of gyri and sulci, comparable to what can be achieved at the autopsy table in a postmortem brain after the meninges have been removed. The technique permits the accurate marking of such structures in coronal axial or parasagittal slices, with the advantage that the extension of lesions into the depths of sulci can also be determined (Fig. 2-1).

Other advantages of the new technique are as follows. First, the identification of anatomic structures is based on each individual brain rather than on an idealized "average" brain. The standard landmarks of each area of interest can be localized in the brain of each individual subject rather than on a template. Although templates use anatomic constants, they cannot account for individual variation and thus introduce an error of measurement, albeit small in some cases. Second, because each area of interest has been customized for each subject, it is possible to determine with considerable rigor the proportion of a given area that has been destroyed by a lesion as well as the proportion of subjacent white matter that has been involved by the lesion (Fig. 2-2). Again, error is reduced.

This new technique requires a T1-weighted MRI scan with contiguous thin slices (1.5 mm). For best results, the scan should be performed in the chronic stage. Regular MRI scans obtained for diagnostic purposes with thicker slices, interslice gaps, and other pulse specifications are not adequate for reconstruction. Furthermore, application of this elaborate procedure to acute lesions would be a waste of effort.

The Template Technique

Whenever MRI or CT scans are obtained with regular parameters (thick slices, and, in the case of MRI, interslice gaps), anatomic analyses must rely on the template technique.

The template technique relies on film transparencies of MRI or CT. For research purposes, it is advisable to have a technician collect all the films for a given case, mask the subject identification in all of them, and substitute a numerical entry code on the basis of which imaging data can be stored. This step ensures that the investigator performing the anatomic study is blind to the neurologic and neuropsychological data available for the same subject.

Figure 2-1

Three-dimensional reconstruction (obtained from 124 contiguous thin coronal MRI slices) of the brain of a subject with an infarct in the left frontal lobe. Acutely, the subject had a nonfluent aphasia and mild paresis of the right face and arm. At the time of the MRI (1 year later), both language deficit and paresis had improved.

Several sulci were identified and color-coded on the 3D reconstructed brain: central sulcus (red), precentral sulcus (green), inferior frontal sulcus (yellow), superior frontal sulcus (brown), and sylvian fissure (magenta).

Inspection of the left lateral and top views of the brain shows that the area of infarct is centered on the precentral sulcus, which is clearly visible only in the top view. The most anterior sector of the precentral gyrus is damaged, as well as the posterior sector of the middle frontal and inferior frontal gyrus.

The brain volume was also resectioned in axial (ax), coronal (co), and parasagittal (ps) slices (as shown in the three rows of brain slices in the lower segment of the image). Whenever any of the slices intersected a color-coded sulcus, the color automatically appeared on the slice, thus permitting an accurate identification of sulci and of gyri. Resectioning allowed us to inspect the lesion in depth and show that it extended all the way to the insula, which is compromised in its most superior sector (best seen in slice ps-3).

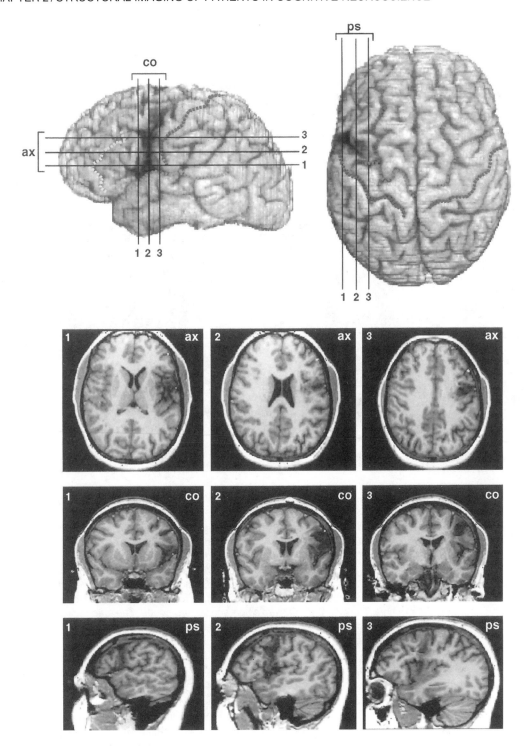

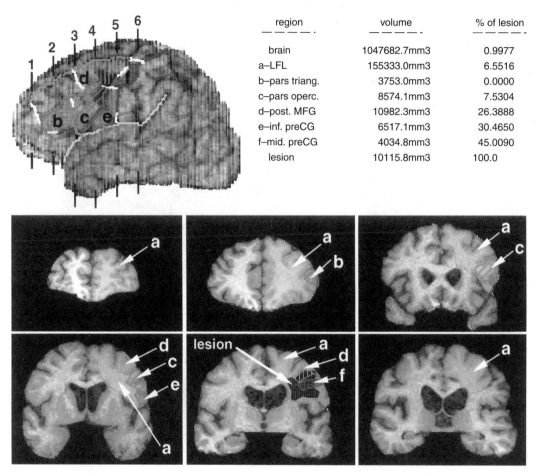

region	volume	% of lesion
brain	1047682.7mm3	0.9977
a–LFL	155333.0mm3	6.5516
b–pars triang.	3753.0mm3	0.0000
c–pars operc.	8574.1mm3	7.5304
d–post. MFG	10982.3mm3	26.3888
e–inf. preCG	6517.1mm3	30.4650
f–mid. preCG	4034.8mm3	45.0090
lesion	10115.8mm3	100.0

Figure 2-2

Three-dimensional reconstruction of a human brain with a lesion in the left frontal lobe. The questions addressed here concerned the size of the lesion and the percentage of volume it occupied in the whole brain, in the left frontal lobe (LFL), and in some subdivisions of the frontal lobe: the pars triangularis (pars triang.) and the pars opercularis (pars operc.), the posterior half of the middle frontal gyrus (post. MFG), and the precentral gyrus in its inferior (inf. preCG) and middle thirds (mid. preCG). The limits of all of these regions of interest (ROI) were marked on the 3D reconstructed brain. On all coronal slices, the several ROIs are individually traced, as is the contour of the lesion. Six coronal slices are shown as an example. The different ROIs are color- and texture-coded. The automatically calculated absolute volumes and the percentage of damage in each of them are recorded on the top right-hand corner.

As with the previous technique, detailed knowledge of human neuroanatomy is indispensable. Needless to say, the investigator must be conversant with the imaging techniques themselves. The template technique relies on the availability of brain templates of the normal brain such as those published by us in 1989 and 1995. The key steps are as follows:

1. Determine the angle of incidence in which CT or MRI were obtained. This can be achieved on the

basis of a pilot scan or by inspection of the lower axial slices in which the relative positions of structures in the three main cranial fossae can be observed.

2. On the basis of the above determination, select the set of templates that best fits the subject's films.

3. Chart the lesion on the templates at every level at which it occurs, using an *X/Y* plotting strategy.

4. Superimpose over the template an appropriate "in register" transparency that contains anatomic cells representing neural "areas of interest" in both gray and white matter structures. Each of those cells is limited by a linear boundary and has a letter and number code on the basis of which it can be anatomically identified.

5. Assign the area of damage charted in the template to the cells that encompass the abnormal images.

6. Assign the estimation of the amount of involvement within target cells. We usually code this 0 when there is less than 25 percent involvement of the total, 1 if the involvement is between 25 and 75 percent; and 2 if more than 75 percent of the total area is damaged. This step can be achieved in two ways: (a) using a transparent square grid and counting the number of units involved by the lesion at each level, then calculating the percentage in relation to the total number of units encompassed by each area of interest (which is the sum of units occupied by the region at each template level); or (b) transferring the template system into computer software, tracing the lesion's limits as marked on the template with a digitizer, and then using automated determination of the percentage of area involved.

The number of cuts in the scan and in the correctly chosen set of templates may not coincide for two reasons: varied thickness of cuts and variations in individual brain size. Therefore, the investigator must search for the most appropriate scan/template matches, on a cut-by-cut basis, using all available anatomic constants—for example, ventricular system and prominent sulci. Fortunately, current MRI resolution provides such a wealth of landmarks that finding appropriate correspondences is no longer a daunting task. Correspondences are a necessary complement to the *X/Y* plotting approach. The results of *X/Y* plotting should be counterchecked by inspection of identifiable landmarks, since "blind" plotting may produce an inaccurate chart. This is why we do not advocate the use of fully automated lesion analysis with the template technique.

The major source of error in the template technique is the choice of the wrong template set. The key to the correct choice of templates is the inspection of *all* available brain cuts, especially the lower ones, which contain crucial landmarks for the determination of the incidence of a particular scan. In practical terms, it is necessary to compare the proportion of frontal lobe, temporal lobe, and posterior fossa structures shown in the scan with those seen in the various template sets and to select the best match. It is not possible to find the right match based on the inspection of high cuts alone, because in high-lying cuts, the cues from anatomic constraints such as the ventricular system or bony landmarks are lost.

Improved Template Technique

The availability of BRAINVOX and of 3D reconstructed normal brains has allowed us to improve the template technique. It is now possible to create "customized templates" for any set of CT or MRI slices. Instead of using published templates, a 3D reconstructed normal brain can be resliced so as to match the incidence of cut and the level of slices in the CT or MR images to the analyzed (Fig. 2-3). The key steps are as follows:

1. All major sulci are identified and color-coded in the 3D reconstructed normal brain.

2. The normal brain is resliced on the computer screen so as to match the slice orientation and thickness of the 2D images of the brain to be analyzed, creating an equal number of brain slices (the "customized template set"). The color codes generated in (1) are automatically transferred onto the single brain slices.

3. On each matched pair of normal/abnormal brain slices, the lesion is transferred in much the same manner as described for the basic template technique.

4. The result is a 3D transfer of the lesion, which can then be "read off" the normal 3D reconstructed brain.

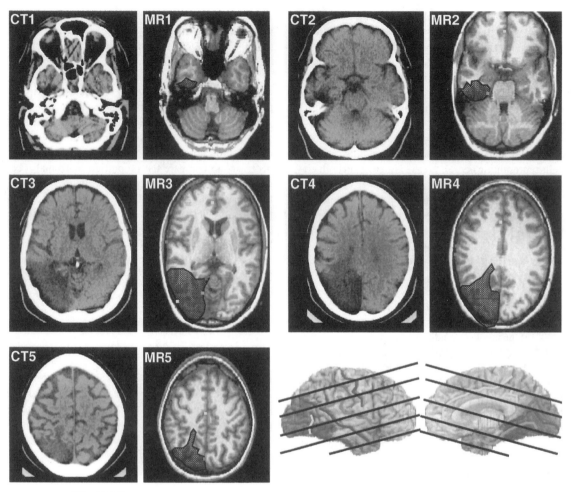

Figure 2-3

Demonstration of the improved template method. Brain CT (CT 1–5) of a subject who could not undergo an MRI study. A normal 3D reconstructed brain was resliced so as to match the orientation and level of the CT slices (MR 1–5). The lesion seen on the CT slices was transferred onto each matched MR slice, taking into account all identifiable sulci and gyri. Once the sulci were color-coded on the 3D reconstruction, the lesion could be read off each individual slice. The object defined by the transferred traces could be fused with the normal brain to visualize the lesion's surface extent (right lower corner).

Analysis of Groups of Subjects

Whenever a study involves a large number of subjects, it may be advantageous to create maps of lesion overlap. For this purpose we have developed a technique that permits the determination of the region of maximal overlap in terms of brain surface ("Map-2," a 2D map),

or in volumetric terms ("Map-3," a 3D map). Each of these techniques entails the transfer of all individual lesions onto a normal reference brain.

For Map-2, the steps are as follows:

1. For each case, each view of the 3D brain showing the lesion is matched with the corresponding

view of the normal reference brain, in terms of spatial coordinates.

2. The surface contour of the lesion is transferred from the subject's brain and fitted onto the normal reference brain, taking into account its relation to sulcal and gyral landmarks.

3. The lesions are then superimposed to form a surface map. A region of maximal lesion overlap is determined on the basis of the superimpositions and assigned a numerical weight based on the number of contributing lesions.

To obtain a Map-3, we transfer and fit the limits of all the target lesions onto the normal reference brain reconstructed in 3D (by transferring the contour of each lesion as seen in each slice into the corresponding slices of the reference brain in the way described above). The sum total of lesion contours for each case constitutes a 3D object. Given the collection of such objects, we then determine the intersection of their volumes in whatever plane we prefer. This allows us to determine overlap in both cortical "surface" and white matter "depth." We refer to the area of maximal overlap as the "center of volume."

Identifying Lesions with Computed Tomography and Magnetic Resonance Imaging

The identification of neuropathologic changes using CT depends on the detection, within a given brain region, of an x-ray absorption that departs from the norm. The presence of cerebral infarction, edema, or tumor at a specified anatomic location alters the standard x-ray absorption for that region and produces an abnormal image.

In the case of MRI, the identification of neuropathologic changes depends on the production of a locally different rate of hydrogen proton spinning, within the affected brain region, after the brain is exposed to a magnetic field. In other words, after the brain is subjected to a magnetic field, with varied magnetic pulse sequence parameters, the presence of a pathologic brain region due to edema, infarction, or tumor will determine hydrogen proton spinning rates within the area that are different from what normally would be expected for the given anatomic structure subjected

to the same magnetic pulse sequence. Lesion-detection sensitivity with either method varies according to the specific procedure, the nature of the pathology, the stage at which the imaging measurement is made in relation to the onset of the pathologic process, and the quality of the equipment and proficiency of the technique.

The potential for false negatives or false positives is considerable, their magnitude depending on the factors listed above. For example, CT is often negative in the first 24 h following an infarct but is usually positive in the days after. However, in the second and third weeks after an infarct, because the infarcted tissue absorbs x-rays at the same rate as normal tissue, the CT may become negative again if not performed after the injection of a contrast-enhancing substance. Contrast seeps out of damaged vessels in the damaged region and increases the density of the area.

Neuroanatomic Resolution

The limits of resolution in the lesion method are set by the state of the technology. Current-generation CT and MRI scanners detect lesions as small as 1 mm on the plane of section. From the perspective of microstructure, these seemingly astounding resolutions are actually modest, since such small areas contain so many neurons and connections. Nonetheless, from the perspective of cytoarchitecture or of cortical regions defined neurophysiologically, this resolution is quite respectable. In short, current imaging technology visualizes neural structure at a level that permits the neuroanatomic definition of most lesions resulting from acquired neurologic disease or neurosurgical ablations.

Neither CT nor MRI can detect discrete cellular pathology except when a fairly large cortical region or subcortical nucleus is affected over a sizable surface or volume that turns out to be, in the aggregate, larger than the lower limit of resolution discussed above. This is why, in the early stages of degenerative dementia of either the Alzheimer or Pick types, when neuropsychological assessment already reveals marked cerebral dysfunction, CT and MRI studies may be so deceptively normal. At the same stage, however, dynamic neuroimaging using emission tomography procedures, of either the SPECT or PET types, may show changes in cerebral blood flow or metabolism.

Decreased radio signal in posterior temporal and temporoparietal regions is quite characteristic of Alzheimer's dementia.[8–11] This is probably the consequence of both local pathologic changes and local physiologic changes brought about by anterior temporal lesions.

In moderate to advanced stages of Alzheimer's disease, CT and MRI often show fairly widespread cerebral atrophy or ventricular enlargement. In addition, MRI studies may also show a reduction in the volume of medial temporal structures, the result of accumulated damage in entorhinal and perirhinal cortices, and subsequent degeneration in hippocampus.[12,13]

In Pick's disease, autopsy studies have shown repeatedly that the characteristic pathology is especially evident in the frontal and anterior temporal cortices,[14] and in moderate to advanced cases, anatomic analysis of CT or MRI of patients with progressive dementia does reveal severe atrophy localized to those regions.[15]

The Choice of Neuropathologic Specimens

The choice of pathologic specimen is a major technical consideration in the lesion method, given that the neuropathologic characteristics of infarctions, intraparenchymal hemorrhages, or varied types of tumor are entirely different.

Nonhemorrhagic infarctions provide the best specimens for neuroanatomic investigation and correlation with neuropsychological findings, because cerebral infarctions actually destroy brain parenchyma. The infarcted area is eventually replaced by scar tissue and by cerebrospinal fluid, and CT or MRI in the chronic state provide a clear demarcation of the infarct. In CT, the damage is depicted as an area of decreased density, seen as a darker area in the gray scale that accompanies the images. In MRI, infarctions show as a dark area in T1-weighted images and a white bright signal region in T2-weighted images.

Herpes simplex encephalitis provides comparable anatomic detail. In adults, the virus has an affinity for a limited set of brain structures, mostly within the limbic system, and it destroys those areas rather completely by a mechanism that includes vascular collapse. In the chronic state, both CT and MRI produce extremely accurate images of the involved territories.

In most other varieties of neuropathologic process, the precise anatomic definition of lesions is less accurate and the functional impact of the lesion itself is less well defined. For instance, earlier in their growth, *gliomas* infiltrate brain tissue by dislocating local populations of neurons but may not destroy them immediately. Moreover, the region of low or high density seen on the CT or MRI of such tumors corresponds not just to the tumor tissue but also to edema surrounding it and to brain tissue that may still be functionally competent. In other words, in such cases it may be impossible to decide that the brain parenchyma is destroyed or that the area is functionally inoperative, or, for that matter, that an area without apparent abnormality is free of tumor. For these reasons, we do not believe that patients with glial tumors are a first choice for the lesion method. This point is made clear in a study by Anderson and coworkers,[16] who compared the neuropsychological profile of patients with confirmed gliomas to that of patients with strokes in the same regions.

Where subjects with glial tumors pose problems for the lesion method, those in whom *meningiomas* have been excised and who have had a circumscribed ablation of brain tissue are actually ideal cases. The images from such cases are entirely appropriate to establish a link between the anatomic site of the ablation and the neuropsychological profile obtained *after* the ablation has taken place.

Patients who have had ablations for seizure treatment also afford a good opportunity for behavioral and anatomic studies. In those cases, MRI obtained with T1-weighted images can help delineate the extent of brain tissue removal with extraordinary precision, although some caution is recommended in the interpretation of neuropsychological data obtained in such patients. Some patients who undergo surgical removal of brain tissue for the treatment of uncontrollable seizures may have developmental brain defects. Those whose seizures began early in life are likely to have had some degree of compensatory brain reorganization before surgery. Frequent and long-standing seizural discharges may also produce changes elsewhere in the brain. The participation of such patients in lesion studies must be evaluated on an individual basis.

The inclusion in lesion method studies of subjects with *metastatic disease, intracerebral hemorrhages,* or *severe head injury* must also be decided on an individual basis, lest it contaminate otherwise valid results. For instance, data from patients with a single brain metastasis, removed surgically and studied in the stable, postoperative state, concomitantly with a good-quality CT or MRI, are quite acceptable.

Intracerebral hemorrhages affect the brain by two different mechanisms. They destroy neural tissue, as nonhemorrhagic infarctions do, and they cause a space-occupying blood collection that displaces neurons, as tumors do. During the acute phase of a hemorrhage, neither CT nor MRI provides an accurate picture of the abnormality, because within the area of abnormal signal some neurons are truly destroyed, whereas others are simply displaced. The amount and location of tissue destruction can be estimated only after the resolution of the hematoma.

In conclusion, the specimen of choice for the purpose of establishing correlates between dysfunction and site of brain destruction are cases of nonhemorrhagic infarction and herpes encephalitis. Surgical ablations performed for the treatment of meningiomas also provide excellent material. Other material should be used on an individual basis, after careful assessment of the dynamics of lesion development.

Timing of Imaging

The timing of CT and MRI data collection is of the essence, especially in relation to subjects with stroke. Both CT and MRI may fail to show *any* abnormality when they are obtained immediately after the occurrence of a stroke. With modern-generation CT and MRI scanners, most images will be positive after 24 h. This is certainly not the case with older scanners, however. It is important to keep in mind that many CT (or even MRI) studies obtained less than 24 h after the onset of a stroke may be negative, especially when a patient with an acute stroke happens to have a CT or MRI that shows a well-demarcated area of low density with sharp margins. Such an image, early after stroke, should suggest a previous infarct, probably unrelated to the new set of symptoms.

Positive CT images obtained in the first week post-onset usually show areas of abnormality that are far larger than the region of actual structural damage because of confounding phenomena—for example, edema. This commonly occurs and means that the results of observations and experiments conducted at later epochs should not be correlated with the anatomic analysis performed in the acute images.

When CT is obtained in the second or third week after a stroke's onset without intravenous infusion of a contrast-enhancing substance, the images are negative in a good number of cases. The image can change even after a previous CT obtained earlier showed a large area of decreased density. During this period, the damaged area can show the same density as the normal tissue. On the other hand, in contrast-enhanced CT images, those normal-looking areas will appear as areas of increased density (primarily due to seepage of contrast substance through the walls of newly formed vessels in the affected region). In the chronic stage, which we define as 3 months post-onset and beyond, most CT studies of infarction are unequivocally positive. Even then, however, when strokes are small and located close to a major sulcus or to the wall of a ventricle, the chronic CT may mislead the observer, resembling images of focal "atrophy" with sulcal enlargement or images of ventricular dilatation. When no previous images are available for comparison with those obtained in the chronic stage, the correct interpretation and the establishment of an adequate behavioral/anatomic correlation may not be possible.

Similar problems befall MRI with images obtained with only one pulse sequence. T1-weighted images obtained with an inversion recovery (IR) pulse sequence provide maximal anatomic detail. With this pulse sequence, however, infarctions appear as dark areas, in precisely the same range of grays used to depict the ventricular system or any region filled with cerebrospinal fluid, such as the cerebral sulci and fissures. When infarcts are small and close to one of these structures, they may not be readily distinguishable. Images obtained with different pulse sequences on MRI (proton density or T2-weighted) show the damaged area as a region of intense bright signal, more easily distinguishable from the bright signals generated by white and even gray matter.

A meaningful relation between an anatomic image and a particular neuropsychological pattern requires reasonable temporal closeness between the epochs at which the image and the neuropsychological data were obtained. Because, during the acute period, edema and brain distortion often occur, it is not easy to define precisely the location and amount of destroyed tissue. The pairing of such images with observations made in the chronic state may lead to error. Likewise for the inverse situation—that is, pairing the results of acute neuropsychological observations obtained in the acute state with the anatomy gleaned during the chronic stage. The most reliable anatomic and neuropsychological data are obviously those obtained in the chronic stage.

Other Considerations

A traditional limitation of the lesion method in humans has been the excessive reliance on single cases. Many of the important observations made in the past were uncontrolled and went unreplicated, the significance of the results being thus diminished. Notable exceptions—for instance, Milner's collection of epileptic patients with surgical ablations in temporal and frontal lobe, Newcombe's head injury project, or Gazzaniga's group of epileptics with split brain interventions—simply confirm the rule. In our laboratory, we have obviated this limitation by creating a continuously renewed population of patients with lesions in varied neural systems who would be willing to participate in neuropsychological experiments. The goal was to conduct multiple single-subject studies in target patients and in controls with an approach as rigorous as the one used in the traditional experimental setting and to make it possible to design and carry out experiments in which certain hypotheses regarding anatomy and function could be probed comprehensively, using many individual data sets.

It goes without saying that, given optimal neuroanatomic analysis, the lesion method will be only as successful as the quality of the cognitive tasks used in the experiments and the quality of the theoretical framework and hypotheses being tested. The rapidly evolving fields of cognitive science and experimental neuropsychology have provided investigators with many useful tasks applicable to most aspects of cognition and behavior likely to be studied with the lesion method. There are also many relevant theoretical developments concerning the conceptualization of both the cognitive and neural architectures in humans. The traditional divisions between behaviorist and cognitivist views seem to have been largely overcome by theoretical positions that combine the best of both (see, for examples, Refs. 17 to 19). The conceptualization of neural structures and of their operations, insofar as mental processes and behaviors are concerned, has also changed radically, as indicated at the beginning of this chapter. Neural signaling is seen as both massively parallel and massively sequential, and, no less importantly, massively recurrent. The prevalence of feedforward and feedback loops disposed along as well as across neural streams has been duly noted, and so has the convergent/divergent nature of those neuron streams. The dependence on timing mechanisms for the normal operations of these networks is well accepted.[20–24]

REFERENCES

1. Ungerleider LG, Mishkin M: Two cortical visual systems, in Ingle DJ, Mansfield RJW, Goodale MA (eds): *The Analysis of Visual Behavior.* Cambridge, MA: MIT Press, 1982.

2. Newcombe F, Russell WR: Dissociate visual, perceptual and spatial deficits in focal lesions of the right hemisphere. *J Neurol Neurosurg Psychiatry* 332:73–81, 1969.

3. Damasio A, Tranel D, Damasio H: Face agnosia and the neural substrates of memory. *Annu Rev Neurosci* 13:89–109, 1990.

4. Damasio AR, Damasio H, Tranel D, Brandt JP: Neural regionalization of knowledge access: Preliminary evidence. *Symposia on Quantitative Biology* 55:1039–1047, 1990.

5. Tranel D, Damasio H, Damasio AR, Brandt JP: Separate concepts are retrieved from separate neural systems: Neuroanatomical and neuropsychological double dissociations (abstr). *Soc Neurosci* 21:1497, 1995.

6. Damasio H, Damasio A: *Lesion Analysis in Neuropsychology.* New York, Oxford University Press, 1989; Japanese edition, Tokyo: Igaku-Shoin, 1992.

7. Damasio H: *Human Brain Anatomy in Computerized Images.* New York: Oxford University Press, 1995.

8. Chase TN, Foster NL, Fedio P, et al: Regional cortical dysfunction in Alzheimer's disease as determined by positron emission tomography. *Ann Neurol* 15(suppl): S170–S174, 1984.

9. Foster NL, Chase TN, Mansi L, et al: Cortical abnormalities in Alzheimer's disease. *Ann Neurol* 16:649–654, 1984.

10. Friedland RP, Budinger TF, Ganz E, et al: Regional cerebral metabolic alterations in dementia of the Alzheimer

type: Positron emission tomography with (18F) flu-orodeoxyglucose. *J Comp Assist Tomogr* 7:590–598, 1983.

11. Rezai K, Damasio H, Graff-Radford N, et al: Regional cerebral blood flow abnormalities in Alzheimer's disease. *J Nucl Med* 26(5):105, 1985.

12. Hyman BT, Damasio AR, Van Hoesen GW, Barnes CL: Cell specific pathology isolates the hippocampal formation in Alzheimer's disease. *Science* 225:1168–1170, 1984.

13. Van Hoesen GW, Damasio A: Neural correlates of the cognitive impairment in Alzheimer's disease, in Plum F (ed): *The Handbook of Physiology.* Bethesda, MD: American Physiological Society, 1987, pp 871–898.

14. Escourelle R, Poirier J: *Manual of Basic Neuropathology.* Philadelphia: Saunders, 1978.

15. Graff-Radford NR, Damasio AR, Hyman BT, et al: Progressive aphasia in a patient with Pick's disease: A neuropsychological, radiologic and anatomic study. *Neurology* 40:620–626, 1990.

16. Anderson SW, Damasio H, Tranel D: The use of tumor and stroke patients in neuropsychological research: A methodological critique. *J Clin Exp Neuropsychol* 10:32, 1988.

17. Kosslyn SM: *Image and Brain: The Resolution of the Imagery Debate.* Cambridge, MA: Bradford Books/MIT Press, 1994.

18. Damasio AR: *Descartes' Error: Emotion, Reason and the Human Brain.* New York: Grosset/Putnam, 1994.

19. Churchland PS, Sejnowski JF: *The Computational Brain: Models and Methods on the Frontiers of Computational Neuroscience.* Cambridge, MA: Bradford Books/MIT Press, 1992.

20. Damasio AR: The brain binds entities and events by multiregional activation from convergence zones. *Neural Comput* 1:123–132, 1989.

21. Damasio AR, Damasio H: Cortical systems for retrieval of concrete knowledge: The convergence zone framework, in Koch C (ed): *Large-Scale Neuronal Theories of the Brain.* Cambridge, MA: MIT Press, 1994, pp 61–74.

22. Crick F: *The Astonishing Hypothesis: The Scientific Search for the Soul.* New York: Scribner's, 1994.

23. Edelman G: *Neural Darwinism.* New York: Basic Books, 1987.

24. Rockland KS (ed): Special issue: Local cortical circuits. *Cerebral Cortex* 3:361–498, 1993.

Chapter 3

FUNCTIONAL IMAGING IN COGNITIVE NEUROSCIENCE I: BASIC PRINCIPLES

Geoffrey Karl Aguirre

The methods of behavioral neurology and neuropsychology fall into two broad categories, each of which has a long history. The first category includes manipulations of the neural substrate itself. Such an intervention might inactivate a brain area, perhaps through a lesion, with Paul Broca's 1861 observation of the link between language and left frontal lobe damage providing a prototypical example. The effects of stimulation of brain areas can also be studied, as Harvey Cushing did with the human sensory cortex in the early twentieth century. In the second category, observation techniques relate a measure of neural function to behavior. Hans Berger's work in the 1920s on the human electroencephalographic response is a good starting point.

Impressive refinements and additions to both of these categories have taken place over the last century. For example, beyond the static lesions of "nature's accidents" that have been the mainstay of cognitive neuropsychology for many years, it is now possible to reversibly inactivate areas of human cortex using transcranial magnetic stimulation (see Chap. 5 for additional details). The realm of "observational" methodology has also grown dramatically in the last few decades, with the development of functional neuroimaging.

In this chapter we concern ourselves with the theoretical and practical properties of functional neuroimaging techniques in general and with blood oxygen level–dependent (BOLD) functional magnetic resonance imaging (fMRI) in particular. We begin with a brief consideration of the nuts-and-bolts physics and physiology that underlie common imaging methods. Next, we consider several aspects of the inferential basis of neuroimaging. Our deliberations here include a "two-systems" model of neuroimaging inference and three general types of hypotheses that can be tested

using these methods. We also explore the relationship between neuroimaging and lesion studies and describe different methods for behaviorally isolating cognitive processes of interest within a neuroimaging experiment. Finally, we discuss some idiosyncratic properties of BOLD fMRI as they relate to different categories of temporal organization of experiments (e.g., blocked, event-related, etc.). Except for a few glancing references, the subject of the statistical analysis of neuroimaging data in general and BOLD fMRI in particular is avoided.

PROPERTIES OF FUNCTIONAL NEUROIMAGING DATA

In general, functional neuroimaging can be defined as the class of techniques that provide volumetric, spatially localized measures of neural activity from across the brain and across time—in essence, a three-dimensional movie of the active brain. Importantly, functional imaging data have a particular order in time that cannot be changed without fundamentally altering the nature of the original data. Virtually all neuroimaging experiments vary an experimental condition over time and evaluate the relationship between the experimental manipulation and the observed time series.

Relatively noninvasive measurements of blood flow in the human brain were first accomplished in 1963 by Glass and Harper by measuring the decay of inhaled, radioactive xenon gas. This method could provide only global measurements of blood flow within the head, so it could not be used to generate images. This was to change soon after the introduction of computed tomography (CT) in the 1970s. Developed for use with x-ray images, CT methods allowed the reconstruction of a volumetric image of the body by passing x-rays through the subject from multiple directions. These ideas were soon applied to measurements of metabolic function in the human brain, with the twist that instead of directing radiation energy through the body, the source of radiation was located within the subject. In positron emission tomography (PET), the subject is injected with a radioisotope that, as it decays, produces positrons. These are immediately annihilated by joining with electrons, producing two photons that travel outward in opposite directions. An array of sensors located around the subject's head uses "coincidence detection" to determine the source of the radioactive decay in space.

Using radiolabeled water, PET was initially applied as a method of measuring local cerebral tissue perfusion. In the 1980s, functional changes in blood flow became the object of study, by comparing the distribution of cerebral perfusion during different cognitive states. In the following decades, PET techniques were used extensively in the service of research in cognitive neuropsychology. While PET provides for a spatial resolution on the order of a few millimeters, temporal resolution is limited by the half-life of the radioisotope used. Practically, PET images can be obtained only every few minutes, limiting the ability of the method to dynamically track changes in neural activity related to cognitive processes. It is this limitation in temporal resolution, coupled with the invasive and expensive need for radioisotope injection, that ultimately led fMRI methods to supplant PET as the primary tool of investigation in cognitive neuroscience.

The use of MRI to assay neural function was initiated by Belliveau and his colleagues in 1991, who used an injected contrast agent (gadolinium) to obtain perfusion MR images of the occipital cortex during visual stimulation. The widespread application of fMRI awaited the development of a noninvasive endogenous tracer method, subsequently introduced by Ogawa and colleagues in 1993 (see Ref. 26). Fortuitously, hemoglobin, the primary oxygen-carrying molecule in the blood, has different magnetic properties when bound and unbound to oxygen, and this serves as the agent of contrast in BOLD fMRI. Local changes in neural activity give rise to a chain of physiologic and imaging events, many of the details of which are still under study. In brief, increases in neural activity produce local increases in blood flow,[1] which in turn

engender a delayed decrease in local deoxyhemoglobin concentration.[2] This is sometimes referred to as a paradoxical change, as increased metabolic activity leads to a decrease in deoxyhemoglobin. Because deoxyhemoglobin has stronger magnetic properties than oxyhemoglobin, a decrease in the deoxyhemoglobin concentration results in a decreased perturbation of the local magnetic field (referred to as a *susceptibility* gradient). This increases the $T2^*$-weighted fMRI signal[3] from the area, which serves as the dependent data for fMRI. Several excellent reviews of the physics and physiology underlying BOLD fMRI are available for the interested reader (e.g., Moonen and Bandettini[4]).

Unlike PET, where the signal measured can be expressed as a physical quantity (e.g., milliliters of blood per grams of tissue per minute), the BOLD fMRI signal has no simple, absolute interpretation. This is because the particular signal value obtained is not *exactly* a measure of deoxyhemoglobin concentration but is instead a measure that is *weighted* by this concentration (i.e., is $T2^*$-weighted) and is also influenced by a number of other factors that can vary from voxel to voxel, scan to scan, and subject to subject. As a result, experiments conducted with BOLD fMRI generally test for differences in the magnitude of the signal between different conditions within a scan. One could not, for example, directly contrast the absolute level of the BOLD fMRI signal obtained within the temporal lobe of schizophrenic patients with that from controls with much hope of obtaining a reliable or unbiased statistical test. Notably, recent developments in perfusion imaging offer the ability to obtain an fMRI signal that can be interpreted in concrete physical units.[5,6]

The spatial and temporal resolution of BOLD fMRI is limited by the neurovascular coupling that is the source of contrast. While MR images can readily be obtained every 100 ms and with spatial resolution in the tenths of a millimeter, this fine resolution has little practical advantage. Changes in neural activity give rise to a change in BOLD fMRI signal that evolves over seconds (described in detail below). As a result, BOLD fMR images are seldom acquired more frequently than once a second. Additionally, a point of neural activity engenders a change in BOLD signal that spreads over several millimeters; thus BOLD images are typically composed of voxels (the smallest-volume "pixel" of which the image is composed) no smaller than 1 mm on a side.

THE "TWO-SYSTEMS" MODEL OF FUNCTIONAL NEUROIMAGING EXPERIMENTS

Engineers frequently find it convenient to discuss an object of study as a *system*. Simply defined, a system is something that takes input and provides output. One can imagine many different examples of systems, such as a car, where the pressure upon the gas pedal is the input and the speed of the car is the output. Certain types of systems are particularly amenable to study and characterization.

What is the system under study in functional neuroimaging experiments of cognitive neuropsychology hypotheses? A profitable way of answering this question is with a *two-systems* model, in which the domain of mental operations and cognitive processes is held separate from vascular physiology and imaging physics (Fig. 3-1).

The first system is that of cognition, in which the inputs are the instructions, stimuli, and tasks presented to the subject by the experimenter and the output is the pattern of neural activity evoked within the brain. The second system is the domain of physiology

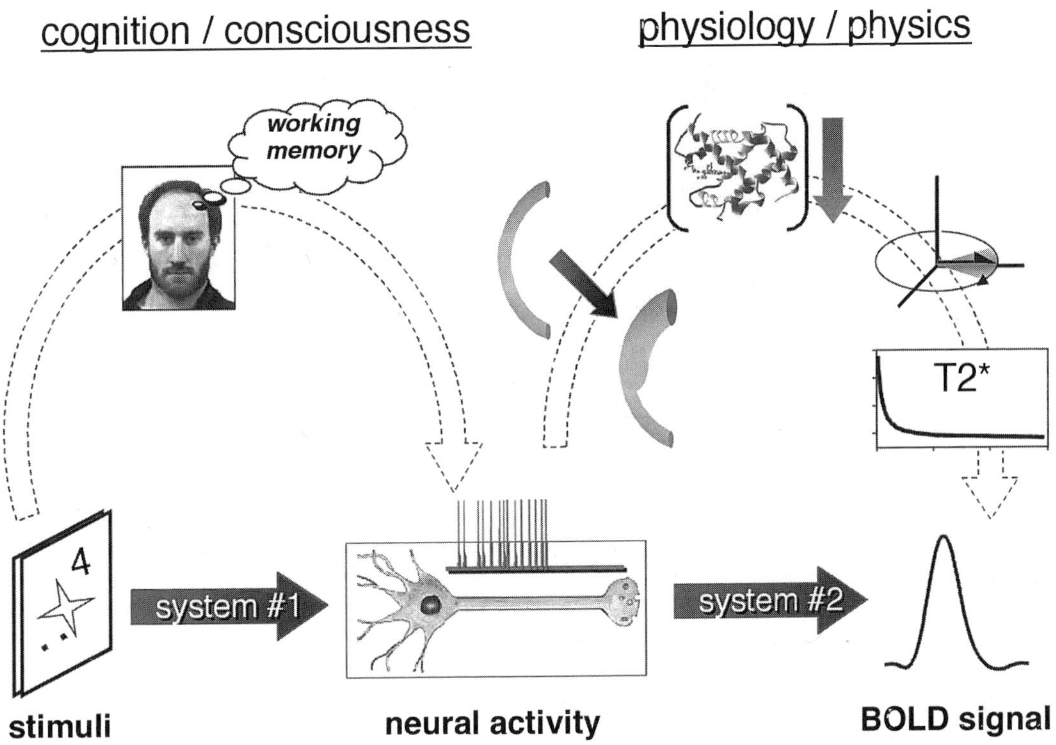

Figure 3-1

Depiction of the "two-systems" model of BOLD fMRI experiments. The left side of the figure represents the system that mediates the transformation of stimuli and instructions into neural activity. The cognitive processes that mediate this transformation are typically the subject of study of neuropsychology experiments. The right side of the figure depicts the system that transforms neural activity into BOLD fMRI signal. Following along the curved arrow on the right, the chain of events that follows an increase in neural activity includes dilatation of local vasculature, a decrease in the concentration of deoxyhemoglobin, and an alteration in local magnetic field inhomogeneity, impacting T2* signal and ultimately BOLD fMRI signal. As is described in the text, the complicated sequence of events that take place under the "system #2" label can be efficiently modeled by a linear system.

and physics; it mediates the transformation of neural activity inputs into blood-flow responses and imaging signal. In most cognitive neuroscience experiments, the hypotheses of interest concern the patterns of neural activity that are evoked by cognitive processes and therefore chiefly concern the first of these two systems. Of course, many scientists have great interest in the exact physical mechanisms that mediate the neurovascular response; the second system is therefore a frequent target of experiments that do not strictly fall within the realm of cognitive neuroscience.

If it were the case that the properties of both systems were unknown, then it would be a daunting (if not impossible) task to study cognition using functional neuroimaging. This is because one would not be able to assign a given change in imaging signal to cognition or neurovascular coupling. Fortunately the properties of the second system are lawful and well described, even if the exact mechanisms of the transformation are still not well understood. Therefore one is able to state what changes in neural activity are implied by a given pattern of imaging signal. After deriving the implied pattern of neural activity from the observed signal, inferences can be drawn regarding the relationship between cognition and neural activity. This is the process that we effortlessly (and frequently unconsciously) engage when we look at a neuroimaging statistical map.

It is essential to keep the distinction between these two systems clear in considering functional neuroimaging experiments and their interpretation, as there are properties that can be ascribed to one system that are clearly not appropriate for the other. For example, and as discussed in greater depth below, it has been demonstrated that the system that transforms neural activity into BOLD fMRI signal is nearly *linear*. For example, twice the neural input leads to twice the BOLD fMRI signal output. This is obviously not a property that can be readily assumed to be true of the cognition system—presenting twice as many words to be remembered is not a priori assumed to produce twice as much neural activity (although this is a property of the system that might be tested).

What aspect of the first system is studied in a neuroimaging experiment? Typically, these experiments involve a subject in the scanner performing a task of the design of the experimenter. (Although there are certainly exceptions: consider studies of seizure activity

Table 3-1

Examples of cognitive processes and tasks purported to evoke them

Task	Cognitive process
Determine if a stimulus is the same as one seen several seconds earlier	Working memory
Match rotated figures	Mental rotation
Generate a verb for a supplied noun	Semantic recall

or rapid-eye-movement sleep.) As depicted, it is the stimuli and instructions from the task that constitute the inputs to the first system. Ultimately, the purpose of the experiment is to state some relationship between the neural activity observed and the behavior in which the subject engaged. Therefore the researcher often seeks to control not only the *task* that the subject performs but also the *mental states* that the subject enters. The internal mental states of the subject are typically referred to as the cognitive processes. Importantly, a cognitive process is distinct from a task in that multiple tasks might be thought to be able to evoke a single cognitive process (Table 3-1).

Note that simply stating that something is a cognitive process does not make it so! The notion of a cognitive process has a fairly rigorous instantiation within psychology, and the demonstration of the existence of a particular cognitive process is often the target of much behavioral research. For example, Sternberg's additive factors method is a logical system used to identify task manipulations that can demonstrate the existence of independent cognitive processes.[7]

BASIC TYPES OF NEUROIMAGING INFERENCE

Although there are many neuroimaging methods and a seemingly limitless number of applications, the basic type of question being asked usually fits within one of a few categories. Each type of approach makes different assumptions and permits different inferences about the relationship between the brain and behavior. Worth noting now and developed below, an experiment that tries to fit into more than one category at once is likely on shaky logical ground.

By far the most common application of neuroimaging methodology is to *localization* questions, which ask: "what are the neural correlates of a given cognitive process?" Generally, the subject is presented with a task designed to selectively evoke a particular cognitive state of interest, and the neuroimaging method identifies whether and where bulk changes in neural activity accompany that cognitive process. The key assumption for this type of design is that a given cognitive process exists and that the task isolates only that cognitive process. Various techniques are used (such as cognitive subtraction or parametric manipulation, discussed below) to isolate the mental operation of interest from the other processes that invariably are present (e.g., button pushing, preparing responses, etc.).

It is important to understand what these types of experiments *cannot* conclude. Activity evoked by a particular cognitive process cannot be taken as evidence that the activated cortical region is necessary for the cognitive process (in the sense that a lesion of the area would impair the subject's ability to perform the task). If the assumptions of the localization framework are perfectly met, the strongest inference that can be made is that the region is *activated* by the cognitive process. Demonstration of necessity requires a lesion study (or some other method of inactivating neural structures, such as transcranial magnetic stimulation; see below).

In contrast, *implementation* studies ask about the computational mechanisms of a cognitive process within a cortical region. This type of study begins with the assumption that a cortical region is involved in a particular cognitive process. The purpose of the study is then to determine the neurocomputational parameters that mediate the area's participation in that process. For example, one might know that area MT is involved in the cognitive process of motion detection. However, what is the relationship between speed of motion and the MT response? Does motion directed toward the viewer, as opposed to motion directed across the visual field, change the magnitude of neural activity? As another example, consider a region of prefrontal cortex assumed to be involved in the cognitive process of working memory. Does this region change its bulk level of neural activity with increasing memory load (i.e., remember four items instead of two)?

Finally, an *evocation* design turns the familiar direction of neuroimaging inference on its head and asks: "What cognitive process does a given task evoke? Also termed "reverse inference," this framework is used to make inferences about cognition as opposed to neural activity; i.e., the behavior of the subject is the unknown variable. One begins by assuming that a particular cortical region is activated by a *single cognitive process.* This mapping must be unique, in that one and only one cognitive process is capable of activating a particular region. The subject performs a task that may or may not evoke the cognitive process of interest. The fMRI data are then examined to determine whether increased neural activity was present within the specified region during the task; if so, the conclusion is drawn that the subject recruited the cognitive function. In other words, the evocation paradigm may be used to test hypotheses regarding the engagement of cognitive processes during a behavioral state in which the cognitive processes need not be under experimental control.

Suppose, for example, we assume that neural activity in area MT indicates the presence of the cognitive process of motion perception. By examining the neural activity within this area, it becomes possible to learn how unrelated distractors affect motion perception.[8] In another example, we might assume that activity in the "fusiform face area" indicates the cognitive process of face perception. We can then monitor the responses of this area during a binocular-rivalry paradigm that pits face stimuli against house stimuli to learn about the time course of perceptual switching.[9]

What provides the evidence that a particular region is uniquely activated by a specific cognitive process? Logically, only an exhaustive neuroimaging examination of every possible cognitive process under every possible circumstance could provide the necessary evidence. This is obviously impractical, so a series of neuroimaging experiments that demonstrate activation of a particular region during a given cognitive process and no other usually suffices to support the assumption (a logical inference termed *enumerative induction*).

It is worth noting that a common logical error in neuroimaging studies is to try to conduct both evocation *and* localization inferences at the same time. Often, the discussion section of a paper will identify activity in one cortical area as the consequence of a cognitive process the experimenter intended to manipulate in the task and then, in the next paragraph, suggest that activity in some other location (e.g., the frontal lobe) is the result of some other behavior in which the subject engaged (e.g., working memory). This is an error, because the assumptions of each type of inferential framework contradict the other. The localization framework assumes that only a single cognitive process is being manipulated, while the evocation framework assumes that multiple, unspecified mental states are in play.

These three categories of neuroimaging inference should be taken as guidelines and do not exhaust the realm of possible designs. For example, studies of effective connectivity[10] examine the relationship of neural activity in different areas of the brain and are often used to support inferences about implementation, although other applications are certainly possible as well. The primary use of this tripartite division is to help organize one's thinking about the assumptions that underlie a particular experiment.

THE RELATIONSHIP BETWEEN LESION AND NEUROIMAGING STUDIES

Although perhaps counterintuitive, lesion and neuroimaging studies provide for very different and nonoverlapping inferences about the relationships between the brain and behavior. One way to think about these differences is in terms of the logical construct of *necessity*. A common neuropsychological hypothesis states that a particular brain region is necessary for the performance of a particular mental operation. If the region in question is removed (perhaps through a lesion) and the cognitive process is impaired, the hypothesis has been affirmed. While this seems straightforward, several inferential complications can ensue, and the interested reader is directed to Chaps. 2 and 4 for further discussion. One wrinkle discussed here is the possibility that more than one region is capable of supporting the process of interest (perhaps working in parallel, or one serving as a "backup" for the other). In this case, the region still plays an interesting role in the cognitive process, although it is not strictly *necessary* in that a lesion of only that region will not impair the cognitive

process. Therefore an alternate relationship between a neural substrate and a behavior that might be sought is *involvement* (I am indebted to my colleague Eric Zarahn for this particular construct and to his general contribution to the ideas in this chapter). A region is *involved* in a cognitive process if it is necessary under some circumstance (the circumstance being that all the other potential "backup" regions have also been damaged).

Does finding activation of a cortical region in a functional neuroimaging study imply that the region is necessary (or even just involved) in the cognitive process? In short, the answer is no; not only for functional neuroimaging but for all "observation" methods mentioned at the outset (electroencephalography, depth electrode recording, etc.). The primary cause of this state of affairs is the observational, correlative nature of neuroimaging. Although we make inferences regarding cognitive processes, these processes are not themselves directly subject to experimental manipulations. Instead, the investigator controls the presentation of stimuli and instructions, with the hope that these circumstances will provoke the subject to enter a certain cognitive state and *no other.* Careful consideration reveals how this assumption might fail. Although cooperative, the subject may unwittingly engage in confounding cognitive processes in addition to that intended by the experimenter or, alternatively, may fail to differentially engage the process. For example, a subject might constantly engage in the process of declarative memory formation, even during periods of time when he or she is "supposed" to be performing some other control behavior. It is therefore not possible to know if observed changes in neural activity in a brain region are the result of the evocation of the cognitive process of interest or an unintended, confounding process. Negative results (even in the face of arbitrarily high statistical power) are also not conclusive, not only because of the failure of perfect control of evocation of cognitive processes but also because of the possibility that the neuroimaging method employed is not sensitive to the critical change in metabolic activity (e.g., pattern of neuronal firing as opposed to bulk, integrated synaptic activity).

What about the converse inference? If a region is involved in a cognitive process, may we deduce that it would be activated by that cognitive process in a neuroimaging experiment? Again, the answer is no.

Consider the situation in which two cortical regions are both involved in the same cognitive process. One is the "primary" region and the other is the "backup" region. As long as the primary region is functioning, the backup region is quiescent. Thus, a neuroimaging study might fail to demonstrate activation of the backup region even though it is involved in the cognitive process. Interestingly, one might study a patient with a lesion of the primary region and thereby demonstrate activation of the backup region by the cognitive process of interest under that circumstance (see Chap. 4).

What about the case in which a region is actually *necessary* for a cognitive process? Can we now expect that the region will be activated by the cognitive process? The answer is yes, but with a number of caveats. For example, we must be able to assume that the necessity of the region is not some side effect of the lesion method itself—for example, damaging axons that simply passed through the area ("fibers of passage"[11]) or affecting the metabolic activity of remote areas (causing, for example, diaschisis[12]). Also, we must assume that our neuroimaging method is sensitive to all possible changes in neural activity that might be induced by the cognitive process (not just bulk neural activity but synchronicity of firing). If not, then it is possible that the necessary cortical region undergoes a change in state associated with the cognitive process that our technique is unable to observe.

The upshot is that caution should be exercised in applying neuroimaging results to the clinical interpretation of the necessity of a cortical region for behavior. For example, there has been interest in using BOLD fMRI to replace the "Wada" or intracarotid amobarbital test.[13] When this test is performed to guide surgical resection of epileptic foci, each internal carotid artery is in turn catheterized and instilled with anesthetic to determine which hemisphere is dominant for language. The hope is that BOLD fMRI can be used to determine which hemisphere responds to language tasks and thus to replace this invasive procedure. While results so far have indicated a good correlation between the two methods, there is no logical requirement that this be the case. In fact, counterexamples have been presented in which neuroimaging has demonstrated activation in frontal cortical areas not subsequently found to be necessary for language function, and vice versa.[14] Further discussion of the inferences possible from the

joint consideration of imaging data and neurologic patients is deferred until the next chapter.

MANIPULATION OF THE COGNITIVE PROCESS

As was discussed in the setting of inferential framework, many neuroimaging experiments depend upon the isolation of a particular cognitive process for study. Specifically, the fundamental assumption of the localization category of neuroimaging inference is that the cognitive process of interest can be isolated from other mental operations so that the neural correlates of that solitary process can be observed. Here we consider several broad classes of manipulations designed to do this. Note that any of these techniques for evoking a particular cognitive process can be coupled with different temporal structures of designs, described in the next section.

Cognitive subtraction is the prototypical neuroimaging method for putative isolation of cognitive processes, the logic of which derives from similar arguments made in the study of reaction times (e.g., Donders[15]). One condition of the experiment is designed to engage a particular cognitive process, such as face perception, episodic encoding, or semantic recall. This "experimental" condition is contrasted with a "control" condition that is designed to evoke all of the cognitive processes present in the experimental period except for the cognitive process of interest. Under the assumptions of "cognitive subtraction,"[16] differences in neural activity between the two conditions can be attributed to the cognitive process of interest.

Cognitive subtraction assumes, as do the other manipulations described below, that the particular cognitive process of interest can be evoked uniquely. This is a fundamental inferential weakness of many cognitive neuroimaging studies. As has been discussed, although we make inferences regarding cognitive processes, these processes are not themselves directly subject to experimental manipulations. Even the cooperative subject might engage other, confounding mental operations unintentionally, rendering this assumption invalid.

Cognitive subtraction (in neuroimaging) relies upon two additional assumptions: "pure insertion" and linearity. Pure insertion is the idea that a cognitive process can be *added* to a preexisting set of cognitive processes without affecting them. This assumption is difficult to prove, because one would need an independent measure of the preexisting processes in the absence and presence of the new process. If pure insertion fails as an assumption, a difference in neuroimaging signal between the two conditions might be observed not because of the simple addition of the cognitive process of interest, but because of an interaction between the added component and preexisting components. For example, the act of pressing a button to signal a semantic judgment may be different from pressing a button in response to a visual cue. Effects upon the imaging signal that result from this difference would be erroneously attributed to semantic judgment per se.

A second assumption of cognitive subtraction is that the transformation of neural activity into fMRI signal is linear. While the BOLD fMRI system has been shown to exhibit behavior close to that of a linear system, there is some evidence for systematic departures.[17] Failures of linearity can cause adjacent neural events to produce more or less signal than those events would in isolation, rendering subtraction approaches invalid. In fact, failures of cognitive subtraction along these lines have been empirically demonstrated for working memory experiments.[18]

Several other cognitive process manipulations have as their goal a reduction in the reliance upon the assumption of pure insertion. *Factorial* experiments[19] are designed to examine the interactions of two different candidate cognitive processes. The scheme of the design involves (in the simplest case) four conditions, during which two different processes are evoked individually and then jointly. The proposed advantage of the design is that interactions between the two processes can be examined. The presence of an interaction is indicated if the difference in imaging signal between the presence and absence of cognitive process A is itself different when cognitive process B is present or absent. While factorial designs do provide a compelling method for gaining greater insight into the neural implementation of cognitive processes, it is a mistake to claim that such designs obviate the need for the pure insertion assumption. Interpretation of the design requires the assumption that the two cognitive processes have indeed been isolated. The logic by which this

isolation is to occur is the same as that outlined for cognitive subtraction above. That is, process A and process B must be purely inserted into the other cognitive components that allow the experiment to evoke these processes.

The *cognitive conjunction* design[20] has also been proposed to reduce reliance upon the assumption of pure insertion. The logic of the approach is that, if one wishes to discount the possibility of an interaction (i.e., a failure of pure insertion) between the cognitive component to be added and the set of preexisting processes, one should repeat the experiment with a different set of preexisting processes and replicate the result. A rigorous implementation of this notion involves conducting a series of categorical subtraction experiments that all aim to isolate the same cognitive process. The novel twist is that the subtractions need not be complete; that is, the experimental and control conditions can differ in several cognitive processes in addition to the one of interest. The imaging data are then analyzed to identify areas that have a significant, consistent response to the putatively isolated process (i.e., a significant main effect across subtractions in the absence of any significant interactions). Again, while this design reduces the plausibility of some failures of cognitive subtraction, it does not eliminate the possibility. In particular, some cognitive processes by their very nature require the evocation of an antecedent process. For example, can working memory be meaningfully present if not preceded by the presentation of a stimulus to be remembered? If not, then any cognitive conjunction design that attempts to demonstrate the presence of neural activity during a delay period will be susceptible to erroneous results due to interactions between the task manipulation and preexisting task components.

Finally, *parametric* designs offer an attractive alternative to cognitive subtraction approaches. In a parametric design, the experimenter presents a range of different levels of some parameter and seeks to identify relationships (linear or otherwise) between imaging signal and the values that the parameter assumes. This can be done to identify the neural correlates of straightforward changes in stimulus properties or manipulations of a cognitive process. Unlike cognitive subtraction methods, parametric designs do not rely as heavily upon the assumption of pure insertion, as the cognitive process is present during all conditions.

PROPERTIES OF THE BOLD fMRI SYSTEM THAT AFFECT EXPERIMENTAL DESIGN

So far we have described properties of all neuroimaging techniques and considered the inferential consequences of different ways of influencing a subject's mental state. We now turn our attention to the idiosyncratic properties of one particular neuroimaging method: BOLD fMRI. We focus here on two key properties of BOLD fMRI data that fundamentally affect the design of BOLD fMRI experiments: the hemodynamic response function and the presence of low-frequency noise.

As was mentioned earlier, the cascade of neurovascular events that ensue following changes in neural activity and produce changes in BOLD fMRI signal are still under investigation. Fortunately, the BOLD fMRI system has properties of a *linear system,* allowing us to ignore for the most part the messy details of physics and physiology. Like any other system, a linear system takes input and provides output (in this case, neural activity in, BOLD fMRI signal out). Importantly, a linear system can be completely characterized by a property called the impulse response function (IRF), which is the output of the system to an infinitely brief, infinitely intense input. In the context of BOLD fMRI, the hemodynamic response function (HRF) is taken as an estimate of the IRF of the BOLD fMRI system and is the change in BOLD fMRI signal that results from a brief (< 1 s) period of neural activity. Knowledge of the IRF can be used to predict the output of the system to any arbitrary pattern of input by a mathematical process called *convolution.* Therefore knowledge of the shape of the HRF allows one to predict the BOLD fMRI signal that will result from any pattern of neural activity.

The HRF itself can be empirically measured from human subjects by studying the BOLD fMRI signal that is evoked by experimentally induced, brief periods of neural activity in known cortical areas (e.g., neural activity in the primary motor cortex in response to a button press). The shape of the HRF reflects its vascular origins (Fig. 3-2) and rises and falls smoothly over a period of about 16 s. While the shape of the HRF varies significantly across subjects, it is very consistent within a subject, even across days to months.[21] There is some

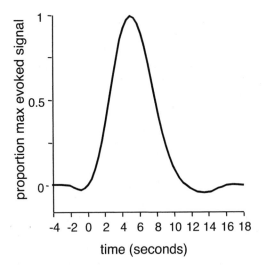

Figure 3-2
An average, across-subject hemodynamic response function. The brief period of neural activity that produced this signal change took place at time zero.

evidence that the shape of the HRF varies from one region of the brain to another (perhaps from variations in neurovascular coupling), but this is a difficult notion to test, as it is necessary to induce patterns of neural activity in disparate areas of the brain that can be guaranteed to be very similar.

The temporal dynamics of neural activity are quite rapid, on the order of milliseconds, but changes in blood flow take place over the course of seconds. One consequence of this, as demonstrated by the smooth shape of the HRF, is that rapid changes in neural activity are not well represented in the BOLD fMRI signal. The "temporal blurring" induced by the HRF leads to many limitations placed on the types of experiments that can be conducted using BOLD fMRI. Specifically, the smooth shape of the HRF makes it difficult to discriminate closely spaced neural events. Despite this, it is still possible to detect (1) brief periods of neural activity; (2) differences between neural events in a fixed order, spaced as closely as 4 s apart; (3) differences between neural events, *randomly* ordered and closely spaced (e.g., every second or less); and (4) neural onset asynchronies on the order of 100 ms. The reason that these seemingly paradoxical experimental designs can work is that some patterns of events that occur rapidly or switch rapidly create a low-frequency "envelope"—a larger structure of pattern of alternation that can pass through the hemodynamic response function. In the next section, several types of temporal structures for BOLD fMRI experiments are discussed as well as how the shape of the HRF dictates the properties of these designs.

Another important property of BOLD fMRI data is that greater power is present at some temporal frequencies than others under the null hypothesis (i.e., data collected without any experimental intervention). The power spectrum (a frequency representation) of data composed of independent observations (i.e., white noise) should be "flat," with equal power at all frequencies. When calculated for BOLD fMRI, the average power spectrum is found to contain ever-increasing power at ever lower frequencies (Fig. 3-3), often termed a 1/frequency distribution. This pattern of noise can also be called "pink," named for the color of light that would result if the corresponding amounts of red, orange, yellow, etc., of the visible light frequency spectrum were combined. The presence of noise of this type within BOLD fMRI data has two primary conse-

quences. First, traditional parametric and nonparametric statistical tests are invalid for the analysis of BOLD fMRI data, which is why much of such analysis is conducted using Keith Worsley and Karl Friston's "modified" general linear model[22] as instantiated in SPM and other statistical packages. The second impact is upon experimental design. Because of the greater noise at lower frequencies, slow changes in neural activity are more difficult to distinguish from noise.

The astute reader might note that the consequences of the shape of the hemodynamic response function and the noise properties of BOLD fMRI are at odds. Specifically, the shape of the HRF would tend to favor experimental designs that induce slow changes in neural activity, while the presence of low-frequency noise would argue for experimental designs that produce more rapid alterations in neural activity. As it happens, knowledge of the shape of the HRF and the distribution of the noise is sufficient to provide a principled answer as to how best balance these two conflicting forces.

It is worth noting that other neuroimaging methods have different data characteristics, with different consequences for experimental design. For example, perfusion fMRI is a relatively new approach that provides a noninvasive, quantifiable measure of local cerebral tissue perfusion.[5] Perfusion data do not suffer from the elevated, low-frequency noise present in BOLD, and as a result, perfusion fMRI can be used to detect extremely long time-scale changes in neural activity (over minutes to hours to days) that would simply be indistinguishable from noise using BOLD fMRI.[6]

DIFFERENT TEMPORAL STRUCTURES OF BOLD fMRI EXPERIMENTS

As BOLD fMRI experiments by necessity include multiple task conditions (prototypically, an "experimental" and "control" period), several ways of ordering the presentation of these conditions exist. Different terms are used to describe the pattern of alternation between experimental conditions over time; they include such familiar labels as *blocked* or *event-related*. While these are often perceived as rather concrete categories, the distinction between blocked, event-related, and other

Figure 3-3

The power spectrum representation of the "pink," or "1/frequency" noise present in BOLD fMRI data under the null hypothesis. Data composed of independent observations over time is termed "white" noise and would have a flat line in this representation.

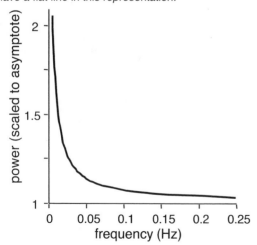

sorts of designs is actually fairly artificial. These may be better considered as extremes along a continuum of arrangements of stimulus order. Consider every period of time during an experiment as a particular experimental condition. This includes the "intertrial interval" or "baseline" periods between stimulus presentations. In this setting, blocked and event-related designs are viewed simply as different ways of arranging periods of "rest" (or no stimulus) with respect to other sorts of conditions. (For a more complete exploration of these concepts, see Friston.[23])

The prototypical fMRI experiment is a blocked approach in which two conditions alternate over the course of a scan. For most hypotheses of interest, these periods of time will not be utterly homogeneous but will consist of several trials of some kind presented together. For example, a given block might present a series of faces to be passively perceived, or a sequence of words to be remembered, or a series of pictures to which the subject must make a living/nonliving judgment and press a button to indicate the response. Blocked designs have superior statistical power compared to all other experimental designs. This is because the fundamental frequency of the boxcar can be positioned at an optimal location with respect to the filtering properties of the hemodynamic response function and the low-frequency noise.

Event-related designs model signal changes associated with individual trials as opposed to blocks of trials. This makes it possible to ascribe changes in signal to particular events, allowing one to randomize stimuli, assess relationships between behavior and neural responses, and engage in retrospective assignment of trials. Conceptually, the simplest type of event-related design to consider is one which uses only a single stimulus type and uses sufficient temporal spacing of trials to permit the complete rise and fall of the hemodynamic response to each trial; a briefly presented picture of a face once every 16 s, for example. Importantly, while this prototypical experiment has only one stimulus, it has *two* experimental conditions (the stimulus and the intertrial interval). If one is willing to abandon the fixed ordering and spacing of these conditions, more complex designs become possible. For example, randomly ordered picture presentations and rest periods could be presented as rapidly

as once a second. The ability to present rapid alternations between conditions initially seems counterintuitive, given the temporal smoothing effects of the hemodynamic response function. While BOLD fMRI is insensitive to the particular high-frequency alternation between one trial and the next, it is still sensitive to the low-frequency "envelope" of the design. In effect, with closely spaced, randomly ordered trials, one is detecting the low-frequency consequences of the random assortment of trial types.

The discussion thus far regarding event-related designs has assumed an ability to randomize perfectly the order of presentation of different event types. There are certain types of behavioral paradigms, however, that do not permit a random ordering of the events. For example, the delay period of a working memory experiment always follows the presentation of a stimulus to be remembered. In this case, the different events of the trial cannot be placed arbitrarily close together without risking the possibility of false-positive results that accrue from the hemodynamic response to one trial event (e.g., the stimulus presentation) being interpreted as resulting from neural activity in response to another event (e.g., the delay period). It turns out that, given the shape typically observed for hemodynamic responses, events within a trial as close together as 4 s can be reliably discriminated.[18] Thus, event-related designs can be used to examine directly, for example, the hypothesis that certain cortical areas increase their activity during the delay period of a working memory paradigm without requiring the problematic assumptions traditionally employed in blocked, subtractive designs.

As a final example of event-related design, consider an experiment that aims to identify a neural onset asynchrony. As noted above, the hemodynamic response observed for a subject during a scanning session is highly reliable in its shape and is relatively smooth (i.e., is not composed of high-frequency components). As a result, it might be possible to use fMRI to detect small neural onset asynchronies. Such a design might present one of two different behavioral trials (in a random order) every 16 s. Because of the reliability of the hemodynamic transformation, differences in the mean time to peak of the responses to the two different types of stimuli could be identified and ascribed to an asynchrony in onset of neural activity.[24] Such a design might allow one, for example, to test the hypothesis that a cortical area that responds to pictures of faces responds with a slightly longer latency (on the order of 100 ms) to pictures of inverted faces.

CONCLUSION

There is an enormous variety of experimental designs that may be used to ask cognitive neuropsychology questions with neuroimaging methods. I have provided here frameworks for organizing these approaches into inferential categories, methods of manipulating evoked cognitive processes, and ways of arranging different experimental conditions in time. Hopefully, the general principles enumerated here will be of use not only for BOLD fMRI, the preeminent neuroimaging method of today, but also for whatever leap in neuroimaging methodology awaits us tomorrow.

REFERENCES

1. Leniger-Follert E, Hossmann K-A: Simultaneous measurements of microflow and evoked potentials in the somatomotor cortex of the cat brain during specific sensory activation. *Pflugers Arch* 380:85–89, 1979.
2. Malonek D, Grinvald A: Interactions between electrical activity and cortical microcirculation revealed by imaging spectroscopy: implications for functional brain mapping. *Science* 272:551–554, 1996.
3. Jezzard P, Song A: Technical foundations and pitfalls of clinical fMRI. *Neuroimage* 4:S63–S75, 1996.
4. Moonen CTW, Bandettini PA (eds): *Functional MRI*. Berlin: Springer-Verlag, 1999.
5. Detre JA, Alsop DC: Perfusion fMRI with arterial spin labeling. In: Bandettini PA, Moonen C (eds): *Functional MRI*. Berlin: Springer-Verlag, 1999, pp 47–62.
6. Aguirre GK, Detre JA, Alsop DC: Experimental design and the relative sensitivity of BOLD and perfusion fMRI. *Neuroimage* 15:488–500, 2002.
7. Sternberg S: The discovery of processing stages: extensions of Donder's method. *Acta Psychol* 30:276–315, 1969.
8. Rees G, Frith CD, Lavie N: Modulating irrelevant motion perception by varying attentional load in an unrelated task. *Science* 278:1616–1619, 1997.
9. Tong F, Nakayama K, Vaughan JT, Kanwisher N: Binocular rivalry and visual awareness in human extrastriate cortex. *Neuron* 21:753–759, 1998.
10. Buchel C, Friston K: Assessing interactions among neural systems using functional neuroimaging. *Neural Networks* 13:871–882, 2000.
11. Jarrard LE: On the role of the hippocampus in learning and memory in the rat. *Behav Neural Biol* 60:9–26, 1993.
12. Feeney DM, Baron J-C: Diaschisis. *Stroke* 17:817–830, 1986.
13. Binder JR, Swanson SJ, Hammeke TA: Determination of language dominance using functional MRI: a comparison with the Wada test. *Neurology* 46:978–984, 1996.
14. Jayakar P, Bernal B, Medina LS, Altman N: False lateralization of language cortex on functional MRI after a cluster of focal seizures. *Neurology* 58:490–492, 2002.
15. Donders FC: On the speed of mental processes. *Acta Psychologia* 30:412–431, 1969.
16. Posner MI, Petersen SE, Fox PT, Raichle ME: Localization of cognitive operations in the human brain. *Science* 24:1627–1631, 1988.
17. Boynton G, Engel S, Glover G, Heeger D: Linear systems analysis of functional magnetic resonance imaging in human V1. *J Neurosci* 16:4207–4221, 1996.
18. Zarahn E, Aguirre GK, D'Esposito M: A trial-based experimental design for fMRI. *Neuroimage* 6:122–138, 1997.
19. Friston KJ, Price CJ, Fletcher P, et al: The trouble with cognitive subtraction. *Neuroimage* 4:97–104, 1996.
20. Price CJ, Friston KJ: Cognitive conjunctions: a new experimental design for fMRI. *Neuroimage* 5:261–270, 1997.
21. Aguirre GK, Zarahn E, D'Esposito M: The variability of human BOLD hemodynamic responses. *Neuroimage* 8:360–369, 1998.
22. Worsley KJ, Friston KJ: The analysis of fMRI time-series revisited—again. *Neuroimage* 2:173–182, 1995.
23. Friston KJ, Zarahn E, Josephs O, et al: Stochastic designs in event-related fMRI. *Neuroimage* 10:607–619, 1999.
24. Menon RS, Luknowsky DC, Gati JC: Mental chronometry using latency-resolved functional MRI. *Proc Natl Acad Sci USA* 95:10902–10907, 1998.
25. Engel S, Zhang X, Wandell B: Colour tuning in human visual cortex measured with functional magnetic resonance imaging. *Nature* 388:68–71, 1997.
26. Ogawa S, Menon RS, Tank DW, et al: Functional brain mapping by blood oxygenation level–dependent contrast magnetic resonance imaging. A comparison of signal characteristics with a biophysical model. *Biophys J* 64:803–812, 1993.

Chapter 4

FUNCTIONAL IMAGING IN COGNITIVE NEUROSCIENCE II: IMAGING PATIENTS

Cathy J. Price
Karl J. Friston

In this chapter, we consider the types of questions that can be addressed with functional neuroimaging investigations of neuropsychologically impaired patients. In particular, we consider the contributions that can be made to normal and abnormal cognitive and anatomic models of behavior. To this end, Sec. I starts with a brief overview of the advantages of functional imaging relative to behavioral measures. Section II highlights the constraints functional imaging places on cognitive models of normal and abnormal processing. Sections III and IV describe how functional imaging studies of neurologically impaired patients can contribute to models of normal functional anatomy and recovery; and Sec. V concludes by emphasizing some of the critical limitations related to patient studies.

SECTION I: ADVANTAGES OF FUNCTIONAL IMAGING STUDIES OF PATIENTS

Relative to behavioral measurements—which usually rely on the accuracy or speed of vocal responses and finger movements—PET and fMRI have several advantages. The first advantage is that neurophysiologic changes at the neural level always precede the motor output/muscular activity required for vocal responses and finger movements. Thus, PET and fMRI can detect significant responses even when there are no behavioral manifestations. The obvious benefit with neuropsychologically impaired patients is that neural activity can be measured in patients who are unable to make vocal or manual responses. For example, a patient could be scanned with PET or fMRI while listening to stories, a task that does not involve behavioral responses. If

semantic areas activate normally, some residual semantic processing might be implied. Another advantage of PET and fMRI is that the hemodynamic response is multidimensional, measured in thousands of voxels across the brain, irrespective of whether the brain regions are involved in task performance or not. By simultaneously recording thousands of data sequences across the whole brain, abnormal effects can be categorized in terms of which neural area or cognitive stage they arise in. For instance, a patient listening to stories may show normal responses in auditory processing areas but no activation in semantic areas.

Multidimensional recordings also have the advantage of tapping into processing that is superfluous to task requirements times. For instance, face naming may elicit emotional responses that do not affect naming times but do change the distribution and composition of hemodynamic responses. Functional imaging can therefore detect activation related solely to changes in facial expression.[1] In this context, we argue that the effect of facial expression is not involved in the task but induced by the stimulus change. It is therefore incidental to the task requirements. Detecting incidental processing of this sort can be particularly useful in the study of patients with limited behavioral responses. For example, Morris et al.[2] have recently reported a functional imaging study of a patient with blind sight. Although the patient was not aware that fearful faces were being presented, discriminatory amygdala responses were detected with functional imaging.

In summary, PET and fMRI provide a measure of cognitive function that is independent of behavioral responses because condition effects are measured by hemodynamic changes (blood flow or deoxyhemoglobin content) rather than the speed and accuracy of overt motor responses. Whereas behavioral measurements are primarily determined by factors that affect task performance (response time and accuracy), functional imaging can reveal significant effects in the absence of any task or when the task/stimulus change has no effect on reaction times and accuracy.

SECTION II: THE CONSTRAINTS THAT FUNCTIONAL NEUROIMAGING PLACES ON COGNITIVE MODELS

The contribution that PET and fMRI provide for understanding the functional anatomy of cognitive processes is undisputed. What is often less clear is how an understanding of normal and abnormal functional anatomy contributes to the corresponding cognitive models. The answer is that functional imaging provides physiologic constraints on cognitive models. In particular it distinguishes between functions associated with specific neural areas from those that emerge from changes in the way a set of areas interact with one another. Without neuroanatomic constraints, an infinite number of cognitive modules can be hypothesized. Although computational approaches have emphasized the explanatory power and biological efficiency associated with implementing functions via changes in connection strengths, connectionist models seldom conform to biological constraints. A classic illustration of the importance of this issue is provided by cognitive models of reading. In the 1980s, the most influential cognitive models of reading (e.g., Patterson and Shewell[3]) emphasized multiple cognitive modules including (1) orthographic analysis, (2) an orthographic input lexicon, (3) a phonologic output lexicon, (4) an orthographic output lexicon, (5) semantic processing, and (6) a subword orthographic to phonologic conversion route. In the 1990s, connectionist models emphasized that the same set of functions could be implemented by only three modules (orthography, semantics, and phonology) and changes in the interactions between these modules (see Seidenberg and McClelland[4]). Functional neuroimaging can evaluate the validity of these models by identifying which neural areas are activated for reading and what the functions of these regions correspond to. For instance, is reading implemented by interactions between neural systems specialized for orthography, semantics, and phonology or are there also neural areas that can be associated with the input and output lexicons?

Studies of neuropsychologically impaired patients can also establish the physiologic validity of cognitive models of normal and abnormal function. Returning to cognitive models of reading, a key factor in their formulation was the observation that brain damage can have remarkably selective effects on reading ability. The well-documented double dissociation[5] is between patients (e.g., surface dyslexics) who have less difficulty reading words and pseudowords with regular/consistent spelling to sound relationships (e.g., *pond* and *yeeping*) than words with irregular spellings (e.g., *yacht*). These patient sometimes attempt to read on the basis of sublexical spelling to sound relationships (e.g., pronouncing *yacht* as *yatched*). In contrast, other patients (e.g., phonologic dyslexics) have more difficulty reading pseudowords (e.g., *yeeping*) that rely on sublexical spelling to sound relationships but are relatively better at reading familiar words with strong semantic associations even when the spelling is irregular (e.g., *yacht* and *choir*). To account for this double dissociation in function, all cognitive models of reading include two or more possible reading routes: one that incorporates sublexical spelling to sound relationships and one that can retrieve the sounds linked to familiar words irrespective of their spelling.

The potential that functional imaging studies of dyslexia offer can be appreciated in light of a limitation with functional imaging studies with normal subjects. The limitation is that irrespective of whether normal subjects are engaged in reading pseudowords or words with regular and irregular spellings, the same set of reading areas are activated with very little effect of word type.[6–12] The most likely explanation is that, irrespective of word type, normal subjects engage all potential reading systems to ensure robust and veridical lexical processing. Scanning patients, with brain damage to one or another reading route, provides a means to segregate these different pathways. An example of such a study is provided by Small and Flores,[13] who report that the left angular gyrus was activated in a patient who presented with "phonologic dyslexia"; after therapy, however, when the patient had learned to read words on the basis of sublexical spelling to sound relationships, there was increased activation in the left lingual gyrus. Further studies of this sort may help to segregate the different reading strategies and explain how they are compromised and then recover following brain damage.

Another way that functional imaging can contribute to abnormal models of cognitive function is through a clear understanding of the role that the damaged area normally plays. Neuropsychological assessments of patients usually focus on deficits that interfere with a normal lifestyle or deficits that the investigator has particular interest in. Understanding normal functional anatomy can motivate and guide other behavioral assessments. Thus, if a patient has a lesion in an area that is known to participate in a particular function, then assessment of that function would be indicated. For example, functional imaging has shown that the right cerebellum is engaged by verbal fluency tasks, although patients with right cerebellar damage do not present with behavioral deficits on standardized language tasks. Motivated by this discrepancy, Feiz et al.[14] investigated the verbal fluency performance of a patient with a right cerebellar infarct and revealed that the patient had subtle deficits learning and completing the task. However, as described in the next section, damage to an area activated in normal subjects does not always impair the patient's performance on the activating task.

SECTION III: NORMAL FUNCTIONAL ANATOMY

In the previous sections, we described how the multidimensional measurements afforded by functional imaging make it sensitive to processes that are "incidental" to task requirements. Incidental processing reflects processes that are elicited in parallel with the task. This may arise because there are multiple routes for performing the same task (e.g., semantic and sublexical word processing) or because the stimuli trigger processing that is not involved in the task (e.g., the effects of facial expression during face naming). Incidental processing has advantages when the aim of the experiment is to detect cognitive responses in patients who have limited motor output (see Sec. I) but disad-

vantages when the aim is to segregate processes that are either necessary or not necessary for intact task performance (see Sec. II). The problem disentangling "necessary" and "incidental" activation can be partially resolved by investigating the effect of damage to areas that activate in normal subjects. In the example given above, Feiz et al.[14] demonstrated that damage to the right cerebellum (activated by verbal fluency tasks) did impair verbal fluency performance. However, if the right cerebellar activation in normal subjects was incidental to task requirements, then no effect of damage would have been detected. Thus, the combination of (1) functional imaging studies of normal subjects and (2) neuropsychological studies of patients with damage to the activated areas should help to refine our models of normal functional anatomy by distinguishing "necessary" from "incidental" activations.

The combination of functional imaging and neuropsychological studies can also help to distinguish different types of incidental processing. Incidental processing can be of two types: (1) involved in the task but "not necessary" because there are other systems/areas that can subserve the same function and (2) not involved in the task but triggered by the same stimuli. Although impaired performance may not be detectable following selective damage to areas involved in either type of incidental processing, damage to an area that is involved in the task would change the necessity of the remaining intact areas. For example, if there are two possible neural mechanisms for the same function, damage to one mechanism should not impair performance but would result in increased reliance on the surviving mechanism. In other words, the surviving mechanism would become necessary for the function. A second lesion affecting the surviving system (or a large lesion incorporating both) would then be expected to impair performance. Incidental processing that is involved in the task can therefore be identified by the differential effects of selective and multiple lesions.[15]

The segregation of different types of activation involved in a task is facilitated in two important ways by functional imaging studies of patients.[16] First, functional imaging studies of patients can identify neural systems that are not activated by normal subjects. For instance, it may be the case that a patient may retain task performance despite damage to all the areas activated by normal subjects. This situation could arise if the patient engaged neural systems that are not normally involved because they are either "inhibited" or "untrained." Functional imaging studies of patients with damage to areas that activate in normal subjects are therefore important for revealing alternative neural systems for the same task. Once a neural system becomes involved in a function, it may also become "necessary" even if it was not necessary in the normal system. This has been demonstrated using the Wada test following lesions to the right hemisphere in the context of a previous lesion to the left hemisphere. For example, injection of sodium amytal in the right hemisphere does not normally disrupt language, but Kinsbourne[19] reported impaired language capabilities in patients who had recovered from aphasia following a left hemisphere lesion.

Functional imaging studies of patients are also required to moderate conclusions that an area is not necessary to complete the task. This is because functional imaging allows pathologic damage to be characterized in a way that cannot be deduced from structural scans (e.g., CT and conventional use of MRI). Residual responsiveness within or around the site of brain damage (i.e., perilesional activation; see Heiss et al.,[17] Warburton et al.[18]) can therefore be detected and indicates that the damaged area may retain some functionality. It would therefore be wrong to conclude that the damaged area was not required for performing the task.

In summary, behavioral studies of patients cannot detect when patients are using atypical neural mechanisms when there are alternative systems for performing the same task. By contrast, functional imaging studies of normal subjects can not distinguish whether activation is (1) necessary to complete the task; (2) involved in the task but "not necessary" because there are other systems/areas that can subsume the same function; or (3) not involved in the task but triggered by the same stimuli. Functional imaging studies of patients with selective and multiple lesions to each component of the normal system can help to overcome these limitations by revealing alternative neural systems for the same task and discriminating among the different types of activation observed in normal subjects.

Another contribution that functional imaging studies of patients can provide for normal models of functional anatomy concerns our understanding of "functional integration" or "functional connectivity" among brain regions. This is because, unlike structural imaging (CT and conventional MRI), functional imaging can detect abnormal neuronal responses distant to the site of brain damage. These distant effects can either be expressed as an under- or an overactivation relative to normal. In either case, we assume that the cause of the abnormality relates to the damaged area perturbing responses elsewhere in the system. The distant effect of lesions has been referred to as "diaschisis." Classical diaschisis, demonstrated by early anatomic studies and more recently by neuroimaging studies of resting brain activity, refers to regionally specific reductions in metabolic activity at sites that are remote from damaged regions but connected to them. The clearest example is "crossed cerebellar diaschisis," in which abnormalities of cerebellar metabolism are characteristically seen following cerebral lesions involving the motor cortex.[20] Crossed cerebellar diaschisis highlights the strong connections between the (e.g., right) cerebellum and the (e.g., left) motor cortex.

We have introduced the term *dynamic diaschisis*[21] to refer to the context-sensitive and task-specific effects that a lesion can have on the *evoked* responses of distant cortical regions. The basic idea is that an undamaged area can have abnormal responses when it relies on interactions with the damaged area but normal responses when neural dynamics depend only upon integration with undamaged regions. This effect can arise because normal responses in any given region depend upon driving and modulatory inputs from many other regions and reciprocal interactions with them. The regions involved will depend on the cognitive and sensorimotor operation engaged at any particular time. For example, we report a patient with left frontal damage who activated the left posterior temporal cortex normally during a semantic task but abnormally during a reading task.[21] These results suggest that left posterior temporal activation depended on interaction with the damaged area during the reading task but not during the semantic task. Thus, dynamic diaschisis can contribute to our understanding of normal functional anatomy, connectivity, and functional integration among brain regions. Critically, abnormal activation distant to the site of brain damage can only be fully characterized with whole-brain functional neuroimaging studies of patients.

SECTION IV: COGNITIVE AND ANATOMIC MODELS OF RECOVERY

The clinical literature[22,23] offers several popular theories of recovery (see Chaps. 6 and 18) that can be tested with functional neuroimaging studies of patients. These theories have been referred to as (1) redundancy, (2) unmasking, (3) vicarious redundancy, (4) perilesional activation, (5) reversal of diaschisis, and (6) compensatory cognitive strategies. Each of these is considered in turn.

Redundancy

The term *redundancy* has been used to refer to the availability of more than one neural mechanism for performing the same function/task. More recently, however, Edelman and colleagues have emphasized the distinction between redundancy and degeneracy.[24,25] The term *degeneracy* has been defined as "the ability of elements that are structurally different to perform the same function or yield the same output." In contrast, *redundancy* refers to the same structures performing the same function. Since neuropsychological and neuroimaging studies are concerned with cortical and subcortical structures that have a spatial scale of millimeters or centimeters, there will be no redundancy because no two areas have the same structure. Nevertheless, irrespective of terminology, if there are several neural systems for the same task with each being able to substitute for another, functional competence will be protected from selective damage to any one system. Functional imaging studies of patients who recover solely by virtue of the availability of redundant or alternative systems should reveal activation in only a subset of the normally activated regions. There may also be enhanced activation in undamaged areas of the normal system because, if one neuronal system engaged by a task is damaged, intact task performance may become increasingly dependent on the surviving systems.

Unmasking

The term *unmasking* has been used in the clinical literature to refer to neural systems that are "inhibited" in normal subjects but "disinhibited" following damage to the inhibiting system or its adaptation. Functional imaging studies of patients who recover by virtue of "unmasking" or "disinhibition" should reveal activation in regions that are not normally observed. The most likely systems to be disinhibited are those in regions of the contralateral hemisphere that are homologous to the damaged areas. This is because the functional role played by any brain component (cortical area, subarea, neuronal population, or neuron) is defined by the connections and interactions it has with other cortical areas. Therefore, functional similarities between neuronal systems depend on the similarity in their connection profiles. These similarities are likely to be greatest within a cytoarchitectonic region or in the homologous area of the contralateral hemisphere (by virtue of transcollosal interhemispheric connections). Although there is empiric evidence for inhibition in the motor system,[26,27] the role it plays in other neuronal systems is less clear. Some functional imaging studies have revealed right hemisphere activation during language tasks following recovery from left hemisphere damage,[28–31] but the role of disinhibition in these studies is not clear because right hemisphere activation may also be seen following compensatory cognitive strategies (below). Nevertheless, it might be expected that disinhibition would occur earlier in the reorganization process than learning-related compensatory strategies and be less dependent on rehabilitation therapy.

Vicarious Redundancy

Vicarious redundancy has been used to imply that patients might recover by engaging neural systems that were previously unrelated to the task (i.e., "equipotential" systems). This would necessitate the growth of new neuronal processes (neurogenesis). Recently it has been demonstrated that even in the adult brain, there are mitotically competent cells that can divide and create new cells.[32,33] However, despite these recent observations, it is still generally accepted that long-range extrinsic axonal connections do not form de novo in the mature brain. This means that it is unlikely that patients recover by engaging neural systems that were previously unrelated to the task. Demonstrating vicarious redundancy with functional imaging studies of patients would involve demonstrating that abnormal neural systems were engaged by the patient and that normal subjects did not activate these neural systems under any other conditions. In other words, an infinite number of experiments with normal subjects would be required.

Perilesional Activation

Perilesional activation has already been discussed in Sec. III above. It refers to residual functional responsiveness at the site of damage and indicates that the damaged area may retain some functionality. This residual function may emerge during the acute stages of recovery when edema is controlled and circulation is reestablished in areas subject to partial ischemia. Functional neuroimaging of the patient would demonstrate normal activation everywhere except at the site of lesion where it is "patchy."[17,18]

Reversal of Diaschisis

Reversal of diaschisis results when basal activity in an undamaged area is reestablished following a temporary lesion-dependent reduction (see Sec. III for a definition of diaschisis). If evoked responses return to normal, activation in the patient should be normal after recovery and, indeed, monitored with longitudinal studies.

Compensatory Cognitive Strategies

A compensatory cognitive strategy may involve either learning a new strategy or using a preestablished strategy. Learning a new strategy is mediated by changes in the function or number of synapses (i.e., synaptic plasticity) that follow attempts to perform the task. With respect to functional neuroimaging, compensatory cognitive strategies could change activation patterns in contralateral, ipsilateral, or subcortical brain systems. An example of how activation can change with relearning is provided by Small and Flores[13] and described in Sec. II above. They demonstrate how the activation pattern for reading changed after the patient was taught a sublexical phonologic reading strategy. Critically, to demonstrate the involvement of a compensatory cognitive strategy, functional imaging of the patient is required before and after retraining.

In summary, there are several different theories of functional recovery that can be tested with functional imaging studies of neurologically impaired patients.

These theories emphasize differential effects from (1) reestablishing the normal neuronal system (periinfarct activation and the reversal of diaschisis), (2) neuronal reorganization (e.g., following disinhibition, or neuroplasticity), and (3) cognitive reorganization (following learning-related synaptic changes). However, it should be emphasized that distinguishing among cognitive or neuronal reorganization is not always easy. This is because to infer neuronal reorganization, one has to demonstrate that the cognitive processes are the same; to infer that a patient is using a different cognitive strategy, one has to demonstrate that the neuronal processing for this cognitive strategy is normal. These inferences rest on (1) a detailed cognitive analysis of the task, (2) a detailed assessment of the patient's and normal subjects' strategies during the task, and (3) neuroimaging experiments to identify the neuronal systems engaged. For instance, abnormal cognitive processing might be assumed if (1) extensive behavioral testing suggested abnormal cognitive processes, (2) normal subjects could be enticed to use the same cognitive processes as the patient, and (3) the normal subjects activated the same set of brain regions as the patient when using this abnormal cognitive strategy. On the other hand, neuronal reorganization in the absence of abnormal cognitive processing might be assumed if the criteria outlined above were not evident—i.e., that there was no evidence that the patient was performing the task differently from normals and no evidence that normal subjects could ever use the alternative neuronal system to perform the task.

SECTION V: LIMITATIONS

In the previous sections, we focused on the advantages of functional imaging studies of neurologically impaired patients. There are, however, two critically important limitations of such studies that have led to many misguided applications. The first limitation is that the interpretation of abnormal activations relies upon our understanding of normal activation patterns. Thus, patient studies will inevitably lag behind and will depend upon developments made in the normal domain. In particular, we need a good understanding of normal variability before inferring patient activation profiles are abnormal. The second limitation is that to make inferences about abnormal neuronal responses, the patient must enact the same set of cognitive, sensory, and motor processes as normal subjects do. Obviously, this is not possible if the processes engaged by the task are impaired. For example, if a patient cannot make speech production responses, the corresponding neuronal correlates will not be expressed. It may be tempting to infer that reduced activation relative to normals is the physiologic cause of the deficit (e.g., with speech production), but fully functional areas may simply not activate when the task is not being performed.

Debate in the current functional imaging literature about developmental dyslexia highlights the issues discussed above. For example, most functional imaging studies of developmental dyslexia have reported abnormal activation in a posterior region of the left temporoparietal junction, in the vicinity of the left angular gyrus.[34–36] Consequently, it has been argued that developmental dyslexics have a dysfunctional or "disconnected" left angular gyrus.[37,38] However, in all of these studies, the developmental dyslexics had reduced accuracy and slower response times than the normal subjects. In contrast, when response accuracy for the dyslexics and controls is matched, no abnormality in the left angular gyrus has been detected.[9,39] Furthermore, functional imaging studies of normal subjects suggest that the left posterior temporoparietal junction is involved in semantic processing (see Price[40] for a review). An alternative interpretation of the abnormal temporoparietal responses in developmental dyslexia could therefore be that there was less semantic activation consequent on less accurate reading.

In summary, when performance is impaired, the neuronal and cognitive abnormalities are confounded and we cannot determine whether abnormal neuronal responses are (1) the physiologic cause or (2) the consequence of impaired performance. Functional imaging studies of patients therefore require that the patients perform the task with the same level of performance as the normal controls. This is counterintuitive from the perspective of neuropsychological studies, where the focus is usually on testing selective deficits in cognitive function. Some functional imaging studies of patients have attempted to match performance by using different experimental parameters for the patients and the normals. For example, stimulus presentation can be made slower for the patient than the normal controls.

However, this only substitutes one problem for another, because even subtle changes in stimulus parameters can have highly significant effects on the pattern of activation.[41,42]

In conclusion, although functional imaging studies of neurologically impaired patients are limited to paradigms that the patient can perform, they offer several advantages relative to behavioral tests and functional imaging studies of normals. This chapter has focused on the contributions that imaging studies of patients offer normal and abnormal cognitive and anatomic models, particularly the insights afforded to the mechanisms that sustain functional recovery.

REFERENCES

1. Morris JS, Ohman A, Dolan RJ: Concious and unconscious emotional learning in the human amygdala. *Nature* 93:467–470, 1998.
2. Morris JS, DeGelder B, Weiskrantz L, Dolan RJ: Differential extrageniculostriate and amygdala responses to blind field presentation of emotional faces. *Brain* 124:1241–1252, 2001.
3. Patterson K, Shewell C: Speak and spell: Dissociations and word class effects, in Coltheart M, Sartori G, Job R (eds): *The Cognitive Neuropsychology of Language.* London: Erlbaum, 1987, pp 273–294.
4. Seidenberg MS, McClelland JL: Distributed developmental model of word recognition and naming. *Psychol Rev* 96:523–568, 1989.
5. Marshall JC, Newcombe F: Patterns of paralexia: A psycholinguistic approach. *J Psycholinguist Res* 2:175–199, 1973.
6. Price CJ, Wise RJS, Frackowiak RSJ: Demonstrating the implicit processing of visually presented words and pseudowords. *Cerebr Cortex* 6:62–70, 1996.
7. Herbster AN, Mintun MA, Nebes RD, Becker JT: Regional cerebral blood flow during word and nonword reading. *Hum Brain Map* 5:84–92, 1997.
8. Rumsey JM, Horwitz B, Donohue C, et al: Phonologic and orthographic components of word recognition: A PET-rCBF study. *Brain* 120:739–759, 1997.
9. Brunswick N, McCrory E, Price CJ, et al: Explicit and implicit processing of words and pseudowords by adult developmental dyslexics: A search for Wernicke's Wortschatz. *Brain* 122:1901–1917, 1998.
10. Fiez JA, Balota DA, Raichle ME, Petersen SE: Effects of lexicality, frequency, and spelling-to-sound consistency

on the functional anatomy of reading. *Neuron* 24:205–218, 1999.

11. Hagoort P, Indefrey P, Brown C, et al: The neural circuitry involved in the reading of German words and pseudowords: A PET study. *J Cogn Neurosci* 11(4):383–398, 1999.

12. Tagamets MA, Novick JM, Chalmers ML, Friedman RB: A parametric approach to orthographic processing in the brain: An fMRI study. *J Cogn Neurosci* 12:281–297, 2000.

13. Small SL, Flores DK: Different neural circuits subserve reading before and after therapy for acquired dyslexia. *Brain Lang* 62:298–308, 1998.

14. Fiez JA, Petersen SE, Cheney, MK, Raichle ME: Impaired nonmotor learning and error detection associated with cerebellar damage. *Brain* 115:155–178, 1992.

15. Price CJ, Friston KJ: Functional imaging studies of neuropsychological patients: Applications and limitations. *Neurocase*. In press.

16. Price CJ, Mummery CJ, Moore CJ, et al: Delineating necessary and sufficient neural systems with functional imaging studies of neuropsychological patients. *J Cogn Neurosci* 11(4):371–382, 1999.

17. Heiss WD, Karber H, Weber-Luxenburger G, et al: Speech-induced cerebral metabolic activation reflects recovery from aphasia. *J Neurol Sci* 145(2):213–217, 1997.

18. Warburton EA, Price CJ, Swinburn K, Wise RJS: Mechanisms of recovery from aphasia: evidence from positron emission tomography studies. *J Neurol Neurosurg Psychiatry* 66:155–161, 1999.

19. Kinsbourne M: The minor cerebral hemisphere as a source of aphasic speech. *Arch Neurol* 15:530–535, 1971.

20. Feeney DM, Baron JC: Diaschisis. *Stroke* 17:317–377, 1986.

21. Price CJ, Warburton EA, Moore CJ, et al: Dynamic diaschisis: Context sensitive human brain lesions. *J Cogn Neurosci* 13:419–429, 2001.

22. Kertesz A: Recovery and treatment, in Heilman KM, Valenstein E (eds): *Clinical Neuropsychology,* 3d ed. New York: Oxford University Press, 1993.

23. Hallett M: Plasticity, in Frackowiak RSJ, Mazziotta JC, Toga A (eds): *Mapping: The Disorders*. San Diego, CA: Academic Press, 2000, pp 569–585.

24. Edelman GM, Gally JA: Degeneracy and complexity in biological systems. *Proc Natl Acad Sci U S A* 98:13763–13768, 2001.

25. Tononi G, Sporns O, Edelman GM: Measures of degeneracy and redundancy in biological networks. *Proc Natl Acad Sci U S A* 96:3257–3262, 1999.

26. Geffen GM, Jones DL, Geffen LB: Inter-hemispheric control of manual motor activity. *Behav Brain Res* 64:131–140, 1994.

27. Meyer BU, Roricht S, Woiciechowsky C: Topography of fibres in the human corpus callosum mediating inter-hemispheric inhibition between the motor cortices. *Ann Neurol* 43:360–369, 1998.

28. Weiller C, Isenee C, Rijntjes M, et al: Recovery from Wernicke's aphasia: A positron emission tomography study. *Ann Neurol* 37:723–732, 1995.

29. Gold BT, Kertesz A: Right hemisphere semantic processing of visual words in an aphasic patient: An fMRI study. *Brain Lang* 73:456–465, 2000.

30. Miura K, Nakamura Y: Functional magnetic resonance imaging to word generation task in a patient with Broca's aphasia. *J Neurol* 246:939–942, 1999.

31. Calvert GA, Brammer MJ: Using fMRI to study recovery from acquired dysphasia. *Brain Lang* 71:391–399, 2000.

32. Barinagh M: No-new-neurons dogma loses ground. *Science* 279:2041–2042, 1998.

33. Gross CG: Neurogenesis in the adult brain: Death of a dogma. *Nat Neurosc Rev* 1:67–73, 2000.

34. Rumsey JM, Nace K, Donohue BC, et al: A positron emission tomographic study of impaired word recognition and phonological processing in dyslexic men. *Arch Neurol* 54:562–573, 1997.

35. Shaywitz SE, Shaywitz BA, Pugh KR, et al: Functional disruption in the organization of the brain for reading in dyslexia. *Proc Natl Acad Sci U S A* 95:2636–2641, 1998.

36. Temple E, Poldrack RA, Protopapas A, et al: Disruption of the neural response to rapid acoustic stimuli in dyslexia: Evidence from functional MRI. *Proc Natl Acad Sci U S A* 97:13907–13912, 2000.

37. Horwitz B, Rumsey JM, Donohue BC: Functional connectivity of the angular gyrus in normal reading and dyslexia. *Proc Natl Acad Sci U S A* 95:8939–8944, 1998.

38. Rumsey JM, Horwitz B, Donohue BC, et al: A functional lesion in developmental dyslexia: Left angular blood flow predicts severity. *Brain Lang* 70:187–204, 1999.

39. Paulesu E, Demonet JF, Fazio F, et al: Dyslexia: Cultural diversity and biological unity. *Science* 291:2165–2167, 2001.

40. Price CJ: The anatomy of language: Contributions from functional neuroimaging. *J Anat* 197:335–359, 2000.

41. Price CJ, Moore CJ, Frackowiak RSJ: The effect of varying stimulus rate and duration on brain activity during reading. *Neuroimage* 3:40–52, 1996.

42. Price CJ, Friston KJ: The temporal dynamics of reading: A PET study. *Proc R Soc Lond Ser B* 264:1785–1791, 1997.

Chapter 5

ELECTROPHYSIOLOGICAL METHODS, INCLUDING TRANSCRANIAL MAGNETIC STIMULATION, IN COGNITIVE NEUROSCIENCE*

Leon Y. Deouell
Richard B. Ivry
Robert T. Knight

Electrophysiologic recording techniques are widely employed to study cognitive processing in normal and clinical populations.[1–3] Frequency analysis of the ongoing electroencephalogram (EEG) and extraction of event-related potentials (ERPs) embedded in the ongoing EEG provide information on tonic and phasic changes in brain activity during cognitive processing. Analysis of EEG frequencies is particularly valuable for the study of alterations in regional neural activity in a time domain extending from one to several seconds, approximating the time scale of blood-flow–based physiologic techniques described in Chap. 3, such as positron emission tomography (PET) or functional magnetic resonance imaging (fMRI). Metabolic techniques such as PET and fMRI currently provide better spatial resolution of cognitive activity, but their temporal resolution is limited to the second (fMRI) or minute (PET) range.

ERP methods can extract stimulus, response, or cognition-related neural activity from the ongoing EEG in the millisecond-to-second range, providing a method for real-time assessment of changes in neural activity during cognitive processing. Recent efforts to record EEG and fMRI simultaneously represent a promising approach to linking neuronal and regional blood-flow changes during mental activity.[4–8] Converging data from ERP, PET, and fMRI will likely provide the strongest insights into the neural regions and mechanisms involved in mental activity. This review focuses predominantly on the use of event-related potentials in behavioral neurology (for discussions of frequency-based methods, see, for example, Refs. 9 to 15).

While metabolic and electrophysiologic measurements allow researchers to "eavesdrop" on neural activity, it has long been recognized that an alternative physiologic approach to understanding the function of specific brain regions would be to manipulate neural activity directly. By applying an electrical current, neural discharge can be induced, and the effects of this stimulation can be observed in the resulting behavior. The classic example of this approach is Penfield's work in the 1950s, in which the somatotopic organization of sensorimotor cortex was revealed through direct cortical stimulation applied during the course of neurosurgery.[16] The direct stimulation of human neural tissue is naturally limited to relatively rare situations, however—surgical situations in which the individuals suffer from neurologic conditions such as epilepsy, Parkinson's disease, or tumors.

Transcranial magnetic stimulation (TMS) allows either activation or disruption of activity in neural tissue through the intact skull, providing a more widely applicable method. Rapid improvements in the methodology and safety of these methods provide an exciting way for testing the integrity of neural pathways[17] and for testing hypotheses regarding the role of cortical areas in sensory, motor, and higher cognitive functions.[18] By

* **ACKNOWLEDGMENTS:** Special thanks to Clay C. Clayworth for skillful technical assistance. Supported by NINDS Grants NS21135, NS30256, and NS33504.

producing brief deactivation of cortical areas, TMS results in highly selective "virtual lesions" within healthy brains. It thus has the potential to pinpoint the critical areas responsible for specific functional deficits found in patients with naturally occurring (and permanent) lesions.

EVENT-RELATED POTENTIALS

Neural activity in axonal pathways and inhibitory (IPSPs) and excitatory (EPSPs) postsynaptic potentials on the soma and dendrites of active neurons contribute to scalp-recorded field potentials, with the brunt of scalp EEG activity due to summed IPSPs and EPSPs. A major limitation of scalp electrical and (to a lesser degree) magnetic recording is uncertainty about the precise brain locations of the signal sources. However, intracranial source localization is improved by using mathematical dipole modeling constrained by information obtained from intracranial recordings in surgical patients, event-related fMRI studies, the study of brain-damaged patients, and animal models (see Refs. 19 to 21 for reviews).

ERPs are classified as either exogenous (sensory) or endogenous (cognitive). The latency and amplitude of exogenous responses are determined predominantly by stimulus parameters such as intensity and rate. Examples of exogenous responses include the brainstem auditory evoked response (BAEP), the pattern shift P100 visual evoked potential (VEP), and primary somatosensory evoked potentials (SEP). Since these responses are largely resistant to cognitive influences, they are widely employed in a variety of neurologic conditions to measure neural activity in sensory pathways.

In contrast, endogenous potentials are sensitive to the cognitive parameters of the task. The degree of attention [P300 (P for positive, 300 for latency in milliseconds)], effort [contingent negative variation (CNV)], movement preparation [movement-related potentials (MRPs)], and linguistic analysis [N400 (N for negative, 400 for latency in milliseconds)] are examples of cognitive factors determining the amplitude, latency, and scalp distribution of different types of endogenous brain potentials (see Refs. 22 to 24 for reviews). Since endogenous potentials reflect mental processes not im-

mediately evoked by an external stimulus, the term *evoked potentials* has been replaced by the term *event-related potentials* in describing these signals. However, the borderline between a truly exogenous (presumably sensory, data-driven, hard-wired, and automatic) response and one involving higher cognitive functions is frequently blurred, as several "exogenous" components are modulated by top-down processes (see below). Moreover, some potentials may be regarded as being "exogenous" in some respects and "endogenous" in others [e.g., the mismatch negativity (MMN); visual N170]. Therefore the term *event-related potential* (ERP) may be used for all time-locked scalp potentials, as is done in this chapter.

General Technical Considerations

The local intracranial geometry of intracranial neural sources places an important constraint on scalp or extracranial EEG or magnetoencephalography (MEG) recording. Neural sources must have an open-field configuration to generate dipole sources recordable at a distance.[19,25] Simply put, an open-field geometry occurs when neurons assume a local organized cellular structure wherein neurons are oriented in the same direction. Examples of open-field geometry would include the laminar structure of the cortex or the hippocampus where electromagnetic fields of synchronously active pyramidal neurons are aligned and sum to produce a dipole field recordable at the scalp. A closed-field geometry occurs when a neuronal structure lacks a clear local cellular anatomic substructure (e.g., the intralaminar thalamic nuclei). In this situation, neurons may fire synchronously but the local extracellular fields are not well aligned, and the dipoles will cancel out locally and not generate a summed dipole field recordable at a distance.

This constraint of open-versus closed-field geometry is shown schematically in Fig. 5-1. On the left are two neurons that are aligned in the same direction in an open-field configuration. If these neurons fire synchronously, their extracellular fields will sum and this activity can be propagated by volume conduction and recorded at a distant site such as the scalp. On the right are the same two neurons firing synchronously but aligned 180 degrees out of phase in a closed-field configuration. In this situation their extracellular fields

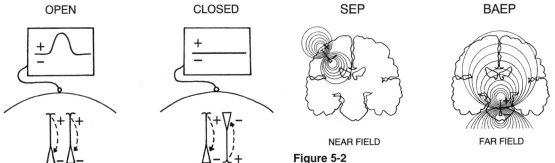

Figure 5-1
Schematic of an idealized open- and closed-field neuronal configuration. In the open-field situation, extracellular fields sum and can be recorded at a distance. In the closed-field condition, the extracellular fields of the two synchronously active neurons cancel and no evoked field is recorded at a distance.

Figure 5-2
On the left is the near field of the primary SEP. The evoked field changes rapidly over small distances on the scalp. On the right is an example of the far-field response of the BAEP. Note that the field is broadly distributed over the scalp, since the neural source is deep in the brainstem. See text for details. (Modified from Knight,[53] with permission.)

would cancel and no electrical field would be recorded at a distance. A single-unit recording electrode would record equivalent activity in both the open- and closed-field condition, and metabolic techniques would also record comparable activity in each situation.

The distance of an active neuronal source from the recording site has a major influence on the strength of the signal recorded at the scalp. This is due to the fact that electric and magnetic fields drop in amplitude as an inverse power function of the distance of the active neuronal elements from a recording site. Intracranial neuronal generators can be classified as near- or far-field sources. An example of a near-field source would be the primary SEP generated in the depths and crown of the postcentral gyrus. Since this neuronal source is on the surface of the hemisphere, the scalp field will be strong and focally distributed in parietal scalp electrodes situated over the postcentral gyrus (Fig. 5-2). A classic far-field source would be the BAEP. The BAEP is generated by sequential activity of auditory structures located in the brainstem extending from the eighth nerve to the inferior colliculus. The dipole field of these generators is broadly distributed over the scalp and small in amplitude due to its distance from the scalp (Fig. 5-2). Because of this biophysical constraint, the brunt of electrical activity recorded at scalp sites arises in near-field generators in neocortical regions. This selectivity for near-field sources may be sharpened us-

ing scalp current-density (SCD) derivations of scalp potentials.[26] The SCD is calculated by taking the second spatial derivative (the Laplacian) of the potential distribution over the scalp. Therefore it reflects the rate of change of potential between nearby electrodes. Since far-field sources will not result in large differences between adjacent electrodes (Fig. 5-2), their contribution will be effectively filtered out, providing a finer resolution of more superficial (cortical) sources. Figure 5-3 provides a demonstration of potential maps and SCD maps from the same data set.[103] Whereas the potential maps reveal a broad frontocentral negativity and posterior positivity which is quite similar across conditions, the SCD maps reveal more localized foci of activity, highlighting differences between the conditions (see legend for Fig. 5-3).

Event-related potentials range in amplitude from 0.5 μV for the exogenous BAEP to 10 to 20 μV for longer-latency endogenous potentials such as the P300, N400, and CNV. These signals are buried in the ongoing EEG, which typically varies from 10 to 200 μV, depending in large part on the arousal state of the subject. In order to extract these signals from the ongoing EEG, the event-related response to a discrete sensory stimulus or cognitive manipulation must be averaged over multiple trials. Since the background EEG can be approximated as random noise, the average of repetitive EEG epochs will approximate zero.

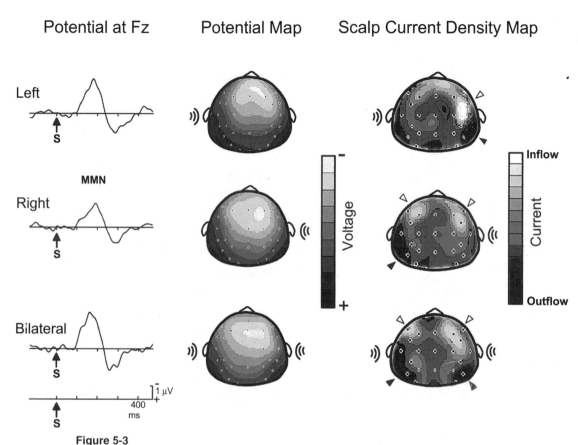

Figure 5-3

Waveforms, potential maps, and scalp current density (SCD) maps for the same data. Fifteen subjects heard sequences of two different tones presented simultaneously, one to each ear. The waveforms show the difference, at the Fz site, between the event-related potential (ERP) elicited by a standard pair and the ERP elicited by a change in the pitch of the left, right, or both tones. The deviants elicited the typical mismatch negativity. The potential maps around the peak of the MMN for each condition show a broad frontocentral negativity, skewed rightward, regardless of the side of deviation, and a bilateral temporal positivity. The SCD maps, which are the laplacian derivations of the same data, show more circumscribed foci of activity with different patterns dependent on side of deviation. The temporal foci (black arrowheads) were significantly stronger contralateral to the side of deviation (symmetrical for the bilateral condition). The frontal scalp foci (open arrowheads) were significantly right lateralized in the left-deviant condition but were symmetrical when the deviant was on the right or bilateral (see Deouell et al.[103] for details).

Conversely, the event-related response, time-locked to a specific stimulus or response, is assumed to repeat itself across trials and therefore emerges by averaging from the background EEG. The signal-to-noise ratio, which can be viewed as a measure of the ability to confidently identify the evoked signal in the background

EEG "noise," is proportional to the square root of the number of epochs averaged. Consequently, smaller signals require many more trials before a reliable potential is seen. The effects of signal averaging for the small, far-field, exogenous BAEP is shown in Fig. 5-4. Note that no signal is apparent in the evoked potential

BAEP AVERAGING

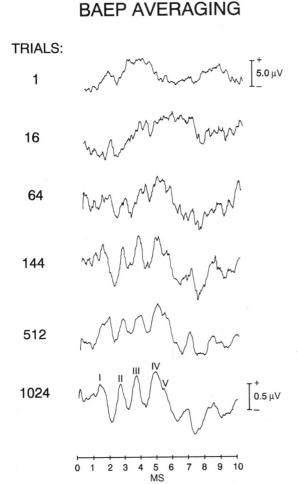

Figure 5-4
The signal averaging of the BAEP. Note that a clear signal is not observable for at least 144 trials, since the BAEP is small (~0.5 μV) and buried in the background EEG activity.

P300 AVERAGING

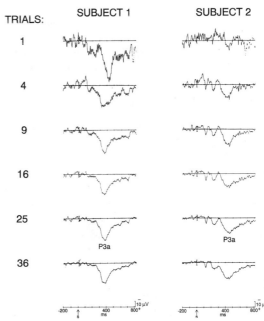

Figure 5-5
The signal averaging of novelty P3a responses in two subjects. Since the P3a amplitude is large (~10 μV), the signal is well seen in only a few trials.

average of the first 16 trials. A clear but noisy signal is seen after 144 trials. By 1024 trials, a clean signal is obtained, revealing the principal five components of the BAEP as well as two additional potentials that reflect thalamocortical activity projecting from the inferior colliculus to primary auditory cortex. A different pattern is seen in Fig. 5-5, which shows the averaging of a P300 response to unexpected novel sounds over 1 to 36 trials in two subjects. Since the P300 to these

unexpected sounds is in the range of 10 to 30 μV for a single stimulus, it can be readily distinguished from the background EEG noise after just a few trials. Indeed, it can be seen after a single trial in subject 1 and after four trials in subject 2. Note that the superimposed EEG noise continues to flatten out with repetitive trials, especially apparent in the prestimulus epoch. Several techniques have been developed to extract single trials from the ongoing EEG during cognitive tasks that generate large responses (see Refs. 19 and 27 for reviews of signal processing techniques).

Special Considerations in Studying Brain-Damaged Patients with ERPs

Chapter 4 reviews some of the advantages and special challenges of functional neuroimaging with brain-damaged patients. Many of these special considerations arise with the use of ERPs with neurological populations, along with others unique to electrophysiologic methods.

The recording of ERPs requires considerable cooperation from the subject, both in minimizing artifacts and, in some cases, in complying with the task requirements. These limitations may be especially pronounced for brain-damaged patients, particularly when studied in relative proximity to the onset of their illness. The difficulties result from several factors. First, it is often difficult to make sure that the patient fully understands the procedure, aim, and significance of the test, especially when he or she manifests language disturbances (aphasia), disorientation, or confusion. Under these circumstances, the environment and equipment used in an ERP study may also be particularly intimidating. Second, with or without psychoactive medications, patients frequently undergo significant fluctuations in their arousal. This may cause both problems in performance and interference from slow waves (in the alpha band or slower) in the EEG. Third, patients with motor weakness may have difficulty sitting quietly in their chairs for the entire test duration, causing excessive artifacts of muscular activity. Fourth, patients may suffer from general attention deficits, making it difficult for them to stay alert, focused, and compliant throughout a prolonged testing session. The last problem is especially evident in patients with right hemisphere damage (RHD).

The above difficulties require the adjustment of experimental paradigms to shorten the testing sessions as much as possible and to minimize the patient's discomfort and apprehension. Alternatively, patients can be tested in a more chronic phase, when many of the above concerns are alleviated. However, if the goal is to correlate ERPs with behavioral deficits that may subside with time (e.g., unilateral neglect or aphasia), one must attempt to deal with the problems inherent in studying acute patients. Unfortunately, even if these precautions are taken, patients are occasionally excluded a priori from ERP studies because of failure to cooperate fully, and considerable amounts of data may often have to be discarded because of excessive noise (cf. Ref. 28). Of course, this procedure increases the risk of a selection bias toward less severely affected patients.

An additional problem (not unique to ERPs) is that the comparison of patients with normal controls is confounded by many factors other than the phenomenon under investigation. Such factors are, for example, the hospitalization, the use of medications, concomitant affective components such as depression, and the level of alertness. In fact, even the comparison between patients is complicated by inescapable variability in lesion sites and volumes, general medical condition, and uncontrolled premorbid differences. A possible partial remedy is to prefer designs in which each patient serves as his or her own control ("within subject" designs; see, for example, the studies of neglect patients below).

A major methodologic concern involves the interpretation of scalp-recorded ERPs in brain-damaged patients. The amplitude and spatial distribution of the ERP signals may be altered by the lesion in at least three ways: (1) there may be direct damage to the electrical source generating the ERP, (2) the damaged area may modulate the activity of an electrical source distant from the lesion, and (3) altered electrical conduction in the damaged tissue may diminish or augment the amplitude of scalp-recorded potentials over the damaged hemisphere even if the underlying generators are functioning normally[29] (Fig. 5-6). There is no simple solution to these problems, and the best approach (as is the case in almost any method in neuroscience) may be awareness of these potential caveats and reliance on converging information from several methodologies.

Despite these difficulties, ERPs have been applied to the study of almost every functional problem covered in this volume, providing invaluable data in many cases. This endeavor has benefited from the convergence of better understanding of the cognitive correlates and anatomic substrate of different ERP components (e.g., Refs. 20, 22, and 30), improved localization of lesions with the advent of MRI and computerized reconstructions (e.g., Refs. 31 to 33), and increasingly refined neuropsychological methods. This combination of ERPs, lesion analysis, and cognitive neuropsychology is informative in at least two complementary ways. First, by examining the effect of discrete lesions on specific components of ERPs, it is possible to discern the neural elements of large-scale networks controlling, for example, attention and memory in the healthy brain.[34] Second, by using electrophysiologic components whose correlation with specific cognitive operations is reasonably clear, it is possible to shed light on the cognitive, anatomic, and physiologic mechanisms

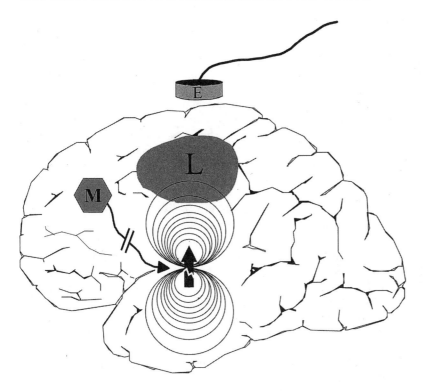

Figure 5-6
Schematic model depicting three possible ways in which a lesion can change the pattern of a scalp recorded potential: (1) The lesion destroys the neural generator (broken arrow); (2) the conductivity of the damaged parenchyma (L) is altered, distorting the amplitude recorded at the scalp electrode (E); (3) The lesion is remote from the neural generator of the recorded potential, but it disrupts modulatory input (M) to the generator by ablating the source of the modulatory input or by disconnection.

of specific functional deficits, information that cannot be obtained by traditional behavioral methods.[35,36]

In the following, we attempt to demonstrate some of these insights through examination of three cardinal neurobehavioral domains—prefrontal damage, unilateral neglect following right hemisphere damage, and aphasia following left hemisphere damage.

Prefrontal Damage and Executive Control

As discussed in Chap. 23, prefrontal cortex is crucial for executive control and efficient goal-directed activity. Through its attentional, inhibitory and/or working memory functions, prefrontal cortex enables us to suppress irrelevant information and facilitate the processing of relevant information. These functions may be bound under the headings of sustained and selective attention. For attention to be flexible, we must also be able to respond to potentially important events (e.g., a threat) outside the focus of attention and to detect and further process targets within the focus of attention (phasic attention). Lateral prefrontal cortex is crucial for the control of sustained and phasic attention

to environmental events, as well as to novelty and target detection.[37,38] Attention and orienting ability have been studied using ERP techniques in neurologic patients with damage centered in Brodmann's areas 9 and 46 and in patients with posterior cortical and mesial temporal damage. Both the electrophysiologic and behavioral data from these patients have indicated that problems with inhibitory control of sensory inputs, reduced facilitation of processing of relevant information (sustained attention), and abnormalities in the detection of novel events are central concomitants of prefrontal disease.[39] At the same time, these data reveal the dynamic interaction between bottom-up and top-down processes that is necessary for normal function.

Inhibitory Modulation and Sensory Gating

The attention deficits of patients with prefrontal lesions and the behavioral phenomena of perseveration in advanced prefrontal disease have been linked to problems with inhibitory control of posterior sensory and perceptual mechanisms.[40,146] Inability to inhibit internal representations of previous responses that are now incorrect, coupled with random inappropriate shifts of attention, contributes to the poor performance of patients with prefrontal damage on the Wisconsin Card Sorting Task and on the Stroop task.[41,77] Problems with tasks involving "working memory" (operationally defined as the holding of information needed for the execution of action over short delays) may be due to intrusion of irrelevant information coupled with failures to sustain neural activity in distributed task-dependent neural circuits.[43] Physiologic data indicates that this lack of inhibitory control may extend to early sensory processing in primary cortical regions.

Neural inhibition by prefrontal regions has been reported in a variety of mammalian preparations. A net inhibitory output to both subcortical[44] and cortical regions has been documented.[45] Cryogenic blockade of a prefrontal-thalamic gating system in cats results in enhancement of amplitudes of primary sensory cortex evoked responses.[46,47] This system is modulated by an excitatory lateral prefrontal projection to the nucleus reticularis thalami, although the precise course of anatomic projections between these structures is not well understood. The nucleus reticularis thalami, in turn, sends inhibitory GABAergic projections to sensory relay nuclei, providing a neural substrate for selective sensory suppression.[48]

This prefrontal-thalamic inhibitory system provides a potential mechanism for modality-specific suppression of irrelevant inputs at an early stage of sensory processing. Support for a similar mechanism in humans has been obtained from the observation of patients with prefrontal damage due to stroke.[49,50] Task-irrelevant auditory and somatosensory stimuli were delivered to patients with damage to lateral prefrontal cortex (PFC) and to others with comparably sized lesions in the temporoparietal junction or the lateral parietal cortex. Evoked responses from primary auditory and somatosensory cortices were recorded in these patients and in age-matched controls (Fig. 5-7). The stimuli consisted of either monaural clicks or brief electric shocks to the median nerve, eliciting a small opponens pollicis twitch.

Lesions of the posterior association cortex invading either the primary auditory or somatosensory cortex reduced early latency (20 to 40 ms) evoked responses generated in these regions. Lesions in posterior association cortex, sparing primary sensory regions, had no effects on the amplitudes or latencies of the primary

cortical evoked responses; such patients served as a brain-lesioned control group. Lateral prefrontal damage resulted in enhanced amplitude of both the primary auditory and somatosensory evoked responses generated from 20 to 40 ms poststimulation.[43,49–51] Spinal cord and brainstem potentials were unaffected by prefrontal damage, indicating that amplitude enhancement of primary cortical responses was due to abnormalities in either prefrontal-thalamic or direct prefrontal-sensory cortical mechanisms. Chronic disinhibition of sensory inputs may contribute to many of the behavioral sequelae of prefrontal damage. For instance, decision confidence is decremented by a noisy internal milieu, and the orienting response would be expected to habituate.[52,53] A direct correlation between disinhibition and decreased performance in a delayed matching to sample task has been now demonstrated in a group of prefrontal patients, required to compare two sounds separated by a 5-s delay.[43,54] Patients' performance was significantly degraded when the delay period was filled with tone pips, and these tone pips, in turn, elicited an augmented primary auditory potentials (Na, Pa) relative to normals. The enhancement of Pa in response to the distracting tones also correlated with the number of delay errors. Similarly, in patients with right prefrontal damage, sounds presented to an unattended ear in a dichotic paradigm reduce the attentional enhancement (see next section) of subsequent to-be-attended sounds. The unattended sounds have no such effect in healthy controls.[55]

Attentional Facilitation In addition to suppressing irrelevant information, normal function involves facilitation of processing of relevant information. A "biased competition" model suggests that excitatory signals to neurons result in inhibition of nearby task-irrelevant neurons, resulting in a sharpening of the attentional focus.[56] Selective attention to a sensory channel such as an ear, a portion of the visual field, or a finger increases the amplitude of evoked potentials generated to all stimuli delivered to that region[57–60] and induces a slow negative potential spanning several hundreds of milliseconds following the presentation of the stimulus [known, in different contexts, as negative difference (Nd), selection negativity (SN), or processing negativity (PN)].[22] There is evidence that attention reliably modulates neural activity at early sensory

Frontal Gating

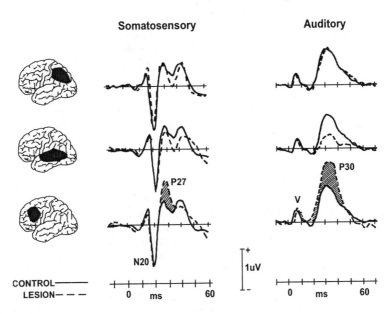

Figure 5-7

Primary cortical auditory and somatosensory event-related potentials are shown for controls (solid line) and patients (dashed line) with focal damage in the lateral parietal cortex (top, n =8), temporoparietal junction (middle, n =13), or dorsolateral prefrontal cortex (bottom, n =13). Reconstructions of the center of damage in each patient group are shown on the left. Somatosensory event-related responses were recorded from area 3b (N20) and areas 1 and 2 on the crown of the postcentral gyrus (P26). Stimuli were square-wave pulses of 0.15 ms duration delivered to the median nerve at the wrist. Stimulus intensity was set at 10 percent above opponens twitch threshold, and stimuli were delivered at a rate of 3/s. Damage in posterior cortical regions sparing primary somatosensory cortex had no effect on the N20 or earlier spinal cord potentials. Prefrontal damage resulted in a selective increase in the amplitude of the P26 response (hatched area). Auditory stimuli were clicks delivered at a rate of 13/s at intensity levels of 50 dB HL. Unilateral damage in the temporoparietal junction extending into primary auditory cortex reduces P30 responses. Lateral parietal damage sparing primary auditory cortex has no effect on P30 responses. Dorsolateral prefrontal damage results in normal inferior collicular potentials (wave V) but an enhanced P30 primary cortical response (hatched area). The shaded area in each modality indicates the area of event-related potential amplitude enhancement.

cortices, including secondary and perhaps primary sensory cortex.[61–65] Visual attention involves modulation in the excitability of extrastriate neurons through descending projections from hierarchically ordered brain structures.[66] Single-cell recordings in monkeys,[67,68] lesion studies in humans[34,39,42] and monkeys,[69] and blood-flow data[70–76] have linked PFC to control of extrastriate cortex during visual attention.

ERP studies in patients with lateral PFC damage suggests that human lateral PFC regulates extrastriate neural activity through three distinct mechanisms: (1) by enhancement of extrastriate cortex response to attended information; (2) through a tonic excitatory influence on ipsilateral posterior areas for all sensory information, including attended and nonattended sensory inputs; and (3) by a phasic excitatory influence of ipsilateral posterior areas to correctly perceived task relevant stimuli. In a series of ERP studies, patients with unilateral PFC lesions (centered in Brodmann's areas 9 and 46) were required to detect inverted triangles (targets) among a series of upright triangles (distractors). In one experiment, patients and age-matched controls were asked to press a button whenever a target appeared

at fixation.[34] In another, the target appeared in either visual field[42] while both visual fields were similarly attended. In a third experiment, subjects were instructed to attend to only one visual field.[79]

An interesting pattern of results emerged from these experiments (Figs. 5-8 and 5-9). First, the experiments revealed that lateral PFC provides a tonic excitatory influence to ipsilateral extrastriate cortex. When the stimuli appear centrally the PFC patients showed a significant reduction of the extrastriate N1 component (with a latency of 170 ms).[34,78] When the

Figure 5-8

*Visual event–related potentials in patients with lateral frontal lobe damage and healthy controls. Patients with dorsolateral prefrontal cortex lesions and controls had to detect upright triangles in a series of inverted triangles (standards, 70 percent), upright triangles (targets, 20 percent), and novel stimuli (10 percent) presented one at time to either side of fixation. Patients (n = 8) and controls (n = 11) were instructed to attend and respond to targets on the left or on the right of fixation. **A:** The ERPs elicited by the contralesional standard stimuli elicited significantly reduced P1 responses in the patients whether the standards were in the attended or the unattended side. **B:** The attention effect (extracted by subtracting the response to unattended standards from the response to the attended ones) reveals a significantly smaller effect for contralesional standards in patients relative to controls, starting around 200 ms postonset. POi = The ipsilesional of P7 and P8. POc = The contralesional of the two. For controls POi/POc = P7/P8, respectively. (Modified from Yago and Knight.[79])*

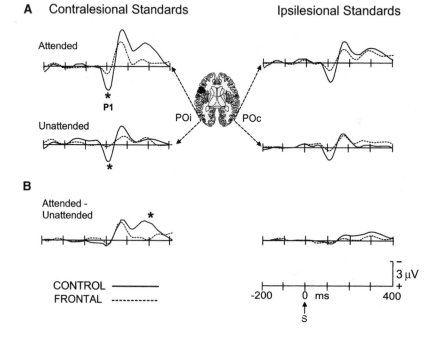

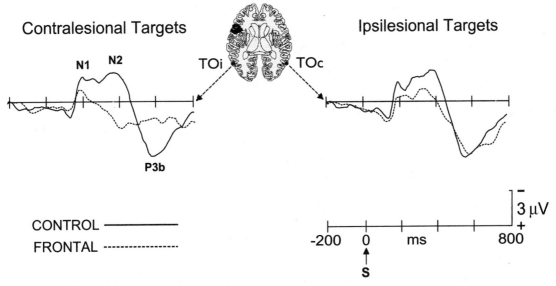

Figure 5-9

Same paradigm as Fig. 5–8, only that the patients (n = 10) and controls (n = 10) were attending to both right and left sides in this case. The N1, N2, and P3b peaks, seen in the controls' waveform, were significantly reduced in the patients in response to contralesional targets but not for ipsilesional targets (see Ref. 42 for more details). TOi = T5 or T6, the one ipsilateral to the lesion in patients; T5 in controls. TOc = T5 or T6, the one contralateral to the lesion in patients, T6 in controls.

stimuli were lateralized, the P1 component of the visual ERP was markedly reduced in amplitude for all stimuli presented to the contralesional field.[42,79] Importantly, this tonic influence was attention-independent, since a reduced P1 potential in extrastriate cortex was found ipsilateral to PFC damage for all visual stimuli (attended and nonattended targets and nontargets) presented to the contralesional field (Fig. 5-8a.).[79] This tonic component may be viewed as a modulatory influence on extrastriate activity. In the auditory modality, the patients elicited a reduced N1 component peaking 100 ms after the onset of the stimulus.[43] The auditory N1 has several sources in the superior temporal plane[20] providing additional evidence or prefrontal modulation of early sensory processing. Second, when the attention was directed to only one visual field, attention effects on extrastriate cortex were normal in the first 200 ms for the PFC patients and severely disrupted after 200 ms (Fig 5-8b).[79] This finding suggests that other cortical areas, possibly the posterior parietal cortex,

are responsible for attention-dependent regulation of extrastriate cortex in the first 200 ms. The PFC facilitation appears to begin after 200 ms. It is conceivable that inferior parietal cortex is responsible for the early reflexive component of attention, whereas PFC is responsible for more controlled and sustained aspects of visual attention beginning after the parietal signal to extrastriate cortices.

Third, in addition to the observation of channel-specific enhancement, another distinct electrophysiologic event (including the N2-P3b complex) was observed when a relevant target event was detected in an attended channel (Fig. 5-9).[79] The latency of this top-down signal was about 200 ms after a correct detection, and it extended throughout the ensuing 500 ms, superimposed on the channel-specific ERP attention enhancement.[80] Damage to lateral PFC results in marked decrements in the top-down signal, accompanied by behavioral evidence of impaired detection ability.[42] The N2, a component which is generated in the inferior temporal lobe in response to targets and which is therefore assumed to reflect postselection processing, was abolished over the lesioned hemisphere for targets in both visual fields. Behaviorally, the patients reacted more slowly to targets in the contralesional visual field and missed more targets than the controls did. The frontal patients also showed reduced P3b over the temporooccipital electrodes, but not at parietal sites.[42]

The P3b has been proposed to underlie a range of cognitive processes. One proposal is that the P3b is generated during closure of a perceptual task.[81] According to this theory, the P3b represents inhibition of a discrete epoch of stimulus processing. More precisely, this theory posits that the P3b is generated by inhibition of regional negativity in activated neocortex or mesial temporal sites associated with the termination of voluntary processing of an expected stimulus.[82,83] Alternatively, the P3b may index the updating of information in working memory.[84] Other proposals, such as those linking P3b and template matching, may be subsumed under the concept of context updating in working memory.[85] Most likely, the P3b includes contributions from multiple intracranial sources and processes (for reviews see Refs. 30, 86, and 87), which may include also modality-specific components.[88] This is highlighted by the fact that, in the PFC patients, the parietal P3b was intact, but at the same latency positivity was reduced over ipsilateral occipitotemporal sites.

Auditory selective attention capacity has also been examined in patients with lateral PFC lesions. In dichotic selective attention tasks, normal subjects generate an enhanced ("selection") negativity to all stimuli in an attended channel with onset from 25 to 50 ms after delivery of an attended auditory stimulus. Prefrontal patients generated reduced attention effects depending on the side of the lesion. Patients with left hemisphere lesions showed a reduced attention effect regardless of which ear was attended. In contrast, patients with right prefrontal damage showed reduced enhancement effect mainly when the contralateral ear was to be attended, consistent with the symptoms of unilateral neglect (see below).[89] Posterior association cortex lesions in the temporoparietal junction have comparable attention deficits for left- and right-sided lesions.[90] This suggests that some aspects of hemineglect subsequent to temporoparietal damage may be due to remote effects of disconnection from asymmetrically organized prefrontal regions.

The CNV is a negative-polarity brain potential maximal over frontal-central scalp sites generated during a delay period initiated by a warning stimulus. The CNV is terminated by a behavioral response that is contingent on information delivered in the warning stimulus.[91] The behavioral structure of tasks that generate a CNV shares attributes with paradigms associated with working memory in monkeys and humans.[92,93] The CNV potentials are focally reduced by discrete prefrontal damage, supporting a generator of the CNV in prefrontal cortex[94–96] (Fig. 5-10). These data provide a further link between prefrontal regions and sustained attention and working memory capacity.

Novelty Detection   The earliest brain potential directly reflecting the detection of deviance is the mismatch negativity (MMN). The MMN[97] is elicited in response to small deviations from regularities in the acoustic environment (e.g., a pitch change in a series of tones). The MMN can be observed for events outside the focus of attention and peaks 100 to 250 ms following the deviant event. It reflects an "error signal" generated automatically by a neural mechanism comparing a perceived stimulus to a sensory "memory trace" formed by the standard stimuli[98] or the updating of the existing model of the environment.[99] The mismatch response is presumed to trigger an involuntary reorientation of attention.[98,100] The MMN is generated mainly in the secondary auditory cortex (see Ref. 101 for review) but may have a second frontal generator, presumably related to the triggering of an attention switch.[102,103] The distribution of this frontal generator is reminiscent of the distribution of the visual attention mechanism, whereby the left frontal generator is active in response to contralateral deviancies while the right frontal generator responds to events on either side (Fig. 5-3).[103,104]

The MMN in response to pitch and pattern changes[51,105] is reduced in patients with prefrontal lesions, indicating an early deficit in automatic detection of deviance outside the focus of attention. Whereas temporoparietal lesions caused an MMN reduction

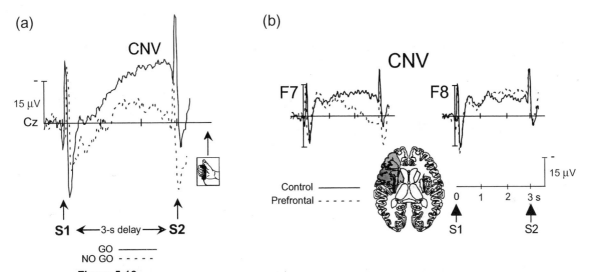

Figure 5-10

This figure shows the results of a classic auditory contingent negative variation (CNV) experiment in patients with focal prefrontal (PFCx) damage. On the left (a) are the results of a CNV task in normals. A warning stimulus (S1) triggers either a GO or NO/GO trial, which is terminated by the imperative S2 stimulus. GO trials generate a large DC shift maximal over frontocentral scalp sites, referred to as the CNV. Damage to the PFCx results in severe attenuation in the CNV over lesioned cortex (b), reductions observed throughout the lesioned hemisphere (see Rosahl and Knight[95] for details). On the bottom right are the group-averaged lesion reconstructions in 10 patients with prefrontal damage. Posterior lesions focally reduce the CNV over lesioned cortex but do not result in widespread hemispheric declines. These data provide evidence of PFCx involvement in sustaining distributed neural activity during delay periods.

mainly to contralesional stimuli, dorsolateral prefrontal lesions elicited comparable deficits regardless of stimulus side in one study[105] and more to ipsilesional sounds in another.[51] In addition, there was a tendency for right prefrontal lesions to be associated with larger MMN reductions than left frontal lesions, while no such asymmetry was found for the temporoparietal lesions.[105] These results suggest different contributions of the temporoparietal region and the prefrontal region to the MMN. It is yet to be determined whether reduced MMN following prefrontal damage reflects a weakened memory trace of the previous regularity due to disinhibition of irrelevant information, reduced frontal facilitation of a comparator mechanism in the secondary auditory cortex, a failure to initiate an attention switch following the detection of the change, or a damage to the postulated frontal generator of MMN.

Delivery of an unexpected and novel stimulus generates a P300 response (P3a) that is observed over widespread anterior and posterior scalp sites. The P3a potential has an earlier latency and a more frontocentral scalp distribution than the P3b in all sensory modalities and has been proposed to be a central marker of the orienting response.[52,53,106,107] Intracranial recordings in the visual, auditory, and somatosensory modalities have shown that multiple neocortical and limbic regions are activated during tasks that generate scalp novelty-dependent P3a potentials.[108–111] Intracranial P3a activity has been recorded in widespread areas of frontal and posterior association cortex in addition to cingulate and mesial temporal regions.[112] These intracranial novelty-related P3a potentials have been proposed to reflect neural activity in a distributed multimodal corticolimbic orienting

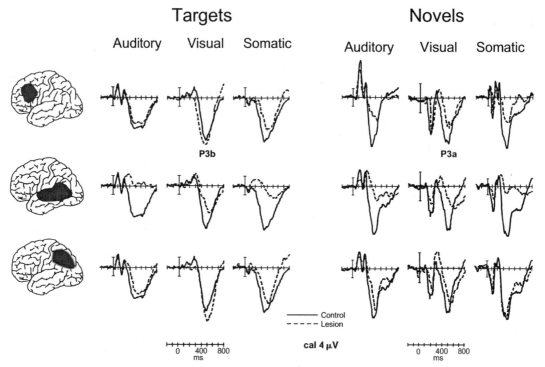

Figure 5-11

Summary of the target P3b and novelty P3a effects in controls and three patient groups with focal cortical damage. The center of the damage in each group is shown on the left. The waveforms from selected electrodes with maximal response amplitude (Pz for targets, Fz for novels) are shown for both target and novel stimuli in the auditory, visual, and somatosensory modalities in patients and controls. Prefrontal and lateral parietal lesions had no significant effect on the latency or amplitude of the target P3b generated in this simple detection task in the auditory, somatosensory, or visual modalities, implying that substantial regions of dorsolateral, prefrontal, and parietal association cortex are not critical for the parietal maximal P3b. Conversely, focal infarction in the temporoparietal junction resulted in marked P3b reductions in the auditory and somatosensory modalities and partial reductions in the visual modality. On the right are the results of the novelty experiments. Lateral parietal damage again had no significant effect on the P3 to novel stimuli and served as a brain lesioned control. Both prefrontal and temporoparietal damage resulted in multimodal reductions of the novelty P3a.

system. Similar theories have been suggested for the scalp P3a response.[53,106,113] fMRI studies using both blocked and event-related designs indicate distributed regions of activation during novelty and target detection, including the inferior frontal gyri, inferior parietal regions, the insula, the lateral temporal lobe,[114,115] and, in certain paradigms, also in the hippocampus.[116]

Novelty P3a responses generated over prefrontal scalp sites to unexpected novel stimuli are reduced by prefrontal lesions, with reductions observed throughout the lesioned hemisphere.[34] Comparable P3a decrements have been observed in the auditory,[53,117] visual,[34] and somatosensory modalities in humans with prefrontal damage[118] (Fig. 5-11). Reductions appear to be more severe after right prefrontal damage.[119]

Galvanic skin response (GSR), a peripheral marker of the orienting response, is also reduced by damage to the prefrontal and posterior association cortex.[120] These findings support a prefrontal source for the frontal scalp component of the novelty P300 and converge with both clinical observations and animal experimentation supporting a critical role of prefrontal structures in the detection of novel stimuli.[121,122] The combination of data from patients with lesions in anterior and posterior lesions suggest distributed interaction between prefrontal and posterior regions during both voluntary and involuntary attention and working memory,[123,124] with a special role for the right prefrontal region.[2]

Unilateral damage centered in the posterior hippocampal region has no effect on parietal P3b activity generated to auditory, visual, and somatosensory stimuli but reduces frontocentral P3 activity to both target and novel stimuli in all modalities. Reductions are most prominent over frontal regions and for novel stimuli[87,126] (Figs. 5-12 and 5-13). These reductions are comparable in amplitude to those observed after focal prefrontal damage. However, unilateral hippocampal damage reduces P300 potentials over both prefrontal cortices, whereas prefrontal damage results in predominantly unilateral reductions over the lesioned hemisphere. Studies with PET have also documented frontal hypometabolism in patients with medial temporal amnesia.[127] These observations support involvement of a prefrontal-hippocampal system in the detection of deviancies in the ongoing sensory stream and indicate that the hippocampal formation has bilateral facilitatory input to prefrontal cortex. Reciprocal pathways coursing through the caudomedial lobule of the mesial temporal lobe provide a potential anatomic substrate for prefrontal-hippocampal interactions during sensory and mnemonic processing.[128]

These results, in conjunction with the data from intracranial and functional imaging studies, provide further evidence that the P300 phenomenon is not a unitary phenomenon but represents distributed neural activity in corticolimbic regions engaged during both voluntary and involuntary response to discrete environmental events. Although this view is more complicated than initial proposals of a unitary nature of P300 activity, it strengthens the potential utility of scalp ERP recording, since it provides a means for the measurement of neural activity in distributed brain regions in the time domain of cognitive processing.

Unilateral Neglect and Extinction after Right Hemisphere Damage

Unilateral neglect (UN) is a frequent sequel of right hemisphere damage. As reviewed in Chaps. 14 and 15, patients suffering from neglect following right hemisphere damage fail to orient and respond to stimuli and events occurring on the left side of their personal or extrapersonal space.[129] In extinction, a related disorder, the failure to notice a contralesional stimulus occurs only when a competing stimulus is simultaneously presented more toward the side of the lesion.[130-132] Unilateral neglect (UN) may manifest itself in the visual, auditory, or tactile modalities.[133-135] Examination of UN patients has been widely used to explore mechanisms of attention and awareness. Yet, despite the ubiquity of such patients and the grave implications for their recovery after stroke, the cognitive and anatomic underpinnings of UN are not clear (see Chaps. 14 and 15). Since UN and extinction may occur in the absence of primary sensory deficits, theoretical accounts of UN have emphasized higher-order processes associated with the allocation of attention, representation of space, or motor preparation. These theories are based almost exclusively on clinical observations and studies employing behavioral methods. Recently, functional neuroimaging methods including ERP and fMRI have begun to provide new insights that might necessitate modification of current theories.

A major question in neglect research is still whether early perceptual processes are really unaltered, as suggested by theories that emphasize higher-order deficits in neglect. Normal SEPs (including N9, N13, P15, N20, and P25) were observed in three UN patients with lesions in the right frontotemporo-parietal regions and in one patient with damage in the right occipital periventricular region, even though the patients were not aware of the electrical shocks applied to the left median nerve.[136,137] Moreover, in two of the patients whose primary visual cortex was largely spared, the visual evoked potentials (VEPs) including N75, P100, and N145 were within normal range.[136] In contrast, SEPs and VEPs were absent or reduced in patients suffering from hemianesthesia or hemianopsia,

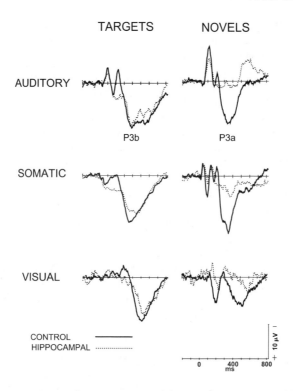

Figure 5-12

Group-averaged event-related potential (ERP) data from controls and patients with hippocampal lesions (n = 7) for auditory, visual, and somatosensory target and novel stimuli. Subjects were seated in a sound-attenuated booth and instructed to press a button upon detection of a designated target stimulus during each experiment. Auditory stimuli consisted of blocks of repetitive standard 1000-Hz monaural tone bursts (60 dB HL; 50 ms duration, 1 s ISI). Tone bursts of 1500 Hz occurred randomly on 10 percent of the trials and served as targets. Unexpected novel tones consisting of complex computer-generated sounds, and environmental noises such as bells or barks were randomly delivered on 10 percent of the trials. A similar paradigm was employed in the visual modality. Visual stimuli consisted of repetitive presentation of triangles. On 10 percent of the trials, inverted triangles served as target stimuli. On an additional 10 percent of trials, random line drawings or pictures of irrelevant stimuli served as novel events. Somatosensory stimuli consisted of repetitive taps to the index finger, with targets being random taps to the ring finger that occurred on 10 percent of the trials. Novel stimuli consisted of brief random shocks to the median nerve on 6 percent of the trials. The ERPs shown are from the electrode where maximal responses were recorded (Pz for targets; Fz for novels). The novelty P3a is markedly reduced at prefrontal sites in all three modalities, and the target P3b is spared.

respectively—syndromes that resulted from damage to the left primary somatosensory and visual cortices, respectively. Analogous results were reported by Viggiano and colleagues, who recorded steady-state VEPs in 10 neglect patients, 10 brain-damaged patients without neglect, and 6 healthy subjects.[138] No differences in right-left amplitude were observed in the neglect patients. These data support the view that the impairment in neglect stems from "defective access of the output of *preserved* primary sensory analyses to successive processes involved in conscious perception and in overt verbal response" (Vallar et al.,[137] p. 1921, our italics). However, more recent findings suggest that early sensory analysis may not be completely intact.

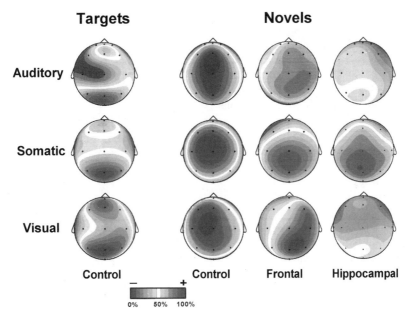

Figure 5-13
This figure shows the scalp voltage topographies for target and novel stimuli in controls. Note the marked increase in prefrontal activity to the novel stimuli in all sensory modalities. The effects of prefrontal or hippocampal lesions on the brain novelty response are shown on the right. Unilateral prefrontal damage results in multimodal decreases in the novelty response. Unilateral hippocampal damage results in severe bilateral reductions in the novelty response, maximal at prefrontal sites. These findings implicate a prefrontal-hippocampal network in the detection of perturbations in the environment (see text for details).

Abnormal sensory function in neglect was found in studies reporting that the visual and auditory N1 components are smaller over the damaged relative to the intact hemisphere of neglect patients regardless of the side of stimulation.[35,139] In contrast, the N1 in normal subjects is larger over the hemisphere contralateral to the stimulus side.[140] The enhanced left hemisphere (relative to right hemisphere) auditory N1, irrespective of the side of the stimuli, may contribute to the tendency of patients with left-side auditory neglect to err localizing auditory stimuli as coming more to the right of their true source.[141]

Drawing from the putative association between the N1 and the orienting response,[142] it has been suggested that the N1 reduction over the damaged hemisphere reflects the patients' difficulty in orienting toward the contralesional side of space.[139] This is consistent with two single-case studies in which the

visual N1 and P1 components were reduced in trials in which the left-sided stimulus was extinguished, but not when it was recognized[143,144] (see also Ref. 145). Recent fMRI studies comparing detected versus extinguished stimuli revealed reduced activation in right occipital cortex (as well as in bilateral fusiform and left parietal sites) when stimuli were extinguished in patients with right hemisphere damage.[144,145] The fact that in these fMRI studies extinguished faces seemed to activate the so-called fusiform face area suggests that the lack of awareness may not result from a breakdown of the object recognition pathway of the visual system but from a failure of its interaction with parietal and frontal mechanisms.[35,144,146,147]

Steady-state VEPs revealed an intriguing pattern in neglect patients. Latencies are increased for steady-state VEPs elicited by stimulation in the neglected side compared with those elicited by similar stimulation in the intact side.[28,148–150] This delay was absent in brain-damaged patients who did not show signs of neglect. Even more revealing is the fact that the latency increase was found with relatively high frequency luminance-contrast gratings but not with chromatically modulated contrasts,[151] suggesting a specific deficit related to the magnocellular system (luminance sensitive but color blind) and sparing the parvocellular part of the visual system.[152] The possibility of a feature specific deficit in preattentive processing has also been investigated in the auditory modality using the MMN.

As noted previously, the MMN is an electrical brain manifestation elicited by infrequently occurring oddball stimuli interspersed among repetitive stimuli. Several characteristics of the MMN make it an especially interesting measure in the study of UN and extinction. First, the MMN is assumed to reflect an automatically elicited preattentive process.[153–155] Second, the process underlying the MMN has a potential role in triggering an involuntary attention switch,[98,156–158] and such a process is likely disrupted in UN. Third, the MMN paradigm allows one to examine separately the feature-specific processing of auditory stimuli[159–162] (see Ref: 163 for a discussion of the feature-specificity). Fourth, elicitation of the MMN does not require the subject to perform a task or impose any attentional requirements. Therefore it is an ideal probe for comparing preattentive processing of left- and right-sided stimuli and for evaluating the processing of different dimensions of the auditory stimulus.

In a study of 10 patients with auditory and visual UN, deviations on either side of space were examined, with the stimulus differences defined in terms of spatial location, duration, or the pitch of sounds presented from loudspeakers.[35] The most robust finding was that the MMN elicited by deviation in sound-source location was considerably reduced when the stimuli were on the left (neglected) compared to the right side. Pitch deviance also tended to exhibit right-side advantage, but this effect was not as robust as for location. In contrast, no right-left difference was found for the MMN elicited by duration deviance (Fig. 5-14). Since the magnocellular visual pathway is the main contributor to the dorsal stream of the visual system, which is involved with the processing of spatial information, the results from the studies in vision[151] and audition[35] suggest a specific, preattentive deficit in encoding spatial attributes of sensory events. A possible reason for the

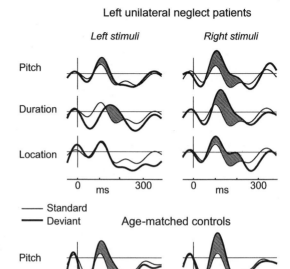

Figure 5-14

Mismatch negativity (hatched area) to deviation in pitch, duration, and location of stimuli in 10 patients with damage to the right hemisphere and with unilateral left visual and auditory neglect and 10 age-matched controls. Stimuli were presented in different blocks 60 degrees to the right or to the left of the subjects through loudspeakers. Standard stimuli were 75-ms-long harmonic tones (600-Hz fundamental). The probability of the pitch deviants (60 Hz lower), duration deviants (50 ms shorter), and location deviants (30 degrees more medial) was 0.1 each. Data presented are for Fz electrode referenced to averaged mastoids. There was a significant decrement in MMN to left location deviants (comparing within patient to the response to right side stimuli). The decrement approached significance for pitch and was not significant for duration (see Ref. 35 for details).

lack of awareness in UN despite implicit processing of the neglected stimuli is that perceived events cannot be placed in a spatial framework, which is necessary for conscious awareness and for adequately shifting attention towards the stimuli.[35]

The "Posner paradigm"[164] was used to explore the effect of neglect on the allocation of attention as reflected by the P3 and Nd.[139] It has been previously shown that in right temporoparietal patients, a misleading (invalid) cue on the ipsilesional side dramatically slows down the reaction time to contralesional targets more than the normal effect of such a cue and more than the effect of a contralesional invalid cue on the reaction time to an ipsilesional target,[164,165] suggesting that patients with these lesions fail to "disengage" from stimuli (e.g., the invalid cue) on the ipsilesional side. This conjecture was corroborated by the finding that in right parietal patients the Nd, an ERP manifestation of selective attention, was significantly smaller following right-sided (invalid) cues than any other cue-target combination.[139] This effect was evident as early as 200 ms after target onset, suggesting that even if the underlying deficit may originate in the higher-order attention mechanism, it affects "the very processing of perceptual input" (Verleger et al.,[139] p. 455).

A more complex pattern of results was obtained regarding the patients' P3 component in the Posner paradigm.[139] The late positive potential (LAP or P3f, denoting a P3 recorded at Fz[166]) was largest for the critical combination of right cue and left target. This pattern resembles the enhanced P3 observed in monkeys with frontoparietal damage and signs of UN.[167] Post hoc, the P3f enhancement was interpreted as reflecting the patients' attempt to reorient attention toward the left-side target following late detection. Direct tests of this hypothesis are needed. In contrast to the P3f, the P3b (recorded at a central parietal site) was reduced in patients irrespective of the cue and target location, corroborating earlier observations.[125] This general reduction was ascribed to damage to P3 generators, especially those centered in the temporoparietal junction.

The use of electrophysiological and hemodynamic functional imaging sheds new light on intact and impaired processes in UN. The extant studies show that the lesion may induce specific impairments in an early stage of processing to which behavioral methods may be blind.

Linguistic Processing in Aphasic Patients

Whereas language deficits following brain damage are traditionally classified into crude clinical syndromes such as Broca's or Wernicke's aphasia, advances in neurolinguistics suggest that a finer-grain analysis, based on individual symptoms, may be more fruitful (see Chap. 12). Distinct ERP components have been linked to stages of language comprehension including (1) early left anterior negativity (ELAN), a marker of syntactic violations[168,169]; (2) The N400, related to lexical/semantic integration (N400)[170]; and (3) the "late positivity" or P600, which has been attributed to reprocessing of linguistic information (P600).[171] The N400 was first described by Kutas and Hillyard as being elicited by violations of semantic expectancies at the end of sentences ("She takes her coffee with cream and *dog*" rather than ". . . cream and *sugar*").[170] The N400 amplitude is modulated by the extent to which a word is related to its prior context ("N400 effect"), being more negative the more unexpected the word is.[172] The effect is not limited to sentences but can be seen both when comparing words primed or not primed by a previous semantically related or associated word[173] or when a word in a sentence is incompatible with the general context of a discourse.[174] In fact, even nonverbal stimuli such as faces,[175] pictures,[176–178] and environmental noises[85] (but not endings of melodies[179,180]) have been reported to elicit N400-type components, suggesting a link to lexical access[181] or postlexical integration of a stimulus into the semantic context.[182] It is conceivable that multiple intracranial regions contribute to the scalp N400 with different subcomponents related to various aspects of cognitive processing, as has been suggested for P300 phenomena.[183] The N400 amplitude was reduced in patients with lesions of the left temporoparietal cortex exhibiting symptoms of Wernicke's aphasia. Conversely, N400 amplitudes were reported to be less affected in patients with frontal lesions exhibiting symptoms of Broca's aphasia.[184] Intracranial recordings in the anterior medial temporal lobe (MTL) have revealed potentials resembling the scalp N400 in verbal recognition memory, lexical decision, semantic priming, and picture-naming tasks.[183,185,186] MTL-N460 amplitudes have been reported to be largest in the left MTL following new words, while an MTL-P620 potential was largest to repeated words and was reduced in a passive condition. Puce and colleagues[187] found similar MTL potentials to both verbal stimuli and abstract "nonverbalizable" patterns during recognition memory. These data suggest that a posterior cortical-mesial-temporal network is engaged during N400 generation.

Elderly controls and patients with Broca's aphasia demonstrated semantic and associative priming effects, manifest by a decreased N400 to related targets versus unrelated targets, while patients with Wernicke's aphasia failed to show this priming effect.[184] However, the N400 effect was found to correlate significantly with the degree of comprehension in a group of aphasic patients irrespective of their diagnosis as Broca's or Wernicke's aphasia.[36,184] Whereas the hallmark of Broca's aphasia is an expressive problem, it is now believed that these patients also have some problems with comprehension. For example, agrammatic nonfluent aphasics have difficulty in understanding sentences involving atypical syntactic constructions.[188] An interesting double dissociation was found between a "Broca" patient with a frontal lesion including the frontal operculum and the insula, and a "Wernicke" patient with posterior-temporal/inferior-parietal lesion.[189] The patient with the frontal lesion failed to elicit the "early left anterior negativity" (ELAN) effect following a phrase structure (grammatical) violation but showed a normal N400 effect for a semantic violation of the sort outlined in the previous paragraph. The patient with the posterior lesion showed the opposite result. This supports the existence of distinct mechanisms for grammatical parsing and lexical-semantic integration, with the former dependent on the inferior frontal and insular cortex and the latter dependent on posterior parietotemporal cortex. Patients with anterior lesions fail to exhibit a differential ERP response to closed-class (e.g., pronouns) and open-class (e.g., nouns) words, possibly reflecting a deficit in the rapid categorization of words into their syntactic roles.[190] However, the semantic processing in patients with anterior lesions may not be completely intact. When an ambiguous word (e.g., *bank*) is placed as the last word in a sentence, the sentence may disambiguate the word in one direction (e.g., "the man called the bank"). In normal controls, a target word (e.g., *river*) following the disambiguated word elicits a smaller N400 if it is associated with the selected meaning than if it is unrelated or is related to the alternative meaning (the N400 effect). The same result was obtained in a group of patients with frontal lesions and Broca's aphasia as long as the time between the disambiguated word and the target

word was long (1250 ms).[190] When this gap was short (100 ms), the alternative meaning primed the target word significantly (although to a smaller degree than the selected meaning). Age-matched controls showed the normal pattern for both gaps. This has been interpreted as a slowing of lexical integration in the aphasic patients, with both meanings of the ambiguous word remaining "active" for a longer time and thus hampering comprehension. In addition to higher-order linguistic deficits, ERP studies using the MMN component revealed a lower level deficit of phonetic discrimination in patients with comprehension deficits following left posterior temporal lesions, including Wernicke's area, but not in patients with anterior lesions and signs of Broca's aphasia.[159,191–193] Thus, some of the deficit in comprehension may reflect difficulty in deciphering the phonetic stream, resulting in degraded input to higher-order linguistic processes.

Although the results of these pioneering studies of language impairment may be open to different interpretations based on competing theories of language processing, they nevertheless demonstrate the potential benefits of using ERPs to investigate normal and impaired language processes. Initial attempts have also been made to use ERPs as a diagnostic aid in examining the comprehension of patients with global aphasia, which cannot be examined behaviorally.[194,195]

TRANSCRANIAL MAGNETIC STIMULATION

Merton and Morton provided the first demonstration of transcranial electrical stimulation (TES) in 1980.[196] By applying a brief, high-voltage electric shock to the scalp over motor cortex, they were able to elicit focal muscle activity, or what has come to be called the motor evoked response (MER). This technique had obvious utility for clinicians, offering a tool for measuring the integrity of efferent pathways in a manner analogous to that provided by the somatosensory evoked potential. However, TES had one serious drawback: the shocks were very painful because the stimulus also activated pain receptors in the scalp. Transcranial magnetic stimulation (TMS) was developed as a painless alternative to TES[197] (for recent reviews, see Refs. 198 and 199).

Technical Considerations

The TMS device consists of a tightly wrapped wire coil that is encased in an insulated sheath and connected to a power source of electrical capacitors. When triggered, the capacitors send a large electric current through the coil, resulting in the generation of a large yet compact magnetic field (up to 3 tesla) with lines of flux perpendicular to the plane of the coil. The magnetic field peaks within about 150 μs and decays within 1 ms. This rapid change induces electric eddy currents in conductive tissue. The skull presents low impedance to magnetic fields of this frequency; thus there is minimal current induction in extracerebral tissue, including pain receptors. However, eddy currents are produced within the brain, thus stimulating neural tissue. The exact mechanism is unknown. It may be that the current leads to the generation of action potentials in the soma; alternatively, the current may directly stimulate axons or involve a mixture of cell body and axonal stimulation.

The current generated is strongest under the edges of the coil; it become weak near the center. Thus, with circular coils, the area of activation is dispersed and not homogenous across the region spanned by the coil. To obtain more focal stimulation, figure-eight coils are commonly employed, with the current strongest at the point where the two circles intersect (Fig. 5-15). With such coils, the primary activation can be restricted to an area of about 1 to 1.5 cm. The extent and intensity of the induced neural activity varies with the intensity of the generated current and falls off fairly rapidly as the distance from the coil increases. As such, TMS is primarily targeted at cortical areas that lie along the gyri, although deeper structures such as the supplementary motor area have been successfully stimulated.[200] In addition, the resistance of white matter is greater than that of gray matter, further reducing the likelihood that TMS can be targeted to deep structures of the cortex or subcortical nuclei.

Applications of TMS

TMS has become a relatively standard clinical tool for evaluating the speed of conduction in motor pathways. For example, activation of the abductor digiti minimi muscle (fifth finger) can be elicited by placing the stim-

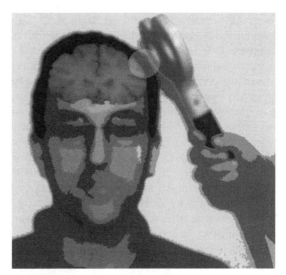

Figure 5-15
Transcranial magnetic stimulation (TMS). The figure shows a figure-eight-shaped TMS stimulator applied to the head; the region of stimulated cortex is indicated schematically.

ulator over the ulnar nerve at the wrist, at the C7 level of the spinal cord, or over the contralateral motor cortex.[17] In this manner, it is possible to determine if abnormal latencies arise from central or peripheral pathology in a disease such as multiple sclerosis or when monitoring corticospinal function during spinal cord surgery. While clinical uses of this kind are primarily diagnostic, TMS has also been studied as a possible therapeutic device. Preliminary studies have indicated that repetitive TMS (rTMS; with rates varying from 0.5 Hz for 10 s to 10 Hz for 5 s) applied over prefrontal cortex may prove effective for treating major depression.[201,202] The mechanism of such treatment is unclear, but it may offer a more focal and less debilitating treatment than electroshock therapy for patients with resistant mood disorders.

TMS offers a new experimental approach for cognitive neuroscience. With this method, an experimenter can disrupt neural function in a selected region of the cortex and, as with lesion studies, the resulting changes in behavior can shed light on the normal function of the targeted tissue. What makes this method appealing is that, appropriately applied, the technique is safe and noninvasive. Moreover, since the principal use is with neurologically healthy individuals, TMS allows for the creation of "virtual" reversible lesions in an otherwise intact brain.[18]

Virtual lesions have been created over a number of disparate cortical areas. A functional scotoma can be created by a single TMS pulse applied over the occipital pole, presumably reflecting the disruption of processing within primary visual cortex.[203,204] An important feature of TMS is that the effect shows a high degree of temporal specificity. Corthout et al.[205] found that performance on a letter-identification task was essentially abolished for one subject when the TMS pulse followed the stimulus onset by about 100 ms. For stimulus-to-TMS intervals less than 60 ms or greater than 140 ms, performance was near perfect.

While it is tempting to conclude that the critical activity within primary visual cortex for letter identification occurs about 100 ms after stimulus presentation, it is also possible that there is a delay between the onset of the TMS-induced activity and the actual neural disruption in task performance. For example, it is quite possible that a silent period follows the TMS volley, and it may be that this silent period is what leads to the scotoma. Nonetheless, TMS can be useful for examining the relative timing of processing within different visual areas. For example, Beckers and Zeki[206] reported that stimulation over either V1 or V5 (MT) impaired performance on a motion discrimination task. Interestingly, the disruptive effects in V1 occurred with much longer stimulus-to-TMS intervals than found for V5, a result that would seem at odds with conventional notions that processing proceeds in a serial manner from V1 to higher visual areas. The TMS results would suggest that back projections from V5 to V1 might be an important part of the discrimination process (see also Ref. 207).

A second example of the use of TMS for exploring functional connectivity comes from a study in which subjects were trained to perform sequential finger movements.[200] When the coil was centered over the hand area of motor cortex, the next response in the sequence was frequently disturbed, either because the movement was halted in midstream or because the wrong key was pressed. The subjects perceived the problem as a temporary loss of coordination, commenting that the finger suddenly seemed to jerk in the wrong direction. In contrast, when the coil

was targeted to affect the supplementary motor area (SMA), the effects were delayed, occurring about three key presses after the TMS pulse. Here, the subjects reported that they lost track of their place in the sequence or that they temporarily forgot the order of responses. Thus, TMS demonstrated the differential role of supplementary motor area and primary motor cortex in motor planning and execution, respectively. It is important to note that TMS pulses in this study were applied in a rapid series (3 Hz). It is unclear whether measurable effects on higher-level aspects of cognition such as motor programming can be obtained with single-pulse TMS. Unfortunately, there have been a few reported cases of induced seizure activity with rapid TMS (>1 Hz), thus limiting the use of this method.[216]

There have recently been a number of impressive reports in which TMS and functional neuroimaging have been used in combination. A long-standing debate in cognitive neuroscience has centered on the question of whether visual imagery requires the engagement of neural regions involved in visual perception. Evidence in favor of a shared medium for imagery and perception comes from imaging studies; as measured by PET, activation in visual areas including primary visual cortex have been reported when subjects were asked to image visual patterns and then make judgments about properties such as length and orientation.[208]

However, as with all imaging studies, the evidence is correlational, making it difficult to draw conclusions about causation. Connections from higher-order visual areas (or even nonvisual areas) to primary visual cortex due to long-term perceptual experience may have led to the activation of primary visual cortex even though this activity was not essential for task performance. To test this possibility, Kosslyn and colleagues used a novel TMS method. Prior to performing a second session on the imagery task, 1-Hz TMS was applied over the occipital pole for 10 min.[208] Previous studies had shown that the efficacy of neural activity is depressed for an extended period after such repetitive TMS, allowing performance to be assessed under conditions in which the nonspecific effects such as the noise from the stimulator or muscle twitches are not present.[209] Indeed, performance on the imagery task was impaired following this stimulation in comparison to a sham TMS control condition in which the coil was oriented perpendicular to the skull. Thus it appears that disruption of normal activity in primary visual cortex can impair imagery, providing experimental evidence that converges with the correlational results obtained in the PET phase of the study. In a similar way, TMS over visual cortex has been shown to disrupt tactile perception of shape in both sighted[210] and blind individuals,[211] indicating that the activation observed in these areas during neuroimaging studies[212,213] is not an epiphenomenon.

TMS has recently been used to reproduce phenomena naturally observed after brain damage. The line bisection task is a common test for unilateral neglect (see above and Chap. 14). In a variant of this task known as the landmark task, subjects are asked to judge whether a line is correctly bisected into two equal segments. Single-pulse TMS applied within 200 ms following the stimulus over posterior parietal area of healthy volunteers slowed down reaction times when the bisecting landmark was to the right of the midline[214] and biased perception toward underestimating the left segments.[215] Left-sided pulses or sham pulses did not alter performance. Notably, patients with right parietal lesions bisect lines to the right of the midline. Thus, the posterior parietal region stimulated (corresponding to Brodman's area 7 and the intraparietal sulcus) may indeed have a critical role in this task. In addition, this procedure suggests the possibility of a human model for studying some visuospatial deficits found in unilateral neglect.

CONCLUSIONS

The use of event-related potentials to study patients with localized brain damage and with specific behavioral dysfunctions continues to provide invaluable information on the underlying mechanisms of normal and pathologic cognition and its neural mechanism. TMS provides a new and promising method of inducing virtual lesions in healthy subjects, thus providing a method to test functional hypotheses regarding the contribution of targeted neural areas to particular tasks. The combination of these methods with traditional neuropsychological and hemodynamic imaging methods is likely to transform our understanding of brain function. Hopefully, this will yield better diagnostic as well as restorative procedures for neurologic patients.

REFERENCES

1. Hillyard SA, Picton TW: Electrophysiology of cognition, in Plum F (ed): *Handbook of Physiology: The Nervous System.* Baltimore: American Physiological Society, 1987, pp 519–584.
2. Knight RT: Attention regulation and human prefrontal cortex, in Thierry AM, Glowinski J, Goldman-Rakic P, Christen Y (eds): *Motor and Cognitive Functions of the Prefrontal Cortex: Research and Perspectives in Neurosciences.* Berlin and Heidelberg: Springer-Verlag, 1994, pp 160–173.
3. Egan MF, Duncan CC, Suddath RL, et al: Event-related potential abnormalities correlate with structural brain alterations and clinical features in patients with chronic schizophrenia. *Schizophr Res* 11:259–271, 1994.
4. Bonmassar G, Schwartz DP, Liu AK, et al: Spatiotemporal brain imaging of visual-evoked activity using interleaved EEG and fMRI recordings. *Neuroimage* 13:1035–1043, 2001.
5. Goldman RI, Stern JM, Engel J, et al: Acquiring simultaneous EEG and functional MRI. *Clin Neurophysiol* 111:1974–1980, 2000.
6. Allen PJ, Josephs O, Turner R: A method for removing imaging artifact from continuous EEG recorded during functional MRI. *Neuroimage* 12:230–239, 2000.
7. Kruggel F, Herrmann CS, Wiggins CJ, et al: Hemodynamic and electroencephalographic responses to illusory figures: Recording of the evoked potentials during functional MRI. *Neuroimage* 14:1327–1336, 2001.
8. Lazeyras F, Zimine I, Blanke O, et al: Functional MRI with simultaneous EEG recording: Feasibility and application to motor and visual activation. *J Magn Reson Imaging* 13:943–948, 2001.
9. König P, Engel AK: Correlated firing in sensory-motor systems. *Curr Opin Neurobiol* 5:511–519, 1995.
10. Basar-Eroglu C, Strüber D, Schürmann M, et al: Gamma-band responses in the brain: a short review of psychophysiological correlates and functional significance. *Int J Psychophysiol* 24:101–112, 1996.
11. Llinas R, Ribary U, Contreras D, et al: The neuronal basis for consciousness. *Philos Trans R Soc Lond B Biol Sci* 353:1841–1849, 1998.
12. Pfurtscheller G, Lopes da Silva FH: Event-related EEG/MEG synchronization and desynchronization: Basic principles. *Clin Neurophysiol* 110:1842–1857, 1999.
13. Sannita WG: Stimulus-specific oscillatory responses of the brain: A time/frequency-related coding process. *Clin Neurophysiol* 111:565–583, 2000.

14. Tallon-Baudry C, Bertrand, O, Peronnet F, et al: Induced gamma-band activity during the delay of a visual short-term memory task in humans. *J Neurosci* 18:4244–4254, 1998.

15. Herrmann CS, Knight R: Mechanisms of human attention: event-related potentials and oscillations. *Neurosci Biobehav Rev* 25:465–476, 2001.

16. Penfield W. Jasper H: *Epilepsy and the Functional Anatomy of the Human Brain.* Boston: Little, Brown, 1954.

17. Brunholzl C, Claus D: Central motor conduction time to upper and lower limbs in cervical cord lesions. *Arch Neurol* 51:245–249, 1994.

18. Pascual-Leone A, Bartres-Faz D, Keenan JP: Transcranial magnetic stimulation: Studying the brain-behaviour relationship by induction of "virtual lesions." *Philos Trans R Soc Lond B Biol Sci* 354:1229–1238, 1999.

19. Picton TW, Lins OG, Scherg M: The recording and analysis of event-related potentials, in Boller F, Graffman J (eds): *Handbook of Neuropsychology.* New York: Elsevier, 1995, pp 3–73.

20. Picton TW, Alain C, Woods DL, et al: Intracerebral sources of human auditory-evoked potentials. *Audiol Neurootol* 4:64–79, 1999.

21. Swick D, Kutas M, Neville HJ: Localizing the neural generators of event-related brain potentials, in Kertesz A (ed): *Localization in Neuroimaging in Neuropsychology.* New York: Academic Press, 1994, pp 73–121.

22. Näätänen R: *Attention and Brain Function.* Hillsdale, NJ: Erlbaum, 1992.

23. Knight RT: Electrophysiology in behavioral neurology, in Mesulam M-M (ed): *Principles of Behavioral Neurology.* Philadelphia: Davis, 1985, pp 327–346.

24. Picton TW: Human event-related potentials, in *Handbook of Electroencephalography and Clinical Neurophysiology.* Philadelphia: Elsevier, 1987, vol 3.

25. Klee M, Rall W: Computed potentials of cortically arranged populations of neurons. *J Neurophysiol* 40:647–666, 1977.

26. Pernier J, Perrin F, Bertrand O: Scalp current density fields: Concept and properties. *Electroencephalogr Clin Neurophysiol* 69:385–589, 1998.

27. Gevins A, Smith ME, McEvoy LK, et al: Electroencephalographic imaging of higher brain function. *Philos Trans R Soc Lond B Biol Sci* 354:1125–1133, 1999.

28. Angelelli P, De Luca M, Spinelli D: Early visual processing in neglect patients: A study with steady-state VEPs. *Neuropsychologia* 34:1151–1157, 1996.

29. Aboud S, Bar L, Rosenfeld M, et al: Left-right asymmetry of visual evoked potentials in brain-damaged patients: a mathematical model and experimental results. *Ann Biomed Eng* 24:75–86, 1996.

30. Knight RT, Scabini D: Anatomic bases of event-related potentials and their relationship to novelty detection in humans. *J Clin Neurophysiol* 15:3–13, 1998.

31. Damasio H, Damasio AR: *Lesion Analysis in Neuropsychology.* New York: Oxford University Press, 1989.

32. Fiez JA, Damasio H, Grabowski TJ: Lesion segmentation and manual warping to a reference brain: Intra- and interobserver reliability. *Hum Brain Mapp* 9:192–211, 2000.

33. Brett M, Leff AP, Rorden C, et al: Spatial normalization of brain images with focal lesions using cost function masking. *Neuroimage* 14:486–500, 2001.

34. Knight RT: Distributed cortical network for visual attention. *J Cogn Neurosci* 9:75–91, 1997.

35. Deouell LY, Bentin S, Soroker N: Electrophysiological evidence for an early (pre-attentive) information processing deficit in patients with right hemisphere damage and unilateral neglect. *Brain* 123:353–365, 2000.

36. Swaab T, Brown C, Hagoort T: Spoken sentence comprehension in aphasia: Event-related potential evidence for a lexical integration deficit. *J Cogn Neurosci* 9:39–66, 1997.

37. Knight RT, Stuss DT: Prefrontal cortex: the present and the future, in Stuss DT, Knight RT (eds): *Principles of Frontal Lobe Function.* New York: Oxford University Press, 2002, pp 573–597.

38. Knight RT, D'Esposito M: The lateral prefrontal syndrome: A deficit in executive control, in D'Esposito M (ed): *Neurological Foundations of Cognitive Neuroscience.* Cambridge, MA: MIT Press. In press.

39. Knight, RT, Staines WR, Swick D, et al: Prefrontal cortex regulates inhibition and excitation in distributed neural networks. *Acta Psychol* 101:159–178, 1999.

40. Lhermitte F: Human autonomy and the frontal lobes: Part II. Patient behavior in complex and social situations: The "environmental dependency syndrome." *Ann Neurol* 19:335–343, 1986.

41. Shimamura AP: Memory and the frontal lobe, in Gazzaniga M (ed): *The Cognitive Neurosciences.* Cambridge, MA: MIT Press, 1994, pp 803–813.

42. Barcelo F, Suwazono S, Knight RT: Prefrontal modulation of visual processing in humans. *Nat Neurosci* 3:399–403, 2000.

43. Chao LL, Knight, RT: Contribution of human prefrontal cortex to delay performance. *J Cogn Neurosci* 10:167–77, 1998.

44. Edinger HM, Siegel A, Troiano R: Effect of stimulation of prefrontal cortex and amygdala on diencephalic neurons. *Brain Res* 97:17–31, 1975.
45. Alexander GE, Newman JD, Symmes D: Convergence of prefrontal and acoustic inputs upon neurons in the superior temporal gyrus of the awake squirrel monkey. *Brain Res* 116:334–338, 1976.
46. Skinner JE, Yingling CD: Central gating mechanisms that regulate event-related potentials and behavior, in Desmedt JE (ed): *Progress in Clinical Neurophysiology.* Basel: Karger, 1977, vol 1, pp 30–69.
47. Yingling CD, Skinner JE: Gating of thalamic input to cerebral cortex by nucleus reticularis thalami, in Desmedt JE (ed): *Progress in Clinical Neurophysiology.* Basel: Karger, 1977, vol I, pp 70–96.
48. Guillery RW, Feig SL, Lozsadi DA: Paying attention to the thalamic reticular nucleus. *Trends Neurosci* 21:28–32, 1998.
49. Knight RT, Scabini D, Woods DL: Prefrontal cortex gating of auditory transmission in humans. *Brain Res* 504:338–342, 1989.
50. Yamaguchi S, Knight RT: Gating of somatosensory inputs by human prefrontal cortex. *Brain Res* 521:281–288, 1990.
51. Alho K, Woods DL, Algazi A, et al: Lesions of frontal cortex diminish the auditory mismatch negativity. *Electroencephalogr Clin Neurophysiol* 91:353–362, 1994.
52. Sokolov EN: Higher nervous functions: The orienting reflex. *Annu Rev Physiol* 25:545–580, 1963.
53. Knight RT: Decreased response to novel stimuli after prefrontal lesions in man. *Electroencephalogr Clin Neurophysiol* 59:9–20, 1984.
54. Chao L, Knight RT: Human prefrontal lesions increase distractibility to irrelevant sensory inputs. *Neuroreport* 6:1605–1610, 1995.
55. Woods DL, Knight RT: Electrophysiological evidence of increased distractibility after dorsolateral prefrontal lesions. *Neurology* 36:212–216, 1986.
56. Desimone R: Visual attention mediated by biased competition in extrastriate visual cortex. *Philos Trans R Soc Lond B Biol Sci* 353:1245–1255, 1998.
57. Hillyard SA, Hink RF, Schwent UL, et al: Electrical signs of selective attention in the human brain. *Science* 182:177–180, 1973.
58. Heinze HJ, Mangun GR, Burchert W, et al: Combined spatial and temporal imaging of brain activity during visual selective attention in humans. *Nature* 372:543–546, 1994.
59. Mangun GR: Neural mechanisms of visual selective attention. *Psychophysiology* 32:4–18, 1995.
60. Martínez A, Anllo-Vento L, Sereno MI, et al: Involvement of striate and extrastriate visual cortical areas in spatial attention. *Nat Neurosci* 2:364–369, 1999.
61. Woldorff MG, Gallen CC, Hampson SA, et al: Modulation of early sensory processing in human auditory cortex during auditory selective attention. *Proc Natl Acad Sci U S A* 90:8722–8726, 1993.
62. Grady CL, Van Meter JW, Maisog JM, et al: Attention-related modulation of activity in primary and secondary auditory cortex. *Neuroreport* 8:2511–2516, 1997.
63. Somers DC, Dale AM, Seiffert AE, et al: Functional MRI reveals spatially specific attentional modulation in human primary visual cortex. *Proc Natl Acad Sci U S A* 96:1663–1668, 1999.
64. Steinmetz PN, Roy A, Fitzgerald PJ, et al: Attention modulates synchronized neuronal firing in primate somatosensory cortex. *Nature* 404:187–190, 2000.
65. Roelfsema PR, Lamme VAF, Spekreijse H: Object-based attention in the primary visual cortex of the macaque monkey. *Nature* 395:376–381, 1998.
66. Hillyard SA, Anllo-Vento L: Event-related brain potentials in the study of visual selective attention. *Proc Natl Acad Sci U S A* 95:781–787, 1998.
67. Fuster JM, Bodner M, Kroger JK: Cross-modal and cross-temporal association in neurons of frontal cortex. *Nature* 405:347–351, 2000.
68. Funahashi S, Bruce CJ, Goldman-Rakic PS: Dorsolateral prefrontal lesions and oculomotor delayed-response performance: Evidence for mnemonic "scotomas." *J Neurosci* 13:1479–1497, 1993.
69. Rossi AF, Rotter PS, Desimone R, et al: Prefrontal lesions produce impairments in feature-cued attention. *Soc Neurosci Abstr* 29:2, 1999.
70. McIntosh AR, Grady CL, Ungerleider LG, et al: Network analysis of cortical visual pathways mapped with PET. *J Neurosci* 14:655–666, 1994.
71. Büchel C, Friston KJ: Modulation of connectivity in visual pathways by attention: Cortical interactions evaluated with structural equation modeling and fMRI. *Cereb Cortex* 7:768–778, 1997.
72. Chawla D, Rees G, Friston KJ: The physiological basis of attentional modulation in extrastriate visual areas. *Nat Neurosci* 2:671–676, 1999.
73. Rees G, Frackowiak R, Frith C: Two modulatory effects of attention that mediate object categorization in human cortex. *Science* 275:835–838, 1997.
74. Kastner S, Pinsk MA, de Weerd P, et al: Increased activity in human visual cortex during directed attention in the absence of visual stimulation. *Neuron* 22:751–761, 1999.

75. Corbetta M: Frontoparietal cortical networks for directing attention and the eye to visual locations: Identical, independent, or overlapping neural systems? *Proc Natl Acad Sci U S A* 95:831–838, 1998.

76. Hopfinger JP, Buonocore MH, Mangun GR: The neural mechanisms of top-down attentional control. *Nat Neurosci* 3:284–291, 2000.

77. Barcelo F, Knight RT: Both random and perseverative errors underlie WCST deficits in prefrontal patients. *Neuropsychologia* 40:349–356, 2001.

78. Swick D: Effects of prefrontal lesions on lexical processing and repetition priming: An ERP study. *Brain Res Cogn Brain Res* 7:143–157, 1998.

79. Yago E, Knight RT: Tonic and phasic prefrontal modulation of extrastriate processing during visual attention. *Soc Neurosci Abstr* 30:8397, 2000.

80. Suwazono S, Machado L, Knight RT: Predictive value of novel stimuli modifies visual event-related potentials and behavior. *Clin Neurophysiol* 111:29–39, 2000.

81. Verleger R: Event-related potentials and cognition: A critique of the context updating hypothesis and an alternative interpretation of P3. *Behav Brain Sci* 11:343–356, 1988.

82. Heit G, Smith ME, Halgren E: Neuronal activity in the human medial temporal lobe during recognition memory. *Brain* 113:1093–1112, 1990.

83. Schupp HT, Lutzenberger W, Rau H, Birbaumer N: Positive shifts of event-related potentials: A state of cortical disfacilitation as reflected by the startle reflex probe. *Electroencephalogr Clin Neurophysiol* 90:135–144, 1994.

84. Donchin E, Coles MGH: Is the P300 component a manifestation of context updating? *Behav Brain Sci* 11:357–427, 1988.

85. Chao L, Nielsen-Bohlman L, Knight RT: Auditory event-related potentials dissociate early and late memory processes. *Electroencephalogr Clin Neurophysiol* 96:157–168, 1995.

86. Soltani M, Knight RT. The neural origins of P3. *Crit Rev Neurobiol*. In press.

87. Knight RT, Nakada, T: Cortico-limbic circuits and novelty: A review of EEG and blood flow data. *Rev Neurosci* 9:57–70, 1998.

88. Verleger R, Heide W, Butt C, Kompf D: Reduction of P3b potentials in patients with temporo-parietal lesions. *Cogn Brain Res* 2:103–116, 1994.

89. Knight RT, Hillyard SA, Woods DL, et al: The effects of frontal cortex lesions on event-related potentials during auditory selective attention. *Electroencephalogr Clin Neurophysiol* 52:571–582, 1981.

90. Woods DL, Knight RT, Scabini D: Anatomical substrates of auditory selective attention: behavioral and electrophysiological effects of temporal and parietal lesions. *Cogn Brain Res* 1:227–240, 1993.

91. Walter WG, Cooper R, Aldridge V, et al: Contingent negative variation: An electrical sign of sensorimotor association and expectancy in the human brain. *Nature* 203:380–384, 1964.

92. Levy R, Goldman-Rakic PS: Segregation of working memory functions within the dorsolateral prefrontal cortex. *Exp Brain Res* 133:23–32, 2000.

93. McCarthy G, Puce A, Constable RT, et al: Activation of human prefrontal cortex during spatial and nonspatial working memory tasks measured by functional MRI. *Cereb Cortex* 6:600–611, 1996.

94. Chao LL, Knight RT: Age related prefrontal changes during auditory memory. *Soc Neurosci Abstr* 20:1003, 1994.

95. Rosahl S, Knight RT: Prefrontal cortex contribution to the contingent negative variation. *Cereb Cortex* 5:123–134, 1995.

96. Zappoli R, Versari A, Zappoli F, et al: The effects on auditory neurocognitive evoked responses and contingent negative variation activity of frontal cortex lesions or ablations in man: three new case studies. *Int J Psychophysiol* 38:109–144, 2000.

97. Näätänen R, Gaillard AW, Mäntysalo S: Early selective-attention effect on evoked potential reinterpreted. *Acta Psychol* 42:313–29, 1978.

98. Näätänen R: The role of attention in auditory information processing as revealed by event-related potentials and other brain measures of cognitive function. *Behav Brain Sci* 13:201–288, 1990.

99. Winkler I, Karmos G, Näätänen R: Adaptive modeling of the unattended acoustic environment reflected in the mismatch negativity event-related potential. *Brain Res* 742:239–252, 1996.

100. Schröger E: A neural mechanism for involuntary attention shifts to changes in auditory stimulation. *J Cogn Neurosci* 8:527–539, 1996.

101. Alho K: Cerebral generators of mismatch negativity (MMN) and its magnetic counterpart (MMNm) elicited by sound changes. *Ear Hearing* 16:38–51, 1995.

102. Giard M-H, Perrin F, Pernier J, et al: Brain generators implicated in the processing of auditory stimulus deviance: A topographic event related potential study. *Psychophysiology* 27:627–640, 1990.

103. Deouell LY, Bentin S, Giard M-H: Mismatch negativity in dichotic listening: Evidence for interhemispheric differences and multiple generators. *Psychophysiology* 35:355–365, 1998.

104. Kaiser J, Lutzenberger W, Birbaumer N: Simultaneous bilateral mismatch response to right- but not leftward sound lateralization. *Neuroreport* 11:2889–2892, 2000.

105. Alain C, Woods DL, Knight RT: Distributed cortical network for sensory memory in humans. *Brain Res* 812:23–37, 1998.
106. Courchesne E, Hillyard SA, Galambos R: Stimulus novelty, task relevance, and the visual evoked potential in man. *Electroencephalogr Clin Neurophysiol* 39:131–143, 1975.
107. Yamaguchi S, Knight RT: P300 generation by novel somatosensory stimuli. *Electroencephalogr Clin Neurophysiol* 78:50–55, 1991.
108. Paller KA, McCarthy G, Wood CC: Event-related potentials elicited by deviant endings to melodies. *Psychophysiology* 29:202–206, 1992.
109. Halgren E, Baudena P, Clarke JM, et al: Intracerebral potentials to rare target and distractor auditory and visual stimuli: I. Superior temporal plane and parietal lobe. *Electroencephalogr Clin Neurophysiol* 94:191–220, 1995.
110. Smith ME, Halgren E, Sokolik ME, et al: The intracranial topography of the P3 event-related potential elicited during auditory oddball. *Electroencephalogr Clin Neurophysiol* 76:235–248, 1990.
111. Scabini D, McCarthy G: Hippocampal responses to novel somatosensory stimuli. *Soc Neurosci Abstr* 19:564, 1993.
112. Halgren E, Marinkovic K, Chauvel P: Generators of the late cognitive potentials in auditory and visual oddball tasks. *Electroencephalogr Clin Neurophysiol* 106:156–164, 1998.
113. Squires N, Squires K, Hillyard SA: Two varieties of long-latency positive waves evoked by unpredictable auditory stimuli in man. *Electroencephalogr Clin Neurophysiol* 38:387–401, 1975.
114. Opitz B, Mecklinger A, Friederici AD, et al: The functional neuroanatomy of novelty processing: integrating ERP and fMRI results. *Cereb Cortex* 9:379–391, 1999.
115. Kiehl KA, Laurens KR, Duty TL, et al: Neural sources involved in auditory target detection and novelty processing: An event-related fMRI study. *Psychophysiology* 38:133–142, 2000.
116. Zeineh MM, Engel SA, Bookheimer SY: Application of cortical unfolding techniques to functional MRI of the human hippocampal region. *Neuroimage* 11:668–683, 2000.
117. Scabini D, Knight RT: Frontal lobe contributions to the human P3a. *Soc Neurosci Abstr* 15:477, 1989.
118. Yamaguchi S, Knight RT: Anterior and posterior association cortex contributions to the somatosensory P300. *J Neurosci* 11:2039–2054, 1991.
119. Scabini D: Contribution of anterior and posterior association cortices to the human P300 cognitive event related potential. PhD dissertation. University of California, Davis: University Microfilms International, 1992.
120. Tranel D, Damasio H: Neuroanatomical correlates of electrodermal skin conductance responses. *Psychophysiology* 31:427–438, 1994.
121. Kimble DP, Bagshaw MH, Pribram KH: The GSR of monkeys during orienting and habituation after selective partial ablations of the cingulate and frontal cortex. *Neuropsychology* 3:121–128, 1965.
122. Knight RT, Grabowecky M: Escape from linear time: Prefrontal cortex and conscious experience, in Gazzaniga M (ed): *The Cognitive Neurosciences.* Cambridge, MA: MIT Press, 1995, pp 1357–1371.
123. Mesulam MM: A cortical network for directed attention and unilateral neglect. *Ann Neurol* 10:309–325, 1981.
124. Friedman HR, Goldman-Rakic PS: Coactivation of prefrontal and inferior parietal cortex in working memory tasks revealed by 2DG functional mapping in the rhesus monkey. *Neuroscience* 14:2775–2788, 1994.
125. Lhermitte F, Turell E, LeBrigand D, et al: Unilateral neglect and wave P300. A study of nine cases with unilateral lesions of the parietal lobes. *Arch Neurol* 42:567–573, 1985.
126. Knight, RT: Contribution of human hippocampal region to novelty detection. *Nature* 383:256–259, 1996.
127. Perani D, Bressi S, Cappa SF, et al: Evidence of multiple memory systems in the human brain: A 18F FDG PET metabolic study. *Brain* 116:903–919, 1993.
128. Goldman-Rakic PS, Selemon LD, Schwartz ML: Dual pathways connecting the dorsolateral prefrontal cortex with the hippocampal formation and parahippocampal cortex in the rhesus monkey. *Neuroscience* 12:719–743, 1984.
129. Heilman KM, Watson RT, Valenstein E: Neglect and related disorders, in Heilman KM, Valenstein E (eds): *Clinical Neuropsychology,* 3d ed. New York: Oxford University Press, 1993, pp 279–336.
130. Rapcsak SZ, Watson R, Heilman KM: Hemispace-visual field interactions in visual extinction. *J Neurol Neurosurg Psychiatry* 50:1117–1124, 1987.
131. De Renzi E, Gentilini M, Pattacini F: Auditory extinction following hemispheric damage. *Neuropsychologia* 22:733–744, 1984.
132. Heilman KM, Pandya DN, Geschwind N: Trimodal inattention following parietal lobe ablations. *Trans Am Neurol Assoc* 95:259–261, 1970.
133. De Renzi E, Gentilini M, Barbieri C: Auditory neglect. *J Neurol Neurosurg Psychiatry* 52:613–617, 1989.
134. Soroker N, Calamaro N, Glickson J, et al: Auditory inattention in right-hemisphere-damaged patients with and without visual neglect. *Neuropsychologia* 35:249–256, 1997.

135. Gainotti G, De Bonis C, Daniele A, et al: Contralateral and ipsilateral tactile extinction in patients with right and left focal brain lesions. *Int J Neurosci* 45:81–89, 1989.

136. Vallar G, Sandroni P, Rusconi ML, et al: Hemianopia, hemianesthesia, and spatial neglect: a study with evoked potentials. *Neurology* 41:1918–22, 1991.

137. Vallar G, Bottini MD, Sterzi R, et al: Hemianesthesia, sensory neglect, and defective access to conscious experience. *Neurology* 41:650–652, 1991.

138. Viggiano MP, Spinelli D, Mecacci L: Pattern reversal visual evoked potentials in patients with hemineglect syndrome. *Brain Cogn* 27:17–35, 1995.

139. Verleger R, Heide W, Butt C, et al: On-line correlates of right parietal patients' attention deficits. *Electroencephalogr Clin Neurophysiol* 99:444–457, 1996.

140. Näätänen R, Picton TW: The N1 wave of the human electric and magnetic response to sound: A review and an analysis of the component structure. *Psychophysiology* 24: 375–425, 1987.

141. Bisiach E, Cornacchia L, Sterzi R, et al: Disorders of perceived auditory lateralization after lesions of the right hemispheres. *Brain* 107:37–52, 1984.

142. Luck SJ, Heinze HJ, Mangun GR, et al: Visual event related potentials index focused attention within bilateral stimulus arrays: II. Functional dissociation of P1 and N1 components. *Electroencephalogr Clin Neurophysiol* 75:528–542, 1990.

143. Marzi CA, Girelli M, Miniussi C, et al: Electrophysiological correlates of conscious vision: Evidence from unilateral extinction. *J Cog Neurosci*, 12:869–877, 2000.

144. Vuilleumier P, Sagiv N, Hazeltine E, et al: Neural fate of seen and unseen faces in visuospatial neglect: A combined event-related fMRI and ERP study. *Proc Natl Acad Sci U S A* 98:3495–3500, 2001.

145. Driver J, Vuilleumier P, Eimer M, et al: Functional magnetic resonance imaging and evoked potential correlates of conscious and unconscious vision in parietal extinction patients. *Neuroimage* 14:S68–S75, 2001.

146. Lhermitte F, Pillon B, Serdaru M: Human anatomy and the frontal lobes: Part I. Imitation and utilization behavior: A neuropsychological study of 75 patients. *Ann Neurol* 19:326–334, 1986.

147. Driver J, Vuilleumier P: Perceptual awareness and its loss in unilateral neglect and extinction. *Cognition* 79:39–88, 2001.

148. Pitzalis S, Spinelli D, Zoccolotti P: Vertical neglect: Behavioral and electrophysiological data. *Cortex* 33:679–88, 1997.

149. Spinelli D, Burr DC, Morrone MC: Spatial neglect is associated with increased latencies of visual evoked potentials. *Vis Neurosci* 11:909–18, 1994.

150. Spinelli D, Di Russo F: Visual evoked potentials are affected by trunk rotation in neglect patients. *Neuroreport* 7:553–556, 1996.

151. Spinelli D, Angelelli P, De Luca M, et al: VEP in neglect patients have longer latencies for luminance but not for chromatic patterns. *Neuroreport* 7:815–859, 1996.

152. Doricchi F, Angelelli P, De Luca M, et al: Neglect for low luminance contrast stimuli but not for high colour contrast stimuli: A behavioural and electrophysiological case study. *Neuroreport* 31:1360–1364, 1996.

153. Alho K, Sams M, Paavilainen P, et al: Event related potentials reflecting processing of relevant and irrelevant stimuli during selective listening. *Psychophysiology* 26:514–528, 1989.

154. Alho K, Woods DL, Algazi A, et al: Intermodal selective attention: II. Effects of attentional load on processing of auditory and visual stimuli in central space. *Electroencephalogr Clin Neurophysiol* 82:356–368, 1992.

155. Näätänen R: Mismatch negativity outside strong attentional focus: A commentary on Woldorff et al (1991). *Psychophysiology* 28:478–484, 1991.

156. Alho K, Escera C, Diaz R, et al: Effects of involuntary auditory attention on visual task performance and brain activity. *Neuroreport* 8:3233–3237, 1997.

157. Novak G, Ritter W, Vaughan HG Jr: The chronometry of attention-modulated processing and automatic mismatch detection. *Psychophysiology* 29:412–430, 1992.

158. Schröger E: A neural mechanism for involuntary attention shifts to changes in auditory stimulation. *J Cogn Neurosci* 8:527–539, 1996.

159. Aaltonen O, Tuomainen J, Laine M, et al: Cortical differences in tonal versus vowel processing as revealed by an ERP component called mismatch negativity (MMN). *Brain Lang* 44:628–640, 1993.

160. Deacon D, Nousak JM, Pilotti M, et al: Automatic change detection: does the auditory system use representations of individual stimulus features or gestalts? *Psychophysiology* 35:413–419, 1998.

161. Deouell LY, Bentin S: Variable cerebral responses to equally distinct deviance in four auditory dimensions: A mismatch negativity study. *Psychophysiology* 35:745–754, 1998.

162. Schröger E: Processing of auditory deviants with changes in one versus two stimulus dimensions. *Psychophysiology* 32:55–65, 1995.

163. Ritter W, Deacon D, Gomes H, et al: The mismatch negativity of event-related potentials as a probe of transient auditory memory: A review. *Ear Hear* 16:52–57, 1995.

164. Posner MI, Walker JA, Friedrich FJ, et al: Effects of parietal lobe injury on covert orienting of visual attention. *J Neurosci* 4:1863–1874, 1984.

165. Friedrich FJ, Egly R, Rafal RD, et al: Spatial attention deficits in humans: A comparison of superior parietal and temporal-parietal junction lesions. *Neuropsychology* 12:193–207, 1998.

166. Donchin E, Ritter W, McCallum WC: Cognitive psychophysiology: The endogenous components of the ERP, in Callaway E, Tueting P, Koslow SH (eds): *Event-Related Potentials in Man.* New York: Academic Press, 1978, pp 349–442.

167. Watson RT, Miller BD, Heilman KM: Evoked potential in neglect. *Arch Neurol* 34, 224–227, 1977.

168. Neville H, Nicole JL, Barss A, et al: Syntactically based sentence processing classes: Evidence form event related brain potentials, *J Cogn Neurosci* 3:155–170, 1991.

169. Friederici AD, Pfeifer E, Hahne A: Event-related brain potentials during natural speech processing: Effects of semantic, morphological and syntactic violations. *Brain Res Cogn Brain Res* 1:183–192, 1993.

170. Kutas M, Hillyard SA: Reading senseless sentences: Brain potentials reflect semantic incongruity. *Science* 207:203–205, 1980.

171. Osterhout L, Holcomb PJ: Event-related brain potentials elicited by syntactic anomaly. *J Mem Lang* 31:785–806, 1992.

172. Van Petten C, Kutas M: Influences of semantic and syntactic context on open- and closed-class words. *Mem Cognit* 19:95–112, 1991.

173. Bentin S, McCarthy G, Wood CC: Event-related potentials, lexical decision and semantic priming. *Electroencephalogr Clin Neurophysiol* 60:343–355, 1985.

174. van Berkum JJ, Hagoort P, Brown CM: Semantic integration in sentences and discourse: Evidence from the N400. *J Cogn Neurosci* 11:657–671, 1999.

175. Barrett SE, Rugg MD, Perrett DI: Event-related potentials and the matching of familiar and unfamiliar faces. *Neuropsychology* 26:105–117, 1988.

176. Nielsen-Bohlman LC, Knight RT: Rapid memory mechanisms in man. *Neuroreport* 5:1517–1521, 1994.

177. Friedman D: Cognitive event-related potential components during continuous recognition memory for pictures. *Psychophysiology* 27:136–148, 1990.

178. Nigam A, Hoffman JE, Simons RF: N400 to semantically anomalous pictures and words. *J Cogn Neurosci* 4:15–22, 1992.

179. Paller KA, McCarthy G, Roessler E, et al: Potentials evoked in human and monkey medial temporal lobe during auditory and visual oddball paradigms. *Electroencephalogr Clin Neurophysiol* 84:269–279, 1992.

180. Besson M, Macar F: An event-related potential analysis of incongruity in music and other nonlinguistic contexts. *Psychophysiology* 24:14–25, 1987.

181. Deacon D, Hewitt S, Yang C, et al: Event-related potential indices of semantic priming using masked and unmasked words: evidence that the N400 does not reflect a post-lexical process. *Brain Res Cog Brain Res* 9:137–146, 2000.

182. Brown C, Hagoort P: The processing nature of the N400: Evidence from masked priming. *J Cogn Neurosci* 5:34–44, 1993.

183. Nobre AC, McCarthy G: Language-related ERPs: Scalp distributions and modulation by word type and semantic priming. *J Cogn Neurosci* 6:233–255, 1994.

184. Hagoort P, Brown CM, Swaab T: Lexical-semantic event-related potential effects in left hemisphere patients with aphasia and right hemisphere patients without aphasia. *Brain* 119:627–649, 1996.

185. Smith ME, Stapleton JM, Halgren E: Human medial temporal lobe potentials evoked in memory and language tasks. *Electroencephalogr Clin Neurophysiol* 63:145–159, 1986.

186. McCarthy G, Nobre AC, Bentin S, et al: Language-related field potentials in the anterior-medial temporal lobe: I. Intracranial distribution and neural generators. *J Neurosci* 15:1080–1089, 1995.

187. Puce A, Andrewes DG, Berkovic SF, et al: Visual recognition memory: neurophysiological evidence for the role of temporal white matter in man. *Brain* 114:1647–1666, 1991.

188. Berndt RS, Mitchum CC, Haendiges AN: Comprehension of reversible sentences in "agrammatism": A meta-analysis. *Cognition* 58:289–308, 1996.

189. Friederici AD, Hahne A, von Cramon DY: First-pass versus second-pass parsing processes in a Wernicke's and a Broca's aphasic: Electrophysiological evidence for a double dissociation. *Brain Lang* 62:311–341, 1998.

190. ter Keurs M, Brown CM, Hagoort P, et al: Electrophysiological manifestations of open- and closed-class words in patients with Broca's aphasia with agrammatic comprehension. An event-related brain potential study. *Brain* 122:839–854, 1999.

191. Swaab TY, Brown C, Hagoort P: Understanding ambiguous words in sentence contexts: Electrophysiological evidence for delayed contextual selection in Broca's aphasia. *Neuropsychologia* 36:737–761, 1998.

192. Auther LL, Wertz RT, Miller, et al: Relationships among the mismatch negativity (MMN) response, auditory

comprehension and site of lesion in aphasic adults. *Aphasiology* 14:461–470, 2000.

193. Wertz RT, Auther LL, Burch-Sims GP, et al: A comparison of the mismatch negativity (MMN) event-related potential to tone and speech stimuli in normal and aphasic adults. *Aphasiology* 12:499–507, 1998.

194. Connolly JF, D'Arcy RC, Lynn Newman R, et al: The application of cognitive event-related brain potentials (ERPs) in language-impaired individuals: review and case studies. *Int J Psychophysiol* 38:55–70, 2000.

195. Revonsuo A, Laine M: Semantic processing without conscious understanding in a global aphasic: Evidence from auditory event-related brain potentials. *Cortex* 32:29–48, 1996.

196. Merton PA, Morton HB: Stimulation of the cerebral cortex in the intact human subject. *Nature* 285:227, 1980.

197. Barker AT, Jalinous R, Freeston IL: Noninvasive magnetic stimulation of human motor cortex. *Lancet* 1:1106–1107, 1985.

198. Hallett M: Transcranial magnetic stimulation and the human brain. *Nature* 406:147–150, 2000.

199. Walsh V, Cowey A: Transcranial magnetic stimulation and cognitive neuroscience. *Nat Rev Neurosci* 1:73–79, 2000.

200. Gerloff C, Corwell B, Chen R, et al: Stimulation over the human supplementary motor area interferes with the organization of future elements in complex motor sequences. *Brain* 120:1587–1602, 1997.

201. Loo C, Mitchell P, Sachdev P, et al: Double-blind controlled investigation of transcranial magnetic stimulation for the treatment of resistant major depression. *Am J Psychiatry* 156:946–948, 1999.

202. Menkes DL, Bodnar P, Ballesteros RA, et al: Right frontal lobe slow frequency repetitive transcranial magnetic stimulation (SF r-TMS) is an effective treatment for depression: a case-control pilot study of safety and efficacy. *J Neurol Neurosurg Psychiatry* 67:113–115, 1999.

203. Amassian VE, Cracco RQ, Maccabee PJ, et al: Suppression of visual perception by magnetic coil stimulation of human occipital cortex. *Electroencephalogr Clin Neurophysiol* 74:458–462, 1989.

204. Kastner S, Demmer I, Ziemann U: Transient visual field defects induced by transcranial magnetic stimulation over human occipital pole. *Exp Brain Res* 118:19–26, 1998.

205. Corthout E, Uttl B, Ziemann U, et al: Two periods of processing in the (circum)striate visual cortex as revealed by transcranial magnetic stimulation. *Neuropsychologia* 37:137–145, 1999.

206. Beckers G, Zeki S: The consequences of inactivating areas V1 and V5 on visual motion perception. *Brain* 118:49–60, 1995.

207. Pascual-Leone A, Walsh V: Fast backprojections from the motion to the primary visual area necessary for visual awareness. *Science* 292:510–512, 2001.

208. Kosslyn SM, Pascual-Leone A, Felician O, et al: The role of area 17 in visual imagery: Convergent evidence from PET and rTMS. *Science* 284:167–170, 1999.

209. Pascual-Leone A, Tormos JM, Keenan J, et al: Study and modulation of human cortical excitability with transcranial magnetic stimulation. *J Clin Neurophysiol* 15:333–343, 1998.

210. Zangaladze A, Epstein CM, Grafton ST, et al: Involvement of visual cortex in tactile discrimination of orientation. *Nature* 401:587–590, 1999.

211. Cohen LG, Celnik P, Pascual-Leone A, et al: Functional relevance of cross-modal plasticity in blind humans. *Nature* 389:180–183, 1997.

212. Deibert E, Kraut M, Kremen S, et al: Neural pathways in tactile object recognition. *Neurology* 52:1413–1417, 1999.

213. Sathian K, Zangaladze A, Hoffman JM, et al: Feeling with the mind's eye. *Neuroreport* 8:3877–3881, 1997.

214. Pourtois G, Vandermeeren Y, Olivier E, et al: Event-related TMS over the right posterior parietal cortex induces ipsilateral visuo-spatial interference. *Neuroreport* 12:2369–2374, 2001.

215. Fierro B, Brighina F, Piazza A, et al: Timing of right parietal and frontal cortex activity in visuo-spatial perception: a TMS study in normal individuals. *Neuroreport* 12:2605–2607, 2001.

216. Wasserman EM: Risk and safety of repetitive transcranial magnetic stimulation: Report and suggested guidelines from the International Workshop on the Safety of Repetitive Transcranial Magnetic Stimulation, June 5–7, 1996. *Electroencephalogr Clin Neurophysiol* 108:1–16, 1998.

Chapter 6

STUDYING PLASTICITY IN THE DAMAGED AND NORMAL BRAIN

Albert M. Galaburda
Alvaro Pascual-Leone

PLASTICITY AS AN INTRINSIC PROPERTY OF THE BRAIN

It is not possible to understand psychological function in normal individuals or patients with cognitive or emotional deficits without invoking the concept of brain plasticity. Even though clinicians and researchers in behavioral neurology and cognitive neuroscience know better, discussions of patients with developmental, acquired, or degenerative brain injury affecting behavior often imply that the observed behaviors are the result of simple loss of function from some steady state caused by the injury. In fact, loss of function is not the only and even perhaps not the most important clinical behavioral consequence of brain damage. Injury can lead to changes in behavior by loss of function, by uncovering normally suppressed behaviors, and by the emergence of totally novel behaviors that result from brain remodeling, otherwise known as neural plasticity.

The brain is designed to be able to change in response to changes in the environment. This, in fact, is the mechanism for learning and for growth and development—changes in the anatomy of the input of a particular neural system, or in the information coming in along its afferent connections, or changes in the targets of its efferent connections can lead to system reorganization that can be demonstrable at the level of behavior, anatomy, and physiology, and down to the cellular and molecular levels. Initial damage and plasticity confer either no perceptible change in the behavioral capacity of the brain or can lead to changes that are demonstrated only under special testing conditions and not otherwise clinically significant. Otherwise, behavioral changes will bring the patient to medical attention. There may be loss of a previously acquired behavioral capacity; there may be release of behaviors normally suppressed in the uninjured brain; there may be the takeover of lost function by semiadapted neighboring systems that can complete some of the lost function (albeit perhaps via different strategies or computations); there may be the emergence of new behaviors that are adaptive or maladaptive. Reorganization does not necessarily mean recovery of function. In other words, plasticity at the neural level does not speak to the question of behavioral change and certainly does not necessarily imply functional recovery or even functional change.

It is reasonable to assume that plasticity is a characteristic of the nervous system that evolved for coping with changes in the environment associated with learning and development and that are coopted as a response to brain injury. Yet, as these mechanisms did not specifically evolve to cope with injury, they are not altogether successful in this regard. It is also safe to say, at this stage of our knowledge, that structural plasticity does not predict for behavioral plasticity, even though a fuller understanding will probably lead to such predictions.

The brain has millions of cells that are connected with each other by billions of synapses. In the course of development, very complex processes having to do with the intrinsic properties of neurons, as well as with influences arising either externally to the brain or in one brain region with respect to another, help to establish this intricate and highly specific network. Given that changes in the brain during development serve in part as a record of the history of the interaction between the brain and its environment (and among the different interconnected brain components), it is reasonable to think that the brain would, once development is completed, be resistant to change. Indeed, for many years, this notion of a rather static and unchanging postdevelopmental brain was the pervasive belief. More recently, it has become clear that this notion is wrong. The brain does not only undergo reorganization after injury, but it is in fact constantly reorganizing itself in response to change taking place around and within it.[1-3] The brain's intrinsic capacity to change persists throughout the human life span. A striking example lending support to this claim is witnessed during the acquisition of new skills. Neuroimaging studies have found decreases, increases, and shifts in regional brain activation resulting from task practice as a function of the amount of repetition and priming, level of learning proficiency, and overlearning and automatization.[4-6] Behavioral plasticity requires that structural and physiologic properties of the brain change to permit representation of new knowledge and implementation of new behaviors. As with learning, plasticity is seen in response to pathologic conditions, including injury to the central or peripheral nervous system.[7,8] As in learning, whereby input information into various brain areas changes, thus modifying plasticity, in injury structural changes also change input-output relationships in areas connectionally related to the area of damage and therefore also modify plasticity. In this setting, plasticity is likely to represent the mechanisms by which recovery of function after the injury is possible,[9] but, as already noted, could instead lead to maladaptive remodeling.

Plasticity is not an occasional state of the nervous system; instead, it is the normally ongoing state of the nervous system. A full, coherent account of any sensory or cognitive theory has to build into its framework the ongoing changes that occur as the brain continually learns from and updates its model of the world while reshaping its structure at multiple levels in response to changes in its input afferents and output targets. The need to understand the brain as an intrinsically plastic and hence changing system becomes critical not only for comprehending the effects of injury but also for the interpretation of behavioral, neurophysiologic, and functional imaging studies. Implicit in the commonly held notion of plasticity is the concept that there is a definable starting point after which it may be possible to record and measure change. In fact, there is no such beginning point, since any event, which could be exposure to a new learning situation, a seizure, or an infarct, falls upon a moving target—i.e., a brain that is undergoing constant change triggered by previous events or resulting from intrinsic remodeling activity. We should therefore not conceive of the brain as a stationary object

capable of activating a cascade of changes that we shall call plasticity, nor as an orderly stream of events, driven by plasticity. We might be better served by thinking of the nervous system as a continuously changing structure of which plasticity is an integral property and the obligatory consequence of each sensory input, each motor act, association, reward signal, action plan, or awareness. In this framework, notions such as psychological processes as distinct from organic-based functions or dysfunctions cease to be informative. Behavior will lead to changes in brain circuitry (just as changes in brain circuitry will lead to behavior), hence establishing organic symbiosis between learned attitudes, dispositions, or thinking styles and functional brain circuits.

MECHANISMS OF PLASTICITY

There are a number of mechanisms for plasticity in humans that can be studied at different levels, ranging from systems physiology all the way down to cellular and molecular levels. Thus far, our understanding of these mechanisms remains incomplete. Nonetheless, it can be said that descriptions at the level of large systems of interconnected neurons more specifically characterize human psychological processes than do descriptions at molecular and cellular levels, which seem to be shared not only between human and nonhuman primates but among all vertebrate and invertebrate organisms thus far studied. There are no known molecular mechanisms of learning unique to humans. Therefore, descriptions of plasticity at the systems levels are stressed in this chapter.

Expansion of a specialized cortical area or recruitment of a remote area as a result of learning or brain disease or injury comprises the two most characteristic forms of brain plasticity. The underlying general phenomenon is that neurons in one area assume properties of neurons in an adjacent or remote area. Such remodeling might take place within the cortex but could also implicate related subcortical levels.[10,11] Such remodeling can take place across brain areas within a given modality, for example within visual, tactile, or motor distributed systems (homotypic or intramodal plasticity), or may bridge across modalities (heterotypic or crossmodal plasticity), as in the case of tactile information processing in the occipital ("visual") cortex in the blind.[12,13] The time course of plasticity is extended, with some changes appearing within seconds of the initial event and continuing many years after an intervention or injury.[14,15]

Regardless of the physiologic mechanisms underlying plasticity, a series of principles can be put together. First, changes in the balance between excitatory and inhibitory influences can take place in established connectivity.[10] Such changes can take place in a very short time, because neural connectivity is larger than functional connectivity. Thus, learning- or injury-induced loss of inhibition can quickly expand the functional reach of a neural system. This process is commonly known as "unmasking." The application of the GABA antagonist bicuculline, for demonstrating the effects of unmasking, is a now classic strategy to study mechanisms of plasticity in animal models.[16,17] In humans, magnetic resonance spectroscopy or paired-pulse transcranial magnetic stimulation (TMS) can be used to provide similar insights.

A second process underlying fast-onset plasticity is the modulation (strengthening or weakening) of existing synapses. Processes such as long-term potentiation (LTP) or long-term depression (LTD) are examples of such mechanisms. LTP or LTD occurs following specific patterns of synaptic activity and may last for long periods of time. Such processes have been shown to occur in a variety of brain regions, most notably in the hippocampus, but also in the cortex.[18,19] Thus, in many regions of the cerebral cortex, calcium ion influx through NMDA (N-methyl-D-aspartate)-sensitive glutamate receptors (NMDA receptors) can trigger both LTP or LTD. LTD is induced by low levels of postsynaptic NMDA-receptor activation, for instance in response to low-frequency stimulation, whereas LTP is induced by the stronger activation that occurs following high-frequency stimulation.[20]

A third mechanism playing a role in early plasticity is the change in neuronal membrane excitability.[21] There are multiple described mechanisms for changing membrane excitability; these have been shown with the use of cell and patch clamp techniques and implicate the function of calcium and sodium channels, calcium-dependent potassium channels, and other potassium channels, as well as transmitters like serotonin and genes affecting the function of membrane components.[22,23]

A fourth mechanism is anatomic change demonstrable under the microscope, with axonal and dendritic sprouting and the establishment of new synaptic connections.[24-28] Such anatomic change would take place over a longer time period and may indeed require for its induction the initial activation of one or several of the previously mentioned faster mechanisms of plasticity. Synaptic reorganization and local changes in axonal and dendritic architecture would take less time than changes involving longer corticocortical connections, and some connections acting at greater distances may not be able to regrow and remodel following injury in the mature brain, while this may still be possible in young brains in which excess connectivity, even long connections, has not as yet been pruned. Synaptic changes may take the form of increase or decrease in synaptic density, hence strengthening or weakening preexisting connections, rearrangement of synapses into novel synaptic architectures capable of new functions, or a combination of these, with unpredictable effects on function.

Finally, a fifth process is the generation and maturation of new neurons that can be incorporated into preexisting networks.[29-33] This possibility has generated a great deal of excitement lately, with both supporters and detractors of the idea that new neurons are generated in the cerebral cortex of the mature human brain, which can establish functionally relevant connectivity.

METHODS FOR THE STUDY OF PLASTICITY IN HUMANS

Information about brain plasticity in humans can be gathered using a variety of methods. The rapid development of noninvasive mapping methodologies in the past two decades has greatly accelerated progress in this area of research. The basic approach, common to all methodologies, is to identify, localize, and characterize changes in brain function (e.g., changes in glucose or oxygen utilization, blood flow, electrical activity) in relation to the performance of a specific psychological task, and to document how this brain "representation" changes according to various circumstances. The motor and visual systems have been particularly extensively studied, but the approach is also applicable to regions linked to the performance of cognitive functions, specifically the multimodal areas of the frontal, temporal, and parietal lobes.

Functional neuroimaging with positron emission tomography (PET) or functional magnetic resonance imaging (fMRI) depends on serial changes in regional blood flow, which demarcate a functionally active area or areas (PET can also be used to study specific neurotransmitter activity, including GABA and glutamate, using radioactive tracers). These techniques, discussed in greater detail in Chap. 3, are only indirect measures of synaptic activity, and depend on predictable blood-flow responses to metabolic needs. Signals obtained in optical brain imaging—e.g., near-infrared spectroscopy (NIRS)—are also indirect measures of synaptic activity, but their source is largely limited to the cortex. All of the above methods have relatively good spatial resolution, down to the millimeter or submillimeter range, but poor temporal resolution, on the order of seconds to minutes.

Magnetic resonance spectroscopy (MRS), whereby spectral signatures of brain chemical constituents and metabolites of brain function can be mapped, may eventually allow for the study of behavior as correlations of regional chemical change and specific behaviors are established. The anatomic resolution of MRS would certainly be superior to that of tracer PET, and it would have the additional advantage of not exposing the subjects to radiation.

Electroencephalography (EEG) and magnetoencephalography (MEG) represent direct measures of neuronal activity in real psychological time—that is, on the order of milliseconds. Unfortunately, as discussed in Chap. 5, the anatomic sources of the EEG/MEG signals cannot be accurately determined and thus the topographic organization of the psychological function remains underdetermined. The combined use of EEG/MEG with fMRI will certainly enhance the utility of either method alone.

Transcranial magnetic stimulation (TMS), covered in more detail in Chap. 5, has proven to be a valuable tool for studying brain plasticity.[34] Using repetitive stimulation with a variable, rapidly changing magnetic stimulus, TMS transiently deactivates a region of the brain, thus creating a virtual patient. Cortical areas seen to activate in PET or fMRI images during psychological tasks can be suppressed with TMS and the effects on the behavior noted. Thus, a causal relationship between regional brain activation and behavior can be tested and confirmed.[35] Moreover, TMS can accurately measure changes in cortical excitability, thus providing a way to assess one of the mechanisms by which plasticity takes place in the brain.[36] The technique allows for the exploration of corticocortical interactions, e.g., intracortical inhibition and facilitation, which are likely markers of glutamatergic, dopaminergic, and GABAergic effects. Lesion studies and direct cortical stimulation have hitherto been the only approaches for the study of causal interactions between brain and behavior. TMS allows for the gathering of comparable information in a relatively noninvasive manner, with the additional possibility of the serial testing of normal subjects in carefully designed experimental paradigms. In addition, when appropriately delivered in time and space, TMS can provide information regarding the exact time when activity in a brain area is critical for a given behavior. The combined use of these different methodologies enables us to inquire with exquisite anatomic and temporal resolution about the causal roles of specific brain activities in behavior and hence about the plastic changes resulting from specific circumstances, influences, or dysfunction.

PLASTICITY IS NOT NECESSARILY BENEFICIAL

An intrinsic property of brain function, plasticity during a learning situation and especially after brain damage need not lead to improvement of function. Indeed, plastic changes might result in behavioral gain or loss in normal subjects or in the development or amelioration of symptoms in disease states. The concept of "maladaptive plasticity" was introduced to capture the idea of potentially functionally undesirable consequences of plasticity (see, for instance,[37] in development and[38] in acquired disease). However, we might be better served by discarding the notion of an obligatory link between plasticity and adaptation and rather think of plasticity as a generator of change, some of which may be behaviorally adaptive and some not, much the same as what is seen in the implementation of Darwinian theory. Thus, brain change generated by plasticity is adaptive only if the environment can support and maintain the resultant behavior. For example, imagine a patient who, because of an ankle injury, requires weeks of immobilization of the distal leg and foot. This immobilization leads to diminished activity in the cortical output to the spinal segment subserving the tibialis anterior muscle, which is primarily responsible for the extension of the foot at the ankle. This reduction in efferent demand leads to a reduction in the size of the motor output map of the tibialis anterior muscle in the precentral cortex, and the extent of reduction is correlated with the duration of the immobilization and can be reversed by voluntary muscle contraction.[39] In this case, the plastic changes are adaptive only in relation to the immobilized limb, but the moment the ankle is released from restriction the plasticity is maladaptive and might result in the need for physical therapy of longer duration. Other examples of maladaptive plasticity include the possible exacerbation of cognitive deficits in Alzheimer's disease occasioned by hippocampal sprouting following cell loss[38] and the exacerbation of the distortion of the visual field in hamsters in which a collicular lesion leads to reactive cross innervation.[37]

The role played by plasticity in task-specific dystonia, for example in "pianist's cramp," is another heuristically useful example. A pianist confronted with a new composition, after understanding the task and its demands, develops a cognitive representation of the behavior and initiates an initial, centrally guided response that consists of a sensorimotor feedback and movement correction. At the beginning, the limbs move slowly, with fluctuating accuracy and speed, and success requires visual, proprioceptive, and auditory feedback. Eventually, each single movement is refined, the different movements are chained into the proper sequence with the desired timing, a high probability of stability in the ordered sequence is attained, and a fluidity of all movements is developed. Only then can the pianist shift his or her attention away from the mechanical details of the performance and focus on the emotional content of the task. We can think of the acquisition of such a skill as the conversion of declarative knowledge (facts) into procedural knowledge (actions, skills).

Normal subjects taught to perform with one hand a five-finger exercise on a piano keyboard require several days of practice to acquire proficiency.[40] Over the course of 5 days, and 2 h of practice each day, the number of sequencing errors and unevenness of the intervals separating key presses decrease significantly and accuracy improves. These behavioral gains are associated with changes in the motor output maps to the muscles involved in the task, which can be demonstrated using TMS. As the subjects' performance improve, the thresholds for TMS activation of the finger flexor and extensor muscles (a measure of cortical excitability) decrease steadily and, even taking this change in activation threshold into account, the sizes of the cortical representation for both muscle groups increase significantly (Fig. 6-1).

The plastic reorganization associated with piano practice results from increased demand for sensorimotor integration and poses the risk of unwanted plasticity. One outcome of this unwanted cortical rearrangement can be the development of overuse syndrome and focal, task-specific dystonias. The style of piano playing seems to affect the risk of developing clinical problems. Thus, forceful playing with the fingers held bent and executing hammer-like movements is more frequently associated with overuse syndrome and dystonia than softer playing with extended fingers "caressing" the keys. A guitarist experiencing dystonia during playing shows significantly greater activation of the contralateral primary sensorimotor cortices and lesser bilateral activation of premotor areas as compared with dystonia-free practice[41] (Fig. 6-2). Furthermore, the somatosensory homunculi of patients with focal, task-specific dystonia are abnormal.[42,43] They show distortions in the representation of adjacent fingers and excessive overlap among them, likely reflecting extensive practice of coordinated hand postures in which two or more digits function as a unit, as in arpeggios and chords. The map distortions are more striking when small repeated traumas are added, for example in forceful, "hammer-finger" piano practice. In these cases, the plasticity associated with learning to play a musical instrument can produce abnormal sensorimotor remodeling leading to the development of clinically significant motor problems.

PLASTICITY IN THE PATHOGENESIS OF DISEASE

As suggested by the example of task-specific dystonia during learning in normal subjects, plasticity can in fact be the mechanism underlying the symptomatology of clinical conditions. A case in point is illustrated by developmental dyslexia.

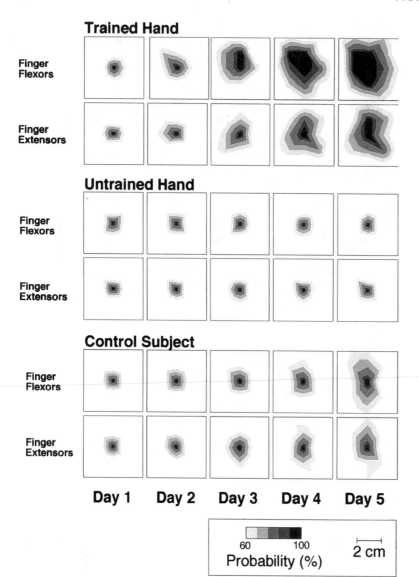

Figure 6-1
Representative examples of the cortical motor output maps for the long finger flexor and extensor muscles on days 1–5 in a test subject (trained and untrained hand) and a control subjects. The maps express the probability of evoking a motor potential with a peak-to-peak amplitude of at least 50,μ181/'b5V in the contralateral muscles with a stimulus intensity of 10% above motor threshold at the optimal scalp position. Eight stimuli were given at each scalp position. Each contour map represents 25 scalp positions (1 cm apart) arranged in a 5 × 5 grid around the optimal positions. (Modified from Pascual-Leone et al.[40] with permission.)

As reviewed in Chap. 37, most dyslexics have difficulties with phonological tasks—e.g., pseudoword reading, rhyming, phoneme deletion tasks.[44] They have also been shown to have problems with sound perception.[45] Dyslexic brains show focal cortical malformations consisting most often of nests of ectopic neurons and glia in the first cortical layer.[46,47] They also show changes in the sizes of neurons in the (auditory) medial geniculate nucleus.[48] Experiments in rats to produce cortical ectopias by early freezing damage to the incipient cortex indicate that the cortical anomalies produce the cell changes in the thalamus as part of developmental plasticity.[49] Moreover, it appears that the plastic changes in the thalamus, and not the cortical malformations themselves, are associated with the sound processing deficits. Female rats, which receive the injury and develop the same cortical malformations, but do not show cell changes in the thalamus, do not

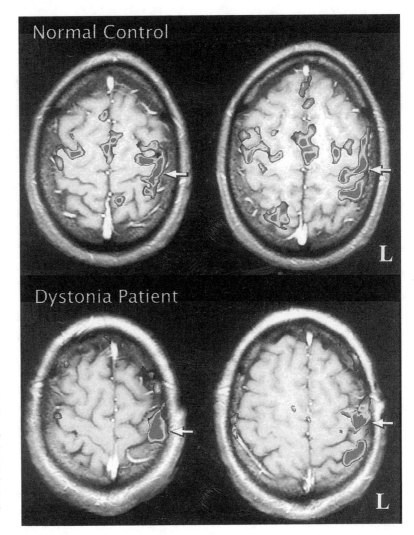

Figure 6-2
The figure displays the fMRI images of a normal and a dystonic guitar player executing right hand arpeggios in the scanner. Note the greater activation of the sensory-motor cortex (arrows) and the lack of activation of premotor and supplementary motor cortices in the dystonic patient. (Modified from Pujol et al,[41] with permission.)

exhibit sound processing problems.[50,51] In other words, developmental plasticity associated with early cortical injury, and not the cortical injury itself, leads to the abnormal behavior.

PLASTICITY IN THE ADAPTATION TO BLINDNESS

The changes in sensorimotor representation of the reading finger of proficient Braille readers and the cross-modal plasticity by which the deafferented "visual" cortex is recruited for processing auditory and tactile information provide useful illustrations of many of the principles of plasticity discussed so far. One may argue that early blindness represents a "pathologic state" resulting in substantial cross-modal brain plasticity.[12,13,52,53] A person who has suffered the total loss of a particular form of sensory input has, in reality, suffered a brain lesion. For example, with blindness, the brain is functionally deprived of approximately 2 million sensory fibers. This deprivation has a bottom-up effect and implicates multiple stages of processing, from the lateral geniculate nucleus in the thalamus,

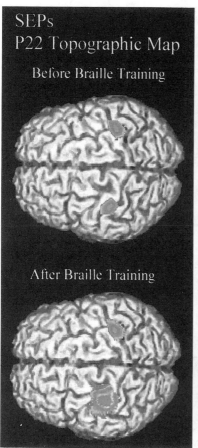
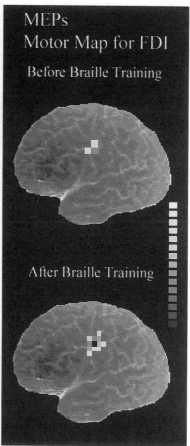

Figure 6-3
Evidence of plasticity in sensory, motor, and occipital cortex in early blind subjects after learning Braille. Representative example of the studies performed before and at the end of one year of learning Braille are shown. The different studies were conducted on different subjects using somatosensory evoked potentials (SEPs) to mechanical stimuli to the index finger pad (adapted from Pascual-Leone and Torres,[54] with permission), motor mapping with transcranial magnetic stimulation of the potentials evoked in the first dorsal interosseus muscle FDI, side-to-side mover of the index finger (adapted from Pascual-Leone et al.,[43] with permission), and functional magnetic resonance imaging (fMRI) while reading Braille characters. (Modified from Hamilton and Pascual-Leone,[12] with permission.)

through the primary visual cortex, to subsequent stations of associative visual processing. This dramatic change in the brain's experience of the outside world is likely to lead to reorganization. Therefore, blindness provides a reasonable model for studying mechanisms underlying brain plasticity in response to sensory deprivation and loss of acquisition of modality specific skills.

Learning Braille poses a logistical challenge, because it demands a marked increase (over normal use) in functional afferent input and efferent demand from a restricted body space (the pads of Braille-reading fingers) not evolutionarily designed for this task. Blind Braille readers must first discriminate, with exquisite sensitivity and accuracy, subtle patterns of raised and depressed dots with the pads of their fingers, after which they must translate this spatial representation

into associative meaning. Faced with the complex cognitive demands of Braille reading, the brain undergoes striking adaptive changes (Fig. 6-3). Recording somatosensory evoked potentials (SEPs) arising in the tips of the reading and nonreading index fingers of blind Braille readers, Pascual-Leone and Torres[54] demonstrated that the sensory map of the reading finger is enlarged as compared with the representation of the contralateral, homologous, nonreading finger or with the finger of a sighted or non-Braille-reading blind control subject. TMS revealed similar enlargement of the Braille-reading finger map.[55] Serial measurements of the cortical output maps of blind subjects learning Braille show that this enlargement seems to develop in two stages: (1) A rapid, dramatic, and transient enlargement that is likely the result of the unmasking of connections or upregulation of synaptic efficacy and

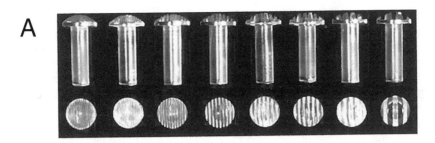

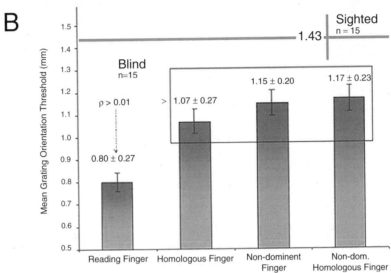

Figure 6-4

A. JVP Domes used for gratings orientations discrimination testing. B. Histogram display-ing the thresholds for grating orientation discrimination in early blind and sighted control subjects. Note the marked superiority (lower thresholds) of the blind subjects in general and in paricular of their dominant Braille reading finger. (Modified from van Boven et al,[58] with permission.)

(2) a slower, less prominent, but more stable enlarge-ment of the cortical representation of the reading finger that may represent structural plasticity.[56] If this find-ing can be extrapolated to other forms of skill learning, we might infer that learning involves a transient rapid change in the efficacy of existing connections, which leads the way to a more enduring structural modifica-tion in the face of continued practice.

Preceding activity affects the size of the motor output maps in Braille readers.[57] A comparison of mo-tor output maps following a day of intensive reading to those obtained after being off for 2 days demonstrates significant differences in the cortical representation of the reading finger of proficient Braille proofreaders.

Disuse, in this case by virtue of the 2 days' respite, re-sults in a measurable decrease in the sizes of the cortical output maps. Vacation consisting of a week of minimal Braille reading leads to an even more dramatic reduc-tion in the motor output maps. These disuse-related changes might underlie the common experience of "rustiness" upon returning to work following a break, and constitute a regressive form of neural plasticity.

In addition to the expanded cortical representa-tion of the fingers used in Braille reading, there is en-hanced fidelity in the neural transmission of spatial details of a stimulus that results in heightened tactile spatial acuity. Using the grating orientation discrimination task (Fig. 6-4), in which threshold performance is accounted for by the spatial resolution limits of the neural image evoked by a stimulus, van Boven et al.[58] quantified the psychophysical limits of spatial resolution at the middle and index fingers of blind Braille readers and sighted control subjects. The mean grating orientation threshold was significantly lower in the blind group compared to the sighted group. The self-reported dominant reading finger in blind subjects had the lowest grating orientation threshold in all subjects and was significantly better than other fingers tested. In this case, neural plasticity is probably causally linked to superior skill.

However, it does not appear that it is just the expansion of the sensorimotor cortical map of the reading finger that confers superior spatial skills to it, because the relative map size does not correlate with Braille reading or sensory discrimination ability. In fact, although appropriate somatosensory cortical representations expand as subjects develop sensorimotor skills, eventually they decrease in size as subjects gain mastery of those skills.[59,60] Instead, there appears to be recruitment of other cortical areas. In the case of Braille learning, the recruitment of parts of the occipital cortex, ordinarily the visual cortex (V1 and V2), for tactile information processing appears to be a critical contributor to the improved tactile acuity.

In blind, proficient Braille readers, the occipital cortex can be shown not only to be associated with tactile Braille reading[61,62] but indeed to be critical for reading accuracy[63] (Fig. 6-5). Peripherally blind subjects have very large areas of their cerebral cortex deafferented from visual input; hence portions of what would have been visual cortex are in principle available to be recruited for processing tactile and auditory information. Indeed, proficient Braille reading by blind subjects activates the dorsal and ventral portion of the occipital cortex.[61,62] Furthermore, there is suppression in the parietal operculum and activation in the ventral portion of the occipital cortex in blind subjects during tactile discrimination tasks, opposite to the pattern of activation and deactivation observed in sighted subjects. Studies using event-related potentials, cerebral blood flow, and magnetoencephalography (MEG) also demonstrate occipital cortex activation by tactile stimuli in persons blind from an early age.[12,13] Participation of the striate cortex in a tactile task seems related to the difficulty of the tactile discrimination regardless

of whether there is a linguistic component.[61,62] These findings suggest that the pathway for tactile discrimination changes with blindness. The interpretation that occipital lobe activation is causally related to the performance of the Braille task in the congenitally blind is supported by findings from a repetitive TMS experiment that found that Braille reading was disrupted by occipital stimulation.[63] Subjects were aware of the presence of Braille characters, but during rTMS to their occipital cortex they were unable to discriminate them. Some of the subjects reported phantom tactile sensations–Braille dots that were not there—or distortions of the Braille symbols. In sighted subjects, rTMS to the visual cortex does not interfere with the ability to detect or discriminate embossed Roman letters by touch. Therefore, it would appear that Braille reading in the blind is an example of true "cross-modal sensory plasticity" by which the deafferented occipital cortex is recruited for demanding tactile tasks.

Cohen et al.[64] argued for a critical time window for the above-mentioned plasticity associated with peripheral blindness, such that beyond the age of age 14 years the striate cortex is no longer recruited for the processing of tactile information. The argument is based on the study of subjects who became blind after age 15, in whom tactile stimulation failed to reveal activation of the striate cortex on PET and rTMS to the striate cortex did not interfere with reading of embossed Roman characters.

Recruitment of occipital cortical areas for processing of auditory information in blind subjects has also been reported.[13,65] The use of transient event-related potentials (ERPs) and the oddball paradigm, which consists of a repeating stimulus (standard) that is replaced occasionally by a physically different (oddball) stimulus, allows the investigation of stimulus discrimination and change detection during passive and active conditions. No significant differences were found between early-blind and sighted individuals in the distribution of brain activity associated with the automatic detection of sound change as indexed by mismatch negativity (usually peaking at about 100 to 200 ms from stimulus change onset). However, when oddball tones had to be detected, they elicited an additional response, one with a scalp distribution that was more posterior in the blind than in the sighted subjects.[13] This effect was observed with sound

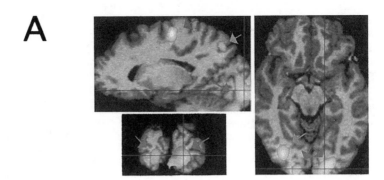

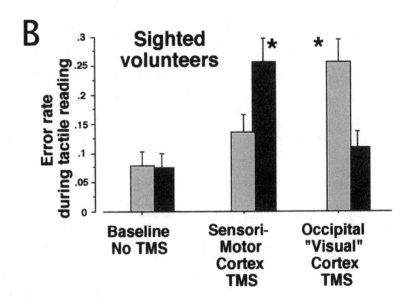

Figure 6-5
A. Activation of the occipital cortex in congenitally and early blind subjects during tactile Braille reading as demonstrated by positron emission tomography (PET). (Modified from Sadato et al,[61] with permission.) B. Effects of repetitive transcranial magnetic stimulation (TMS) to the occipital or somatosensory cortex on tactile Braille reading ability in early blind subjects and on tactile perception of embossed Roman letter in sighted controls. (Modified from Cohen et al.,[63] with permission.)

frequency, amplitude, or location change. Remarkably, and reminiscent of the findings regarding activation of the occipital cortex in tactile tasks, the results in early-blind subjects differed from those found in late-blind subjects. These results indicate that both temporal and occipital brain areas of individuals with early blindness are involved in attentive sound-change detection. Recent work using PET has demonstrated similar findings.[65] During tasks that required auditory localization both the sighted and blind subjects strongly activated posterior parietal areas. In addition, the blind subjects activated association areas in the right occipital cortex, the foci of which were similar to areas

previously identified in visual location and motion detection experiments in sighted subjects. The blind subjects, therefore, demonstrated auditory to "visual" (occipital) cross-modal plasticity with auditory localization activating occipital association areas ordinarily intended for dorsal-stream visual processing. Interestingly, during auditory localization in the blind subjects, regional cerebral blood flow in the right posterior parietal cortex was positively correlated with that in the right occipital region, whereas in sighted subjects correlations were generally nonsignificant. This indicates that in congenitally blind subjects the right occipital cortex participates in a functional network for auditory localization and that this occipital activity is likely to arise from connections with posterior parietal cortex.

SUMMARY

This chapter introduces the notion that plasticity is an intrinsic property of the human nervous system. Changes in the structural and/or functional properties of neuronal circuits subserving perception and cognition occur for many different reasons throughout life and are inseparable from other properties of the brain. Plasticity can be demonstrated in the bench lab in experimental animal model, and a variety of in-vivo techniques can be used to probe brain plasticity in humans. These methods include functional brain imaging, such as positron emission tomography or functional magnetic resonance imaging, evoked potentials, magnetoencephalography, and transcranial magnetic stimulation.

Plasticity changes occur which take place in seconds, while others require years to develop. Changes occur during the normal course of growth and development, during learning, and in response to disease processes. Some changes result in beneficial behavioral consequences, while others produce no clinically detectable behavioral change, and still others lead to worsening of performance. The challenge for the next decade is to learn enough about the details of mechanisms of plasticity in order to manipulate maladaptive toward adaptive plasticity and thus gain a clinical benefit.

REFERENCES

1. Fuster JM: *Memory in the Cerebral Cortex. An Empirical Approach to Neural Networks in the Human and Nonhuman Primate.* Cambridge, MA: MIT Press, 1995.
2. Kaas JH (ed): *Functional Plasticity in Adult Cortex.* Orlando, FL Academic Press, 1997.
3. Merzenich MM: Representational plasticity in somatosensory and motor cortical fields. *Biomed Res* 10(suppl. 2):85–86, 1989.
4. Schachter DL, Buckner RL: On the relations among priming, conscious recollection, and intentional retrieval: Evidence from neuroimaging research. *Neurobiol Learn Mem* 70:284–303, 1998.
5. Poldrack RA: Imaging brain plasticity: Conceptual and methodological issues–a theoretical review. *Neuroimage* 12:1–13, 2000.
6. van Mier H: Human learning, in Mazziotta JC, Toga AW, Frackowiak RS (ed): *Brain Mapping: The Systems.* San Dieg, CAo: Academic Press, 2000, pp 605–620.
7. Kaas JH: The reorganization of somatosensory and motor cortex after peripheral nerve or spinal cord injury in primates. *Prog Brain Res* 128:173–179, 2000.
8. Chollet F: Plasticity of the adult human brain, in Mazziotta JC, Toga AW, Frackowiak RS (ed): *Brain Mapping: The Systems.* San Diego, CA: Academic Press, 2000, pp 621–638.
9. Chollet F, Weiller C: Recovery of neurological function, in Mazziotta JC, Toga AW, Frackowiak RS (ed): *Brain Mapping: The Disorders.* San Diego, CA: Academic Press, 2000, pp 587–597.
10. Donoghue JP: Plasticity of adult sensorimotor representations. *Curr Opin Neurobiol* 5:749–754, 1995.
11. Donoghue JP, Hess G, Sanes JN: Substrates and mechanisms for learning in motor cortex, in Bloedel J, Ebner T, Wise SP (ed): *Acquisition of Motor Behavior in Vertebrates.* Cambridge, MA: MIT Press, 1996, pp 363–386.
12. Hamilton R, Pascual-Leone A: Cortical plasticity associated with Braille learning. *Trends Cogn Sci* 2:168–174, 1999.
13. Kujala T, Alho K, Naatanen R: Cross-modal reorganization of human cortical functions. *Trends Neurosci* 23:115–120, 2000.
14. Gilbert CD: Rapid dynamic changes in adult cerebral cortex. *Curr Opin Neurobiol* 3:100–103, 1993.
15. Gilbert CD: Adult cortical dynamics. *Physiol Rev* 78:467–485, 1998.
16. Lane RD, Killackey HP, Rhoades RW: Blockade of GABAergic inhibition reveals reordered cortical somatotopic maps in rats that sustained neonatal forelimb removal. *J Neurophysiol* 77:2723–2735, 1997.
17. Chagnac-Amitai Y, Connors BW: Horizontal spread of synchronized activity in neocortex and its control by GABA-mediated inhibition. *J Neurophysiol* 61:747–758, 1989.
18. Debanne D: Associative synaptic plasticity in hippocampus and visual cortex: Cellular mechanisms and functional implications. *Rev Neurosci* 7:29–46, 1996.
19. Iriki A, Pavlides C, Keller A, et al: Long-term potentiation in the motor cortex. *Science* 245:1385–1387, 1989.
20. Kirkwood A, Rioult MC, Bear MF: Experience-dependent modification of synaptic plasticity in visual cortex. *Nature* 381:526–528, 1996.

21. Woody CD, Guruen E, Birt D: Changes in membrane currents during pavlovian conditioning of single cortical neurons. *Brain Res* 539:76–84, 1991.

22. Patil N, Cox DR, Bhat D, et al: A potassium channel mutation in weaver mice implicates membrane excitability in granule cell differentiation. *Nat Genet* 11:126–129, 1995.

23. Sarkisian MR, Rattan S, D'Mello SR, et al: Characterization of seizures in the flathead rat: a new genetic model of epilepsy in early postnatal development. *Epilepsia* 40:394–400, 1999.

24. Okazaki MM, Evenson DA, Nadler JV: Hippocampal mossy fiber sprouting and synapse formation after status epilepticus in rats: visualization after retrograde transport of biocytin. *J Comp Neurol* 352:515–534, 1995.

25. Cotman C, Geddes J, Kahle J: Axon sprouting in the rodent and Alzheimer's disease brain: A reactivation of developmental mechanisms? in Storm-Mathisen J, Zimmer J, Ottersen OP (ed): *Progress in Brain Research.* Amsterdam: Elsevier, 1990, pp 427–434.

26. Aigner L, Arber S, Kapfhammer JP, et al: Overexpression of the neural growth-associated protein GAP-43 induces nerve sprouting in the adult nervous system of transgenic mice. *Cell* 83:269–278, 1995.

27. Murakami F, Song WJ, Katsumaru H: Plasticity of neuronal connections in developing brains of mammals. *Neurosci Res* 15:235–253, 1992.

28. Darian-Smith C, Gilbert CD: Axonal sprouting accompanies functional reorganization in adult cat striate cortex. *Nature* 368:737–740, 1994.

29. Alvarez-Buylla A, Lois C: Neuronal stem cells in the brain of adult vertebrates. *Stem Cells* 13:263–272, 1995.

30. Bayer SA: Neurogenesis in the anterior olfactory nucleus and its associated transition areas in the rat brain. *Int J Dev Neurosci* 4:225–249, 1986.

31. Corotto FS, Henegar JA, Maruniak JA: Neurogenesis persists in the subependymal layer of the adult mouse brain. *Neurosci Lett* 149:111–114, 1993.

32. Kempermann G, Kuhn HG, Gage FH: More hippocampal neurons in adult mice living in an enriched environment. *Nature* 386:493–495, 1997.

33. Shankle WR, Landing BH, Rafii MS, et al: Evidence for a postnatal doubling of neuron number in the developing human cerebral cortex between 15 months and 6 years. *J Theor Biol* 191:115–140, 1998.

34. Pascual-Leone A, Tarazona F, Keenan JP, et al: Transcranial magnetic stimulation and neuroplasticity. *Neuropsychologia* 37:207–217, 1999.

35. Pascual-Leone A, Walsh V, Rothwell J: Transcranial magnetic stimulation in cognitive neuroscience—virtual lesion, chronometry, and functional connectivity. *Curr Opin Neurobiol* 10:232–237, 2000.

36. Pascual-Leone A, Tormos JM, Keenan J, et al: Study and modulation of human cortical excitability with transcranial magnetic stimulation. *J Clin Neurophysiol* 15:333–343, 1998.

37. Finlay BL, Wilson KG, Schneider GE: Anomalous ipsilateral retinotectal projections in Syrian hamsters with early lesions: Topography and functional capacity. *J Comp Neurol* 183:721–740, 1979.

38. Geddes JW, Cotman CW: Plasticity in Alzheimer's disease: Too much or not enough? *Neurobiol Aging* 12:330–333, 1991.

39. Liepert J, Tegenthoff M, Malin JP: Changes of cortical motor area size during immobilization. *Electroencephalogr Clin Neurophysiol* 97:382–386, 1995.

40. Pascual-Leone A, Nguyet D, Cohen LG, et al: Modulation of muscle responses evoked by transcranial magnetic stimulation during the acquisition of new fine motor skills. *J Neurophysiol* 74:1037–1045, 1995.

41. Pujol J, Roset-Llobet J, Rosines-Cubells D, et al: Brain cortical activation during guitar-induced hand dystonia studied by functional MRI. *Neuroimage* 12:257–267, 2000.

42. Bara-Jimenez W, Catalan MJ, Hallett M, et al: Abnormal somatosensory homunculus in dystonia of the hand. *Ann Neurol* 44:828–831, 1998.

43. Pascual-Leone A: The brain that plays music and is changed by it, in Zatorre R, Peretz I (ed): *Music and the Brain.* New York: New York Academy of Sciences, 2001.

44. Liberman IY, Shankweiler D: Phonology and the problems of learning to read and write. *Remed Spec Educ* 6:8–17, 1985.

45. Tallal P: Auditory temporal perception, phonics, and reading disabilities in children. *Brain Lang* 9:182–198, 1980.

46. Galaburda AM, Kemper TL: Cytoarchitectonic abnormalities in developmental dyslexia: A case study. *Ann Neurol* 6:94–100, 1979.

47. Galaburda AM, Sherman GF, Rosen GD, et al: Developmental dyslexia: four consecutive cases with cortical anomalies. *Ann Neurol* 18:222–233, 1985.

48. Galaburda AM, Menard MT, Rosen GD: Evidence for aberrant auditory anatomy in developmental dyslexia. *Proc Natl Acad Sci U S A* 91:8010–8013, 1994.

49. Herman AE, Galaburda AM, Fitch HR, et al: Cerebral microgyria, thalamic cell size and auditory temporal processing in male and female rats. *Cereb Cortex* 7:453–464, 1997.

50. Rosen GD, Herman AE, Galaburda AM: Sex differences in the effects of early neocortical injury on neuronal

size distribution of the medial geniculate nucleus in the rat are mediated by perinatal gonadal steroids. *Cereb Cortex* 9:27–34, 1999.

51. Fitch RH, Brown CP, Tallal P, et al: Effects of sex and MK-801 on auditory-processing deficits associated with developmental microgyric lesions in rats. *Behav Neurosci* 111:404–412, 1997.

52. Rauschecker JP: Compensatory plasticity and sensory substitution in the cerebral cortex. *Trends Neurosci* 18:36–43, 1995.

53. Rauschecker JP: Mechanisms of compensatory plasticity in the cerebral cortex. *Adv Neurol* 73:137–146, 1997.

54. Pascual-Leone A, Torres F: Plasticity of the sensorimotor cortex representation of the reading finger in Braille readers. *Brain* 116:39–52, 1993.

55. Pascual-Leone A, Cammarota A, Wassermann EM, et al: Modulation of motor cortical outputs to the reading hand of Braille readers. *Ann Neurol* 34:33–37, 1993.

56. Pascual-Leone A, Hamilton R, Tormos JM, et al: Neuroplasticity in the adjustment to blindness., in Grafman J, Christen Y (ed): *Neuroplasticity: Building a Bridge from the Laboratory to the Clinic.* Munich and New York: Springer-Verlag, 1998.

57. Pascual-Leone A, Wassermann EM, Sadato N, et al: The role of reading activity on the modulation of motor cortical outputs to the reading hand in Braille readers. *Ann Neurol* 38:910–915, 1995.

58. van Boven R, Hamilton R, Kaufman T, et al: Tactile spatial resolution in blind Braille readers. *Neurology* 54:2030–2036, 2000.

59. Pascual-Leone A, Grafman J, Hallett M: Modulation of cortical motor output maps during development of implicit and explicit knowledge. *Science* 263:1287–1289, 1994.

60. Karni A, Bertini G: Learning perceptual skills: Behavioral probes into adult cortical plasticity. *Curr Opin Neurobiol* 7:530–535, 1997.

61. Sadato N, Pascual-Leone A, Grafman J, et al: Activation of the primary visual cortex by Braille reading in blind subjects. *Nature* 380:526–528, 1996.

62. Sadato N, Pascual-Leone A, Grafman J, et al: Neural networks for Braille reading by the blind. *Brain* 121:1213–1229, 1998.

63. Cohen LG, Celnik P, Pascual-Leone A, et al: Functional relevance of cross-modal plasticity in blind humans. *Nature* 389:180–183, 1997.

64. Cohen LG, Weeks RA, Sadato N, et al: Period of susceptibility for cross-modal plasticity in the blind. *Ann Neurol* 45:51–460, 1999.

65. Weeks R, Horwitz B, Aziz-Sultan A, et al: A positron emission tomography study of auditory localization in the congenitally blind. *J Neurosci* 20:2664–2672, 2000.

Chapter 7

COMPUTATIONAL MODELING OF PATIENTS IN COGNITIVE NEUROSCIENCE

Martha J. Farah

COGNITION AS COMPUTATION

If the insights of cognitive psychology had to be boiled down to a single statement, a good candidate would be "cognition is computation." Starting with the work of Allen Newell and Herbert Simon (1972) in the sixties and seventies, psychologists have been able to explain a wide range of human behavior in terms of information encoded from the environment, information stored in memory, and mechanisms for combining these two sources of information to select appropriate actions.

Viewing cognition as computation freed the field of psychology from the constraints of Skinnerian behaviorism, in which all psychological explanation was confined to directly observable entities such as stimulus and response. According to behaviorism, to hypothesize about the internal mental states intervening between stimulus and response was unscientific, non-explanatory, and downright mystical. The information processing of computers provided a concrete demonstration that the states intervening between stimulus and response could also be within the domain of objective science. Hypothesizing about the knowledge that caused a person to act one way rather than another is no more mystical than hypothesizing about the stored data in a computer that caused it to give one output rather than another. The computational view of the mind made it possible to have a *psychological* level of explanation—dealing with entities such as memory, knowledge, inference and decision—that could be understood as a function of perfectly nonmystical *physical* mechanisms.

There are many different ways in which physical mechanisms can process information. The best-known, and in many ways the most powerful, is the way computers work. Symbolically coded information is retrieved from a particular physical memory location, operated upon in a physically distinct central processing unit according to stored instructions, and then reentered into memory. Most of the early theories of cognitive psychology assumed this type of computational architecture. More recently, a very different computational architecture has been explored by computer scientists, psychologists, and neuroscientists, which has more in common with brains than with office computers. This is the parallel distributed processing (PDP) architecture. Because PDP is similar in many ways to neural information processing, PDP models have increasingly come to be used in neuropsychology.

Computation has played two roles in cognitive psychology and neuropsychology. In some cases theories are simply expressed in terms of the concepts of computation: the informational content and format of representations, the parallel or serial nature of searches, and the like. In other cases, researchers implement their theories as running computer simulations. With the advent of the PDP architecture, computer simulation is increasingly used. One reason for this is that the behavior of PDP systems is not always obvious or predictable by intuition alone.

PARALLEL DISTRIBUTED PROCESSING

PDP systems consist of a large number of highly interconnected neuron-like units. These units are connected to one another by weighted connections that determine how much activation from one unit flows to another. There is no central controller governing the behavior of the network. Rather, each part of the network functions locally and in parallel with the other parts, hence the first P in PDP. Representations consist of the pattern of activation distributed over a population of units, and long-term memory knowledge is encoded in the pattern of connection strengths distributed among a population of units, hence the D. Alternative terms for PDP include connectionism (not to be confused with the center-and-pathway approach of Wernicke and his followers, which has also been called connectionism), brain-style computation, and artificial neural networks. For more than the brief overview offered here, the reader is directed to O'Reilly and Munakata's (2000) recent textbook on computational modeling in cognitive neuroscience.

There are many types of PDP networks with different computational properties. Among the features that determine network type are the activation rule, connectivity, and learning rule. The activation rule governs how the activation values of units are updated given a certain input activation. Units' activations can be discrete or continuous, and activations may be increased in direct proportion to the sum of the inputs (a *linear activation function*) or as a nonlinear function of the inputs (generally a sigmoid shaped function). The activation rule has a variety of consequences for network behavior, some of which are not immediately obvious. For example, as noted below, purely linear networks will not be able to learn certain kinds of associations.

A major distinguishing feature is connectivity, which can be unidirectional, in which case the network is called *feedforward,* or bidirectional, in which case it is called *interactive.* Feedforward networks may consist simply of a set of input units and a set of output units. A pattern associator can be made from such a network if the weights between the first and second layer units are set so that each of a set of patterns of activation over the units in the first layer evokes an associated pattern over the units in the second layer. Some feedforward networks have an additional set of so-called *hidden units* interposed between the input and output units. With nonlinear systems, the additional set of units is useful in transforming the input patterns of activation to the desired output patterns; indeed certain types of problems (such as associating input patterns 00 and 11 with one output and 01 and 10 with another, the "XOR" problem) can be solved only with hidden units. In *recurrent networks,* later layers loop back to earlier layers. In interactive networks, some or all connections are bidirectional. In recurrent and interactive networks,

"downstream" units can influence "upstream" units; more than one processing step is therefore needed to arrive at their final activation state. These networks are said to "settle into" a stable state after the addition of an input pattern of activation.

Learning in neural networks consists of adjusting the weights between units so that, given a set of input activation patterns, in each case the network ends up in the desired activation state. For example, for a network to learn that a certain name goes with a certain face, the weights among units in the network are adjusted so that presentation of any one of the face patterns in the units representing faces or any one of the name patterns in the units representing names causes the corresponding other patterns to become activated.

There is a wide variety of learning algorithms; the choice depends in part on the type of network and the task to be learned. A learning rule proposed many decades ago by the neuroscientist Donald Hebb (1949) forms the basis for many current learning algorithms. The gist of the *Hebb Rule* is: Neurons that fire together wire together. In other words, when there is a positive correlation in the activity of two units, their connection should be strengthened, so that future activation of one will be even more likely to activate the other. This form of the rule enables *unsupervised learning,* that is, learning without an external source of feedback about right and wrong performance. Networks that use unsupervised learning are called *self-organizing,* as they develop their own representations of regularities in their input, for example, developing edge representations from center-surround–like inputs (Ritter, 1990), or semantic representations from patterns of word co-occurrence. (See Kohonen, 1995 for additional information on self-organizing systems.)

The Hebb rule can also be used to learn to associate patterns, but only if the input patterns are orthogonal, a rather stringent requirement. When the object is to learn to associate or complete patterns, then *supervised* learning is normally used. The *Delta Rule* is an example of a supervised learning rule that can be viewed as a variant of the Hebb rule. Both learning rules change weights proportionate with a comparison between activation values; in the case of supervised learning, the comparison is between desired activation value and actual activation value, an error measure. Networks with hidden units demand yet a further modification of the learning rule, as the weights to be changed do not directly link the input with the output units from which the error measure is derived. The *Generalized Delta Rule,* or *Backpropagation,* is often used in this case. With this rule the error in the output units is propagated back to alter the weights of the (nonadjacent) input units.

Further discussion of learning rules is beyond the scope of this chapter, except to note that learning in PDP models is often not intended to simulate real learning. Rather, it is frequently used as a tool for setting the weights in a network so that the network can simulate some aspect of cognition in its mature end-state. Backpropagation is sometimes criticized for being physiologically implausible. This may or may not be a valid criticism, depending on the goal of the simulation. For example, if one were interested in studying the effects of damage to the face recognition system, one would need a model of face recognition that embodied a set of associations between facial appearance and other knowledge about people, on which one could inflict damage. As it is virtually impossible to "hand wire" networks of more than a few units, learning rules would be used to build in these associations. However, they would not be simulating the way in which people learn face recognition. For this reason it might be less confusing to refer to learning algorithms for neural networks as weight-setting algorithms, unless the learning process is explicitly being modeled.

How Realistic are PDP Models?

Of course, there are cases when real human learning is the subject of the model, and then we are right to inquire whether or in what sense the model's learning is similar to human learning. More generally, it is important to consider whether PDP is a reasonable model for human brain function.

PDP models differ from real neural networks, including the human brain, in numerous ways: even the biggest PDP networks are tiny compared to the brain, PDP models have just one kind of unit compared to a variety of types of neurons, and just one kind of activation (which can act excitatorily or inhibitorily) rather than a multitude of different neurotransmitters, and so on. Yet these differences are not necessarily a cause to reject the PDP approach. No

model is identical in all respects to the system being modeled; models possess theory-relevant and theory-irrelevant attributes. Furthermore, science must often simplify nature in order to understand it. PDP models should be viewed as simplifications of the brain, possessing enough theory-relevant attributes of the brain to be informative on many questions but clearly leaving out or even contradicting many known aspects of brain function.

Among the theory-relevant aspects of PDP models are the use of distributed representations, the large number of inputs to and outputs from each unit, the modifiable connections between units, the existence of both inhibitory and excitatory connections, summation rules, bounded activations, and thresholds. PDP models allow us to find out what aspects of behavior, normal and pathologic, can be explained by this set of theory-relevant attributes. Of course, some behavior may be explainable only with the incorporation of other features of neuroanatomy and neurophysiology not currently used in PDP models. This seems quite likely, and the discovery of such instances will be extremely informative with respect to the functional significance of these features of our biology. However, note that this problem does not apply to cases in which the current models perform well. In such cases, the only danger associated with nonrealism is that the model's success might depend on a theory-irrelevant simplification. For example, scale is generally treated as theory-irrelevant, but it is possible that certain mechanisms will work only for small networks or small amounts of knowledge. We must be on the lookout for such cases, but also recognize that it is unlikely that the success of most models will happen to depend critically on their unrealistic features.

Spatial Analogies for Understanding the Behavior of PDP Networks

Spatial analogies are useful for visualizing certain aspects of network dynamics, including the way in which the network's patterns of activation change under the influence of an input and the way in which the ensemble of weights changes during learning. The activation state of the network at any point in time can be represented as a point in a high-dimensional space called *activation space.* The dimensions of this space represent the level of activation of each unit in the network, assuming a fixed set of weights. In addition to the dimensions representing the activation levels of the units, there is one additional dimension, representing the overall "fit" between the current activation pattern and the weights.

When units that are both active have a large positive weight between them, so that they reinforce each other's activation, this is an example of a good fit. If both units are active and the weight between them is negative (i.e., inhibitory), the fit would be poor. This measure of fit is called *energy,* with low energy representing a better fit. The energy value associated with each pattern of activation defines a surface in activation space.

When an input pattern is presented to the network, the corresponding initial position in activation space is defined by the activation levels on the input units, along with resting level values for the dimensions representing the other units in the network. The weights in the rest of the network will not fit well with uniform resting level activation values over their portion of the network. Thus, the initial point in activation space will be in a region of high energy. As activation propagates through the network, the pattern of activation changes and the point representing this pattern moves along the energy surface in activation space. The movement will be generally downward, as the network lowers its energy, much as a ball rolls down a hill to lower its potential energy. To see why this would happen in terms of network dynamics, rather than by analogy with rolling balls, consider the examples given earlier of high- and low-energy activation states. For example, active units connected by negative weights (a poor fit, high energy pattern) will tend to change their activations until one is active and the other not (a good fit, low energy pattern).

The energy minima toward which the network tends are termed *attractors*. Attractors are useful in network computation not only for associating patterns and completing partial patterns but also for their ability to "clean up" a noisy input, by transforming a pattern similar to a known pattern into that known pattern (i.e., a pattern just uphill from an attractor will roll down into the attractor). So long as the input is sufficiently similar to (in the spatial analogy, close to) the attractor that it falls within the attractor's "basin," it will be pulled into the attractor.

The shape of the energy landscape is determined by the network's weights. In an untrained network, the landscape will be generally flat, with random hills and valleys. When the network has learned a certain association, its weights will create an energy landscape in activation space in which the point corresponding to the input pattern and the attractor point corresponding to the complete associated pattern are connected by a smoothly and steeply sloping path that causes the one state to "roll" down into the other.

The weights that determine the attractor structure of activation space can themselves be used to define a space, and this space is useful for visualizing the process of learning. In *weight space,* each of the weights in a network corresponds to one dimension of a space, so that we can represent the sum total of the network's knowledge as a point in this high-dimensional space. If one additional dimension is now added to the space, representing the performance of the network at associating names and faces (an error measure of some sort), then there will be a surface defined by each combination of weights and their associated error measure. Learning consists of moving along this surface in weight space and changing weight values until a sufficiently low point has been reached.

APPLICATIONS OF COMPUTATIONAL MODELING TO BEHAVIORAL NEUROLOGY AND NEUROPSYCHOLOGY

For most of the history of behavioral neurology and neuropsychology, the lesion method has been our primary source of insights into human brain organization. Yet the interpretation of lesion effects is not always as transparent as one would like. As early as the nineteenth century, authors such as John Hughlings-Jackson (1873) cautioned that the brain is a distributed and highly interactive system, such that local damage to one part can unleash new modes of functioning in the remaining parts of the system. As a result, one cannot assume that a patient's behavior following brain damage is the direct result of a simple subtraction of one or more components of the mind, with those that remain functioning normally. More likely, it results from a combination of the subtraction of some components, and changes in the functioning of other components that had previously been influenced by the missing components.

PDP provides a conceptual framework and concrete tools for reasoning about the effects of local lesions in distributed, interactive systems. It has already proven helpful in understanding a number of different neuropsychological disorders. Each of the examples reviewed here constitutes a reinterpretation of a well-known disorder, with qualitatively different implications for the normal organization of the brain and the functional locus of damage within that organization.

Neglect Dyslexia: A Pre- or Postlexical Impairment?

Patients with left visual neglect omit or misidentify letters on the left side of letter strings. When the letter string is a word, this pattern of performance is termed *neglect dyslexia* (see Chap. 20). Surprisingly, neglect dyslexics are more likely to report the initial letters of a word than of a nonword letter string, even when the initial letters of the word cannot simply be guessed on the basis of the end of the word (Sieroff et al., 1988). This seems to imply that the breakdown in the processing of neglected stimuli comes at a late stage, after word recognition, for how else could lexical status (word versus nonword) affect performance? Yet there are other good reasons to believe that neglect affects the early stages of visual perception, prior to recognition (see Chaps. 14 and 15).

It is possible to reconcile these two apparently conflicting observations, that neglect is sensitive to lexical status and that neglect affects prerecognition visual processing, within the context of a network model. Mozer and Behrmann (1990) simulated neglect dyslexia with a model in which spatial attention operates at an early stage, prior to visual recognition. Specifically, in this model, attention gates the flow of information out of early visual feature maps into higher-order letter and letter string representations. Neglect consists of an asymmetrical distribution of attention over letter strings; in the case of left neglect, a reduction of the attention normally allocated to the initial letter positions within the string. Neglect therefore results in full

information from the right side of a letter string, but only partial information from the left, being transmitted to word representations.

According to this model, the errors that occur with nonword letter strings result from partial visual information about the letter features on the left side of the string, which is not sufficient to identify precisely which letters are present. In contrast, the same partial information about the initial letters of a word, with good-quality information about the remaining letters of a word, will result in an activation pattern that is similar to the activation pattern for that word. A key aspect of the model, which explains the relative preservation of word reading in neglect, is that known words are attractor states for the network. Therefore, given enough information about the letters in word, even if not complete information, the network will settle into the pattern of the word, including the initial letters. In this way, it is possible to explain why neglect dyslexics read words better than nonwords without giving up the hypothesis that neglect is a disorder of visual perception, affecting stimulus processing prior to the recognition stage.

Computational models make predictions that can be tested empirically. According to this model of neglect dyslexia, if the asymmetry of attention is too extreme, no information about the initial letters will get through to word representations and the resulting activation state will not fall within the basin of attraction for the word. Behrmann and colleagues tested this prediction with a patient who had severe neglect (Behrmann et al., 1990). As predicted, he did not show better perception of the initial letters of words than nonwords. Furthermore, when his attention was drawn to the left, and the attentional asymmetry thereby made less extreme, he then showed the usual difference between word and nonword letter strings. Conversely, a patient who normally showed this difference between words and nonwords was stopped from doing so by attentional manipulations that increased his attentional asymmetry.

In general, this model demonstrates how the interaction between lower- and higher-level representations is influenced by attractors and the implications such interactions have for our interpretation of neuropsychological data. This general approach has been used to interpret other neuropsychological findings. For example, Mozer (2000) has extended his model to account for findings of object-centered neglect (i.e., neglect in which attention appears to be directed to objects rather than spatial locations; see Chap. 15) in terms of a purely spatial attentional process. The attractors representing objects bias the top-down activation to early visual representations in a way that respects the grouping or object information present at the higher levels. Other examples of the explanatory power of top-down effects of attractors can be found in models of reading and reading disorders, in which phenomena such as regularization by surface dyslexics (see Chap. 20) are explained in terms of a weakened attractor structure in the widest and deepest attractors are the most robust to damage (see Plaut et al., 1996, for a review).

Covert Face Recognition: Evidence for a "Consciousness Module"?

Prosopagnosia is an impairment of face recognition that can occur relatively independently of impairments in object recognition (see Chap. 10). A number of recent findings seem to suggest that the underlying impairment, in at least some patients, is not in face recognition per se but in conscious awareness of recognition. This would seem to imply that recognition and consciousness depend on dissociable and distinct brain systems, as shown in Fig. 7-1. My colleagues and I built a computer simulation that is able to account for covert recognition across a number of very different tasks (Farah et al., 1993; O'Reilly and Farah, 1999). The network is shown in Fig. 7-2 and consists of face recognition units, semantic knowledge units, and name units (embodying knowledge of people's facial appearance, general information about them, and their names, respectively). Hidden units were interposed between these layers to assist the network in learning to associate faces and names by way of semantic information. There is no part of the network that is dedicated to awareness.

The first finding to be simulated was that some prosopagnosics can learn to associate facial photographs with names faster when the pairings are true (e.g., Harrison Ford's face with Harrison Ford's name) than when they are false (e.g., Harrison Ford's face

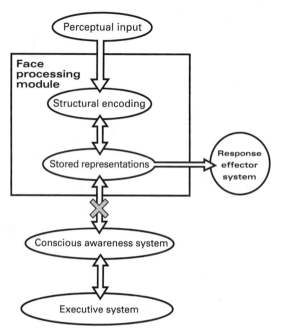

Figure 7-1
A model proposed by De Haan et al. (1992) to account for covert face recognition in prosopagnosia. There is a separate mechanism hypothesized for conscious awareness, distinct from the mechanisms of face recognition, and covert recognition is explained by a lesion at location 1, disconnecting the two parts of the model.

with Michael Douglas's name) (De Haan et al., 1987). This result was initially taken to imply that these patients were recognizing the faces normally, and that the breakdown in processing lay downstream from vision, as shown in Fig. 7-1. However, when some of the face units were eliminated from our model, thus simulating a lesion in the visual system, the network also relearned old face–name pairings faster than new ones. Why should this be? Recall that learning can be viewed as a process of moving through weight space. After damage, the network is in a high-error region of weight space for both old face–name pairings and new ones, and for this reason the network cannot overtly associate any faces with any names. However, that region of weight space is closer to a low-error region for the old pairings than for the new ones, because the residual weights (connecting intact units) have the correct

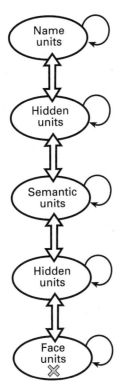

Figure 7-2
A model proposed by Farah et al. (1993) to account for covert face recognition in prosopagnosia. The dissociation between overt and covert face recognition emerges when the face recognition system is damaged.

values for the old pairings, and the learning process is therefore shorter.

A second finding, that previously familiar faces are perceived more quickly in the context of a same/different matching task, has also been interpreted as evidence for intact visual face processing (De Haan et al., 1987). However, after lesions to the face units in our model, the remaining face units settled into a stable state faster for previously familiar face patterns. This can be understood in terms of the distortion of the network's attractor structure after damage. The original structure was designed to take familiar face patterns as input and settle quickly to a stable state. After damage, these patterns will still find themselves on downward sloping parts of the energy landscape more often than

novel patterns, even if the energy minima into which they roll have changed.

In yet another task, which requires classifying a printed name as belonging to an actor or a politician, a face from the opposite occupation category shown in the background has been found to slow the responses of both normal subjects and a prosopagnosic (De Haan et al., 1987). This seems to imply that the face is recognized despite prosopagnosia. In simulating this finding, face units were removed until the network's overt performance at classifying faces according to occupation was as poor as the patient's. At this level of damage, wrong-category faces slowed performance in the name classification task. This can be understood in terms of the distributed nature of representation in neural networks, which allows for partial representation of information when some but not all units representing a face have been eliminated. The partial information generally raises the activation of the appropriate downstream occupation units, thus biasing their responses to the printed names, but is not generally able to raise their activations above threshold to allow an explicit response to faces.

The basic principle at work in this model of covert recognition is that neural network representations are graded in quality, not all-or-none, and that the representations remaining in a damaged network may be sufficient to support performance in some tasks but not others. This principle has also been used to explain dissociations within the realm of visual word recognition (Mayall and Humphreys, 1996), and wide range of other behavioral dissociations in developmental psychology as well as neuropsychology (Munakata, 2001).

Optic Aphasia: How Many Semantic Modules are There?

Optic aphasia is a puzzling disorder in which patients cannot name visually presented objects despite demonstrating good visual recognition nonverbally (e.g., by pantomiming the use of a seen object or sorting semantically related objects together) and good naming (e.g., by naming palpated objects or objects they hear described verbally). If they can get from vision to semantics (intact visual recognition) and from semantics

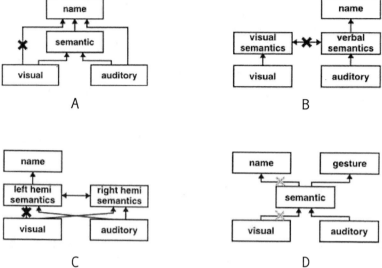

Figure 7-3
Four different models intended to account for optic aphasia. See text for explanation.

to naming (intact object naming of nonvisual inputs), why can they not name visually presented objects?

In response to this counterintuitive dissociation among tasks, traditional accounts of optic aphasia in cognitive neuropsychology have invoked additional processing components for visual naming, beyond vision, semantics, and name retrieval. For example, Ratcliff and Newcombe (1982) hypothesized a system for accessing names from vision directly, shown in Fig. 7-3A, which they proposed might be needed to supplement the semantically mediated processing. Beauvois (1982) hypothesized two separate semantic systems, as shown in Fig. 7-3B, one used for visual input and the other used for verbal input and output. Coslett and Saffran (1989) proposed separate right and left hemisphere semantic systems, with only the latter accessing verbal output, as shown in Fig. 7-3C. On the face of things, it seems that optic aphasia requires additions of one sort or another to the simplest model of visual naming, whereby visual inputs activate a unified semantic system, which in turn activates verbal output.

An alternative account of optic aphasia preserves this simple model, by adding a hypothesized second lesion instead of adding components to the brain's functional architecture. Sitton and coworkers (2000) showed that multiple lesions can have synergistic effects, resulting in impaired performance only when more than one lesioned component is required for a task. Specifically, we simulated visual naming and the other tasks used in studies of optic aphasia with the simple model shown in Fig. 7-3D. When a small lesion is introduced into one of the pathways, the system's attractors are able to "clean up" the resulting noisy representations; the representations are still within the system's basins of attraction. However, two lesions' worth of damage to the representations exceed the system's clean-up abilities and performance suffers. Given that visual naming is the only task requiring both the vision-to-semantics pathway and the semantics to naming pathway, small lesions in these two parts of the system will result in a selective impairment in visual naming.

Many dissociations in neuropsychology have been interpreted as evidence for highly specific modules, yet the possibility of multiple synergistic lesion effects suggests that simpler interpretations may be possible. For example, Young et al. (1990) report a case of neglect confined to faces. The most straightforward interpretation of this case involves a specialized spatial attention module that is dedicated to face processing. However, a pair of small but synergistic lesions in a general spatial attention module and in face processing will also produce this effect (Mozer and Farah, 2001). In principle this same approach could be taken to the explanation of highly specific neurolinguistic dissociations, such as the case of impaired verb production in the face of preserved verb comprehension and preserved production of other parts of speech (Caramazza and Hillis, 1991).

REFERENCES

Beauvois MF: Optic aphasia: A process of interaction between vision and language. Philos Trans R Soc Lond Ser B 298:35–47, 1982.

Behrmann M, Moscovitch M, Black S, Mozer M: Perceptual and conceptual mechanisms in neglect dyslexia: Two contrasting case studies. *Brain*113:1163–1183, 1990.

Caramazza A, Hillis A: Lexical organization of nouns and verbs in the brain. *Nature* 349:788–790, 1991.

Coslett HB, Saffran EM: Preserved object recognition and reading comprehension in optic aphasia. *Brain* 112:1091–1110, 1989.

De Haan EHF, Bauer RM, Greve KW: Behavioral and physiological evidence for covert recognition in a prosopagnosic patient. *Cortex* 28:77–95, 1992.

De Haan EHF, Young AW, Newcombe F: Face recognition without awareness. *Cogn Neuropsychol* 4:385–415, 1987.

Farah MJ, O'Reilly RC, Vecera SP: Dissociated overt and covert recognition as on emergent property of lesioned attractor networks. *Pychol Rev* 100:751–788, 1993.

Hebb DO: *Organization of Behavior.* New York: Wiley, 1949.

Hinton GE, Shallice T: Lesioning an attractor network: Investigations of acquired dyslexia. *Psychol Rev* 98:96–121, 1991.

Jackson JH: On the anatomical and physiological localization of movements in the brain. *Lancet* 1:84–85, 162–164, 232–234, 1873.

Kohonen T: *Self-Organizing Maps.* New York: Springer-Verlag, 1995.

Linsker R: From basic network principles to neural architecture: Emergence of orientation-selective cells. *Proc Natl Acad Sci U S A* 83:8390–8394, 1986.

Mozer MC, Behrmann M: On the interaction of selective attention and lexical knowledge: A connectionist account of neglect dyslexia. *J Cogn Neurosci* 2:96–123, 1990.

Mozer M, Farah MJ: Content-specific neglect syndromes and the modularity of attention. *J Cogn Neurosci* 2001 Suppl.

Munakata Y: Graded representations in behavioral dissociations. *Trends Cogn Sci* 5:309–314, 2001.

Newell A, Simon HA: *Human Problem Solving.* Englewood Cliffs, NJ: Prentice-Hall, 1972.

O'Reilly RC, Farah MJ: Simulation and explanation in neuropsychology and beyond. *Cogn Neuropsychol* 16:1–48, 1999.

O'Reilly RC, Munakata Y: *Computational Explorations in Cognitive Neuroscience.* Cambridge, MA: MIT Press, 2000.

Plaut DC: Understanding normal and impaired word reading: Computational principles in quasi-regular domains. *Psychol Rev* 103:56–115, 1996.

Plaut DC, Shallice T: Deep dyslexia: A case study of connectionist neuropsychology. *Cogn Neuropsychol* 10:377–500, 1993.

Ritter H: Self-organizing maps for internal representations. *Psychol Res* 52:128–136, 1990.

Sieroff E, Pollatsek A, Posner MI: Recognition of visual letter strings following injury to the posterior visual spatial attention system. *Cogn Neuropsychol* 5:427–449, 1988.

Sitton M, Mozer MC, Farah MJ: Superadditive effects of multiple lesions in a connectionist architecture: implications for the neuropsychology of optic aphasia. *Psychol Rev* 107:709–734, 2000.

Young AW, De Haan EH, Newcombe F, Hay DC: Facial neglect. *Neuropsychologia* 28:391–415, 1990.

Part II

PERCEPTION AND ATTENTION

Chapter 8

VISUAL PERCEPTION AND VISUAL IMAGERY

Martha J. Farah

Primates are visual creatures, and humans are no exception to this generalization. If one surveys our cortex and asks which areas are either partially or exclusively devoted to processing information from our eyes, one finds that about half of the cortex is involved in vision. Vision is the main function of occipital cortex and occupies much of parietal and temporal cortex as well. Even the most anterior parts of the brain include areas dedicated to eye-movement programming and visual working memory. One consequence of having this far-flung visual network is that lesions to many different parts of the brain can affect vision. The nature of the visual disturbance depends on the particular contribution that the damaged area would normally have made to vision.

Several chapters in this book are devoted to specific visual disorders that result from damage to high-level visual areas—that is, visual areas that are several synapses past primary visual cortex. These disorders include visual object agnosia (Chap. 9); prosopagnosia (Chap. 10); certain disorders of reading (Chap. 20), neglect (Chaps. 14 and 15), and visuo, spatial disorders (Chap. 11). The goal of this chapter is to review cortical visual processing at stages prior to these high-level functions. The chapter also considers cognitive disorders of mental imagery, or the activation of these visual representations endogenously as a medium of thought. In each case, the disorders arising from damage to these stages of vision is reviewed with respect to their main behavioral features, associated lesion sites, and implications for our understanding of normal vision.

VISUAL PERCEPTION

Damage to Primary Visual Cortex and Its Afferents

Although considerable information processing is carried out in the retina and thalamus, the visual disorders relevant to behavioral neurology generally involve brain damage at the level of primary visual cortex and beyond. Because the vast majority of visual information is processed through primary visual cortex on its way to higher-level perceptual areas, destruction of primary visual cortex causes cortical blindness. Partial destruction causes partial blindness, and the location of the lesion within primary visual cortex corresponds to the location of the blind spot, or visual field defect, in a highly systematic way that reflects the retinotopy of primary visual cortex. With vascular lesions, it is common for some or all of the primary cortex in one hemisphere to be damaged while the opposite hemisphere is unaffected. This results in blindness restricted to one-half of the visual field, or *hemianopia*. It is sometimes called *homonymous hemianopia* to indicate that the blind regions are the same regardless of which eye is used to see.

As shown in Fig. 8-1, visual field defects can be used to deduce the location of the lesion and were regularly used in this way before the days of computed tomography (CT). Homonymous visual field defects imply that the lesion is posterior, because input from the two eyes merges anteriorly. Because the left optic radiation projecting to left visual cortex represent only the right visual field, and vice versa, visual field

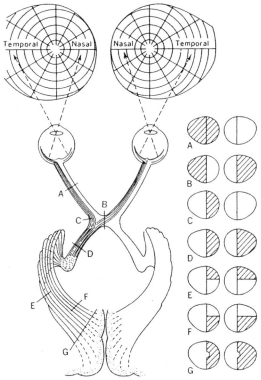

Figure 8-1

Correspondences between location of lesion within the visual system and pattern of visual field defects. (From Homans J: A Textbook of Surgery. Springfield, IL: Charles C Thomas, 1945, with permission.)

defects also reveal the side of the lesion. The altitude of the visual field defect is also informative, with lower-quadrant blindness, or *quadrantanopia,* suggesting a parietal or superior occipital lesion, because of the dorsal course of the pathways from thalamus to cortex, and upper quadrantanopia suggesting a temporal or inferior occipital lesion, because of the ventral course.

Prosopagnosia (see Chap. 10) was first localized on the basis of the visual field defects reported in a large set of cases (Meadows, 1974). Most cases reported a upper-left quadrantanopia, some with defects in the upper right as well. From this, Meadows was able to infer that the critical substrates for face recognition are in the right temporal cortex or bilateral temporal cortices in most people—a conclusion that has withstood the

tremendous increase in localizing capability as structural and functional brain imaging became available.

Although hemianopia and quadrantanopia are, by definition, blindness in the regions of the visual field represented by damaged visual cortex or its afferents, there are patients who retain some visual functions in these regions. *Blindsight* is the appropriately oxymoronic term applied to this puzzling phenomenon. The preserved perceptual abilities may be limited to localization of light and movement, but in some cases the limitations go well beyond this.

In one very thoroughly studied case of blindsight, Weiskrantz and colleagues (1986) found relatively preserved ability to point to the locations of visual stimuli, to detect movement, to discriminate the orientations of lines and gratings, and to discriminate large shapes such as X and O despite the patient's denial that he could see anything. The mechanism of blindsight has been a controversial topic. One possibility is that it simply reflects incomplete damage to visual cortex (see, e.g., Fendrich and coworkers, 2001), although this seems unlikely given that hemidecorticate patients have shown blindsight. Other explanations involve pathways to visual association cortex that bypass primary visual cortex. One such possibility is that blindsight is mediated by the subcortical visual system, which consists of projections from the retina to the superior colliculus and pulvinar and its projections to secondary cortical visual areas (e.g., Rafal et al., 1990). Alternatively, there may be sparse projections within the cortical visual system, from the lateral geniculate nucleus directly to visual association cortex (Stoerig and Cowey, 1997).

Damage to Surrounding Association Cortex

Surrounding primary visual cortex is additional modality-specific visual cortex that receives its input principally from primary visual cortex. From single-cell recording and other invasive measures used in animals, it is known that this region is functionally a mosaic of areas, each of which represents the visual field with some degree of retinotopy and has largely reciprocal projections to particular sets of other visual areas (see Zigmond et al., 1999). It is assumed that this multiplicity of areas is there for some purpose and that each area probably analyzes different aspects of the input, although this assumption has been fully validated in only a couple of cases—areas that subserve color vision and motion vision.

Primate neurophysiology has shown that neurons in area V4 of the monkey brain are highly selective for color and indeed respond to color per se rather than wavelength (Zeki, 1983). (The difference can be appreciated by considering that the green color of a plant, for instance, remains at least roughly constant across ambient lighting conditions containing widely differing wavelengths, which result in different wavelengths reflecting off the plant's surface and stimulating the retina.) That a homologous area exists in humans and is vulnerable to damage is suggested by the disorder *cerebral achromatopsia,* color blindness due to brain damage. Achromatopsic patients report that the world seems drained of color, like a black-and-white movie. In other respects, their vision may be at least roughly normal. For example, they may have good acuity, motion and depth perception, and object recognition. It should be added that problems with face, object and printed word recognition do sometimes accompany achromatopsia, but they are often transient and are likely to be caused by impairment to areas neighboring the color area. Cases in which the color vision impairment is truly selective imply that there is a brain region dedicated to color perception—that is, necessary for color perception and not for other aspects of vision.

In some cases, a unilateral lesion will result in color loss in just one hemifield, consistent with retinotopic mapping of the area responsible for color vision. A particularly selective and well-studied case of this was described by Damasio et al. (1980). Although acuity, depth perception, motion perception, and object recognition was normal in both hemifields, they differed strikingly for color perception:

> *He was unable to name any color in any portion of the left field of either eye, including bright reds, blues, greens and yellows. As soon as any portion of a colored object crossed the vertical meridian, he was able instantly to recognize and accurately name its color. When an object such as a red flashlight was held so that it bisected the vertical meridian, he reported that the hue of the right half appeared normal while the left half was gray.*

He was also unable to match colors in the left visual field.

The lesions in achromatopsia are usually on the inferior surface of the temporooccipital region, in the lingual and fusiform gyri. In full achromatopsia they are bilateral, and in hemiachromatopsia they are confined to the hemisphere contralateral to the color vision defect. This localization accords well with functional neuroimaging studies in which the substrates of color perception have been isolated by comparing cerebral activation patterns while subjects view colored displays to patterns resulting when gray-scale versions of the same displays are viewed (e.g., Zeki et al., 1991). Chapter 20 reviews achromatopsia in further detail, as well as distinguishing it from a number of other disorders of color cognition.

Single-cell recording has also been used to elucidate the neural systems of motion perception in the monkey. Area MT (for middle temporal) contains neurons whose response properties suggest a primary role in motion perception. Consistent with this, humans with damage in the homologous region have developed *cerebral akinotopsia* (see Zeki, 1993, for a review). By far the best-studied case is that of Zihl et al. (1983). This was case L.M., a 43-year-old woman who, following bilateral strokes in the posterior parietotemporal and occipital regions, was left with but one major impairment, namely the complete inability to perceive visual motion. Zihl et al. (1983) tested L.M.'s visual perception in a variety of simple experimental tasks and compared her performance with that of normal subjects. In her color and depth perception, object and word recognition, and a variety of other visual abilities tested by these authors, L.M. did not differ significantly from normal subjects. In addition, her ability to judge the motion of a tactile stimulus (wooden stick moved up or down her arm) and an auditory stimulus (tone-emitting loudspeaker moved through space) was also normal. In contrast, her perception of direction and speed of visual motion in horizontal and vertical directions within the picture plane and in depth was grossly impaired.

In her everyday life she was profoundly affected by her visual impairment. When she was pouring tea or coffee, the fluid appeared to be frozen, like a glacier. Without being able to perceive movement, she could not stop pouring at the right time and frequently filled the cup to overflowing. She found it difficult to follow conversations without being able to see the facial and mouth movements of each speaker, and gatherings of more than two other people left her feeling unwell and insecure. She complained that "People were suddenly here or there but I have not seen them moving." The patient could not cross the street because of her inability to judge the speed of a car. "When I see the car at first, it seems far away. But then, when I want to cross the road, suddenly the car is very near." She gradually learned to estimate the distance of moving vehicles by means of the sound as it became louder.

As with achromatopsia, the existence of akinotopsia implies a high degree of cerebral specialization, with one cortical area being necessary for motion perception and not necessary for other aspects of perception. Although L.M.'s lesions were fairly large and encompassed both parietal and temporal cortex, the critical lesion site has been inferred to be the posterior middle temporal gyrus. Functional neuroimaging studies of motion perception, comparing brain activation patterns to moving and static displays, show their maximum in this same region (Zeki et al., 1991).

An Organizing Framework for Higher-Level Visual Disorders

Vision has two main goals, the identification of stimuli and their localization. Although a bit of an oversimplification, this dichotomy has provided a useful organizing framework for the neuropsychology of high-level vision. The two goals, sometimes abbreviated as *what* and *where,* are achieved by relatively independent and anatomically separate systems, located in ventral and dorsal visual cortices, respectively, as shown in Fig. 8-2. These have been termed *the two cortical visual systems* (Ungerleider and Mishkin, 1972).

Note that the color and motion disorders discussed in the previous section fit naturally into this framework: color is an aspect of appearance that is useful for object recognition but plays little role in spatial function. The critical lesion site for achromatopsia

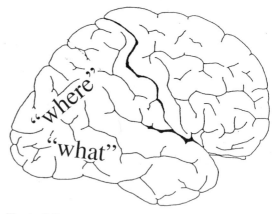

Figure 8-2
The two cortical visual systems: Dorsal visual areas are particularly important for spatial or "where" processing, and ventral visual areas are particularly important for appearance or "what" processing.

lies on the ventral surface of the brain. Motion is, by its very nature, a spatial property—change of location over time—and is one of the most powerful cues for summoning spatial attention. The critical lesion site for akinotopsia is dorsolateral to this, in the posterior temporal lobe.

Damage further along the dorsal and ventral visual streams is responsible for a variety of neurobehavioral syndromes. The disorders of spatial perception and attention discussed in Chaps. 11, 14, and 15 result from damage to posterior parietal cortex, part of the dorsal *where* route, whereas the disorders of object and face recognition discussed in Chaps. 9 and 10 result from damage to inferior temporal cortex, part of the ventral *what* route.

VISUAL MENTAL IMAGERY

The most obvious function of the cortical visual system is the analysis of retinal inputs. Yet under some circumstances it is also used in thinking, as when we generate a visual image from memory. Brain damage can affect the process of generating a visual mental image in two ways: by impairing the visual representations themselves or by impairing the process of activating those representations in the absence of a stimulus.

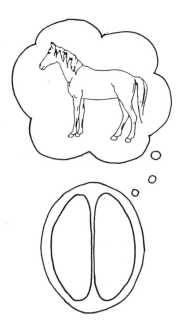

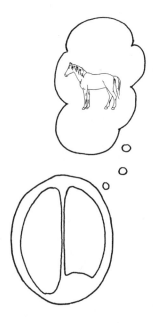

"I can get to within 15 feet of the horse in my imagination before it starts to overflow"

"The horse starts to overflow at an imagined distance of about 35 feet"

Figure 8-3

Depiction of the effects of unilateral occipital lobectomy on the visual angle of the mind's eye. (From Farah MJ, in Gazzaniga MS (ed): The Cognitive Neurosciences. *Cambridge, MA: MIT Press, 1996, with permission.)*

Disorders of Image Representation

If imagery and perception are both impaired after brain damage, this suggests that the functional locus of damage is the representations of visual appearance used by both. There are many reports of parallel impairments of imagery and perception, and these have attracted interest for what they can tell us about mental image representation. Specifically, they imply that mental imagery shares representations with the cortical visual system.

A clear-cut example of parallel imagery-perception impairment comes from a study comparing visual and "imaginal" fields. We were able to test an epileptic woman before and after a right occipital lobectomy. If mental imagery consists of activating representations in the occipital lobe, then it should be impossible to form images in regions of the visual field that are blind due to occipital lobe destruction. This predicts that after surgery, she should have both a narrower visual field and a narrower imaginal field. By asking her to report the distance of imagined objects such as a horse, breadbox, or ruler when they are visualized as close as possible without "overflowing" her imaginal field, we could compute the visual angle of that field. We found that the size of her biggest possible image was reduced after surgery, as represented in Fig. 8-3. Furthermore, by measuring maximal image size in the vertical and horizontal dimensions separately, we found that only the horizontal dimension of her imaginal field was significantly reduced. These results provide strong evidence for the use of occipital visual representations during imagery.

Other parallels have been noted as well—for example, between disorders of color perception and disorders of color imagery, between left visual neglect and inattention to the left sides of mental images, and between the ability to recognize objects from their visual appearance and the ability to imagine their appearance. A fuller discussion of these findings, as well as cases of visual impairment in which imagery ability is not affected, may be found in Farah (2000).

Disorders of Image Generation

In the absence of visual perceptual disorder, visual imagery may be impaired because of damage affecting image generation ability. Patients with an image generation deficit are disproportionately impaired at answering questions such as "Which is bigger, a grapefruit or a cantaloupe?" or "Does a kangaroo have a short or a long tail?" compared to questions that do not evoke imagery such as "Do kangaroos wash their food before eating it?" Other indications are that their drawing from memory is sketchy despite good copying ability, and their ability to report the color of objects from memory depends upon the availability of verbal associations (e.g., the colors of the sky, lemons, and fire engines can be retrieved without imagery, but the color of a coke can, a mailbox, or a peanut cannot). Some typical cases include those of Farah and coworkers (1988), Goldenberg (1992), Grossi and colleagues (1986), and Riddoch (1990). The critical lesion site in these cases appears to be left temporooccipital cortex (see Farah, 1995, for a review of lesion and neuroimaging data).

REFERENCES

Damasio AR, Yamada T, Damasio H, et al: Central achromatopsia: behavioral, anatomic, and physiologic aspects. *Neurology* 30:1064–1071, 1980.

Farah MJ: Current issues in the neuropsychology of mental image generation. *Neuropsychologia* 33:1445–1471, 1995.

Farah MJ: *The Cognitive Neuroscience of Vision.* Oxford, UK: Blackwell, 2000.

Farah MJ, Hammond KL, Levine DN, Calvanio R: Visual and spatial mental imagery: Dissociable systems of representation. *Cogn Psychol* 20:439–462, 1988.

Fendrich R, Wessinger CM, Gazzaniga MS: Speculations on the neural basis of islands of blindsight. *Prog Brain Res* 134:353–366, 2001.

Goldenberg G: Loss of visual imagery and loss of visual knowledge—a case study. *Neuropsychologia* 30:1081–1099, 1992.

Grossi D, Orsini A, Modafferi A: Visuoimaginal constructional apraxia: On a case of selective deficit of imagery. *Brain Cogn* 5:255–267, 1986.

Meadows JC: The anatomical basis of prosopagnosia. *J Neurol Neurosurgery Psychiatry* 37:489–501, 1974.

Rafal R, Smith J, Krantz J, et al: Extrageniculate vision in hemianopic humans: saccade inhibition by signals in the blind field. *Science* 250:118–121, 1990.

Riddoch JM: Loss of visual imagery: A generation deficit. *Cogn Neuropsychol* 7:249–273, 1990.

Stoerig P, Cowey A: Blindsight in man and monkey, *Brain* 120:535–559, 1997.

Ungerleider LG, Mishkin M: Two cortical visual systems, in Ingle DJ, Goodale MA, Mansfield RJW (eds): *Analysis of Visual Behavior.* Cambridge, MA: MIT Press, 1982.

Weiskrantz L: *Blindsight: A Case Study and Implications.* Oxford, UK: Oxford University Press, 1986.

Zeki S: Colour coding in the cerebral cortex: The reaction of cells in monkey visual cortex to wavelengths and colours. *Neuroscience* 9:741–756, 1983.

Zeki S: *A Vision of the Brain.* Oxford, UK: Blackwell, 1993.

Zeki S, Watson JDG, Lueck CJ, et al: A direct demonstration of functional specialization in human visual cortex. *J Neurosci* 11:641–649, 1991.

Zigmond M, Floom FE, Landis SC (eds): *Fundamental Neuroscience.* New York: Academic Press, 1998.

Zihl J, von Cramon D, Mai N: Selective disturbance of movement vision after bilateral brain damage. *Brain* 106:313–340, 1983.

Chapter 9

VISUAL OBJECT AGNOSIA

Martha J. Farah
Todd E. Feinberg

The term *visual object agnosia* refers to the impairment of object recognition in the presence of relatively intact elementary visual perception, memory, and general intellectual function. This chapter reviews the different subtypes of agnosia, their major clinical features and associated neuropathology, and their implications for cognitive neuroscience theories of visual object recognition.

The study of agnosia has a long history of controversy, with some authors doubting that the condition even exists. For example, Bay[1] suggested that the appearance of disproportionate difficulty with visual object recognition could invariably be explained by synergistic interactions between mild perceptual impairments on the one hand and mild general intellectual impairments on the other. The rarity of visual object agnosia has contributed to the slowness with which this issue has been resolved, but several decades of careful case studies have now shown, to most people's satisfaction, that agnosic patients may be no more impaired in their elementary visual capabilities and their general intellectual functioning than many patients who are not agnosic. Therefore, most current research on agnosia focuses on a new set of questions. Are there different types of visual object agnosia, corresponding to different underlying impairments? At what level of visual and/or mnestic processing do these impairments occur? What can agnosia tell us about normal object recognition? What brain regions are critically involved in visual object recognition?

APPERCEPTIVE AGNOSIA

Lissauer[2] reasoned that visual object recognition could be disrupted in two different ways: by impairing visual perception, in which case patients would be unable to recognize objects because they could not see them properly, and by impairing the process of associating a percept with its meaning, in which case patients would be unable to recognize objects because they could not use the percept to access their knowledge of the object. He termed the first kind of agnosia *apperceptive agnosia* and the second kind *associative agnosia*. This terminology is still used today to distinguish agnosic patients who have frank perceptual impairments from those who do not, although the implicit assumption that the latter have an impairment in "association" is now questioned.

Behavior and Anatomy

One might wonder whether apperceptive agnosics should be considered agnosics at all, given that the definition of agnosia cited at the beginning of this article excludes patients whose problems are caused by elementary visual impairments. The difference between apperceptive agnosics and patients who fall outside of the exclusionary criteria for agnosia is that the former have relatively good acuity, brightness discrimination, color vision, and other so-called elementary visual capabilities. Despite these capabilities, their perception of shape is markedly abnormal. For example, in the classic case of Benson and Greenberg,[3] pictures, letters, and even simple geometric shapes could not be recognized. Figure 9-1 shows the attempts of their patient to copy a column of simple shapes. Recognition of real objects may be somewhat better than recognition of geometric shapes, although this appears to be due to the availability of additional cues such as size and surface properties such as color, texture, and specularity rather than object shape. Facilitation of shape perception by motion of the stimulus has been noted in several cases of apperceptive agnosia. In most cases of apperceptive

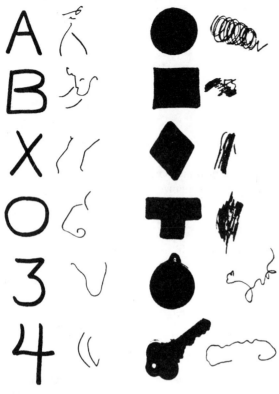

Figure 9-1
The attempts of an apperceptive agnosic patient to copy simple shapes. (From Benson and Greenberg,[3] with permission.)

agnosia, the brain damage is diffuse, often caused by carbon monoxide poisoning. For a review of other cases of apperceptive visual agnosia, see Ref. 4.

Interpretation of Apperceptive Agnosia

One way of interpreting apperceptive agnosia is in terms of a disorder of grouping processes that normally operate over the array of local features representing contour, color, depth, and so on.[4] Outside of their field defects, apperceptive agnosics have surprisingly good perception of local visual properties. They fail when they must extract more global structure from the image. Motion is helpful because it provides another cue to global structure in the form of correlated local motions. The perception of form from motion may also

have different neural substrates from the perception of form from static contour,[5] and may therefore be spared in apperceptive agnosia.

Relation to Other Disorders

Some authors have used the term *apperceptive agnosia* for other, quite different types of visual disorders, including two forms of simultanagnosia and an impairment in recognizing objects from unusual views or under unusual lighting conditions. *Simultanagnosia* is a term used to describe an impairment in perception of multielement or multipart visual displays. When shown a complex picture with multiple objects or people, simulanagnostics typically describe them in a piecemeal manner, sometimes omitting much of the material entirely and therefore failing to interpret the overall nature of the scene being depicted.

Dorsal simultanagnosia is a component of Balint's syndrome in which an attentional limitation prevents perception of more than one object at a time.[4,6-8] Occasionally attention may be captured by just one part of an object, leading to misidentification of the object and the appearance of perception confined to relatively local image features. The similarity of dorsal simultanagnosia to apperceptive agnosia is limited, however. Once they can attend to an object, dorsal simultanagnosics recognize it quickly and accurately, and even their "local" errors encompass much more global shape information than is available to apperceptive agnosics. Their lesions are typically in the posterior parietal cortex bilaterally.

Despite some surface similarity to apperceptive agnosia and dorsal simultanagnosia, *ventral simultanagnosia* represents yet another disorder.[4,9] Ventral simultanagnosics can recognize whole objects, but are limited in how many objects can be recognized in a given period of time. Their descriptions of complex scenes are slow and piecemeal, but unlike apperceptive agnosics their recognition of single shapes is not obviously impaired. The impairment of ventral simultanagnosics is most apparent when reading, because the individual letters of words are recognized in an abnormally slow and generally serial manner (letter-by-letter reading, see Chap. 20). Unlike the case with dorsal simultanagnosics, their detection of multiple stimuli appears normal; the bottleneck is in recognition per se.

Unlike apperceptive agnosics, they perceive individual shapes reasonably well. Their lesions are typically in the left inferior temporooccipital cortex.

Some patients have roughly normal perception and recognition of objects except when viewed from unusual perspectives or under unusual lighting. Their impairment has also been grouped with apperceptive agnosia by some, but for clarity's sake can also be called *perceptual categorization deficit* because they cannot categorize together the full range of images cast by an object under different viewing conditions. This disorder does not have great localizing value, although the lesions are generally in the right hemisphere and frequently include the inferior parietal lobe.[4,10]

ASSOCIATIVE AGNOSIA

Behavior and Anatomy

In associative agnosia, visual perception is much better than in apperceptive agnosia. Compare, for example, the copies made by the associative agnosics shown in Figs. 9-2 and 9-3 with the copies shown in Fig. 9-1. Nevertheless, object recognition is impaired. Associative agnosic patients may be able to recognize an object by its feel in their hand or from a spoken definition, demonstrating that they have intact general knowledge of the object in addition to being able to see it well enough to copy it, but they cannot recognize the same

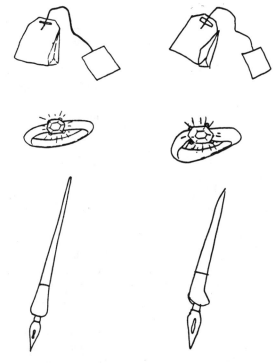

Figure 9-2
The copies of an associative agnosic patient with prosopagnosia and object agnosia. The patient did not recognize any of the original drawings. (From Farah et al.,[31] with permission.)

Figure 9-3
The copies of associative visual agnosic patients with alexia and object agnosia. The patients did not recognize the original drawings. Also shown is a sample of a patient's writing to dictation. After a delay, her own handwriting could not be read. (From Feinberg et al.,[16] with permission.)

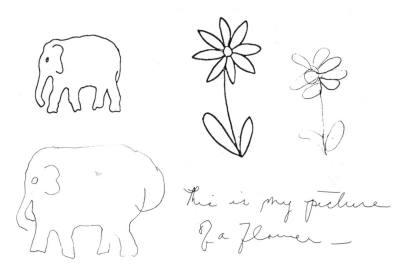

object by sight alone. The impairment is not simply a naming deficit for visual stimuli; associative agnosics cannot indicate their recognition of objects by nonverbal means, as by pantomiming the use of an object or by grouping together dissimilar-looking objects from the same semantic category[11-16] (see Ref. 4 for a review of representative cases).

The scope of the recognition impairment varies from case to case of associative agnosia. Some patients encounter difficulty mainly with face recognition (see Chap. 10), while others demonstrate better face recognition than object recognition. Printed-word recognition is similarly impaired in some cases but not others. The selectivity of these impairments suggests that there is more than one system involved in visual recognition. According to one analysis,[17] there are two underlying forms of visual representation, one of which is required for face recognition, used for object recognition but not for word recognition, and the other of which is required for word recognition, used for object recognition and not required for face recognition. Indeed, if one regards associative agnosia as a single undifferentiated category, it is difficult to make any generalizations about the brain regions responsible for visual object recognition. Although the intrahemispheric location of damage is generally occipitotemporal, involving both gray and white matter, cases of associative agnosia have been reported following unilateral right-hemispheric lesions,[18] unilateral left-hemispheric lesions,[15,16,19,20] and bilateral lesions.[21-23] However, if one considers impairments in face and word recognition as markers for different underlying forms of visual recognition disorder, then a pattern emerges in the neuropathology.

When face recognition alone is impaired or when face and object recognition are impaired but reading is spared, the lesions are generally either on the right or bilateral. De Renzi has proposed that the degree of right-hemispheric specialization for face recognition may normally cover a wide range, such that most cases of prosopagnosia become manifest only after bilateral lesions, but in some cases a unilateral lesion will suffice (see Chap. 10). When reading alone is impaired or when reading and object recognition are impaired but face recognition is spared, the lesions are generally on the left. In a series of patients studied by us and additional cases of agnosia sparing face recognition culled from the literature, the maximum over-

lap in lesion locus was in the left inferior medial region involving parahippocampal, fusiform, and lingual gyri.[16] When recognition of faces, objects, and words is impaired, the lesions are generally bilateral.

The hypothesis of two underlying systems explains the pairwise dissociations among three different stimulus categories—words, objects, and faces—in a parsimonious way, with only two systems. In addition, it reveals a systematicity in lesion sites not previously apparent. Nevertheless, the hypothesis has been questioned following more recent reports of patients with patterns of spared and impaired recognition abilities that are inconsistent with an impairment in one of just two underlying systems. One patient with impaired face and word recognition but relatively less impaired object recognition has been reported.[24] The presence of a degree of object agnosia precludes strong inferences, however. Another patient with an isolated object recognition impairment has also been reported.[25] In this case, however, the object recognition impairment was evident to a degree on purely verbal tasks, limiting its relevance to visual agnosia.

Functional neuroimaging of normal subjects has largely supported the idea of a bilateral- or right-lateralized system for face recognition and a left-lateralized system for word recognition, with object recognition using both,[26] but has also raised the possibility of additional specialization within those systems, for example, specialization for orthography per se.[27]

Interpreting Associative Agnosia

Is associative agnosia a problem with perception, memory, or both? Associative agnosia has been explained in three different ways that suggest different answers to this question. The simplest way to explain agnosia is by a disconnection between visual representations and other brain centers responsible for language or memory. For example, Geschwind[28] proposed that associative agnosia is a visual–verbal disconnection. This hypothesis accounts well for agnosics' impaired naming of visual stimuli, but it cannot account for their inability to convey recognition nonverbally. Associative agnosia has also been explained as a disconnection between visual representations and medial temporal memory centers.[23] However, this would account for a modality-specific impairment in new learning, not the inability to access old knowledge through vision.

The inadequacies of the disconnection accounts lead us to consider theories of associative agnosia in which some component of perception and/or memory has been damaged. Perhaps the most widely accepted account of associative agnosia is that stored visual memory representations have been damaged. According to this type of account, stimuli can be processed perceptually up to some end-state visual representation, which would then be matched against stored visual representations. In associative agnosia, the stored representations are no longer available and recognition therefore fails. Note that an assumption of this account is that two identical tokens of the object representation normally exist, one derived from the stimulus and one stored in memory, and that these are compared in the same way as a database might be searched in a present-day computer. This account is not directly disconfirmed by any of the available evidence. However, there are some reasons to question it and to suspect that subtle impairments in perception may underlie associative agnosia.

Although the good copies and successful matching performance of associative agnosics might seem to exonerate perception, a closer look at the manner in which these tasks are accomplished suggests that perception is not normal in associative agnosia and suggests yet a third explanation of associative agnosia. Typically, these patients are described as copying drawings "slavishly"[29] and "line by line."[30] In matching tasks, they rely on slow, sequential feature-by-feature checking. It therefore may be premature to rule out faulty perception as the cause of associative agnosia.

Recent studies of the visual capabilities of associative agnosic patients confirm that there are subtle visual perceptual impairments present in all cases studied.[4] If the possibility of impaired recognition with intact perception is consistent with the use of a computational architecture in which separate perceptual and memory representations are compared, then the absence of such a case suggests that a different type of computational architecture may underlie object recognition. Parallel distributed processing (PDP) systems exemplify an alternative architecture in which the perceptual and memory representations cannot be dissociated (see Chap. 7; see also Refs. 4 and 5 for discussions of computational approaches to agnosia). In a PDP system, the memory of the stimulus would consist of a pattern of connection strengths among a number of neuronlike units. The "perceptual" representation resulting from the presentation of a stimulus will depend upon the pattern of connection strengths among the units directly or indirectly activated by the stimulus. Thus, if memory is altered by damaging the network, perception will be altered as well. On this account, associative agnosia is not a result of an impairment to perception *or* to memory; rather, the two are in principle inseparable, and the impairment is better described as a loss of high-level visual perceptual representations that are shaped by, and embody the memory of, visual experience. It will thus be of great interest to see whether future studies of associative agnosics will ever document a case of impaired recognition with intact perception.

Relation to Other Disorders

As with apperceptive agnosia, a number of distinct disorders have been labeled associative agnosia by different authors. Visual modality–specific naming disorders exist and are usually termed *optic aphasia* (see Chap. 10), but they may on occasion be called *associative visual agnosia*. *Impairments of semantic memory* (see Chap. 27) will affect object-recognition ability (as well as entirely nonvisual abilities such as verbally defining spoken words) and perhaps for this reason have also sometimes been called *associative visual agnosia*.

REFERENCES

1. Bay E: Disturbances of visual perception and their examination. *Brain* 76:515–530, 1952.
2. Lissauer H: Ein Fall von Seelenblindheit nebst einem Beitrage zur Theori derselben. *Arch Psychiatr Nervenkrankh* 21:222–270, 1890.
3. Benson R, Greenberg JP: Visual form agnosia. *Arch Neurol* 20:82–89, 1969.
4. Farah MJ: *Visual Agnosia: Disorders of Object Recognition and What They Tell Us about Normal Vision*, 2d ed. Cambridge, MA: MIT Press, 2004.
5. Farah MJ: *The Cognitive Neuroscience of Vision*. Oxford: Blackwells, 2000.
6. Williams M: *Brain Damage and the Mind*. Baltimore: Penguin Books, 1970.

7. Girotti F, Milanese C, Casazza M, et al: Oculomotor disturbances in Balint's syndrome: Anatomoclinical findings and electrooculographic analysis in a case. *Cortex* 18:603–614, 1982.

8. Tyler HR: Abnormalities of perception with defective eye movements (Balint's syndrome). *Cortex* 3:154–171, 1968.

9. Kinsbourne M, Warrington EK: A disorder of simultaneous form perception. *Brain* 85:461–486, 1962.

10. Warrington EK: Agnosia: The impairment of object recognition, in Vinken PJ, Bruyn GW, Klawans HL (eds): *Handbook of Clinical Neurology.* Amsterdam: Elsevier, 1985.

11. Rubens AB, Benson DF: Associative visual agnosia. *Arch Neurol* 24:305–316, 1971.

12. Bauer RM, Rubens AB: Agnosia, in Heilman KM, Valenstein E (eds): *Clinical Neuropsychology,* 2d ed. New York: Oxford University Press, 1985.

13. Albert ML, Reches A, Silverberg R: Associative visual agnosia without alexia. *Neurology* 25:322–326, 1975.

14. Hécaen H, de Ajuriaguerra J: Agnosie visuelle pour les objets inanimés par lesion unilateral gauche. *Rev Neurol* 94:222–233, 1956.

15. McCarthy RA, Warrington EK: Visual associative agnosia: A clinico-anatomical study of a single case. *Neurol Neurosurg Psychiatry* 48:1233–1240, 1986.

16. Feinberg TE, Schindler RJ, Ochoa E, et al: Associative visual agnosia and alexia without prosopagnosia. *Cortex* 30:395–412, 1994.

17. Farah MJ: Patterns of co-occurrence among the associative agnosias: Implications for visual object representation. *Cognit Neuropsychol* 8:1–19, 1991.

18. Levine DN: Prosopagnosia and visual object agnosia: A behavioral study. *Neuropsychologia* 5:341–365, 1978.

19. Pilon B, Signoret JL, Lhermitte F: Agnosie visuelle associative rôle de l'hemisphere gauche dans la perception visuelle. *Rev Neurol* 137:831–842, 1981.

20. Feinberg TE, Heilman KM, Gonzalez-Rothi L: Multimodal agnosia after unilateral left hemisphere lesion. *Neurology* 36:864–867, 1986.

21. Alexander MP, Albert ML: The anatomical basis of visual agnosia, in Kertesz A (ed): *Localization in Neuropsychology.* New York: Academic Press, 1983.

22. Benson DF, Segarra J, Albert ML: Visual agnosia-prosopagnosia: A clinicopathologic correlation. *Arch Neurol* 30:307–310, 1973.

23. Albert ML, Soffer D, Silverberg R, Reches A: The anatomic basis of visual agnosia. *Neurology* 29:876–879, 1979.

24. Buxbaum LJ, Glosser G, Coslett HB: Relative sparing of object recognition in alexia-prosopagnosia. *Brain Cognit.*

25. Humphreys GW, Rumiati RI: Agnosia without prosopagnosia or alexia. *Cognit Neuropsychol* 15:243–277, 1998.

26. Farah MJ, Aguirre GK: Imaging visual recognition. *Trends Cognit Sci* 3:179–186, 1999.

27. Polk TA, Stallcup M, Aguirre G et al: Neural specialization for letter recognition. *J Cognit Neurosci* 14:145–159, 2001.

28. Geschwind N: Disconnexion syndromes in animals and man: Part II. *Brain* 88:585–645, 1965.

29. Brown JW: *Aphasia, Apraxia and Agnosia: Clinical and Theoretical Aspects.* Springfield, IL: Charles C Thomas, 1972.

30. Ratcliff G, Newcombe F: Object recognition: Some deductions from the clinical evidence, in Ellis AW (ed): *Normality and Pathology in Cognitive Functions.* New York: Academic Press, 1982.

31. Farah MJ, Hammond K, Levine DN, et al: Visual and spatial mental imagery. *Cognit Neuropsychol* 20:439–462, 1988.

Chapter 10

PROSOPAGNOSIA

Martha J. Farah

Visual object agnosia, discussed in the previous chapter, does not always affect the recognition of all types of stimuli equally. Quite often, the recognition of faces seems disproportionately or even exclusively impaired, a condition known as *prosopagnosia*. Prosopagnosia can be so severe that the patient cannot recognize close friends, family members, or even his or her own face in a photograph. Yet nonfacial knowledge of people is preserved, and prosopagnosics typically resort to recognizing individuals by their voices or even by nonfacial visual cues such as clothing. Of course, such strategies have only very limited effectiveness. Prosopagnosia is therefore a serious problem for patients and is usually discovered because of the patient's complaint rather than by testing or examination.

The most straightforward explanation of prosopagnosia is that a specialized brain system for recognizing faces has been damaged. In recent years, much of the research on prosopagnosia has been aimed at testing this explanation against various alternative explanations. The reason that so much attention has been paid to this issue is that it bears directly on a larger controversy in cognitive science concerning the unity versus modularity of cognitive processes (e.g., Fodor, 1982). Does the brain support intelligent behavior with a relatively small set of general-purpose information processing mechanisms, or has it evolved to carry out its many functions by the use of dedicated, special-purpose mechanisms?

THE FUNCTIONAL DEFICIT IN PROSOPAGNOSIA: FACE-SPECIFIC?

The most straightforward interpretation of prosopagnosia is consistent with anatomically separate recognition systems for faces and objects. More precisely, prosopagnosia suggests that there is some system that is necessary for face recognition and either unnecessary or less important for object recognition. An alternative interpretation is that faces and all other types of objects are recognized using a single recognition system and that faces are simply the most difficult type of object for the recognition system. Prosopagnosia can then be explained as a mild form of agnosia, in which the impairment is detectable only on the most taxing form of recognition task.

The first researchers to address this issue directly were McNeil and Warrington (1993). They studied case W.J., a middle-aged professional man who became prosopagnosic following a series of strokes. After becoming prosopagnosic, W.J. made a career change and went into sheep farming. He eventually came to recognize many of his sheep, although he remained unable to recognize most humans. The authors noted the potential implications of such a dissociation for the question of whether human face recognition is "special" and designed an ingenious experiment exploiting W.J.'s new-found career. They assembled three groups of photographs—human faces, sheep faces of the same breed kept by W.J., and sheep faces of a different breed—and attempted to teach subjects names for each face. Normal subjects performed at intermediate levels between ceiling and floor in all conditions. They performed better with the human faces than with sheep faces, even those who, like W.J., worked with sheep. In contrast, W.J. performed poorly with the human faces and performed normally with the sheep faces.

The issue of whether prosopagnosia is selective for faces relative to common objects was addressed by my colleagues and myself with patient L.H., a well-educated professional man who has been prosopagnosic since an automobile accident in college (Farah et al., 1995). We employed a recognition memory paradigm in which L.H. and control subjects first studied a set of photographs of faces and nonface objects, such as forks, chairs, and eyeglasses. Subjects were then given a larger set of photographs, and asked to make "old"/"new" judgments on them. Whereas normal subjects performed equally well with the faces and nonface objects, L.H. showed a significant performance disparity, performing worse with faces than with objects. In a second experiment, we used a similar method to contrast L.H. and normal subjects' recognition performance with 40 faces and 40 eyeglass frames and again found that L.H. was disproportionately impaired at face recognition. This, as well as the results of testing W.J. with human and sheep faces, implies that prosopagnosia is not a problem with recognizing specific exemplars from any visually homogeneous category but is specific to faces.

Another source of evidence for the independence of face and object recognition comes from patients who show the opposite dissociation—namely, more difficulty with object recognition than with face recognition (Feinberg et al., 1994; Moscovitch et al., 1997). The existence of such cases also supports the interpretation that prosopagnosia is not simply a mild general visual agnosia, because such an interpretation is inconsistent with the possibility of relatively preserved face recognition with object agnosia.

A different kind of alternative interpretation of prosopagnosia does not deny that visual recognition involves some specialized subsystems that are necessary for face recognition. However, according to this alternative, the nature of the specialization is subtly different from that discussed so far. Gauthier and collaborators have proposed that we have a recognition system that is specialized for objects that require expertise to discriminate from one another and which share an overall configuration. Faces fall into this category, but other objects can as well. These include birds or dogs for expert bird watchers and dog show judges (Tanaka and Taylor, 1991) and a set of artificial creatures devised by Gauthier and Tarr (1997) called "greebles." Greeble recognition has been shown to have many similarities to face recognition, and recent efforts to teach a prosopagnosic to recognize Greebles were unsuccessful, adding further support to Gauthier's hypothesis. Of course, it is possible to view such demonstrations as evidence that people occasionally recruit their specialized face recognition system for use with other stimuli.

ANATOMIC BASES OF FACE RECOGNITION

If we are interested in knowing precisely where, in the human brain, face recognition is carried out, individual cases are rarely very informative. L.H. sustained head injuries followed by surgery and W.J. suffered at least three strokes, resulting in widely distributed damage in both cases. Surveys of the lesions in larger groups of prosopagnosics are more helpful for localization, as the regions of overlap among different patients can be identified. Damasio et al. (1982) conducted a survey of the literature for autopsied cases of prosopagnosia, and studied three of their own patients, concluding that the critical lesion site is in ventral occipitotemporal cortex bilaterally. De Renzi and colleagues (1994) reviewed much of the same case material, along with more recent cases and data from living patients whose brain damage was mapped using both structural magnetic resonance imaging (MRI) and positron emission tomography (PET). Their findings supported the ventral localization of face recognition but called for a revision of the idea that bilateral lesions are necessary. Some patients became prosopagnosic after unilateral right hemisphere damage. The possibility of hidden left hemisphere dysfunction in these cases was reduced by the finding of normal metabolic activity in the left hemisphere by PET scan. De Renzi et al. conclude that there is a spectrum of hemispheric specialization for face recognition in normal right-handed adults. Although the right hemisphere may be relatively better at face recognition than the left, most people have a degree of face recognition ability in both hemispheres. Nevertheless, in a minority of cases, face recognition is so focally represented in the right hemisphere that a unilateral lesion will lead to prosopagnosia. The lesion sites associated with prosopagnosia are, as a group, clearly different from the lesions associated with object agnosia in the absence of prosopagnosia. The latter syndrome is almost invariably the result of a unilateral left hemisphere lesion, although confined to roughly the same intrahemispheric region (Feinberg et al., 1994).

Converging evidence about the localization of face recognition in the human brain comes from functional neuroimaging of normal individuals. The most relevant experimental design for comparison with prosopagnosics' lesions is one in which brain activity while viewing faces is contrasted with brain activity while viewing nonface objects. Kanwisher and coworkers (1996) used functional MRI to compare regional brain activity while subjects viewed photographs of faces and of objects. An objects-minus-faces subtraction revealed areas more responsive to objects than faces and the reverse subtraction revealed an area more responsive to faces than objects. Both types of stimuli activated inferior temporooccipital regions, with face-specific activation confined to part of the right fusiform gyrus. A follow-up study identified the same fusiform face area and systematically verified its specificity for faces by comparing its response to faces and to scrambled faces, houses, and hands (Kanwisher et al., 1997). Similar conclusions were reached by McCarthy and coworkers (1997), who found right fusiform activation unique to passive viewing of faces relative to objects or scrambled objects, and left fusiform activation unique to flowers relative to scrambled objects.

REFERENCES

Damasio AR, Damasio H, Van Hoesen GW: Prosopagnosia: anatomic basis and behavioral mechanisms. *Neurology* 32:331–341, 1982.

De Renzi E, Perani D, Carlesimo GA, et al: Prosopagnosia can be associated with damage confined to the right hemisphere—an MRI and PET study and a review of the literature. *Neuropsychologia* 32:893–902, 1994.

Farah MJ, Levinson KL, Klein KL: Face perception and within-category discrimination in prosopagnosia. *Neuropsychologia* 33:661–674, 1995.

Feinberg TE, Schindler RJ, Ochoa E, et al: Associative visual agnosia and alexia without prosopagnosia. *Cortex* 30:395–411, 1994.

Fodor JA: *The Modularity of Mind.* Cambridge, MA: MIT Press, 1983.

Gauthier I, Tarr MJ: Becoming a "greeble" expert: Exploring mechanisms for face recognition. *Vis Res* 37:1673–1682, 1997.

Kanwisher N, Chun MM, McDermott J, Ledden PJ: Functional imaging of human visual recognition. *Cogn Brain Res* 5:55–67, 1996.

Kanwisher N, McDermott J, Chun MM: The fusiform face area: A module in human extrastriate cortex specialized for face perception. *J Neurosci* 17:4302–4311, 1997.

McCarthy G, Puce A, Gore JC, Allison T: Face-specific processing in human fusiform gyrus. *J Cogn Neurosci* 9:605–610, 1997.

McNeil JE, Warrington EK: Prosopagnosia: a face-specific disorder. *Q J Exp Psychol Hum Exp Psychol* 46A:1–10, 1993.

Tanaka JW, Taylor M: Object categories and expertise: Is the basic level in the eye of the beholder? *Cogn Psychol* 23:457–482, 1991.

Chapter 11

VISUOSPATIAL FUNCTION

Martha J. Farah

The integrality of vision and action has recently come to be recognized in vision research (e.g., Milner and Goodale 1995) and is starkly apparent in the behavior of patients with damage to posterior parietal cortex and certain other visual areas. Whereas they may be able to read, recognize faces, perceive colors, and so on, their ability to move through space, reach for objects, or assemble an object from spatially separated parts may be severely impaired. Humans have a constant need to move through space and manipulate the spatial disposition of objects and have evolved a complex system of spatial vision. Damage to any part of this system will result in a visuospatial disorder, the precise nature of which depends on the location of the lesion.

For purposes of organizing a review of these disorders, it is helpful to divide them into two general categories: disorders relating to the space visible at a given moment, in which all relevant stimuli can be perceived from one vantage point given free eye movement, and disorders relating to the topography of an environment, in which multiple views must be integrated into a large-scale spatial representation. These are distinct abilities, although they can, of course, influence one another. For example, certain impairments of the first type of ability will impact a person's ability to learn or navigate a larger-scale environment. The major subtypes of each of these disorders are reviewed in this chapter, including their main features, associated lesion sites, and implications for our understanding of normal vision.

VISIBLE (SMALL-SCALE) SPACE

Impaired Attention to Space

Hemispatial neglect is the most common disorder of visuospatial perception and is mentioned only in passing here because it is the subject of Chaps. 14 and 15. In its most typical manifestation, a patient with neglect will be unaware of the locations and objects contralateral to the brain lesion, which most often affects right posterior parietal cortex. Most authors discuss neglect as a disorder of spatial attention, whereby information from the contralateral hemispace is not fully encoded due to insufficient spatial attention (e.g., Heilman and Valenstein, 1979). Other authors prefer to view it as a disorder of spatial representation, whereby the brain fails to construct a full internal representation of the affected side of space (e.g., Bisiach and Luzzatti, 1978). Still others fail to see the distinction, as one cannot attend to a stimulus without representing it, and one cannot represent it without attending to it (Farah, 2000). Balint's syndrome affects processing of stimuli on both sides of space and is sometimes considered a bilateral neglect syndrome.

Impaired Perception of Location and Orientation

It is difficult to conceive of a person having vision with preserved color and form perception but the inability to perceive location. Yet just such a dissociation, known as *visual disorientation*, exists. Patients with visual disorientation are not only inaccurate in pointing or reaching to an object but also fail at describing its location verbally. For example, they will have difficulty answering whether a pen is above or below a pair of eyeglasses held in front of them by the examiner. Not surprisingly, such patients are severely handicapped in their everyday lives, being effectively blind as far as most visual interactions with the world go. It has been known for many decades that the critical lesion site is the occipitoparietal junction, and in some cases a unilateral form of the disorder is observed after damage to either the left or right hemisphere alone (Riddoch, 1935). Along with visual object agnosia (see Chap. 9), this is probably the strongest evidence for the hypothesis of "two cortical visual systems" in human vision, as it demonstrates the mutual independence (i.e., one can function without the other) of object recognition and spatial localization.

In rare cases, patients may develop an *orientation agnosia,* the selective impairment of orientation perception. Such cases have been described by Turnbull and colleagues (e.g., Turnbull, Beschin, and Della Salla, 1997). One patient's orientation perception was sufficiently compromised that he had hung pictures upside down on the wall of his home.

A subtler impairment of spatial perception, generally brought out by testing, is the impaired perception of line orientation. A widely used test of orientation perception is that of Benton, Varney, and Hamsher (1978), in which diagonal lines of varying orientation are presented and the patient must indicate the identical orientations in an array of oriented lines. The spatial nature of the judgment and the minimal nature of the shape information involved suggests that this ability would depend strongly on parietal cortex, and indeed that is the case. There is also a pronounced asymmetry in favor of greater right hemisphere involvement in this ability (De Renzi, 1982).

Impaired Visually Guided Reaching

Although it can be difficult to disentangle impairments of visual localization from impairments of visually guided reaching, a number of careful studies have done so (DeRenzi, 1982). The latter impairment, also known as optic ataxia, is usually observed in unilateral form, but this generality covers a surprising array of variants. The unilateral aspect may pertain to the hemispace, as when either limb is inaccurate reaching for objects in, for example, the left hemispace. Alternatively, it may pertain to the limb, as when one limb—for example, the left—is inaccurate in reaching for objects at any location. It may even combine these two forms of unilateral selectivity, as when one arm (e.g., the left) is disproportionately inaccurate reaching to the same (left) hemispace compared to other limb-space combinations. Some patients with unilateral lesions show a milder level of optic ataxia on the ipsilateral side of space. Optic ataxia usually follows damage high in the parietal lobe, anterior to the regions most likely to cause visual disorientation. The precise scope of the impairment presumably depends on what parts of parietal gray and underlying white matter are damaged.

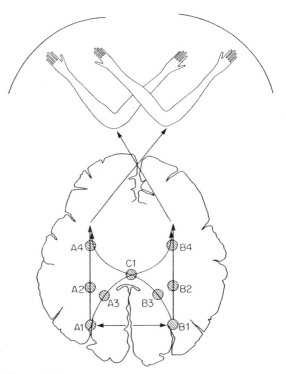

Figure 11-1
Schematic diagram of different possible lesions interrupting visuomotor control, which would result in different patterns of limb and visual field differences in visually guided reaching. Lesions at points marked 1 and 4 would result in pure field selectivity and limb selectivity, respectively. Lesions at points marked 2 and 3 would result in both field and limb selectivity, contralateral and ipsilateral, respectively. A lesion at C would result in a different pattern of field and limb selectivity, with contralateral combinations of limb and field, on either side, impaired (as in callosotomy patients). (From De Renzi E: Disorders of Space Exploration and Cognition, New York: John Wiley, 1982.)

Figure 11-1 shows how different combinations of hemispace and limb selectivity could result from interruption of the pathways from visual to motor cortex at different points.

Impaired Construction: Drawing and Building

Before the days when laptop computers could be carried to patients' bedsides, clinicians relied heavily on construction tasks to assess visuospatial function. These included copying meaningful drawings and arbitrary geometric figures as well as recreating a pattern made from sticks or blocks (the latter either in two or three dimensions). Impairments in construction, known as *constructional apraxia,* were therefore an important topic of study in the neuropsychology of the 1970s and 1980s and continue to be assessed in most mental status exams to this day.

Constructional apraxia differs in two important ways from the other impairments reviewed here. Whereas the perception of object location, navigation through the environment, and so on are basic spatial abilities for which our brains may have evolved specific systems over the course of the millennia, the scope of abilities classified together by the category of constructional apraxia does not seem to instantiate the same kind of basic category. To be sure, the ability to construct complex objects from simple ones would have great

adaptive value. What is in doubt is that a single system is responsible for the ability to draw arbitrary geometric figures, meaningful line drawings, and build block or stick structures.

It seems likely, therefore, that the disorder known as constructional apraxia is many disorders, most of which are secondary to other, more fundamental impairments, including visuospatial perception, visually guided action, and executive function. Sometimes the underlying cause of the constructional impairment is fairly obvious, as when a patient with prefrontal damage and disorganization evident in other tasks produces a disorganized construction. Other times, it is difficult to characterize the underlying impairment. For example, the bicycles shown in Fig. 11-2 were drawn by patients with unilateral posterior brain damage. There is a clear trend for patients with left-sided injuries to produce spare, impoverished constructions and those with right-sided injuries to produce abundantly detailed

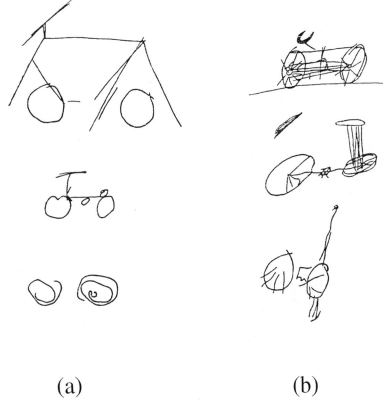

Figure 11-2
Examples of constructional apraxia in a bicycle drawing task following (a) left and (b) right hemisphere lesions. (From McFie J, Zangwill OL: Visual-constructive disabilities associated with lesions of the left cerebral hemisphere. Brain 83:243–261, 1960.)

(a)   (b)

but spatially disorganized constructions. However, the underlying impairment in each case is not clear.

ENVIRONMENTAL (LARGE-SCALE) SPACE

There is relatively little experimental literature on disorders of large-scale spatial cognition. This is undoubtedly due to the practical difficulties of designing "test materials" the size of rooms, houses, or city blocks. Most of what we know about topographic orientation comes from individual case reports of patients with clinically significant topographic disorders. In some of the more recent reports, patients were studied using experimental designs tailored to the patients' own environments.

The one exception to the rule that the neuropsychology of large-scale space has not been studied in any systematic way using experimental tasks originates with the work of Semmes et al. (1955), who developed a locomotor maze. Subjects are given a map showing an array of markers laid out on the floor, and they must walk a path corresponding to the path shown in the map. In an interesting contrast demonstrating the dissociability of small- and large-scale spatial cognition, Ratcliff and Newcombe (1973) administered the locomotor maze and another small tabletop maze task to a group of focally brain-damaged patients. Several of these patients performed well on one task and poorly on the other, suggesting that large- and small-scale spatial cognition is subserved by distinct neural systems.

In addition to parietal cortex, which plays many roles in spatial cognition, certain other brain regions have also been associated with processing of large-scale space. Patients can lose the ability to navigate their environment following damage to posterior parietal cortex as well as posterior cingulate, parahippocampal, and lingual gyri. Not surprisingly, the nature of their impairments can also vary. A recent review by Aguirre and D'Esposito (1999) used cognitive theories of topographic orientation and information about lesion localization to arrive at a useful taxonomy of topographic disorders, which is summarized here. The different forms of topographic disorientation are informative about the organization of topographic knowl-

edge in the normal brain. The patterns of preserved and impaired abilities described below suggest that spatial orientation in the environment involves both specialized topographic representations and more general spatial abilities, that spatial and landmark knowledge of the environment are subserved by different systems, and that the acquisition of topographic knowledge may be carried out by a specialized learning system.

Egocentric disorientation is the term used to describe patients whose topographic disorientation is secondary to visual disorientation, discussed earlier. Not surprisingly, patients who cannot localize seen objects in space are severely handicapped in navigating both familiar and unfamiliar terrain. Of course, this form of topographic impairment is not specific to topographic knowledge. A representative patient, described by Levine, Warach, and Farah (1985), was unable to find his way even around his own home, despite intact recognition of objects and landmarks, and showed spatial impairment on even the simplest small-scale spatial tasks. The critical lesion site, as noted earlier, is the posterior parietal cortex bilaterally, often right at the boundary with occipital cortex.

Heading disorientation is a more specific impairment in large-scale spatial representation, consisting of the inability to perceive and remember the spatial relations among landmarks in the environment and one's orientation relative to them. These patients, who are rare in the literature, do not have a more global form of visual disorientation but are selectively impaired at way finding, map use, and other tests of orientation in the environment. Three cases described by Takahashi et al. (1997) illustrate this disorder. The critical lesion site appears to be the posterior cingulate gyrus.

Landmark agnosia is an impairment of visual recognition that is selective or disproportionate for objects in the environment that normally serve as landmarks. These include buildings, monuments, squares, and so on. Patients with landmark agnosia, such as Pallis's (1955) case, retain their spatial knowledge of the environment, as evidenced by good descriptions of routes, layouts, and maps. However, without the ability to discriminate one building from another, they cannot apply this knowledge. The typical lesions in landmark agnosia are similar to those of other visual agnosias, especially prosopagnosia—that is, the inferior surface of

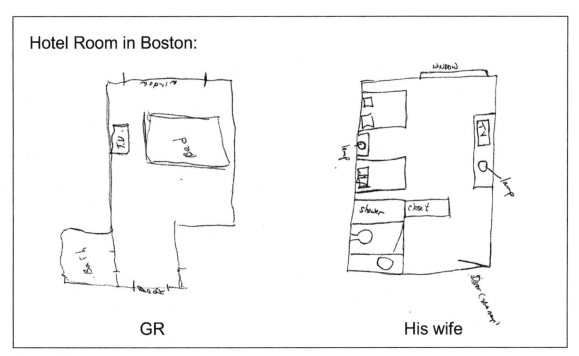

Figure 11-3
Maps of a hotel room drawn by a patient with anterograde topographic disorientation and by his neurologically normal wife.

the occipitotemporal regions, either bilateral or right-sided.

Anterograde disorientation refers to a topographic impairment that encompasses both spatial and landmark knowledge and is selective for the acquisition of this knowledge. Such patients show normal topographic abilities for environments that were familiar before their brain injury, but cannot learn to navigate new environments. The critical lesion site for anterograde disorientation appears to be the right parahippocampal gyrus. Epstein et al. (2001) describe a patient who provides a dramatic example of a selective impairment in learning new environments. Although able to draw an accurate map of the house in which he lived years earlier, the map of his current house was drawn with great difficulty and some inaccuracy, and, as shown in Fig. 11-3, he was completely unable to draw a map of the hotel room in which he had just spent 2 days. He was also unable to learn new landmarks despite good recognition of famous landmarks.

Such cases suggest a heretofore unsuspected form of specialization within memory systems for learning the spatial environment.

REFERENCES

Aguirre GK, D'Esposito M: Topographical disorientation: A synthesis and taxonomy. *Brain* 122:1613–1628, 1999.

Benton AL, Varney NR, Hamsher KD: Visuospatial judgement: A clinical test. *Arch Neurol* 35:364–367, 1978.

Bisiach E, Luzzatti C: Unilateral neglect of representational space. *Cortex* 14:129–133, 1978.

De Renzi E: *Disorders of Space Exploration and Cognition.* New York: John Wiley, 1982.

Epstein R, DeYoe EA, Press DZ, et al: Neuropsychological evidence for a topographical learning mechanism in parahippocampal cortex. *Cognit Neuropsychol* 18: 481–508, 2001.

Farah MJ: *The Cognitive Neuroscience of Vision.* Oxford: Blackwell, 2000.

Heilman KM, Valenstein E: Mechanisms underlying hemi-spatial neglect. *Ann Neurol* 5:166–170, 1979.

Levine DN, Warach J, Farah MJ: Two visual systems in mental imagery: Dissociation of "What" and "Where" in imagery disorders due to bilateral posterior cerebral lesions. *Neurology* 35:1010–1018, 1985.

Milner AD, Goodale MA (eds): *The Visual Brain in Action.* Oxford, UK: Oxford Science Publications, 1995.

Pallis CA: Impaired identification of faces and places with agnosia for colors. *J Neurol Neurosurg Psychiatry* 18:218–224, 1955.

Ratcliff G, Newcombe F: Spatial orientation in man: Effects of left, right, and bilateral posterior cerebral lesions. *J Neurol Neurosurg Psychiatry* 36:448–454, 1973.

Riddoch G: Visual disorientation in homonymous half-fields. *Brain* 58:376–382, 1935.

Semmes J, Weinstein S, Ghent L, Teuber HL: Spatial orientation in man: I. Analyses by locus of lesion. *J Psychol* 39:227–244, 1955.

Takahashi N, Kawamura MKS, Kasahata N, Hirayama K: Pure topographic disorientation due to right retrosplenial lesion. *Neurology* 49:464–469, 1997.

Turnbull OH, Beschin N, Della Sala S: Agnosia for object orientation: Implications for theories of object recognition. *Neuropsychologia* 35:153–163, 1997.

Chapter 12

AUDITORY AGNOSIA AND AMUSIA

Russell M. Bauer
Carrie R. McDonald

Auditory agnosia refers to an impaired capacity to recognize sounds in the presence of otherwise adequate hearing as measured by standard audiometry. Historically, the term has been used broadly to refer to impaired capacity to recognize sounds in general and in a narrow sense to refer to a selective deficit in recognizing nonverbal sounds only. Terminological confusion abounds, with such terms as *cortical auditory disorder,*[1,2] *auditory agnosia,*[3,4] and *auditory agnosia and word deafness*[5] all being used to describe similar phenomena. In most cases, impairment in the recognition of both speech and nonspeech sounds is present to some degree. The relative severity of these impairments depends on lesion localization, on premorbid lateralization of linguistic and nonlinguistic skills in the individual patient, and on which hemisphere is first or more seriously damaged[6] (but see Ref. 7). Complicating the picture even further is the fact that many patients evolve from one disorder to another as recovery takes place.[8]

In regard to generalized auditory agnosia, we prefer the theoretically neutral term *cortical auditory disorder,* and we first discuss this entity together with *cortical deafness.* We then discuss more "selective" deficits, including *pure word deafness* (a selective impairment in speech-sound recognition), *auditory sound agnosia* (selective impairment in recognizing nonspeech sounds), and *paralinguistic agnosias* (in which recognition of prosodic features of spoken language is impaired). We then describe patients with *receptive (sensory) amusia,* loss of the ability to appreciate various characteristics of heard music. Table 12-1 lists the major clinical features of each syndrome. In the final section of the chapter, we consider recent functional neuroimaging studies that have begun to shed important new light on the functional neuroanatomy of auditory abilities and disorders.

CORTICAL DEAFNESS AND CORTICAL AUDITORY DISORDER

Patients with cortical deafness show profound impairments in processing auditory stimuli of any kind and often have electrophysiologic signs of primary impairment in auditory-perceptual acuity. The behavior of patients with cortical auditory disorders is similar, though auditory evoked responses are more often normal in this population. Both groups show a range of impairments in auditory perception, discrimination, and recognition that affect verbal and nonverbal material.[9,10] Aphasic signs, if present, are mild and do not prevent the patient from identifying visual or somesthetic stimuli. Difficulties in elementary auditory function, including temporal auditory analysis and localization of sounds in space, are common.

In our view, cortical auditory disorders and cortical deafness are related in much the same way as visual agnosia is related to cortical blindness. If so, then cortical auditory disorders can take apperceptive or associative[11] forms, though some degree of perceptual deficit is apparent in nearly all cases where the evaluation of auditory abilities has been sufficiently comprehensive. This statement is true even in cases where pure tone audiometry is relatively normal. Jerger and coworkers[12,13] reported impairments in auditory perception (ear suppression in dichotic listening, abnormal click fusion thresholds, and impaired discrimination of basic sound attributes) in patients with cortical auditory disorders. It is important to note that cortical auditory disorders sometimes evolve from a state of cortical deafness, and it is difficult to distinguish between the two entities. Michel and colleagues[14] argued that the cortically deaf patient looks and feels deaf, whereas the patient with cortical auditory disorders insists that he or she is not deaf. This turns out

Table 12-1

Clinical features of various forms of auditory agnosia

	Cortical deafness	Cortical auditory disorder	Pure word deafness	Auditory sound agnosia	Sensory/ receptive amusia
Audiometric sensitivity	−	+/−	+	+	+
Speech comprehension	−	−	−	+	+
Speech repetition	−	−	−	+	+
Spontaneous speech	+	+*	+*	+	+
Reading comprehension	+	+	+	+	+
Written language	+	+	+	+	+
Recognition of familiar sounds	−	−	+	-	?
Musical perception	−	−	−†	−	+/−
Recognition of vocal prosody	−	−	+	?	−

Key: + = spared ability; − = impaired ability; ? = insufficient information in literature to generalize.

*May be some paraphasia.

†When tested (rarely), musical perception has been shown to be impaired in these patients.

Sources: Adapted from Buchman et al.[7] and Oppenheimer and Newcombe,[3] with permission.

to be a poor criterion, because the subjective experience of deafness in the former condition is typically so transient, and patients in both groups are "deaf" when subjected to appropriate tests. Although it was once believed that bilateral cortical lesions involving primary auditory cortex resulted in total hearing loss, evidence from animal experiments,[15,16] cortical mapping of the auditory area,[17] and clinicopathologic studies in humans[18,19] indicate that complete destruction of primary auditory cortex does not lead to permanent loss of audiometric sensitivity. Thus, clinical, pathologic, and electrophysiologic data question the distinctive nature of cortical deafness[1,9,10] and suggest that it is one of a spectrum of auditory impairments that runs from generalized disturbances in detecting and discriminating basic sound attributes to more complex and selective impairments in auditory recognition.

Recent behavioral studies of cortical deafness focused on deficits in attention and behavioral response, rather than entirely on perceptual deficits, as underlying the disorder. Engelien and colleagues[20] studied "deaf behavior" in a patient diagnosed with cortical deafness and found that under conditions of selective attention to audition, their patient achieved normal awareness of sounds, despite persistent impairment in sound lo-

calization and identification. In addition, the patient showed no orienting or startle response to unexpected, sudden sounds unless attention was focused exclusively on audition. This patient, however, had damage to the frontal operculum, in addition to bilateral lesions of the superior temporal gyri, which may have contributed to his auditory attentional deficits. Garde and Cowey[21] described a cortically deaf patient following pontine and bitemporal cortical lesions whose detection *and* localization of auditory stimuli both improved when attention was directed on audition. Their patient, unlike the patient of Engelien et al.,[20] responded reflexively to sounds that she denied hearing.

Cortical deafness is most often seen in bilateral cerebrovascular disease. A recent case of cortical deafness resulting from moyamoya disease (a vascular disorder in which the main cerebral arteries at the base of the brain are replaced by a fine network of vessels) has been reported in the Japanese literature.[22] The course is usually biphasic, with an initial deficit (often aphasia and hemiparesis) related to unilateral damage, followed by a second (contralateral) deficit associated with sudden transient total deafness.[12,13,20,21] A biphasic course is also typical of cortical auditory disorders. In cortical deafness, bilateral destruction of the auditory radiations or the primary auditory cortex (Heschl's gyrus) has been a constant finding.[20] Bilateral temporal lobe damage is generally reported, which in most cases involves the primary auditory cortex, although this area may be partially or completely spared. When the cortex is spared, underlying white matter pathology is a consistent finding.[25] Several researchers[26,27] have claimed that true "cortical" deafness does not result from isolated lesions of the cortex, but more often results from bilateral disconnection of the pathway to the auditory cortices. To date, the importance of cortical versus subcortical involvement in the etiology of cortical deafness is unclear, although this controversy will likely be resolved by studies using detailed MRI and comparison with probabilistic atlases.[28] The anatomic basis of cortical auditory disorder is more variable. Lesions can be quite extensive,[3] though the superior temporal gyrus and efferent connections of Heschl's gyrus are aften involved. Several case reports[29–31] suggest that cortical auditory disorder can result from bilateral lesions sparing the cortex entirely. Thus, the lesions in cortical auditory disorder seem to involve either intrinsic or disconnecting lesions involving the auditory association cortex, with relative sparing of Heschl's gyrus. A recent report[32] suggests that a generalized auditory agnosia may even result from circumscribed bilateral damage to the inferior colliculi.

PURE WORD DEAFNESS (AUDITORY AGNOSIA FOR SPEECH, AUDITORY VERBAL AGNOSIA)

The patient with pure word deafness is unable to comprehend spoken language although he or she can read, write, and speak in a *relatively* normal manner.[7] As such, it can be discussed as a form of aphasia (as in Chap. 16) as well as an impairment of high-level auditory function. Writing to dictation is typically impaired, though copying of written material is not. By definition, comprehension of nonverbal sounds is *relatively* spared, but nonverbal auditory recognition is impaired in the majority of cases in which it has been evaluated.[7] Thus, the syndrome is "pure" in that (1) the patient is *relatively* free of signs of posterior aphasia (see Chap. 16) and (2) the impairment in speech sound recognition is disproportionately severe. The disorder was first described by Kussmaul.[33] Lichteim[34]

later defined it as an isolated deficit and postulated a bilateral subcortical interruption of fibers from ascending auditory projections to the left "auditory word center." With few exceptions, pure word deafness has been associated with bilateral, symmetric cortical-subcortical lesions of the anterior part of the superior temporal gyri with some sparing of Heschl's gyrus, particularly on the left. Some patients have subcortical lesions of the dominant temporal lobe only, presumably destroying the ipsilateral auditory radiation as well as callosal fibers from the contralateral auditory region.[35–37] It is generally agreed that the lesion profile results in a bilateral disconnection of Wernicke's area from auditory input.[38] The fact that it involves an unusually placed, circumscribed lesion explains the low incidence of pure word deafness. In the review performed by Buchman and colleagues,[7] the lesions in 30 of 37 reviewed cases were of cerebrovascular origin. Other etiologies include encephalitis[39] and neoplasm.[40] Childhood forms of pure word deafness have also been associated with Landau-Kleffner syndrome,[41,42] although the course and prognosis in patients with Landau-Kleffner syndrome are highly variable. Kaga[41] reports that patients with Landau-Kleffner syndrome often show a sequential and hierarchical language disorder that commonly begins with sensory aphasia, followed by generalized auditory agnosia, and finally pure word deafness. Language disturbances in Landau-Kleffner syndrome may improve with anticonvulsant medication[43] or may be long lasting.[44]

When first seen, the patient is often recovering from a Wernicke's aphasia, though occasionally pure word deafness may actually give way to a Wernicke's aphasia.[45–48] As the paraphasias and writing and reading disturbances disappear, the patient still does not comprehend spoken language but can communicate by writing. Deafness can be ruled out by normal audiometric pure-tone thresholds. In some cases, however, mild bilateral neurosensory hearing loss is detected in patients with pure word deafness.[49,50] At this point, the patient may experience auditory hallucinations[51] or may exhibit transient euphoric[52] or paranoid[53,54] ideation. The inability to repeat poorly comprehended speech stimuli distinguishes pure word deafness from transcortical sensory aphasia; the absence of florid paraphasia and of reading and writing disturbance distinguishes it from Wernicke's aphasia. This having been said, it should be recognized that "aphasic" and "agnosic" symptoms may both be present, though different in degree, in the individual case.[7]

Many patients are responsive to speech input but complain of dramatic, sometimes aversive changes in their subjective experience of speech sounds.[8] The pure word deafness patient may complain that speech is muffled or sounds like a foreign language. Hemphill and Stengel's[55] patient stated that "voices come but no words." Klein and Harper's[46] patient described speech as "an undifferentiated continuous humming noise without any rhythm" and "like foreigners speaking in the distance." Albert and Bear's[30] patient said "words come too quickly" and, "they sound like a foreign language." The patient of Wee and colleagues[56] described voices as "distorted and cartoonlike." The speech of these patients is often slightly louder than normal and can be dysprosodic. Performance on speech perception tests is inconsistent and highly dependent upon context[57] and linguistic complexity.[58]

Many studies of pure word deafness have emphasized the role of auditory-perceptual processing in the genesis of the disorder.[1,8,12,45,58] Problems with temporal resolution[45] and phonemic discrimination[59–61] have also received attention. Auerbach and coworkers[58] suggest that the disorder may take two forms: (1) a prephonemic temporal auditory acuity disturbance associated with bilateral temporal lesions or (2) a disorder of phonemic discrimination attributable to left temporal lesions and closely linked to Wernicke's aphasia. Wang and colleagues[62] have challenged this division and suggested that prephonemic processing may also be affected following left unilateral lesions with subcortical involvement in patients with pure word deafness. Albert and Bear[45] suggested that the problem in pure word deafness is one of temporal resolution of auditory stimuli rather than specific phonetic impairment. Their patient demonstrated abnormally long click-fusion thresholds, and improved in auditory comprehension when speech was presented at slower rates. Wang et al.[62] provided additional support for impaired temporal processing in the genesis of pure word deafness. They described a patient with a lesion involving the cortical and subcortical white matter of the left temporal lobe who was unable to process sound elements or dynamic acoustic changes that occurred in a short period of time (less than 300 ms). They concluded that the inability to detect even moderately rapid acoustic

changes make it unlikely that these patients can process syllables in speech (which last only several hundred milliseconds) in any meaningful way.

Other researchers have also emphasized the role of poor temporal resolution in pure word deafness associated with Landau-Kleffner's syndrome[42] and progressive neuropathology.[49,63] Klein and others[42] studied electrophysiological abnormalities in six young adults who exhibited "verbal auditory agnosia" associated with Landau-Kleffner syndrome. They found that, compared to a control group, the cortical evoked potentials (CEPs) of their patient group were characterized by a delay in the N1 component to both tones and to speech sounds. This delay in N1 was consistently found over the lateral temporal cortex, despite a normal latency of the N1 component recorded over the frontocentral region of the scalp. These results suggest slowed processing of auditory stimuli within the secondary auditory cortex of the lateral temporal lobes for both speech and tones. The authors concluded that the perceptual impairment associated with verbal auditory agnosia is not speech-specific, rather speech is disproportionately affected since perception of speech sounds involves the analysis of brief acoustic transients that rapidly change in their spectral content. Otsuki et al.[49] described a patient with pure word deafness associated with generalized, progressive cortical atrophy, particularly in the left superior temporal region. Similar to the patient of Albert and Bear, this patient exhibited abnormally long click-fusion thresholds suggestive of an impairment in the temporal processing of auditory information.

Saffran, Marin, and Yeni-Komshian,[61] on the other hand, showed that informing their patient of the nature of the topic under discussion significantly facilitated comprehension. Thus, the disorder appeared to arise at different levels in these two patients. Other researchers have suggested that aside from deficits in temporal resolution and phonemic discrimination, a deficit in the processing of syllable sequences may contribute to pure word deafness.[64] This variability supports Buchman et al.'s[7] contention that pure word deafness describes a spectrum rather than an individual disorder.

On tests of phonemic discrimination, patients with bilateral lesions tend to show distinctive deficits for the feature of place of articulation.[58,59,65] Those with unilateral left hemispheric disease (LHD) show either impaired discrimination of voicing[41] or no distinctive pattern.[60] In dichotic listening, some patients show extreme suppression of right-ear perception,[45,61] suggesting the inaccessibility of the left hemispheric phonetic decoding areas (Wernicke's area) to auditory material that had already been acoustically processed by the right hemisphere. Several studies have reported brainstem and cortical auditory evoked responses in pure word deafness patients.[14] Brainstem auditory evoked potentials (BAEPs) are almost always normal, suggesting intact processing up to the level of the auditory radiations.[42,45,56,58,62,64,66] One study of progressive pure word deafness, however, reported normal amplitudes, but prolonged brainstem auditory evoked response latencies after wave.[63] Results from studies of cortical auditory evoked potentials (AEPs) are more variable, consistent with variable pathology.[58] For example, the patient of Jerger and colleagues[12] had no appreciable AEP, yet heard sounds. The patient of Auerbach and associates[58] showed normal P1, N1, and P2 responses to right-ear stimulation but had minimal response over either hemisphere to left-ear stimulation. A recent study measuring auditory evoked magnetic fields[67] revealed no N100 m detected in the left temporal lobe with the right ear stimulation in two patients with putaminal hemorrhages: one bilateral, the other only on the left. However, normal N100 m was obtained in the right hemisphere with the left ear stimulation in both cases. The location of the equivalent current dipole (ECD) of the intact N100 m in the right hemisphere was superimposed on the Heschl gyrus in brain MRI. These results are consistent with other studies[40] that support the disconnection view of pure word deafness.

Although patients with pure word deafness are supposed to perform relatively well with environmental sounds, many show subnormal performances when such abilities are formally tested.[7] Similarly, the appreciation of music is often disturbed.[7,56] Some patients may recognize foreign languages by their distinctive prosodic characteristics, and others can recognize *who* is speaking, suggesting preserved ability to comprehend paralinguistic aspects of speech. Coslett and associates[68] described a word-deaf patient who showed a remarkable dissociation between the comprehension of neutral and affectively intoned sentences. He was

asked to point to pictures of males and females depicting various emotional expressions. When instructions were given in a neutral voice, he performed poorly, but when instructions were given with affective intonations appropriate to the target face, he performed normally (at a level commensurate to his performance with written instructions). This patient had bilateral destruction of primary auditory cortex with some sparing of auditory association cortex, suggesting at least some direct contribution of the auditory radiations directly to association cortex without initial decoding in Heschl's gyrus.[68] It has been found that patients with pure word deafness generally comprehend better when they can lip-read, although isolated cases have been reported in which lipreading did not improve performance.[62] Coslett and others[68] speculate that one reason why patients with pure word deafness improve their auditory comprehension with lipreading is that face-to-face contact allows them to take advantage of visual cues (gesture and facial expression that are processed by different brain systems). Another explanation is that lipreading provides visual information about place of articulation, a linguistic feature that is markedly impaired at least in the bilateral cases.[58] In either case, the preserved comprehension of paralinguistic aspects of speech in pure word deafness patients further reinforces the widely held belief that comprehension of speech and nonspeech sounds are dissociable abilities.

Although distinctions have been made between basic defects in auditory perception vs. defects in linguistic processing, few studies of pure word deafness have analyzed the defect in terms of the apperceptive-associative distinction so prominent in discussing visual agnosia (see Chap. 9).[69] It has been suggested that word deafness may represent the apperceptive counterpart of a very rare and ill-defined disorder called "pure word meaning deafness," in which the patient can hear and repeat words, but do not know their meaning.[70,71] Franklin and others[71] suggest that in "classic" cases of word meaning deafness, patients present with preserved repetition, phoneme discrimination, and lexical decision, but with impaired comprehension of spoken words alone. This "associative" form of the disorder results in errors that are generally semantic in nature and patients show poorer comprehension of abstract compared to concrete words. While an abstract/concrete dissociation suggests a "language-specific" explanation of word meaning deafness, Tyler and Moss[72] proposed an account of how a more general impairment in auditory processing would affect abstract words more than concrete words. Therefore, apperceptive and associative forms of verbal auditory agnosia have yet to be clearly delineated.

AUDITORY SOUND AGNOSIA (AUDITORY AGNOSIA FOR NONSPEECH SOUNDS)

Patients with auditory sound agnosia have selective difficulty recognizing and identifying nonverbal sounds. The disorder is rare, less common by far than pure word deafness, but its existence has raised interest because it suggests the same type of "domain-specificity" in the auditory system that has received much recent attention in the study of visual recognition disorders.[45–47,74,75] The lower incidence of auditory sound agnosia may be due in part to the fact that such patients are less likely seek medical advice than are those with a disorder of speech comprehension and also because on specific auditory complaints may be discounted when pure tone audiometric and speech discrimination thresholds are normal. This is unfortunate, since normal audiometry does not rule but the possibility of primary auditory perceptual defects.[76,77]

Vignolo[9] argued that there may be two forms of auditory sound agnosia: (1) a perceptual-discriminative type associated mainly with right hemisphere damage and (2) an associative-semantic type associated with left hemisphere damage and linked with posterior aphasia. The former group makes predominantly acoustic (e.g., "man whistling" for birdsong) errors on picture-sound matching tasks, while the latter makes predominantly semantic (e.g., "train" for automobile engine) errors. This division follows the original classification of Kliest,[78] who distinguished between the ability to detect/perceive isolated sounds or noises and the inability to understand the meaning of sounds. In the verbal sphere, the analogous distinction (at least on the input side) is between pure word deafness (perceptual-discriminative) and transcortical sensory aphasia (semantic-associative). Relatively few cases of "pure" auditory sound agnosia have been reported.[79–84] Sometimes a patient's condition evolves into auditory

sound agnosia from a more generalized agnosia for both verbal and nonverbal sounds,[85–87] and occasionclly this evolves from an auditory sound agnosia into an auditory recognition defect that encompasses speech sounds and other auditory stimuli.[41]

The patient of Spreen and colleagues[83] is a paradigm case. He was a 65-year-old right-handed male who complained of "nerves" and headache when seen 3 years after a left hemiparetic episode. Audiometric testing revealed moderate bilateral high-frequency loss and speech reception thresholds of 12 dB for both ears. The outstanding abnormality was the inability to recognize common sounds. There was neither aphasia nor any other agnosic deficit. Sound localization was normal, but scores on the pitch subtest of the Seashore Tests of Musical Talent were at chance level. The patient performed well on a matching-to-sample test, suggesting that his sound recognition disturbance could not be attributed to serious acoustic disturbance. He claimed no musical experience or talent and refused to cooperate with further testing of musical ability. Postmortem examination revealed a sharply demarcated old infarct of the right hemisphere centering around the parietal lobe and involving the superior temporal and angular gyri as well as a large portion of the inferior parietal, inferior, and middle frontal gyri and the insula. Other cases with unilateral pathology were reported by Clark and associates[80] (four patients with variable left temporal lobe lesions), Fuji and coworkers[81] (small posterior right temporal hemorrhagic lesion of the middle and superior temporal gyri), Neilsen and Sult[82] (right thalamus and parietal lobe), and Wortis and Pfeffer[84] (large lesion of the right temporoparietooccipital junction).

These data suggest that an inability to recognize environmental sounds can occur after unilateral right hemisphere damage. Such a defect is less commonly seen in the context of bilateral disease,[79] but these cases are less "pure" at least in the acute stage. The association of auditory sound agnosia with right hemisphere damage implies that acoustic processors within the right hemisphere are preferentially involved in dealing with nonlinguistic sounds. The left hemisphere is likely involved in providing linguistic labels for identified sounds, and in performing semantic-associative functions supporting sound recognition and identification.

Other cases of auditory sound agnosia have been reported following bilateral subcortical lesions[30,87] and bilateral ventricular enlargement[86] in the absence of cortical pathology. The patient of Motomura et al.[30] presented following a thalamic hemorrhage with a generalized auditory agnosia that evolved to an auditory sound agnosia. Their patient showed a temporal discrimination impairment on click fusion tests that is often described in patients following bilateral temporal lobe lesions. Tanawaki and colleagues[87] describe a patient who presented initially with generalized cortical deafness, which then evolved to a generalized auditory agnosia, and finally to an auditory sound agnosia. Neuroradiological examination of their patient revealed bilateral subcortical lesions involving the acoustic radiations following a bilateral putaminal hemorrhage. This patient made errors on tests of sound recognition that were discriminative rather than associative in nature. An unusual case of auditory sound agnosia following head injury was reported by Lambert and others.[86] In their patient, CT and MRI did not provide evidence of cortical or subcortical pathology, but CT showed an intraventricular hemorrhage without parenchymal lesion, resulting in ventricular enlargement. The patient showed deficits on a loudness discrimination test with no deficit observed in temporal auditory acuity.

Clarke and associates[80] described four patients with unilateral, left hemisphere damage who had deficits in auditory recognition, sound localization, or both. Based on lesion analysis, they propose that two anatomically distinct pathways exist for auditory sound recognition and auditory sound localization. The authors suggest that auditory recognition is mediated by the lateral auditory cortex and temporal convexity, whereas auditory localization is mediated by posterior auditory areas, the insula, and the parietal convexity. These anatomically distinct pathways parallel the distinctions made of distinct "what" and "where" pathways described in the human visual system. Additional support for anatomically distinct auditory systems comes from a functional MRI study with healthy individuals which showed greater activation in the auditory cortex and inferior frontal gyrus during sound identification tasks (pitch processing) and greater activation in bilateral posterior temporal, and inferior and superior parietal regions during sound localization tasks.[88]

These studies and others provide convincing evidence that auditory pattern and object recognition are processed along the temporal lobes—specifically, the anterior superior temporal gyrus and sulcus and parts of the middle temporal gyrus.[89]

In summary, case studies of auditory sound agnosia have suggested significant variability in both the localization and lateralization of neuropathology. As with pure word deafness, perceptual and associative forms of the disorder have been proposed, although these subtypes are not well defined. Evidence for distinct "what" and "where" pathways in the auditory modality is increasing with the use of functional imaging techniques.[88] In addition, recent neuroimaging studies have revealed that both the primary auditory cortex and the auditory association cortex may be needed to integrate environmental sounds, with a strong rightward asymmetry,[89] whereas the left temporal and frontal cortical regions are necessary for the analysis of speech information.[90] A review of recent neuroimaging studies of human audition will be presented at the end of this chapter.

"PARALINGUISTIC AGNOSIAS": AUDITORY AFFECTIVE AGNOSIA AND PHONAGNOSIA

The auditory speech signal conveys not only linguistic meaning but also—through variations in volume, timbre, pitch, and rhythm—information about the emotional state of the speaker (see Chap. 21). Recent clinical evidence suggests that comprehension of affective tone can be selectively impaired. Heilman and coworkers[91] showed that patients with hemispatial neglect from right temporoparietal lesions were impaired in the comprehension of affectively intoned speech (a deficit they called "auditory affective agnosia") but showed normal comprehension of linguistic speech content. Patients with left temporoparietal lesions and fluent aphasia showed normal comprehension of both linguistic and affective (paralinguistic) aspects of speech. Whether this defect is "agnosic" in nature remains to be seen, since auditory sensory/perceptual skills were not assessed. It is possible that auditory affective agnosia is a subtype of auditory sound agnosia (i.e., that it represents a category-specific auditory agnosia), but further studies are necessary before this can be asserted with any certainty.

Studies by Van Lancker and associates[92–94] have revealed another type of paralinguistic deficit after right hemisphere damage. In these studies, patients with unilateral right hemisphere damage showed deficits in discriminating and recognizing familiar voices, while patients with left hemisphere damage were impaired only on a task that required a discrimination between two famous voices. Although the exact nature of this distinction is elusive, it seems to parallel that between episodic (personally experienced) versus semantic (generally known) memory in amnesia research. Evidence from computed tomography (CT) suggested that right parietal damage resulted in voice-recognition impairment, while temporal lobe damage in either hemisphere led to deficits in voice discrimination. The authors refer to this deficit as "phonagnosia," but, like auditory affective agnosia, it remains to be seen whether it is truly agnosic in nature.

SENSORY (RECEPTIVE) AMUSIA

The subject of amusia has been reviewed in detail by Wertheim,[95] Critchley and Henson,[96] and Gates and Bradshaw.[97] *Sensory amusia* refers to an inability to appreciate various characteristics of heard music. Impairment of music perception occurs to some extent in all cases of auditory sound agnosia and in the majority of cases of aphasia[97] and pure word deafness, though its exact prevalence in such populations is unknown. Loss of musical perceptual ability is probably underreported because a specific musical disorder rarely interferes with everyday life.

Wertheim[95] believed that receptive amusia occurs more frequently with left hemisphere damage, while expressive musical disabilities are more apt to be associated with right hemisphere damage. More recent evidence suggests that music perception is a multicomponent process to which both hemispheres contribute in complex ways. Dichotic listening studies show that the right hemisphere plays a more important role than the left in the processing of musical and nonlinguistic sound patterns.[98,99] However, the left hemisphere appears to be important in the processing of sequential (temporally organized) material of any kind, including musical series. The dominant hemisphere may process

heard music more analytically or with more attention to specific features of the music, such as temporal order or rhythm.[97,100] According to Gordon,[99] melody recognition becomes more dependent on sequential processing as time and rhythm factors become more important for distinguishing tone patterns (see Ref. 101).

Many clinical studies distinguish between "instant" perceptual processes governing judgments of pitch, harmony, timbre, and intensity (loudness) and more "sequential," time-dependent processes governing melody recognition and judgments of rhythm and duration. Tentative clinical support for this kind of distinction exists in a double dissociation between the perceptual processing of pitch and the processing of temporal sequences,[102] dissociations that also hold true for reading music and for singing. There is further evidence that aspects of musical denotation (the "real-world" events referred to by lyrics) and musical connotation (the formal expressive patterns indicated by pitch, timbre, and intensity) are selectively vulnerable to focal brain lesions.[103,104] Gordon and Bogen[105] reported that during the right hemispheric anesthesia by the Wada procedure, singing was impaired with disrupted pitch production but preserved rhythmic expression. Hallucinations of voices and musical sounds have been reported with electrical stimulation of the lateral and superior surfaces of the first temporal convolutions in either hemisphere with more frequent occurrence on the nondominant side.[106] These complexities make it difficult to define receptive amusia and to localize the deficit to a particular brain region. Further complicating the picture is the fact that pitch, harmony, timbre, intensity, and rhythm may be affected to different degrees and in various combinations in the individual patient.

Peretz and colleagues[103] applied comprehensive nonverbal auditory testing to two patients with bilateral lesions of auditory cortex. In their patients, the perception of speech and environmental sounds was spared, but the perception of tunes, prosody, and voice was impaired. Based on these behavioral dissociations, they argue that music processing is distinct from the processing of speech or environmental sounds. Their data led them to argue for a task- and process-specific approach to the analysis of cases of auditory agnosia. They suggest that nominally "auditory" tasks should be broken down into their functional subcomponents and that more extensive component-based analysis of auditory processing deficits is warranted. For example, they distinguish between processes involved in the recognition of specific voices or musical instruments (which is timbre-dependent), and processes involved in recognition of tunes (which is pitch-dependent). The notion that nominally distinct classes of auditory material (e.g., melodies, prosody, and voice) share common processes may be critically important in developing a functional taxonomy of auditory recognition disorders in general and of amusia in particular.

This suggestion points out certain significant deficiencies in the evaluation of amusic patients. Although theories linking brain function to music perception have long been available,[95,107,108] such theories do not often contain sufficient process specificity to guide the clinical evaluation of amusic patients. Thus, for example, relatively little is known regarding which musical features will be most informative in constructing a neuropsychological model of music perception. Another obstacle to systematic study of acquired amusia is the variability of preillness musical abilities, interests, and experience (see Wertheim[95] for a system of classifying musical ability level). The cerebral organization of musical perception has been suggested to be dependent upon the degree of these preillness characteristics.[107]

NEUROIMAGING THE FUNCTIONAL ANATOMY OF AUDITORY PROCESSING

Recent advances in neuroimaging have contributed significantly to our understanding of auditory processing in both healthy and neurologically impaired individuals. While a thorough review of neuroimaging studies is beyond the scope of this chapter, an overview of the methods can be found in Chaps. 3 to 5, and an excellent review of recent positron emission tomography (PET), functional magnetic resonance imaging (fMRI), and magnetoencephalogram (MEG) studies of human auditory perception has been provided by Engelien and colleagues.[89] In addition, studies of human audition using EEG techniques have been reviewed in detail by Nuwer.[109] Here, we briefly describe some of the recent neuroimaging studies of auditory processing as they relate to our understanding of the cortical auditory disorders presented in this chapter. These studies provide evidence for specific neural networks that underlie the

clinical dissociations observed in patients with selective impairments in speech versus nonspeech sounds as well as those with impairments in attention to auditory information. In addition, we discuss neuroanatomical changes that may underlie recovery from auditory agnosia.

Tzourio and associates[110] used PET to investigate the functional anatomy of auditory selective attention in healthy males. Evoked response potentials were simultaneously recorded with PET, with regional cerebral blood flow (rCBF) measurements obtained during tasks of both passive listening and auditory selective attention to tones. Analysis of the results revealed that two different networks were recruited during passive listening and auditory selective attention. When passively listening to tones, bilateral activations were observed in Heschl's gyrus and the planum temporale, with a strong rightward asymmetry, and in the posterior part of the superior temporal gyrus. In addition, right precentral and right anterior cingulate rCBF increases were observed in the frontal lobe. A second "attentional" network was activated during selective attention to tones, which was composed of the anterior cingulum, the right precentral gyrus, and the right prefrontal cortex. These findings are consistent with studies of auditory sound agnosia which emphasize bilateral involvement, with a disproportionate contribution of the right temporal cortex in the processing of nonspeech sounds.[81] In addition, right frontal activations appear to comprise an auditory "attentional network" which may be additionally impaired in patients with cortical deafness whose performance is aided when attention is directed to auditory stimuli.[89]

Other researchers have used PET to identify the distributed neuronal systems activated by words, syllables, and environmental sounds in healthy individuals. Using this method, Giraud and Price[111] found that central regions in the superior temporal sulcus were equally responsive to speech (words and syllables) and environmental sounds, whereas the posterior and anterior regions of the left superior temporal gyrus were more active for speech. This study is consistent with other neuroimaging studies that have implicated the left temporal and frontal cortical regions in the analysis of speech information, and with clinical studies of patients with pure word deafness who generally have bilateral cortical-subcortical lesions involving the superior temporal gyrus and/or sulcus or unilateral damage to superior temporal regions on the left.

While many functional imaging studies have focused on identifying hemispheric and site-specific processing of verbal and nonverbal information, few studies have focused on the basis of this specialization. Zatorre and Belin[112] used PET to examine the response of human auditory cortex to spectral and temporal variations. They found that distinct subareas of auditory cortex respond to spectral and temporal features, with a leftward and rightward bias, respectively. Temporal changes recruited Heschl's gyrus in both hemispheres, with a greater activation on the left. Spectral changes recruited anterior superior temporal gyrus regions bilaterally, with greater activations on the right. The authors conclude that the left hemisphere's predominant role in complex linguistic function may be related to its ability to process the rapidly changing acoustic features involved in decoding speech sounds. As discussed above, impaired temporal processing of auditory information is one of the prevailing theories of pure word deafness.

Alternatively, Zatorre and Belin suggested that the role of the right hemisphere in spectral processing may underlie its importance in many aspects of musical perception and decoding affectively intoned speech which could explain some accounts of amusia, sound agnosia, and affective agnosia. These findings support a unified theory of complex sound processing disorders proposed by Griffiths and colleagues.[25] These authors suggested that the marked overlap observed among the various auditory agnosias may not be related to impairments in sound perception at the level of words, environmental sounds, or music. Rather, they propose that the auditory agnosias may best be described as "spectrotemporal disorders" in which there is a disruption in the interaction among temporal, spectral, and spatial properties of auditory stimuli. Additional neuroimaging and lesion studies designed to isolate spectral and temporal processing in healthy individuals and in patients are needed to clarify this issue.

Finally, studies examining the functional anatomy associated with recovery from auditory disorders are beginning to advance our understanding of cortical reorganization that may correspond to symptom resolution in many patients. Engelien and others[113] used PET to study the recovery from generalized auditory agnosia in a patient with bilateral perisylvian lesions who partially recovered the ability to recognize environmental sounds. During passive listening to sounds, activations were observed in the spared auditory cortex and in the right inferior parietal lobe and regions adjacent to the perisylvian lesion in the left hemisphere. During sound categorization (the "recovered function"), activations were observed in a bilateral distributed neural network comprising prefrontal, middle temporal, and inferior parietal cortices. In normal controls, sound categorization was associated with activation of a left network alone. This study suggests that bilateral activation and the recruitment of perilesional regions may constitute a functional recovery, or an attempt to compensate for, auditory processing deficits in patients recovering from auditory agnosia and auditory spectrum disorders.

SUMMARY

In this chapter, we have briefly reviewed major types of auditory recognition disorders. Although certain identifiable syndromes exist, our review suggests a bewildering array of clinical symptoms and assessment methods. A fundamental problem concerns the lack of a comprehensive theory of auditory cognition. Compared to vision, for example, we know relatively little about the cognitive architecture underlying auditory identification of voices or environmental sounds. This theoretical anarchy has led to terminologic confusion and has slowed development of a cognitive taxonomy of auditory disorders because it has been unsafe to assume that different authors are using such terms in the same way. Another problem is that relatively little agreement exists regarding necessary and sufficient methods of testing in patients with auditory recognition disturbances. Thus, for example, it is not uncommon for claims of a specific defect in one area of auditory processing to be made when, in fact, such specificity is a spurious result of incomplete testing. This problem has been noted by others,[9] and it is obvious that further theoretical development in the area of auditory recognition disturbances will depend on the ability of researchers to devise more comprehensive and theoretically driven assessments of auditory function.[103]

Despite these problems, some progress has been made in identifying potentially important dissociations within auditory recognition disturbances that may eventually reveal the underlying structure of higher auditory processes. Dissociations between verbal (pure word deafness) and nonverbal (auditory sound agnosia) deficits and between perceptual-discriminative and semantic-associative forms of recognition disturbance have been described. Recent findings of impairments in recognizing affective prosody, tunes, and voice are exciting because they raise the further possibility of "category-specificity"[75,114,115] (or process-specificity) in auditory recognition, as has been described for vision (see Chap. 10).

It seems clear at this point that further divisions within the concept of auditory agnosia are necessary and that a more comprehensive, process-based approach to evaluating auditory function is required. If this approach is developed further, the important building blocks in the structure of auditory cognition will eventually become apparent through behavioral dissociations. In our view, the clinical approach to a patient suspected of auditory agnosia should consist, at a minimum, of the following steps. First, extensive testing of nonauditory language functions and of general neuropsychological status should be conducted in order to rule out the contribution of aphasia or dementia to the auditory recognition deficit. Second, detailed testing of auditory-perceptual abilities should be conducted, including but not necessarily limited to pure tone audiometry, speech-detection thresholds, temporal auditory acuity (e.g., click fusion thresholds), auditory discrimination,[116] and sound-localization tasks. When possible, brainstem and cortical auditory evoked responses should be evaluated in order to ascertain the "level" at which the patient's deficit occurs. Third, a broad evaluation of auditory capacities should be conducted, including evaluation of the patient's ability to recognize speech, environmental sounds, and music. Performance in other areas not typically assessed in these patients (e.g., voice recognition, singing and related expressive behavior, and evaluation of the patient's ability to recognize linguistic and nonlinguistic prosody) should be assessed. In order to sharpen the hazy distinctions between auditory agnosia (identification and recognition disturbances) and auditory comprehension deficits associated with aphasia, it might also be fruitful to routinely subject aphasic groups to the same kind of comprehensive auditory testing instead of assuming that their impairment in speech comprehension is a straightforward consequence of linguistic impairment.

REFERENCES

1. Kanshepolsky J, Kelley J, Waggener J: A cortical auditory disorder. *Neurology* 23:699–705, 1973.
2. Miceli G: The processing of speech sounds in a patient with cortical auditory disorder. *Neuropsychologia* 20: 5–20, 1982.
3. Oppenheimer DR, Newcombe F: Clinical and anatomic findings in a case of auditory agnosia. *Arch Neurol* 35:712–719, 1978.
4. Rosati G, DeBastiani P, Paolino E, et al: Clinical and audiological findings in a case of auditory agnosia. *J Neurol* 227:21–27, 1982.
5. Goldstein MN, Brown M, Holander J: Auditory agnosia and word deafness: Analysis of a case with three-year follow up. *Brain Lang* 2:324–332, 1975.
6. Ulrich G: Interhemispheric functional relationships in auditory agnosia: An analysis of the preconditions and a conceptual model. *Brain Lang* 5:286–300, 1978.
7. Buchman AS, Garron DC, Trost-Cardamone JE, et al: Word deafness: One hundred years later. *J Neurol Neurosurg Psychiatry* 49:489–499, 1986.
8. Mendez MF, Geehan GR: Cortical auditory disorders: Clinical and psychoacoustic features. *J Neurol Neurosurg Psychiat* 51:1–9, 1988.
9. Vignolo LA: Auditory agnosia: A review and report of recent evidence. In Benton AL (ed): *Contributions to Clinical Neuropsychology*. Chicago: Aldine, 1969.
10. Lhermitte F, Chain F, Escourolle R, et al: Etudo des troubles per-ceptifs auditifs dans les lesion temporales bilaterales. *Rev Neurol* 128:329–351, 1971.
11. Teuber H-L: Alteration of perception and memory in man, in Weiskrantz L (ed): *Analysis of Behavior Change*. New York: Harper & Row, 1968.
12. Jerger J, Weikers N, Sharbrough F, Jerger S: Bilaeral lesions of the temporal lobe: A case study. *Acoto-Laryngologica,* 258(suppl):1–51, 1969.
13. Jerger J, Lovering L, Wertz M: Auditory disorder following bilateral temporal lobe insult: Report of a case. *J Speech Hearing Dis* 37:523–535, 1972.
14. Michel J, Peronnet F, Schott B: A case of cortical deafness: Clinical and electrophysiological data. *Brain Lang* 10:367–377, 1980.
15. Massopoust LC, Wolin LR: Changes in auditory frequency discrimination thresholds after temporal cortex ablation. *Exp Neurol* 19:245–251, 1967.

16. Dewson JH, Pribram KH, Lynch JC: Effects of ablation of temporal cortex upon speech sound discrimination in the monkey. *Exp Neurol* 24:279–291, 1969.

17. Celesia GG: Organization of auditory cortical areas in man. *Brain* 99:403–414, 1976.

18. Mahoudeau D, Lemoyne J, Dubrisay J, Caraes J: Sur un cas dagnosie auditive. *Rev Neurol* 95:57, 1956.

19. Wohlfart G, Lindgren A, Jernelius B: Clinical picture and morbid anatomy in a case of "pure word deafness." *J Nerv Ment Dis* 116:818–827, 1952.

20. Engelein A, Huber W, Silbersweig D, et al: The neural correlates of 'deaf-hearing' in man: Conscious sensory awareness enabled by attentional modulation. *Brain* 123:532–545, 2000.

21. Garde MM, Cowey A: "Deaf hearing": Unacknowledged detection of auditory stimuli in a patient with cerebral deafness. *Cortex* 36:71–80, 2000.

22. Wakabayashi Y, Nakano T, Isono M, Hori S: Cortical deafness due to bilateral temporal subcortical hemorrhages associated with moyamoya disease: Report of a case. *No Shinkei Geka* 27:915–919, 1999.

23. Leicester J: Central deafness and subcortical motor aphasia. *Brain Lang* 10:224–242, 1980.

24. Earnest MP, Monroe PA, Yarnell PA: Cortical deafness: Demonstration of the pathologic anatomy by CT scan. *Neurology* 27:1172–1175, 1977.

25. Griffiths TD, Rees A, Green GGR: Disorders of human complex sound processing. *Neurocase* 5:365–378, 1999.

26. Mendez MF, Geehan GR: Cortical auditory disorders: Clinical and psychoacoustic features. *J Neurol Neurosurg Psychiatry* 51:1–9, 1988.

27. Tanaka Y, Kamo T, Yoshida M, Yamadori A: "So-called" cortical deafness. Clinical, neurophysiological, and radiological observations. *Brain* 114:2385–2401, 1991.

28. Penhune VB, Zatorre RJ, MacDonald JD, Evans AC: Interhemispheric anatomical differences in human primary auditory cortex: Probabilistic mapping and volume measurement from magnetic resonance scans. *Cereb Cortex* 6:661–672, 1966.

29. Kazui S, Naritomi H, Sawada T, Inque N: Subcortical auditory agnosia. *Brain Lang* 38:476–487, 1990.

30. Motomura N, Yamadori A, Mori E, Tamaru F: Auditory agnosia: Analysis of a case with bilateral subcortical lesions. *Brain* 109:379–391, 1986.

31. Hasegawa M, Bando M, Iwata M, et al: A case of auditory agnosia with the lesion of bilateral auditory radiation. *Rinsho Shinkeigaku* 29:180–185, 1989.

32. Johkura K, Matsumoto S, Hasegawa O, Kuroiwa Y: Defective auditory recognition after small hemorrhage in the inferior colliculi. *J Neurol Sci* 161:91–96, 1988.

33. Kussmaul A: Disturbances of speech, in von Ziemssien H (ed): *Cyclopedia of the Practice of Medicine*. New York: William Wood, 1877.

34. Lichteim L: On aphasia. *Brain* 7:433–484, 1885.

35. Kanter SL, Day AL, Heilman KM, Gonzalez-Rothi LJ: Pure word deafness: A possible explanation of transient-deterioration after extracranial-intracranial bypass grafting. *Neurosurgery* 18:186–189, 1986.

36. Liepmann H, Storch E: Der mikroskopische Gehirnbefund bei dem Fall Gorstelle. *Monatsschr Psychiatr Neurol* 11:115–120, 1902.

37. Schuster P, Taterka H: Beitrag zur Anatomie und Klinik der reinen Worttaubbeit. *Z Neurol Psychiatr* 105:494, 1926.

38. Geschwind N: Disconnexion syndromes in animals and man. *Brain* 88:237–294, 585–644, 1965.

39. Arias M, Requena I, Ventura M, et al: A case of deaf-mutism as an expression of pure word deafness: Neuroimaging and electrophysiological data. *Eur J Neurol* 2:583–585, 1995.

40. Karibe H, Yonemori T, Matsuno F, et al: A case of tentorial meningioma presented with pure word deafness. *No To Shinkei* 52:997–1001, 2000.

41. Kaga M: Language disorders in Landau-Kleffner syndrome. *J Child Neurol* 14:118–122, 1999.

42. Klein SK, Kurtzberg D, Brattson A, et al: Electrophysiologic manifestations of impaired temporal lobe auditory processing in verbal auditory agnosia. *Brain Lang* 51:383–405, 1995.

43. Pearce PS, Darwish H: Correlation between EEG and auditory perceptual measures in auditory agnosia. *Brain Lang* 22:41–48, 1984.

44. Baynes K, Kegl JA, Brentari D, et al: Chronic auditory agnosia following Landau-Kleffner syndrome: A 23 year outcome study. *Brain Lang* 63:381–425, 1988.

45. Albert ML, Bear D: Time to understand: A case study of word deafness with reference to the role of time in auditory comprehension. *Brain* 97:373–384, 1974.

46. Klein R, Harper J: The problem of agnosia in the light of a case of pure word deafness. *J Mental Sci* 102:112–120, 1956.

47. Gazzaniga M, Glass AV, Sarno MT: Pure word deafness and hemispheric dynamics: A case history. *Cortex* 9:136–143, 1973.

48. Ziegler DK: Word deafness and Wernicke's aphasia: Report of cases and discussion of the syndrome. *Arch Neurol Psychiatry* 67:323–331, 1942.

49. Otsuki M, Soma Y, Sato M, et al: Slowly progressive pure word deafness. *Eur Neurol* 39:135–140, 1988.

50. Yaqub BA, Gascon GG, Al-Nosha M, Whitaker H: Pure word deafness (acquired verbal auditory agnosia) in an Arabic speaking patient. *Brain* 111:457–466, 1988.

51. Anegawa T, Hara K, Yamamoto K, Matsuda M: Unilateral auditory hallucinations due to left temporal lobe ischemia: A case report. *Rinsho Shinkeigaku* 35:1137–1141, 1995.

52. Shoumaker RD, Ajax ET, Schenkenberg T: Pure word deafness (auditory verbal agnosia). *Dis Nerv Sys* 38:293–299, 1977.

53. Mendez MF, Rosenberg S: Word deafness mistaken for Alzheimer's disease: Differential characteristics. *J Amer Geriat Soc* 39:209–211, 1991.

54. Reinhold M: A case of auditory agnosia. *Brain* 73:203–223, 1950.

55. Hemphill RC, Stengel E: A study of pure word deafness. *J Neurol Psychiatry* 3:251–262, 1940.

56. Wee J, Menard MR: "Pure word deafness": Implications for assessment and management in communication disorder—a report of two cases. *Arch Phys Med Rehabil* 80:1106–1109, 1999.

57. Caplan LR: Variability of perceptual function: The sensory cortex as a categorizer and deducer. *Brain Lang* 6:1–13, 1978.

58. Auerbach SH, Allard T, Naeser M, et al: Pure word deafness: Analysis of a case with bilateral lesions and a defect at the prephonemic level. *Brain* 105:271–300, 1982.

59. Chocholle R, Chedru F, Bolte MC, et al: Etude psychoacoustique d'un cas de surdite corticale. *Neuropsychologia* 13:163–172, 1975.

60. Denes G, Semenza C: Auditory modality-specific anomia: Evidence from a case of pure word deafness. *Cortex* 11:401–411, 1975.

61. Saffran EB, Marin OSM, Yeni-Komshian GH: An analysis of speech perception in word deafness. *Brain Lang* 3:255–256, 1976.

62. Wang E, Peach RK, Xu Y, et al: Reception of dynamic acoustic patterns by an individual with unilateral verbal auditory agnosia. *Brain Lang* 73:442–455, 2000.

63. Croisile B, Laurent B, Michel D, et al: Different clinical types of degenerative aphasia. *Rev Neurol* 147:192–199, 1991.

64. Nakakoshi S, Kashino M, Mizobuchi A, et al: Disorder in sequential speech perception: A case study on pure word deafness. *Brain Lang* 76:119–129, 2001.

65. Naeser M: The relationship between phoneme discrimination, phoneme/picture perception, and language comprehension in aphasia. Presented at the Twelfth Annual Meeting of the Academy of Aphasia, Warrenton, Virginia, October 1974.

66. Stockard JJ, Rossiter VS: Clinical and pathologic correlates of brainstem auditory response abnormalities. *Neurology* 27:316–325, 1977.

67. Makino M, Takanashi Y, Iwamoto K, et al: Auditory evoked magnetic fields in patients of pure word deafness. *No To Shinkei* 50:51–55, 1998.

68. Coslett HB, Brashear HR, Heilman KM: Pure word deafness after bilateral primary auditory cortex infarcts. *Neurology* 34:347–352, 1984.

69. Polster MR, Rose SB: Disorders of auditory processing: Evidence for modularity in audition. *Cortex* 34:47–65, 1998.

70. Corballis MC: Neuropsychology of perceptual functions, in Zaidel E (ed), *Neuropsychology*. New York: Academic Press, 1994, pp 83–104.

71. Franklin S, Turner J, Ralph M, Morris J, Bailey PL: A distinctive case of word-meaning deafness. *Cognit Neuropsychol* 13:1139–1162, 1996.

72. Tyler LK, Moss HE: Imageability and category specificity. *Cognit Neuropsychol* 14:293–318, 1977.

73. Bauer RM: Agnosia, in Heilman KM, Valenstein E (eds): *Clinical Neuropsychology,* 3d ed. New York: Oxford University Press, 1993, pp 215–278.

74. Farah MJ: *Visual Agnosia: Disorders of Object Vision and What They Tell Us about Normal Vision,* 2d ed. Cambridge, MA: MIT Press/Bradford, 2003.

75. Farah MJ, Meyer M, McMullen PA: The living/nonliving dissociation is not an artifact. *Cognit Neuropsychol* 13:137–154, 1996.

76. Buchtel HA, Stewart JD: Auditory agnosia: Apperceptive or associative disorder? *Brain Lang* 37:12–25, 1989.

77. Goldstein MN: Auditory agnosia for speech ("pure word deafness"): A historical review with current implications. *Brain Lang* 1:195–204, 1974.

78. Kliest K: Gehirnpathologische und Lokalisatorische Ergebnisse uber Horstorungen, Geruschtaubheiten und Amusien. *Monatsschr Psychiatr Neurol* 68:853–860, 1928.

79. Albert ML, Sparks R, von Stockert T, Sax D: A case study of auditory agnosia: Linguistic and nonlinguistic processing. *Cortex* 8:427–433, 1972.

80. Clarke S, Bellmann A, Meuli RA, Assal, et al: Auditory agnosia and auditory spatial deficits following left hemispheric lesions: Evidence for distinct processing pathways. *Neuropsychologia* 38:797–807, 2000.

81. Fujii T, Fukatsu R, Watabe S, et al: Auditory sound agnosia without aphasia following a right temporal lobe lesion. *Cortex* 26:263–268, 1990.

82. Nielsen JM, Sult CW Jr: Agnosia and the body scheme. *Bull LA Neurol Soc* 4:69–81, 1939.

83. Spreen O, Benton AL, Fincham R: Auditory agnosia without aphasia. *Arch Neurol* 13:84–92, 1965.

84. Wortis SB, Pfeffer AZ: Unilateral auditory-spatial agnosia. *J Nerv Ment Dis* 108:181–186, 1948.

85. Habib M, Daquin G, Milandre L, et al: Mutism and auditory agnosia due to bilateral insular damage—role of the insula in human communication. *Neuropsychologia* 33:327–339, 1995.

86. Lambert J, Eustache F, Lechevalier B, et al: Auditory agnosia with relative sparing of speech perception. *Cortex* 25:71–82, 1989.

87. Taniwaki T, Tagawa K, Sato F, Iino K: Auditory agnosia restricted to environmental sounds following cortical deafness and generalized auditory agnosia. *Clin Neurol Neurosurg* 102:156–162, 2000.

88. Alain C, Arnott, SR, Hevenor S, et al: "What" and "where" in the human auditory system. *Proc Natl Acad Sci U S A* 98:12301–12306, 2001.

89. Engelien A, Stern E, Silbersweig DA: Functional neuroimaging of human central auditory processing in normal subjects and patients with neurological and neuropsychiatric disorders. *J Clin Exp Neuropsychol* 23:94–120, 2001.

90. Binder JR: Neuroanatomy of language processing studied with functional MRI. *Clin Neurosci* 4:87–94, 1997.

91. Heilman KM, Scholes R, Watson RT: Auditory affective agnosia. Disturbed comprehension of affective speech. *J Neurol Neurosurg Psychiatry* 38:69–72, 1975.

92. Van Lancker DR, Kreiman J: Unfamiliar voice discrimination and familiar voice recognition are independent and unordered abilities. *Neuropsychologia* 25:829–834, 1988.

93. Van Lancker DR, Kreiman J, Cummings J: Voice perception deficits: Neuroanatomical correlates of phonagnosia. *J Clin Exp Neuropsychol* 11:665–674, 1989.

94. Van Lancker DR, Cummings JL, Kreiman J, Dobkin BH: Phonagnosia: A dissociation between familiar and unfamiliar voices. *Cortex* 24:195–209, 1988.

95. Wertheim N: The amusias, in Vinken PJ, Bruyn GW (eds): *Handbook of Clinical Neurology.* Amsterdam: North-Holland, 1969, vol 4.

96. Critchley MM, Henson RA: *Music and the Brain: Studies in the Neurology of Music.* Springfield, IL: Charles C Thomas, 1977.

97. Gates A, Bradshaw JL: The role of the cerebral hemispheres in music. *Brain Lang* 4:403–431, 1977.

98. Blumstein S, Cooper W: Hemispheric processing of intonation contours. *Cortex* 10:146–158, 1974.

99. Gordon HW: Auditory specialization of the right and left hemispheres, in Kinsbourne M, Smith WL (eds): *Hemispheric Disconnection and Cerebral Function.* Springfield, IL: Charles C Thomas, 1974.

100. Krashen SD: Mental abilities underlying linguistic and nonlinguistic functions. *Linguistics* 115:39–55, 1973.

101. Mavlov L: Amusia due to rhythm agnosia in a musician with left hemisphere damage: A nonauditory supramodal defect. *Cortex* 16:331–338, 1980.

102. Peretz I: Processing of local and global musical information by unilateral brain-damaged patients. *Brain* 113:1185–1205, 1990.

103. Peretz I, Kolinsky R, Tramo M, et al: Functional dissociations following bilateral lesions of auditory cortex. *Brain* 117:1283–1301, 1994.

104. Gardner H, Silverman H, Denes G, et al: Sensitivity to musical denotation and connotation in organic patients. *Cortex* 13:242–256, 1977.

105. Gordon HW, Bogen JE: Hemispheric lateralization of singing after intracarotid sodium amylobarbitone. *J Neurol Neurosurg Psychiatry* 37:727–738, 1974.

106. Penfield W, Perot P: The brain's record of auditory and visual experience. *Brain* 86:595–696, 1963.

107. Bever TG, Chiarello RJ: Cerebral dominance in musicians and nonmusicians. *Science* 185:137–139, 1974.

108. Hecaen H: Clinical symptomotology in right and left hemispheric lesions, in Mountcastle VB (ed): *Interhemispheric Relations and Cerebral Dominance.* Baltimore: Johns Hopkins University Press, 1962.

109. Nuwer MR: Fundamentals of evoked potentials and common clinical applications today. *EEG Clin Neurophysiol* 106:142–148, 1998.

110. Tzourio N, Massioui FE, Crivello F, et al: Functional anatomy of human auditory attention studied with PET. *Neuroimage* 5:63–77, 1997.

111. Giraud AL, Price CJ: The constraints functional neuroimaging places on classical models of auditory word processing. *J Cogn Neurosci* 13:754–765, 2001.

112. Zattore RJ, Belin P: Spectral and temporal processing in human auditory cortex. *Cereb Cortex* 11:946–953, 2001.

113. Engelien A, Silbersweig D, Stern E, et al: The functional anatomy of recovery from auditory agnosia. A PET study of sound categorization in a neurological patient and normal controls. *Brain* 118:1395–1409, 1995.

114. Warrington EK, Shallice T: Category-specific semantic impairments. *Brain* 107:829–854, 1984.

115. Damasio AR: Category-related recognition defects as a clue to the neural substrates of knowledge. *Trends Neurosci* 13:95–98, 1990.

116. Chedru F, Bastard V, Efron R: Auditory micropattern discrimination in brain damaged subjects. *Neuropsychologia* 16:141–149, 1978.

Chapter 13

DISORDERS OF BODY PERCEPTION AND REPRESENTATION

Georg Goldenberg

In classic neuropsychology, disorders of the perception and of the mental representation of one's body have been conceptualized as being due to the breakdown of a mental "body schema." The body schema has been a central concept to neuropsychological thinking for many years (see reviews in Refs. 1 to 3). It has been attacked as being ill-defined and as narrowing the view to isolated aspects of more general disorders of language and spatial perception, respectively.[4] However, recent research in normal psychology and physiology has brought forward experimental evidence for the contention that perception and representation of one's body are distinct psychological functions[5–8] and has revived interest in their neuropsychological disturbances.

LEVELS OF INFORMATION ABOUT ONE'S BODY

In this chapter, three levels are distinguished at which information about one's body is processed and represented in the cognitive architecture of the human:

A Body-Centered Reference System for Motor Actions

Information about the current configuration and position of one's body is a necessary prerequisite for the planning and execution of most movements aimed at external targets. Muscles move limbs relative to the body and hence within a body-centered frame of reference. The simple motor act of reaching with the hand for a visually presented object requires that the retinotopic coordinates of the perceived object are transformed into body-centered coordinates. This transformation has to take into account the current position of the eyes relative to the head and of the head relative to the trunk. In addition to the representation of the target in body-centered coordinates, the brain must also represent the initial arm configura-

tion in order to plan the trajectory. Single-cell recordings in monkeys have provided evidence that cells in the intraparietal sulcus and adjacent areas 7 and 5 of the posterior parietal lobe are informed about the current position and configuration of the eyes, the head, the body, and the limbs and perform the computations necessary for transforming visually perceived locations into body-centered coordinates.[9,10]

Reaching for an object is a highly automatized task. One need not pay attention to the position and configuration of one's body in order to accurately reach for a seen object. Assessment of the body-centered reference frame and computation of the target's location in body-centered coordinates take place automatically and without necessitating conscious awareness of one's body. The body-centered reference frames used for the planning of movements are implicitly involved in movement planning but do not regularly enter into explicit awareness.

Awareness of One's Own Body

One can pay attention to the position and configuration of one's own body. One can use vestibular, kinesthetic, tactile, and to a limited degree also visual perceptions for inferring the actual position and configuration of one's body. Even in the absence of distinct afferents from these channels, one has a basic "feeling" of where one's body parts are. One can point to the tip of one's nose without a mirror even if the nose does not itch. It is this basic awareness of the limits and of the spatial layout of one's own body which has originally been conceptualized as the "body schema."[11]

General Knowledge about the Human Body

General knowledge about the human body and body parts can have two basically different forms.[12] On the one hand, there is lexical and semantic knowledge, which defines the names, categories, and functions of body parts. This knowledge base specifies, for example, that the wrist and ankle are both articulations, or that the mouth is for speaking and the ear for hearing. On the other hand, there is knowledge about the spatial structure of body parts. This knowledge base specifies the position of individual body parts, the proximity relations that exist between them, and the boundaries that define each body part. For example, it specifies that the nose is in the middle of the face and that its upper end is contiguous to the forehead, with the line of the eyebrows marking the border between them. Furthermore, it defines the back of the nose as an entity that is different from the tip or from the flanks. Hence, the small spatial distance between back and flank is significant, whereas larger distances within the back are not significant for the definition of these body parts.

This knowledge applies equally to one's own or another person's body as well as to sculptural and pictorial representations of the human body. It may also be needed for successful performance of tasks intended to test awareness of one's own body. When given the order "point to the back of your nose," one must have a general concept of what and where the back of the nose is before one can search for it.

With this schematic division of the "body schema" in mind, seven neuropsychological symptoms are treated here: optic ataxia, body-part phantoms, unilateral neglect, awareness of one's own body, autotopagnosia, finger agnosia, and impaired imitation of gestures.

OPTIC ATAXIA

Optic ataxia was originally described in association with apraxia of gaze and simultanagnosia,[13] but it has since then been recognized as an independent symptom that can occur without the other elements of Balint's syndrome.[14-18] Patients with optic ataxia cannot accurately reach for visually perceived external targets. They move their hands into the approximate vicinity of the target and then start searching movements with the widely opened hand. By contrast, they can reach without hesitation or error to parts of their own body. Asked to touch the tip of the nose, they do so as fast and accurately as do controls. A patient who was unable to grasp the outstretched finger of the examiner could accurately touch her own finger placed passively

in the same location.[14] Pointing to auditorily perceived locations can be preserved as well.[15] Misreaching may be confined to the periphery of the visual field, leaving patients able to reach accurately for external targets when they are allowed to fixate them visually before moving the hand.[18]

Many patients with optic ataxia also have difficulties when asked to explore, compare, and estimate spatial positions without reaching for them, but there is no correlation between the severity of this general visuospatial disorder and the severity of visual misreaching. Single patients with optic ataxia pass all tests of visuospatial estimation and exploration perfectly,[14,15] and many patients with severe visuospatial problems can accurately reach for visually presented targets.[19-21]

One interpretation of optic ataxia is that the basic disorder concerns the transformation of retinotopic locations into a body-centered reference frame necessary for movement planning. The patients can accurately reach for parts of their own bodies because body parts are a priori coded in body-centered coordinates. At the same time, successful pointing to body parts indicates that awareness of the patient's own body is preserved as well as general conceptual knowledge about the human body.

Single-cell recordings in monkeys have provided ample evidence that neuronal networks in parietal area 5 and 7 are capable of transcoding visual locations from retinotopic to body-centered reference frames.[9,10,22] The lesions causing optic ataxia are centered around the intraparietal sulcus too and regularly affect area 5 or 7.[15]

With unilateral lesions, optic ataxia can be restricted to the hand or the hemifield opposite the lesioned hemisphere or even only to their combination.[15,16] As already mentioned, manual misreaching may contrast with accurate fixation by saccades.[18] These dissociations indicate that transformations from retinotopic to body-centered coordinates are made by mechanisms dedicated to single body parts and restricted sectors of the visual field.

BODY-PART PHANTOMS

The occurrence of phantom limbs has been among the first[11] and continues to be among the most impressive arguments for the contention that the brain houses a mental body schema that underlies and modifies the way in which we experience our own bodies. After amputations, about 90 percent of adults experience a phantom of lost limbs.[23–25] Phantom experiences have also been reported after loss of eyes, teeth, external genitalia, and the female breast.[24] Phantoms of the amputated breast occur less regularly than phantoms of amputated limbs; still, they occur in about 40 percent of women after mastectomy.[26,27]

Limb phantoms occur not only after amputation but can also be caused by nervous system lesions provided that all afferents from the affected body part are interrupted. This may be the case with lesions of the peripheral nerves, the plexus, and the spinal cord but also with subcortical cerebral lesions.[23,24,28] If the deafferented limb is still present and visible, the phantom may be experienced as an additional, supernumerary limb,[24,28] thus violating the anatomic constraints of the normal body.

Initially, most limb phantoms are experienced in the same way as the true limb was experienced before amputation, but over time the experience may become less natural. Particularly in upper limb phantoms, the representation of the proximal portions may become weaker and eventually vanish, leading to the strange sensation of a hand belonging to one's own body but being disconnected from it. Alternatively, a shrinking of the proximal portions may lead to "telescoping" and give rise to the belief that the phantom arm is shorter than the other arm. Telescoping causes a severe deformation of size and shape of phantoms and may result in the anatomically impossible location of fingers inside the stump.[11,24,29] Full-sized phantoms may be in unnatural positions, violating anatomic constraints. For example, the hand of a phantom arm may penetrate into the chest.[30]

Visual and Somatosensory Influences on Phantom Sensation

Although the very existence of a phantom contradicts the visual evidence for absence of the limb, the phantom experience can be shaped by visual experience. In patients fitted with prostheses, phantoms frequently adapt to their shape.[31,32] Some amputated patients integrate the prosthesis into their body and identify it with the phantom. They feel touch directly at the surface of the prosthesis rather than deducing it from the prosthesis's pressure on the stump.[33] Visual influence on phantom sensations has also been demonstrated in a series of elegant experiments on patients with upper limb phantoms by Ramachandran and coworkers.[25,34] They "resurrected" vision of the phantom arm by means of a mirror reflecting the patient's opposite arm. Movement of the mirror image induced a feeling of phantom movement and touch of the intact arm a sensation at the mirror location on the phantom.

It has been established for about 50 years that touch of the stump can evoke referred sensations in phantoms of amputated limbs,[29,35] but only recently has it been shown that referred sensations can originate in body parts that have no anatomic proximity to the amputated body part. In patients with upper limb amputations, referred sensations have been evoked from both sides of the chest, both sides of the face, and the contralateral arm.[25,36–40] Sensations in phantoms of amputated breasts have been evoked by touch of both sides of the back and the ipsilateral pinna.[41] The presence, extent, and localization of referred sensations vary greatly between patients. In some an exact and reproducible topographic remapping from stimulated to referred locations has been demonstrated, which remained stable for up to several weeks. Reexaminations after longer delays, however, have documented radical changes or even complete breakdown of topographic referral without accompanying changes of the phantom's size and shape.[6,36,38]

Phantoms in Congenital Absence of Limbs

The possibility of phantom limbs in persons with congenital absence or very early amputation of limbs has been reliably established,[31–33,42–46] but their frequency is substantially lower than after later amputation. Permanent phantoms are reported by some 10 percent of persons with congenital absence or very early amputation of limbs as compared to about 90 percent of persons amputated after the age of 10 years.[31,33] The incidence rises to some 20 percent when temporary phantom sensations are considered.[32,42] Some persons report to have had phantoms as long as they can remember,[46,47] but in the majority phantoms occur only after a delay. The mean time to phantom onset has been calculated to be 9 years in congenital absence and 2.3 years in early amputation.[32] The emergence of the phantom may be triggered by minor trauma to the stump.[31]

As the affected children had no or only rudimentary opportunity to experience the presence of the now missing limb, the phantom has been said to testify a genetic prefiguration of the mental representation of body shape.[32,43] There is, however, evidence that experience does shape phantoms in children. In children with early amputation of congenitally deformed limbs, the phantom may replicate the initial deformation rather than a normal limb.[32,42] This shaping by early experience may contrast with an inability to consciously remember the deformation. Like phantoms of adult patients, those of children may be triggered or shaped by prostheses: phantoms of congenitally absent or early lost limbs are more frequent in children who had been fitted with prostheses than in those without,[31,42] and they usually adapt their size and shape to the prosthesis.[31,44,47]

The Cerebral Substrate of Phantom Experience

Plasticity of somatotopic organization of primary sensory cortex in patients with phantoms after amputation of the lower arm and hand has been demonstrated by functional imaging with magnetoencephalography.[38,39,45,48,49] The receptive fields of adjacent regions, devoted to the face on one side and to the upper arm on the other, invade the receptive field originally devoted to the hand. The parallel to remapping of sensations from face and stump to the phantom is striking, but a longitudinal study found that the topography of referred sensations can change without correlated changes in cortical remapping.[38] This finding would suggest that some factor other than cortical remapping must contribute to remapping of sensation. Possibly this factor is to be sought in an interpretative activity of higher brain centers that integrate information from sensory cortex with other sensory afferents to produce a coherent body image.

There are a few cases on record where a cerebral lesion abolished a phantom limb. In all of them the clinical evidence pointed to lesion in the parietal lobe of the opposite hemisphere,[30,50,51] and one autopsy confirmed a metastasis in the supramarginal gyrus. In a further case, clinical evidence strongly suggested sparing of primary sensory cortex.[51] A recent study by functional magnetic resonance imaging [46] found activations in inferior parietal and premotor but not in primary motor or sensory cortex of a patient with phantoms of congenitally absent limbs when she moved her phantom arms. Taken together, these findings suggest that the phantom experience is constructed in the parietal lobe.

NEGLECT OF ONE-HALF OF THE BODY

Patients with hemineglect may neglect not only one-half of external space but also one-half of their own body. They behave as if they had lost one-half of the body. When combing, washing, shaving, and dressing, they restrict grooming to the nonneglected half of their body. When asked to indicate with their normal hand the midline of their body, they deviate to the healthy side[52,53] as if they would bisect only the nonneglected half of their body. When asked to reach with their normal hand to the neglected one, their reaching movement may end at the shoulder or even at the midline of the trunk.[54]

Studies looking for the possibility that neglect of one-half of the body may dissociate from neglect of one-half of external space have yielded inconsistent results. One found personal hemineglect without extrapersonal hemineglect in only 1 out of 97 right brain–damaged patients, while the reverse dissociation occurred in 9 patients.[54] Another study with a smaller sample of patients and more sensitive tests of personal neglect found that one-third of the patients had predominantly extrapersonal, one-third predominantly personal, and one-third combined hemineglect[55]; there also is one report of a patient showing severe personal neglect in testing as well as in spontaneous behavior but no extrapersonal hemineglect at all.[56] On the other hand, there are experimental demonstrations of intricate interactions between personal and extrapersonal neglect in patients who display both. In patients with left hemineglect, blindfolded detection of touch of the left hand improves when the hand is placed across the body midline into the right hemispace.[57] When the ulnar and radial sides of the left hand are touched simultaneously, neglect will affect the side that happens to lie on the left side. Ulnar touch will be neglected when the hand is pronated and radial touch when the hand is supinated.[58,59] The dependence of tactile sensation on hand position suggests an influence of position in peripersonal space on sensations arising from intrapersonal space.

In view of the paucity of systematic observation, it would be premature to offer any speculation as to the location of lesions responsible for personal neglect. It is not even clear whether the preponderance of left-sided hemineglect applies to personal neglect. The large studies that established this hemispheric asymmetry were all restricted to measures of extrapersonal neglect, and the above-mentioned studies that systematically compared personal and extrapersonal neglect were restricted to patients with right brain damage. In clinical practice, right-sided personal neglect following left brain damage may escape observation when there is right-sided hemiplegia and apraxia of the left limbs, as this constellation renders patients unable to groom and dress themselves and thus prevents dramatic manifestations of personal neglect—as, for example, the shaving or dressing of only one-half of the body.

AWARENESS OF ONE'S OWN BODY

Body-part phantoms and neglect of one-half of the body are both disorders that involve the awareness of the patient's own body. In a way, they mirror each other: in body-part phantoms there is awareness of body parts that in reality are absent, while in neglect, body parts that in reality are present are excluded from awareness.

Kinematic analyses revealed abnormalities of reaching in patients with left hemineglect,[19,20,52] but they are different from those shown by patients with optic ataxia. Movements toward targets in the neglected half of space are slowed down and the movement path may deviate toward the nonaffected side of space, but the patients ultimately reach visible targets accurately and without insecurity or searching. Defective awareness of one's own body is usually associated with normal general knowledge about the human body. Patients with phantom limbs or with hemineglect are able to point on command to single parts of their own body provided that these parts are not amputated or, respectively, neglected.[60]

AUTOTOPAGNOSIA

Taken literally, the term *autotopagnosia* would indicate an inablity to recognize locations on one's own body, but it is generally understood as designating the inability to localize body parts on one's own body as well as on another person's body or on a model of the human body. The term *somatotopagnosia*[61] would be more appropriate but has not found wide acceptance.

Earlier case reports of autotopagnosia have been criticized as demonstrating nothing more than the effects of general mental deterioration or of aphasia on the task of pointing to body parts on verbal command; since then, however, several carefully conducted single-case studies have established the independence of autotopagnosia from aphasia and dementia and have drawn a consistent clinical picture of "pure" autotopagnosia.[12,62–68] When asked to point to body parts on themselves, another person, or a model of the human body, these patients commit errors. The majority of these errors are "contiguity" errors: the patients search in the vicinity of the designated body part. Less frequent are "semantic" errors that confuse body parts of the same category, as, for example, the elbow and the knee. These errors occur not only when the body parts are designated by verbal command but also when they are shown on pictures or even when the examiner demonstrates correct pointing and the patient tries to imitate. Most of the patients were able to name the body parts when they were pointed at by someone else or shown on pictures, and although they invariably had left-sided brain lesions (see below), several of them were not aphasic at all.[12,62,63,65,68] Some patients were asked to give verbal descriptions of body parts. They could describe the function and the individual visual appearance of body parts but got lost when asked to describe their location.[12,62,65]

The inability to locate a body part need not affect all body parts nor must it be restricted to the human body. There are patients with autotopagnosia in whom localizing of individual fingers was found to be preserved,[62–64] while some patients had problems not only with pointing to body parts but also with pointing to single parts of other multipart objects like bicycles.[62,63,69] There are, however, other patients with autotopagnosia who could locate the parts of bicycles or animals.[65–67] The conclusion that their disturbance is restricted to the topography of only the human body remains nonetheless arguable. It may be questioned whether the structure of other multipart objects involves, to a similar degree, subtle distinctions between easily confusable and adjacent parts as the structure of the human body. If such distinctions exist, their cognizance is reserved to experts and falls outside the scope of neuropsychological examination. By contrast, subtle distinctions between easily confusable parts of the human body are tested in autotopagnosia and account for the majority of errors. Knowledge about the structure of the human body may be more vulnerable to brain damage because it is more fine-grained and diversified than knowledge about other multipart objects. Few persons have expert knowledge about bicycles but all have expert knowledge about the human body.

Awareness of the patient's own body seems to be preserved in autotopagnosia: Such patients can reach body parts accurately when asked to indicate the typical location of accessories (e.g., a wristwatch) or the location of objects which had been temporarily fixed to a body part.[12,66,67] Apparently they can orient themselves on their own body, and their autotopagnosia stems from the inability to link preserved spatial orientation on their own body with conceptual knowledge about the human body.

The lesions in "pure" cases of autotopagnosia are remarkably uniform and always affect the posterior parietal lobe of the left hemisphere.[62–68] In a group study of patients with left or right brain damage, errors in pointing to body parts occurred only in left brain–damaged patients.[70] In this unselected sample there were no "pure" cases of autotopagnosia. The patients who committed errors in localizing body parts were all aphasic and had on average larger lesions than patients who performed without error.

FINGER AGNOSIA

Finger agnosia was originally described as part of the "Gerstmann syndrome,"[71] which is a combination of finger agnosia with right-left confusion, acalculia, and agraphia, but it has been demonstrated that these symptoms can occur independently of each other.[72]

The value of verbal tasks of finger identification has been called in question because they may be more sensitive to language disorders than to defective orientation on the body.[70,73] However, a considerable number of brain-damaged patients fail on nonverbal tasks of finger localization such as pointing on a drawing of a hand to fingers touched on the own hand[70,73–75] or indicating how many fingers lie between two fingers touched simultaneously by the examiner.[76]

Finger agnosia has been considered as a minor form of autotopagnosia,[71] but we have already mentioned that there are patients with autotopagnosia in whom identification of fingers is preserved. Whereas autotopagnosia has been observed exclusively in patients with left brain damage, finger agnosia occurs with approximately equal frequency in patients with left and right brain damage.[70,73,74,76] There is thus no regular association of finger agnosia with autotopagnosia. Another association has hitherto been examined only in a few patients and may turn out to be more regular: these patients had similar difficulties with selection of toes as with selection of fingers.[75,77]

IMITATION OF MEANINGLESS GESTURES

Defective imitation of meaningless gestures has been recognized as a symptom of apraxia following left brain damage.[78–80] Other symptoms of apraxia are disturbed production and imitation of meaningful gestures, like waving good-bye or miming the use of a hammer, and disturbed use of real objects. There are, however, patients with pure "visuoimitative apraxia" in whom defective imitation of meaningless gestures contrasts with preservation of production and imitation of meaningful gestures and object use.[81,82] It thus seems justified to discuss defective imitation of meaningless gestures as a disorder on its own.

Defective imitation of meaningless gestures affects not only the translation of gestures from a model to the patient's own body but also translation to other instances of human bodies. Patients who commit errors when imitating with their own bodies also commit errors when asked to replicate the demonstrated gesture on a mannikin[83] or to select the gesture from an array of photographs showing gestures performed by different persons and seen under different angles of view.[84]

Like the dissociation between autotopagnosia and finger agnosia, defective imitation of meaningless gestures can affect imitation of gestures defined by

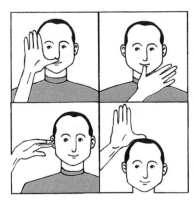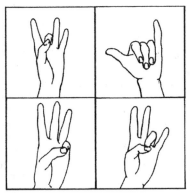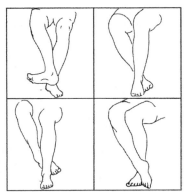

Figure 13-1
Examples of hand, finger, and foot posture used for assessing imitation of meaningless gestures.

proximal body parts differently from finger configurations. Figure 13-1 shows three types of meaningless gestures that have been used to explore these differences: Hand postures specify a position of the hand relative to face and head while the internal configuration of the hand remains invariant. Finger postures specify different configurations of the fingers while the position of the hand is not considered for scoring. Foot postures specify a position of one foot relative to the other foot and leg.[85] Patients with left brain damage have problems with all kind of gestures, but the impairment is distinctly less severe for finger than for hand and foot postures. There are even single apraxic patients in whom defective imitation of hand postures contrasts with completely normal imitation of finger configurations.[82] By contrast, patients with right brain damage have the most difficulties with finger postures and imitate hand postures nearly as perfectly as controls.[84–86]

The dissociation between imitation of hand and finger postures is very similar to the dissociation between autotopagnosia and finger agnosia. Indeed, nonverbal testing for autotopagnosia and finger agnosia may be conceptualized as being a variant of imitation of hand positions and finger configurations.

BODY-PART SPECIFICITY OF KNOWLEDGE ABOUT THE HUMAN BODY

A possible explanation for body-part specificity of disturbed imitation starts from the assumption that imitation of meaningless gestures is accomplished by body-part coding based on general knowledge about the human body.[82,84,85,87] Body-part coding reduces the multiple visual details of the demonstrated gesture to simple relationships between a limited number of well-defined body parts and produces an equivalence between demonstration and imitation that is independent of the different modalities and perspectives of perceiving one's own and other persons' bodies. It accommodates novel and meaningless gestures to combinations of familiar elements. Demands on body-part coding increase with increasing number and diversity of body parts involved in the gesture.

The body-part specificity of autotopagnosia, finger agnosia, and disturbed imitation of meaningless gestures could be accommodated by the assumption that access to knowledge needed for body-part coding is bound to integrity of the left hemisphere but that an additional right hemisphere contribution is needed when demands on perceptual discrimination of body parts increase. Finger configurations pose exceptionally low demands on access to knowledge because they are constituted by one set of uniform elements that differ only in their serial position; however, for the same reasons, their perceptual discrimination is difficult. By contrast, hand postures demand consideration of a variety of different body parts—like forehead, eyebrows, eyes, nose, cheeks, lips and chin on the face, or shoulder, upper arm, elbow, lower arm, wrist, back, and palm of the hand on the upper extremity. Most of them are, however, perceptually salient and hence easy to discriminate. Imitation of foot postures also involves a number of conceptually different parts—like ankle, heel, calf, big toe, and little toe—several of which are perceptually less salient than the parts of the face that have been used to determine hand postures. The different distribution of demands on body-part coding and perceptual discrimination can account for the predominant affection of hand postures in left brain damage and of finger postures in right brain damage and possibly also for disturbed pointing to proximal body parts in autotopagnosia and disturbed selection of single fingers in finger agnosia.

CONCLUSION

We have postulated that information about one's body is represented at three levels. The review of clinical disorders of body perception confirmed the validity of the classification by demonstrating that distinct disorders arise from disturbances at each level. It did not yield evidence for the existence of a unitary "body schema" underlying all forms of body perception. Body perception for different purposes employs different representations. It is questionable whether some of these representations are specifically dedicated to body perception or are applications of more general mechanisms and representations to perception of that highly familiar but intricate mechanical device that is the human body.

REFERENCES

1. Frederiks JAM: Disorders of the body schema, in Frederiks JAM (ed): *Handbook of Clinical Neurology.* Amsterdam: Elsevier, 1985, vol 1, pp 373–393.
2. Denes G: Disorders of body awareness and body knowledge, in Boller F, Grafman J (eds): *Handbook of Neuropsychology.* Amsterdam, New York, Oxford: Elsevier, 1990, vol 2, pp 207–228.
3. Goldenberg G: Body perception disorders, in Ramachandran VS (ed): *Encyclopedia of the Human Brain.* San Diego, CA: Academic Press; 2002, vol 1, pp 443–458.
4. Poeck K, Orgass B: The concept of the body schema: A critical review and some experimental results. *Cortex* 7:254–277, 1971.
5. Reed CL, Farah MJ: The psychological reality of the body schema: A test with normal participants. *J Exp Psychol Hum Percept Perform* 21:334–343, 1995.
6. Berlucchi G, Aglioti S: The body in the brain: neural bases of corporeal awareness. *Trends Neurosci* 20:560–564, 1997.
7. Buccino G, Binkowski F, Fink GR, et al: Action observation activates premotor and parietal areas in a somatotopic manner: an fMRI study. *Eur J Neurosci* 13:400–404, 2001.
8. Grossman E, Donelly M, Price R, et al: Brain areas involved in perception of biological motion. *J Cogn Neurosci* 12:711–720, 2000.
9. Stein JF: The representation of egocentric space in the posterior parietal cortex. *Behav Brain Sci* 15:691–700, 1992.
10. Milner AD, Goodale MA: *The Visual Brain in Action.* Oxford, New York, Tokyo: Oxford University Press; 1995.
11. Pick A: Zur Pathologie des Bewußtseins vom eigenen Körper—Ein Beitrag aus der Kriegsmedizin. *Neurol Zentralbl* 34:257–265, 1915.
12. Sirigu A, Grafman J, Bressler K, Sunderland T: Multiple representations contribute to body knowledge processing. *Brain* 114:629–642, 1991.
13. Balint R: Seelenlaehmung des "Schauens," optische Ataxie, raeumlice Stoerung der Aufmerksamkeit. *Monatschr Psychiatr Neurol* 25:51–81, 1909.
14. Rondot P, De Recondo J, Dumas JLR: Visuomotor ataxia. *Brain* 100:355–376, 1977.
15. Perenin MT, Vighetto A: Optic ataxia; a specific disruption in visuomotor mechanisms: I. Different aspects of the deficit in reaching for objects. *Brain* 111:643–674, 1988.
16. Rizzo M, Rotella D, Darling W: Troubled reaching after right occipito-temporal damage. *Neuropsychologia* 30:711–722, 1992.
17. Jeannerod M, Decety J, Michel F: Impairment of grasping movements following a bilateral posterior parietal lesion. *Neuropsychologia* 32:369–380, 1994.
18. Buxbaum LJ, Coslett HB: Subtypes of optic ataxia: Reframing the disconnection account. *Neurocase* 3:159–166, 1997.
19. Chieffi S, Gentilucci M, Allport A, et al: Study of selective reaching and grasping in a patient with unilateral parietal lesion. *Brain* 116:1119–1137, 1993.
20. Mattingley JB, Phillips JG, Bradshaw JL: Impairment of movement execution in unilateral neglect: A kinematic analysis of directional bradykinesia. *Neuropsychologia* 32:1111–1134, 1994.

21. Hermsdörfer J, Ulrich S, Marquardt C, et al: Prehension with the ipsilesional hand after unilateral brain damage. *Cortex* 35:139–162, 1999.

22. Andersen RA: Visual and eye movement functions of the posterior parietal cortex. *Annu Rev Neurosci* 12:377–403, 1989.

23. Poeck K: Zur Psychophysiologie der Phantomerlebnisse. *Nervenarzt* 34:241–256, 1963.

24. Frederiks JAM: Phantom limb and phantom limb pain, in Frederiks JAM (ed): *Handbook of Neurology*. Amsterdam: Elsevier, 1985, vol 1, pp 395–404.

25. Ramachandran VS, Hirstein W: The perception of phantom limbs—the D.O. Hebb lecture. *Brain* 121:1603–1630, 1998.

26. Kroner K, Krebs B, Skov J, Jorgensen HJ: Immediate and long-term phantom breast syndrome after mastectomy: Incidence, clinical characteristics and relationship to pre-mastectomy breast pain. *Pain* 36:327–334, 1989.

27. Christensen K, Blichert-Toft M, Giersing U, et al: Phantom breast syndrome in young women after mastectomy for breast cancer. *Acta Chir Scand* 148:351–354, 1982.

28. Halligan PW, Marshall JC, Wade DT: Three arms: a case study of supernumerary phantom limb after right hemisphere stroke. *J Neurol Neurosurg Psychiatry* 56:159–166, 1993.

29. Haber WE: Observations on phantom-limb phenomena. *Arch Neurol Psychiatry* 75:624–636, 1956.

30. Bornstein B: Sur le phénomène du membre fantome. *Encéphale* 38:32–46, 1949.

31. Saadah ESM, Melzack R: Phantom limb experiences in congenital limb-deficient adults. *Cortex* 30:469–478, 1994.

32. Melzack R, Israel R, Lacroix R, Schultz G: Phantom limbs in people with congenital limb deficiency or amputation in early childhood. *Brain* 120:1603–1620, 1997.

33. Poeck K: Phantome nach Amputation und bei angeborenen Gliedmaßenmangel. *Dtsch Med Wochenschr* 46:2367–2374, 1969.

34. Ramachandran VS, Rogers-Ramachandran D: Synaesthesia in phantom limbs induced with mirrors. *Proc R Soc Lond B* 263:377–386, 1996.

35. Cronholm B: Phantom limbs in amputees: Study of changes in integration of centripetal impulses with special reference to referred sensation. *Acta Psychiatr Neurol Scand Suppl* 72:1–310, 1951.

36. Halligan PJ, Marshall JC, Wade DT: Sensory disorganization and perceptual plasticity after limb amputation: A follow-up study. *Neuroreport* 5:1341–1345, 1994.

37. Halligan PJ, Marshall JC, Wade DT, et al: Thumb in cheek? Sensory reorganization and perceptual plasticity after limb amputation. *Neuroreport* 4:233–236, 1993.

38. Knecht S, Henningsen H, Höhling C, et al: Plasticity of plasticity? Changes in the pattern of perceptual correlates of reorganization after amputation. *Brain* 121:717–724, 1998.

39. Knecht S, Henningsen H, Elbert T, et al: Reorganizational and perceptional changes after amputation. *Brain* 119:1213–1219, 1996.

40. Kew JJM, Halligan PW, Marshall JC, et al: Abnormal access of axial vibrotactile input to deafferented somatosensory cortex in human upper limb amputees. *J Neurophysiol* 77:2753–2764, 1997.

41. Aglioti S, Cortese F, Franchini C: Rapid sensory remapping in the adult human brain as inferred from phantom breast sensation. *Neuroreport* 5:473–476, 1994.

42. Weinstein S, Sersen EA, Vetter RJ: Phantom and somatic sensation in cases of congenital aplasia. *Cortex* 1:276–290, 1964.

43. Melzack R: Phantom limbs and the concept of a neuromatrix. *Trends Neurosci* 13:88–92, 1990.

44. Lacroix R, Melzack R, Smith D, Mitchell N: Multiple phantom limbs in a child. *Cortex* 28:503–508, 1992.

45. Ramachandran VS: Behavioral and magnetoencephalographic correlates of plasticity in the adult human brain. *Proc Natl Acad Sci U S A* 90:10413–10420, 1993.

46. Brugger P, Kollias S, Müri RM, et al: Beyond remembering: Phantom sensations of congenitally absent limbs. *Proc Natl Acad Sci U S A* 97:6167–6172, 2000.

47. Poeck K: Phantoms following amputation in early childhood and in congenital absence of limbs. *Cortex* 1:269–275, 1964.

48. Flor H, Elbert T, Knecht S, et al: Phantom-limb pain as a perceptual correlate of cortical reorganization following arm amputation. *Nature* 375:482–484, 1995.

49. Pascual-Leone A, Peris M, Pascual AP, Catalá MD: Reorganization of human cortical motor output maps following traumatic forearm amputation. *Neuroreport* 7:2068–2070, 1996.

50. Head H, Holmes G: Sensory disturbances from cerebral lesions. *Brain* 34:102–254, 1911.

51. Appenzeller O, Bicknell JM: Effects of nervous system lesions on phantom experience in amputees. *Neurology* 19:141–146, 1969.

52. Jeannerod M: *The Neural and Behavioural Organization of Goal-Directed Movements*. Oxford: Clarendon Press, 1988.

53. Karnath HO: Subjective body orientation in neglect and the interactive contribution of neck muscle proprioception and vestibular stimulation. *Brain* 117:1001–1012, 1994.

54. Bisiach E, Perani D, Vallar G, Berti A: Unilateral neglect: personal and extrapersonal. *Neuropsychologia* 24:759–767, 1986.

55. Beschin N, Robertson IH: Personal versus extrapersonal neglect: A group study of their dissociation using a reliable clinical test. *Cortex* 33:379–384, 1997.

56. Guariglia C, Padovani A, Pantano P, Pizzamiglio L: Unilateral neglect restricted to visual imagery. *Nature* 364:235–237, 1993.

57. Aglioti S, Smania N, Manfredi M, Berlucchi G: Disownership of left hand and objects related to it in a patient with right brain damage. *Neuroreport* 8:293–296, 1996.

58. Moscovitch M, Behrmann M: Coding of spatial information in the somatosensory system: Evidence from patients with neglect following parietal lobe damage. *J Cogn Neurosci* 6:151–155, 1994.

59. Mattingley JB, Bradshaw JL: Can tactile neglect occur at an intra-limb level? Vibrotactile reaction times in patients with right hemisphere damage. *Behav Neurol* 7:67–77, 1994.

60. Guariglia C, Antonucci G: Personal and extrapersonal space: A case of neglect dissociation. *Neuropsychologia* 30:1001–1010, 1992.

61. Gerstmann J: Problems of imperception of disease and of impaired body territories with organic lesions. Relation to body scheme and its disorders. *Arch Neurol Psychiatry* 48:890–913, 1942.

62. De Renzi E, Scotti G: Autotopagnosia: fiction or reality? *Arch Neurol* 23:221–227, 1970.

63. Poncet M, Pellissier JF, Sebahoun M, Nasser CJ: A propos d'un cas d'autotopagnosie secondaire à une lésion pariéto-occipitale de l'hémisphère majeur. *Encéphale* 61:1–14, 1971.

64. Assal G, Butters J: Troubles du schéma corporel lors des atteintes hémisphériques gauches. *Schweiz Med Rundsch* 62:172–179, 1973.

65. Ogden JA: Autotopagnosia. Occurence in a patient without nominal aphasia and with an intact ability to point to parts of animals and objects. *Brain* 108:1009–1022, 1985.

66. Semenza C: Impairment of localization of body parts following brain damage. *Cortex* 24:443–450, 1988.

67. Denes G, Cappelletti JY, Zilli T, et al: A category-specific deficit of spatial representation: the case of autotopagnosia. *Neuropsychologia* 38:345–350, 2000.

68. Buxbaum LJ, Coslett HB: Specialised structural descriptions for human body parts: Evidence from autotopagnosia. *Cogn Neuropsychol* 18:289–306, 2001.

69. Denes G, Caviezel F, Semenza C: Difficulty in reaching objects and body parts: A sensory motor disconnection syndrome. *Cortex* 18:165–173, 1982.

70. Sauguet J, Benton AL, Hecaen H: Disturbances of the body schema in relation to language impairment and hemispheric locus of lesion. *J Neurol Neurosurg Psychiatry* 34:496–501, 1971.

71. Gerstmann J: Zur Symptomatologie der Hirnläsionen im Übergangsgebiet der unteren Parietal- und mittleren Occipitalwindung. *Nervenarzt* 3:691–696, 1930.

72. Benton AL: The fiction of the "Gerstmann syndrome." *J Neurol Neurosurg Psychiatry* 24:176–181, 1961.

73. Poeck K, Orgass B: An experimental investigation of finger agnosia. *Neurology* 19:801–807, 1969.

74. Gainotti G, Cianchetti C, Tiacci C: The influence of the hemispheric side of lesion on nonverbal tasks of finger localization. *Cortex* 8:364–381, 1972.

75. Mayer E, Martory MD, Pegna AJ, et al: A pure case of Gerstmann syndrome with a subangular lesion. *Brain* 122:1107–1120, 1999.

76. Kinsbourne M, Warrington EK: A study of finger agnosia. *Brain* 85:47–66, 1962.

77. Tucha O, Steup O, Smely C, Lange KW: Toe agnosia in Gerstmann syndrome. *J Neurol Neurosurg Psychiatry* 63:399–403, 1997.

78. De Renzi E, Motti F, Nichelli P: Imitating gestures—a quantitative approach to ideomotor apraxia. *Arch Neurol* 37:6–10, 1980.

79. De Renzi E: Apraxia, in Boller F, Grafman J (eds): *Handbook of Clinical Neuropsychology*. Amsterdam, New York, Oxford: Elsevier, 1990, vol 2, pp 245–263.

80. Rothi LJG, Ochipa C, Heilman KM: A cognitive neuropsychological model of limb praxis. *Cogn Neuropsychol* 8:443–458, 1991.

81. Mehler MF: Visuo-imitative apraxia. *Neurology* 37(suppl):129, 1987.

82. Goldenberg G, Hagmann S: The meaning of meaningless gestures: A study of visuo-imitative apraxia. *Neuropsychologia* 35:333–341, 1997.

83. Goldenberg G: Imitating gestures and manipulating a mannikin—the representation of the human body in ideomotor apraxia. *Neuropsychologia* 33:63–72, 1995.

84. Goldenberg G: Matching and imitation of hand and finger postures in patients with damage in the left or right hemisphere. *Neuropsychologia* 37:559–366, 1999.

85. Goldenberg G, Strauss S: Hemisphere asymmetries for imitation of novel gestures. *Neurology* 59:893–897, 2002.

86. Goldenberg G: Defective imitation of gestures in patients with damage in the left or right hemisphere. *J Neurol Neurosurg Psychiatry* 61:176–180, 1996.

87. Meltzoff AN, Moore MK: Explaining facial imitation: A theoretical model. *Early Dev Parent* 6:179–192, 1997.

Chapter 14

NEGLECT I: CLINICAL AND ANATOMICAL ISSUES

Kenneth M. Heilman
Robert T. Watson
Edward Valenstein

Neglect is a failure to report, respond, or orient to stimuli that are presented contralateral to a brain lesion when this failure is not due to elementary sensory or motor disorders.[1] Many subtypes of neglect have been described. A major distinction is between neglect of perceptual input, termed *sensory neglect* or *inattention*, and neglect affecting response outputs, termed *motor* or *intentional neglect*. Some further distinctions are outlined below.

Sensory neglect involves a selective deficit in awareness, which may apply to all stimuli on the affected side of space (*spatial neglect*) or be confined to stimuli impinging on the patient's body (*personal neglect*). It may even effect awareness of one side of internal mental images (*representational neglect*). The perceptual modalities affected by neglect may also vary: subtypes of sensory neglect exist for the visual, auditory, and tactile modalities. The deficit in awareness is accompanied by an abnormal attentional bias. Attention is usually biased toward the ipsilesional side (*contralateral neglect*) but in rare cases may be contralesional (*ipsilateral neglect*). Once attention is engaged on an ipsilesional stimulus, subjects may have difficulty disengaging their attention to move it to the contralesional side. If the lack of awareness and attentional bias are present only when there is a competing stimulus at a more ipsilateral location, the disorder is termed *extinction*. Many patients with neglect recover and become able to detect isolated contralesional stimuli, but they continue to manifest extinction.

Motor or *intentional neglect* involves a response failure that cannot be explained by weakness, sensory loss, or unawareness. There may be a failure to move a limb (*limb akinesia*), or the limb can be moved but only after a long delay and strong encouragement (*hypokinesia*). Patients with intentional neglect who

can move may make movements of decreased amplitude (*hypometria*). They may also have an inability to maintain posture or movements (*impersistence*). Patients with motor neglect who can move their contralesional limb may fail to move this limb (or have a delay) when they are also required to move their ipsilateral limb (*motor extinction*). Limb akinesia, hypokinesia, hypometria, and motor impersistence can affect some or all parts of the body, including limbs, eyes, or head. The elements of intentional neglect discussed above can be *directional* (toward the contralesional hemispace) or *spatial* (within the contralesional hemispace). Patients with motor neglect may have intentional biases such that there is a propensity to move toward ipsilesional space. There may also be impaired ability to disengage from motor activities (*motor perseveration*).

TESTING FOR NEGLECT

In this brief review we cannot address all aspects of testing; therefore, for a complete discussion and list of references, the reader is referred to Heilman and coworkers.[1]

Inattention or Sensory Neglect

To test for inattention, the patient is presented with unilateral stimuli on either the ipsilesional or contralesional side in random order. If a patient fails to detect more stimuli on the contralesional side than the ipsilesional side, it would suggest that the patient is suffering from inattention. However, if the patient totally fails to detect any stimuli on the contralesional side, it is often difficult to tell whether or not the patient has inattention or a sensory loss. The auditory modality is the least difficult in which to dissociate inattention and sensory loss, because sounds made on one side of the head project to both ears, and each ear projects to both the ipsilateral and the contralateral hemisphere. Therefore, if a patient is unaware of noises made on one side of his or her head, this unawareness cannot be explained by a sensory defect and suggests that the patient has inattention. In the visual modality, because unawareness may be hemispatial (body-centered) rather than retinotopic, having the patient deviate the eyes toward ipsilateral hemispace may allow him or her to become aware of stimuli projected to the contralesional portion of the retina. In regard to tactile neglect, one may have to use caloric stimulation of the ear to see if the patient can detect stimuli during such stimulation. One may also use psychophysiologic techniques such as evoked potentials or galvanic skin responses to see whether patients who are unaware of stimuli demonstrate autonomic signs of stimulus detection.[2]

Extinction

To test for extinction, one may randomly intermix the unilateral stimuli described above with bilateral simultaneous stimuli. The stimuli can be given in any modality (e.g., visual, auditory, tactile). When a subject has hemianopia, extinction may occur even within the ipsilesional visual field.

Intentional or Motor Neglect

Patients who have severe limb akinesia may appear to have a hemiparesis. An arm may flaccidly hang off the bed or wheelchair. Sometimes, with strong encouragement from the examiner, it can be demonstrated that such a patient has normal strength. Some patients, however, will still not move, and one may have to rely on brain imaging to learn whether the corticospinal tract is involved. In patients with motor neglect, the lesion should not involve the corticospinal system. Magnetic stimulation may also be helpful in demonstrating that the corticospinal tract is normal.[3] As discussed, patients with hypokinesia are reluctant to move the affected arm or only move it after delay. However, once they have moved, their strength may be normal. To test for hypometria, the arm is passively moved or the patient is shown a line and asked to make a movement of the same length. Patients with hypometria will undershoot

the target. To test for impersistence, the patient is asked to sustain a posture. Patients with impersistence cannot maintain postures. As mentioned, patients can be tested for forms of motor neglect by using the limbs, eyes, or even head. They can be tested in ipsilateral versus contralateral hemispace and in an ipsilesional versus contralesional direction. For example, patients with right hemisphere lesions might have trouble spontaneously looking leftward (directional akinesia) and even have their eyes deviate to the right (gaze palsy). Other patients might be able to look leftward but make small (hypometric) saccades (directional hypometria). Patients with right hemisphere lesions who are able to look to the left might be unable to sustain gaze in this direction (directional impersistence).

Further Assessments of Spatial Neglect

A more complete assessment of neglect involves additional tests, which require the patient to perform simple tasks that go beyond the reporting of a stimulus or the movement of eyes or limbs toward a target. These tasks can nevertheless be performed at bedside without special equipment. The four most commonly used tests are described here.

In the *line bisection task,* the patient is given a long line and asked to indicate its midpoint (Fig. 14-1). Although horizontal lines are most commonly used (intersection of the coronal and axial planes), neglect has been reported in the vertical dimension (both up neglect and down neglect) and in the radial dimension (near neglect and far neglect). In general, the longer the line, the greater the percentage of error. Placing the line in contralesional hemispace can also increase the severity of the error, as can putting cues on the ipsilesional side.

In performing the *cancellation task,* a sheet of paper that contains targets is placed before the patient and the patient is asked to mark out (cancel) all the targets (Fig. 14-2). Increasing the number of targets can increase the sensitivity of this test. Increasing the difficulty with which one discriminates targets from distractors can also increase the sensitivity of this task.

In testing *drawing,* the patient should be asked to draw spontaneously as well as to copy figures (Figs. 14-3 and 14-4). Copying asymmetrical nonsense figures may be more difficult than copying well-known symmetrical figures.

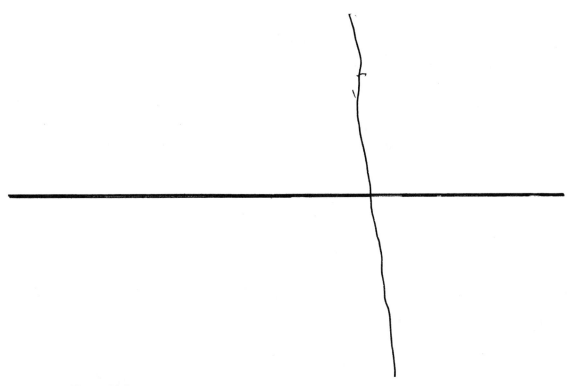

Figure 14-1
Line bisection task performed by a patient with a right hemisphere infarction and left hemispatial neglect. (Courtesy of Dr. Todd E. Feinberg.)

In testing for representational neglect, one should ask a subject to *image a familar scene* and then report what he or she sees. A patient with representational neglect will recall more objects from the ipsilesional than the contralesional part of the image.

Further testing can elucidate the underlying systems of spatial representation, attention, and intention that are affected. For example, it may be difficult to dissociate sensory attentional disorders from motor intentional disorders. In general, the best means of doing this is by performing cross-response tasks where the subject responds in one side of space to a stimulus presented on the opposite side. Video cameras, strings and pulleys, or mirrors can be used in the performance of a cross response task.

To dissociate intentional from representational defects, one can use a fixed-aperture technique. To do this, an opaque sheet with a fixed window is placed over a sheet with targets so that only one target can be seen at a time, thereby reducing attentional demands. In one-half the trials, the subject moves the top sheet; in the other trials, the subject moves the target sheet. A failure to explore one portion of the target sheet in both conditions suggests a representational defect, and a failure to explore opposite sides of the target sheet in direct and indirect conditions suggests a motor intentional deficit.[4]

To dissociate spatial neglect of one side of the environment from neglect of one side of the person, one can ask the patient to lie down on his or her side. This decouples the environmental left and right from the body's left and right. If the patient has a right hemispheric lesion, is lying on the right side, and now fails to detect targets toward the ceiling, the neglect is body-centered. However, if the patient continues to neglect targets on the left side of the room, the neglect is environmentally centered (see Chap. 15).[5,6]

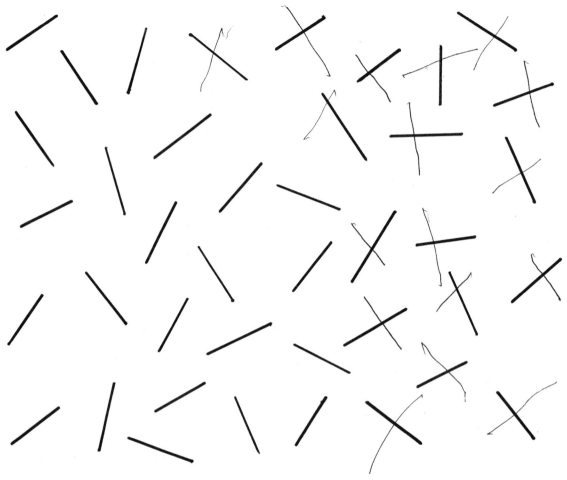

Figure 14-2
Cancellation task of same patient as in Fig. 14-1. (Courtesy of Dr. Todd E. Feinberg.)

PATHOPHYSIOLOGY

As the foregoing review suggests, neglect is not a homogeneous syndrome. The neglect syndrome has not only many manifestations but also many levels of explanation. For a more complete discussion, see Heilman and coworkers.[1] The heterogeneity of neglect is apparent on an anatomic level as well.

In humans, neglect is most often associated with lesions of the inferior parietal lobe (IPL), which includes Brodmann's areas 40 and 39. However, neglect has also been reported from dorsolateral frontal lesions, medial frontal lesions that include the cingulate gyrus, thalamic-mesencephalic lesions, basal ganglia, and white matter lesions. Because there is a limit on the anatomic, physiologic, and behavioral research that can be done in humans, much of what we know about the pathophysiology of the neglect syndrome comes from research on Old World monkeys. Monkeys also have an IPL; however, their IPL is Brodmann's area 7. In humans, the intraparietal sulcus separates the superior parietal area, Brodmann's area 7, from the inferior parietal lobule, Brodmann's areas 40 and 39. Some have thought that the IPL of monkeys is a homologue of the IPL in humans. Others, however, have thought that both banks of the superior temporal sulcus (STS)

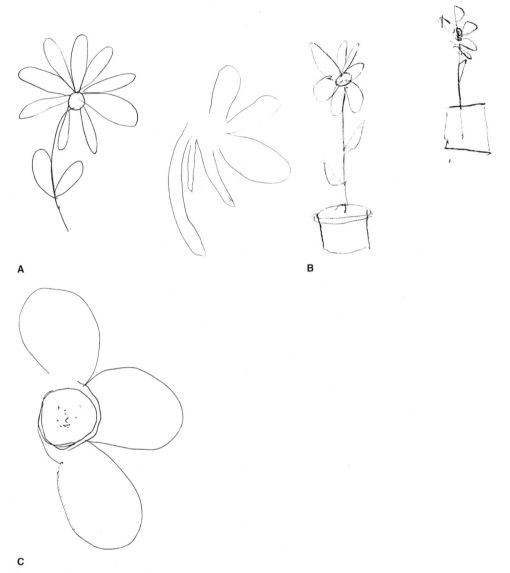

Figure 14-3
Copies of flower demonstrate left hemispatial neglect. A *and* B *provide models on left, patient production on right. (Parts* A *and* B *courtesy of Dr. Todd E. Feinberg; part* C *courtesy of Dr. Robert Rafal.)*

are the homologue of the inferior parietal lobule in humans. We[7] have demonstrated that spatial neglect in monkeys is primarily associated with ablation of the STS region and not the IPL. These results suggest that, in regard to neglect, it is the monkeys' STS that

is the homologue of the temporoparietal junction of humans.

Anatomic studies of the STS of monkeys have provided some information as to why this area produces neglect when ablated. The STS is composed of

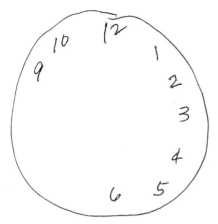

Figure 14-4
Clock drawn by a patient with left hemispatial neglect.
(Courtesy of Dr. Robert Rafal.)

multiple subareas and is one of the sites of multimodal sensory convergence. Visual, auditory, and somatosensory association cortices all project to portions of the STS. In addition, the STS has reciprocal connections to other multimodal convergence areas, such as monkeys' IPL (Brodmann's area 7). Because ablation of area 7 in monkeys, a multimodal convergence area, was not associated with spatial neglect, we do not believe that ablation of a sensory convergence area alone can account for the unawareness that is seen with neglect syndrome. Therefore, we[7] have proposed a role for monkeys' STS in awareness.

Mishkin and colleagues[8] have suggested that the visual system, when presented with stimuli, performs dual parallel processes. Whereas the ventral division is important for determining the type of stimulus ("What is it?"), the dorsal system codes the spatial location of the stimulus ("Where is it?"). In monkeys the "where" system is in part mediated by the posterior portion of Brodmann's area 7 or the monkey's IPL, and the "what" system is in part being mediated by the inferior visual association cortex found in the ventral temporal lobe. It has long been recognized that bilateral ventral temporal lesions in humans and monkeys induce visual object agnosia, a deficit in the "what" system. In contrast, biparietal lesions in monkeys induce deficits of visual spatial localization but not object discrimination. We[7] have posited that these "where" and "what" systems in-

tegrate in the banks of monkeys' STS or in the inferior parietal lobule of humans. According to our research,[7] lesions of monkeys' STS and humans' temporoparietal junction induce unawareness or neglect not only because this is the area that receives polymodal sensory input but also because it is a convergence site of these perceptual-cognitive systems that deal with both the "what" and "where" aspects of environmental awareness. Both anatomic and electrophysiologic data substantiate the hypothesis that monkeys' STS is an area of convergence of these two systems (see Ref. 7). We[7] have also proposed that similar areas important for spatial localization and object identification may also exist in the auditory and tactile systems and that these modalities may also converge in the STS.

Although there is anatomic and physiologic evidence that there is convergence from the Brodmann's area 7 "where" system and the ventral temporal lobes' "what" system, this cannot account for the observation that ablation of the STS induces unawareness. The STS receives input not only from these "what" and "where" systems but also from the cingulate gyrus and the dorsolateral frontal lobe. In earlier studies, we have demonstrated that lesions in both these areas are also able to induce neglect. The dorsolateral prefrontal region is important in the mediation of goal-directed behavior and may provide the STS with information that is not directly stimulus-dependent or related to immediate drives and biological needs but rather directed at long-term goals. The cingulate gyrus is part of the limbic system and may provide the STS with information about biological needs and drives. Because monkeys' STS or humans' temporoparietal junction are supplied with "what" and "where" conative and motivational information, it may be able to make attentional computations.

Monkeys' STS has reciprocal connections with the ventral temporal "what" region and the parietal "where" region. Therefore, after the STS region performs an attentional computation, it may reciprocally influence the neurons in the ventral temporal lobe and Brodmann's area 7 regions.

Electrical stimulation of the STS is capable of activating the midbrain reticular formation more than stimulation of surrounding posterior regions. Therefore, the superior temporal sulcus appears to be important in the cortical control of arousal, and the supermodal synthesis discussed above may also lead to neuronal activation in the ventral temporal "what" and dorsal area 7 "where" systems. Therefore, if the STS in monkeys or the temporoparietal junction in humans is dysfunctional, it not only fails to make attentional computations but also cannot arouse or activate directly or indirectly those areas that determine both location of objects and their identity. This failure of activation may prevent the monkey or human from being aware that there is a stimulus in the space opposite the lesion.

Bisiach and Luzzati[9] have demonstrated that subjects with neglect may have an inability to image those objects in scenes that would fall into contralesional hemispace, and Heilman and coworkers[10] have demonstrated a hemispatial antegrade memory deficit associated with neglect. Therefore, lesions of the IPL in humans may be associated with the inability to activate old memories or form new memories of objects that are located in contralesional hemispace. In monkeys, the STS has strong reciprocal connections with the hippocampus and the hippocampus has been posited to be important in retroactivation of sensory association areas.[11] Thus, a partial (spatial) failure of retroactivation may account for the imagery-memory deficits.

In monkeys and humans, spatial neglect can often be distinguished from deafferentation by observing exploratory behaviors. Deafferented subjects fully explore their environment. However, patients with neglect often fail to fully explore the neglected portion of space. Theoretically, if we ablated both area 7 (the "where" system) and the ventral temporal cortex (the "what" system in monkeys), we suspect that these animals would continue to be able to explore their contralateral hemispace. The failure to explore contralesional space that we observed in animals with STS lesions and humans with IPL lesions may be related to the reciprocal connections that the STS has with the frontal arcuate gyrus region. The frontal arcuate gyrus region or frontal eye field is important for the initiation of purposeful saccades to important visual targets. The periarcuate region is important for the initiation of voluntary arm movements to important visual stimuli. It has been demonstrated that lesions of this region, as well as the basal ganglia and thalamus, which are all part of an intentional functional network, may in-

duce motor intentional neglect. However, exploratory defects may be also seen with posterior STS lesions in monkeys or IPL lesions in humans. In monkeys, the frontal arcuate area and periarcuate regions have strong connections with both area 7 and the STS. Whereas the STS may be critical in activating both periarcuate and arcuate regions, area 7 may be important for providing these frontal regions with the spatial maps needed to make purposeful exploratory limb and eye movements. In addition to the dorsolateral frontal lobe, the motor intentional network also includes the medial frontal lobes, the cingulate gyrus, the basal ganglia, and the thalamic cortical loops as well as input from the STS or IPL. Whereas the attentional and intentional networks are highly interactive, they do not entirely overlap. Therefore one may, as discussed, see neglect fractionate into motor intentional and sensory attentional components.

In humans, neglect can be associated with both right and left hemispheric lesions, but neglect is in general more severe and frequent with right than left hemispheric lesions. These asymmetries appear to be related to asymmetrical representations of space and the body. For example, whereas the left hemisphere primarily attends to the right side, the right hemisphere attends to both sides.[12,13] Similarly, while the left hemisphere prepares for right-side action, the right prepares for both.[12]

TREATMENT AND MANAGEMENT OF NEGLECT

Neglect is a sign and symptom of cerebral disease and thus it is critical to treat the underlying disease and to prevent further insults. Because patients with neglect may be unaware of stimuli, they should avoid both driving and working with tools or machines that might cause injury to themselves or others.

Many patients with neglect have anosognosia; during the acute stages when patients have anosognosia, rehabilitation is often difficult. In most patients, anosognosia is transient; but because patients with neglect remain inattentive to their left side and in general are poorly motivated, training is laborious and in many cases unrewarding. There are, however, some rehabilitation strategies that might be helpful. Diller and Weinberg[14] were able to train patients with neglect to look to their neglected side; however, it was not clear that these top-down attentional-exploratory treatments generalized to other situations. In contrast to this top-down treatment, Butter et al.[15] used a bottom-up treatment, where they used flashing lights to attract attention to the left side and demonstrated that dynamic stimuli presented on the contralesional (left) side reduced neglect. Even patients with hemianopia improved, suggesting that these dynamic stimuli influenced brainstem structures. Robertson and North[16] demonstrated that having patients move their contralesional hand in contralesional hemispace can also reduce the severity of hemispatial neglect.

Rubens[17] induced asymmetrical vestibular activation in patients with left-sided neglect by injecting cold water into the left ear and noting that unilateral spatial neglect abated. Vestibular stimulation can also help sensory inattention.[18] Optokinetic nystagmus and cervical vibration can also reduce neglect.[19,20] Unfortunately, these procedures produce only temporary relief. Rossi et al.[21] used prisms to shift images from the neglected side toward the normal side. Although the treated group performed better than the control group in tasks such as line bisection and cancelation, activities of daily living did not improve. Rossetti et al.[22] had subjects with neglect repeatedly point straight ahead while wearing the prisms. Thereafter, on tests of neglect, these treated patients showed a reduction of their ipsilesional bias, which lasted for 2 h after the prisms had been removed, but it is uncertain how much longer this effect can last.

Some investigators have found that an ipsilesional patching procedure reduces neglect,[23] but others have found that it can make neglect more severe.[24] Thus, when using patching, each eye should be tested before deciding which eye should be patched. Neglect in rats was treated with apomorphine, a dopamine agonist; this treatment significantly reduced neglect in these animals.[25] Fleet et al.[26] treated two neglect patients with bromocriptine, a dopamine agonist. Both showed dramatic improvements. Subsequently, other investigators have also shown that dopamine agonist therapy may be helpful in the treatment of both sensory and motor neglect.[27] Barrett et al.[28] and Grujic et al.[29] found, however, that in some patients, dopamine agonist therapy increased rather than decreased the severity of neglect. Barrett et al.'s patient had striatal injury and suggested that the paradoxical effect seen in their patient may be related to involvement of the basal ganglia. In patients with striatal injury, dopamine agonists may be unable to activate the striatum on the injured side but instead activate the striatum on the uninjured side, thereby increasing the ipsilesional orientation bias.

REFERENCES

1. Heilman KM, Watson RT, Valenstein E: Neglect and related disorders, in Heilman KM, Valenstein E (eds): *Clinical Neuropsychology*. New York: Oxford University Press, 2003.
2. Valler G, Sandroni P, Rusconi ML, Barberi S: Hemianopia, hemianesthesia, and spatial neglect: A study with evoked potentials. *Neurology* 41:1918–1922, 1991.
3. Triggs WJ, Gold M, Gerstle G, et al: Motor neglect associated with a discrete parietal lesion. *Neurology* 44:1164–1166, 1994.
4. Gold M, Shuren J, Heilman KM: Proximal intentional neglect: A case study. *J Neurol Neurosurg Psychiatry* 57:1395–1400, 1994.
5. Mennemeier MS, Wertman E, Heilman KM: Neglect of near peripersonal space: Evidence for multidirectional attentional systems in humans. *Brain* 115:37–50, 1992.
6. Ladavas E: Is the hemispatial deficit produced by right parietal damage associated with retinal or gravitational coordinates. *Brain* 110:167–180, 1987.
7. Watson RT, Valenstein E, Day A, Heilman KM: Posterior neocortical systems subserving awareness and neglect: Neglect after superior temporal sulcus but not area 7 lesions. *Arch Neurol* 51:1014–1021, 1994.
8. Mishkin M, Ungerleider LG, Macko KA: Object vision and spatial vision: Two cortical pathways. *Trends Neurosci* 6:414–417, 1983.
9. Bisiach E, Luzzati C: Unilateral neglect of representational space. *Cortex* 14:129–133, 1978.
10. Heilman KM, Watson RT, Schulman H: A unilateral memory deficit. *J Neurol Neurosurg Psychiatry* 37:790–793, 1974.
11. Damasio AR: Time locked multiregional retroactivation: A systems-level proposal for the neural substrates of recall and recognition. *Cognition* 33:25–62, 1989.
12. Heilman KM, Van Den Abell T: Right hemisphere dominance for attention: The mechanisms underlying

hemispheric asymmetries of inattention (neglect). *Neurology* 30:327–330, 1980.

13. Pardo JV, Fox PT, Raichle ME: Localization of a human system for sustained attention by positron emission tomography. *Nature* 349:61–64, 1991.

14. Diller L, Weinberg J: Hemi-inattention in rehabilitation: The evolution of a rational remediation program, in Weinstein EA, Friedland RR (eds): *Advances in Neurology*. New York: Raven Press, 1977, vol 18.

15. Butter CM, Kirsch NL, Reeves G: The effect of lateralized dynamic stimuli on unilateral neglect following right hemisphere lesions. *Restor Neurol Neurosci* 2:39–46, 1990.

16. Robertson IH, North NT: Spatio-motor cueing in unilateral left neglect: the role of hemispace, hand and motor activation. *Neuropsychologia* 30:553–563, 1992.

17. Rubens AB: Caloric stimulation and unilateral visual neglect. *Neurology* 35(7):1019–1024, 1985.

18. Vallar G, Papagno C, Rusconi ML, Bisiach E: Vestibular stimulation, spatial hemineglect and dysphasia, selective effects. *Cortex* 31(3):589–593, 1995.

19. Pizzamiglio L, Frasca R, Guariglia C, et al: Effect of optokinetic stimulation in patients with visual neglect. *Cortex* 26(4):535–540, 1990.

20. Karnath HO: Transcutaneous electrical stimulation and vibration of neck muscles in neglect. *Exp Brain Res* 105(2):321–324, 1995.

21. Rossi PW, Kheyfets S, Reding MJ: Fresnel prisms improve visual perception in stroke patients with homonymous hemianopia unilateral visual neglect. *Neurology* 40:1597–1599, 1990.

22. Rossetti Y, Rode, G, Pisella L, et al: Prism adaptation to a rightward optical deviation rehabilitates left hemispatial neglect. *Nature* 395:166–169, 1998.

23. Butter CM, Kirsch N: Combined and separate effects of eye patching and visual stimulation on unilateral neglect following stroke. *Arch Phys Med Rehabil* 73(12):1133–1139, 1992.

24. Barrett AM, Crucian GP, Beversdorf DQ, Heilman KM: Monocular patching worsens sensory attentional neglect. *Arch Phys Med Rehabil* 82:516–518, 2001.

25. Corwin JV, Kanter S, Watson RT, et al: Apomorphine has a therapeutic effect on neglect produced by unilateral dorsomedial prefrontal cortex lesions in rats. *Exp Neurol* 36:683–698, 1986.

26. Fleet WS, Valenstein E, Watson RT, Heilman KM: Dopamine agonist therapy for neglect in humans. *Neurology* 37:1765–1771, 1987.

27. Geminiani G, Bottini G, Sterzi R: Dopaminergic stimulation in unilateral neglect. *J Neurol Neurosurg Psychiatry* 65(3):344–347, 1998.

28. Barrett AM, Crucian GP, Schwartz RL, Heilman KM: Adverse effect of dopamine agonist therapy in a patient with motor-intentional neglect. *Arch Phys Med Rehabil* 80(5):600–603, 1999.

29. Grujic Z, Mapstone M, Gitelman DR, et al: Dopamine agonists reorient visual exploration away from the neglected hemispace. *Neurology* 51(5):1395–1398, 1998.

Chapter 15

NEGLECT II: COGNITIVE ISSUES*

Anjan Chatterjee
H. Branch Coslett

As the previous chapter makes clear, unilateral spatial neglect is a fascinating clinical syndrome in which patients are unaware of entire sectors of space on the side opposite to their lesion. These patients may neglect parts of their own body, parts of their environment, and even parts of scenes in their imagination. This clinical syndrome raises several questions, which this chapter addresses. How do humans direct spatial attention? How do humans represent space, and what is meant by a mental representation of space? How do humans direct actions in the environment? Is attention related to perception? Can information be processed without attention? Can information be processed without awareness?

GENERAL THEORIES OF NEGLECT

Spatial Attention

Attention is the process by which some stimuli are selected for privileged processing, presumably because the nervous system has a limited capacity and cannot process all things at all times. Stimuli compete for limited resources and some stimuli may be selected over others for a variety of reasons,[1] among which spatial location seems to be important. Neglect is most often viewed as a disorder of spatial attention. In neglect, spatial attention is biased ipsilesionally so that patients preferentially process stimuli in ipsilesional space over those in contralesional space.

Neglect is more common and severe with right than with left brain damage. Attentional accounts of neglect attempt to explain this hemispheric asymmetry. Kinsbourne postulated that each hemisphere generates

a vector of spatial attention toward contralateral space, and these attentional vectors are inhibited by the opposite hemisphere.[2,3] The left hemisphere's vector of spatial attention is more strongly biased than that of the right hemisphere and, after right brain damage, the left hemisphere's unfettered vector of attention is powerfully oriented to the right. Since the right hemisphere's intrinsic vector of attention is only weakly directed, left brain damage does not produce a similar orientation bias to the left. Thus, neglect of the left side is more common and severe than neglect of the right side.

Heilman and coworkers[4,5] and Mesulam,[6,7] in contrast to Kinsbourne, proposed that the right hemisphere is dominant for arousal and spatial attention. Right brain damage produces greater electroencephalographic slowing than left brain damage. These patients also have decreased galvanic skin responses compared to normal subjects or patients with left hemisphere damage.[8] Behaviorally, they also show a markedly diminished capacity to perform more that one task at a time.[9] Thus, right hemisphere damage diminishes arousal and cognitive capacity, which, combined with hemispheric biases in directing attention, produces the manifestations of left-neglect.[10] The right hemisphere is capable of directing attention into both hemispaces, while the left hemisphere directs attention only into contralateral space. Thus, after right brain damage, the left hemisphere is ill equipped to direct attention into the left hemispace. However, after left brain damage, the right is capable of directing attention in both directions and neglect does not occur with the same severity as after right brain damage.

Posner and colleagues proposed a different model of spatial attention in which spatial attention is decomposed into elementary operations, such as "engage," "disengage," and "shift."[11] They reported that patients with right superior parietal damage are

* **ACKNOWLEDGMENT:** We would like to thank Lisa Santer for helpful editorial suggestions on this chapter.

selectively impaired at disengaging attention from right-sided stimuli before they shift and engage left-sided stimuli. This disengage deficit may contribute to some of the symptoms associated with neglect, most notably visual extinction.

The clearest evidence that these patients have a restricted attentional capacity comes from the phenomenon of extinction. Patients may be aware of single left-sided stimuli but then "extinguish" these stimuli when left-sided stimuli are presented simultaneously with right-sided stimuli.[12] Extinction can occur for visual, auditory, or tactile stimuli[13] and even when patients assess weights placed in their hands simultaneously.[14] Extinction may also be observed with multiple stimuli in ipsilesional space,[15,16] suggesting that the pathologic restriction in processing stimuli is not limited to stimuli competing for processing resources across hemispaces.

Spatial Intention

Spatial intention refers to the cognitive processes by which one selects spatial locations for actions. The selection of locations for action contrasts with their selection for perception[17,18]—a distinction that underlies the notions of intentional and attentional neglect. Some time ago, Watson and colleagues advanced the idea that neglect patients may have an intentional deficit, or a disinclination to initiate movements toward or into contralesional hemispace.[19,20] Similarly, Posner and colleagues proposed an "anterior attentional network" involved in selecting locations for actions. Rizzolatti and coworkers have extended this idea even further by arguing that preparations for actions might be critical to perception.[21]

In most situations, attention and intention are inextricably linked, since attention is naturally directed to objects on which one intends to act. Several experiments have tried to dissociate attention from intention using cameras, pulleys, and mirrors.[22-27] The general strategy in these studies is to disentangle where patients are looking (or attending) from where their limbs are acting (or intending). When patients perform tasks in which attentional and intentional selection are in conflict, some patients' neglect is determined by where they look (attentional neglect) and that of others by where they move their limb (intentional neglect).

Using a different approach, Milner and colleagues[25] introduced the "landmark task." Subjects are asked to point to the end of a pretransected line they think is shorter. Patients with attentional left neglect are biased to think that the left side is shorter for transections close to the objective midpoint and therefore point to the left end of the line. By contrast, patients with intentional neglect are disinclined to move their hand to the left and therefore are more likely to point to the right end of the line. Several studies using the landmark task and its variations have reported dissociations between attentional and intentional neglect.[28,29]

Neglect accompanied by ipsilesional biases in limb movements is sometimes associated with frontal lesions.[22,26,30] However, patients with lesions restricted to the posterior parietal cortex can also have intentional neglect.[31-33] Most patients with neglect probably have combinations of attentional and intentional neglect.[34]

Attention and Intention or Different Perceptual-Motor Systems?

One problem with framing these tasks as probing attentional or intentional systems may be that the attention/intention distinction is not the critical difference being assessed. Instead, the "attention" experimental conditions may reflect the link of visual attention to eye gaze, while the "intention" conditions may reflect the link of visual attention to limb movements.[24,35] The relevant distinction may actually be between two perceptual-motor systems, one driven by direction of gaze and the other by direction of limb movements. Such an interpretation would be consonant with single cell neurophysiologic data from monkeys, which show that visual attentional neurons in the posterior parietal cortex are selectively linked to eye or to limb movements.[36,37]

Spatial Representation

Representational theories of neglect propose that the inability to form adequate contralateral mental representations of space underlies the clinical phenomena.[38] In a classic observation, Bisiach and Luzzatti asked two patients to imagine the Piazza del Duomo in Milan, Italy, from two perspectives: looking across the square toward the cathedral, and looking from the cathedral across the square.[39] In each condition, the patients reported landmarks only to the right of their imagined position in the piazza. In addition to their difficulties with evoking contralateral representations from memory, patients with neglect may also have difficulties with forming new contralateral representations.[40] In sleeping patients with neglect, rapid eye movements are restricted ipsilaterally,[41] raising the intriguing possibility that these patients' dreams are also spatially biased. Neglect for images evoked from memory may dissociate from neglect of stimuli in extrapersonal space.[42,43] Thus, the processes by which spatial representations are formed by memory and those that are derived on line from perception may be selectively damaged.

REGIONS OF SPACE

Brain[44] introduced the idea that space could be viewed as concentric shells around the body's trunk—an idea echoed more recently by Previc.[45] Personal space is the space occupied by the body, peripersonal space is the space surrounding the body but within reach of the limbs, and extrapersonal space is the space beyond that reach. The notion that the nervous system treats these forms of space differently is supported by the observation that neglect in personal space dissociates from neglect in peripersonal and extrapersonal space[46] and that left neglect in peripersonal space also dissociates from neglect in and extrapersonal space.[47]

Personal Neglect

The observation of patients provides a rough indication of personal neglect. They ignore the left side of their body and might not use a comb, use make-up, or shave the left side of their face[48] Patients with personal neglect often deny ownership of their left arm even after this limb is brought into their view. When asked to touch their left arm with their right hand, patients with left personal neglect fail to reach over and touch their left side.[46] They may also fail to explore the left side of their body. Patients may be aware of their contralesional limb but not that it is paralyzed.[38] This phenomenon, called *anosognosia for hemiplegia,* is not an all-or-none phenomenon, with some patients having partial awareness of their contralesional weakness.[49]

Peripersonal and Extrapersonal Neglect

Peripersonal neglect is evident in commonly used bedside tests for neglect, such as line bisection, cancellation, and drawing tasks. On line bisection tasks, patients with left neglect typically place their mark to the right of the true midposition, demonstrating a bias to rightward orientation.[50] When the entire line is placed contralateral to their lesion, patients make larger errors with longer lines.[51,52]

On cancelation tasks, patients demonstrate reluctance to explore contralesional peripersonal space. When asked to "cancel" targets presented in an array, patients typically start at the top right of the display and often search in a vertical pattern.[53] They neglect left-sided targets.[54] Sometimes patients cancel right-sided targets repeatedly. The sensitivity of cancelation tasks can be enhanced by increasing the number of targets[55,56] and presenting arrays in which targets are difficult to discriminate from distracter stimuli.[57]

On drawing tasks, patients copy or draw objects and scenes from memory. When asked to copy drawings with multiple objects or complex objects with multiple parts, patients may omit left-sided objects in the array and/or omit the left side of individual objects.[58,59] In all these tasks, patients demonstrate a lack of awareness of contralesional stimuli located in peripersonal space.

The idea that peripersonal and extrapersonal space are considered different regions by the nervous system is supported by behavioral double dissociations in neglect patients. Halligan and Marshall[47] reported a patient whose severe left neglect for stimuli in peripersonal space was abolished or attenuated for similar stimuli in extrapersonal space. The opposite dissociation of patients with neglect for stimuli in far but not near space has been reported[60,61]

SPATIAL COORDINATES BEYOND LEFT AND RIGHT

Neglect is usually described along the horizontal (left-right) axis. However, our spatial environment also includes radial (near/far) and vertical (up/down) axes. Neglect may be evident in these coordinate systems. Patients with typical left neglect often have subtle neglect for near space. On cancelation tasks, they are most likely to omit targets in the left lower/nearer quadrant.[56,62] Dramatic vertical and radial neglect can occur in patients with bilateral lesions.[63–66] Bilateral lesions to temporoparietal areas may produce neglect for lower and near personal space, whereas bilateral lesions to the ventral temporal structures are associated with neglect for upper and far extrapersonal space. Neglect in the vertical axis probably represents complex interactions of the visual and vestibular influences on spatial attention.[67,68]

ATTENTION AND PERCEPTION

Spatial Anisometry

In patients with neglect, the pathologic capacity limitations and ipsilesional attentional bias result in left-right distortions or "anisometries" of space.[29,69–73] The nature of this anisometry, or distorted perception of spatial extent, can be explored by investigating the relationship between the magnitude of stimuli and the magnitude of patients' representations of these stimuli.[74] It turns out that patients' awareness of stimuli is systematically related to the quantity of stimuli presented.

The evidence that neglect patients are systematically influenced by the magnitude of the stimuli with which they are confronted has been studied most extensively in line bisection tasks.[75] Patients make greater errors on longer lines. Marshall and Halligan[76] described the systematic nature of these performances in psychophysical terms. Following this reasoning, Chatterjee and colleagues showed that patients' performances on a variety of tasks including line bisection, cancellation, single-word reading tasks, and weight judgments can be described mathematically by power functions.[14,51,55,77,78] In these functions, expressed mathematically as $\psi = K\phi^{\beta}$, ψ represents subjective magnitude of the stimuli and ϕ represents the objective magnitude. The constant K and exponent β are derived empirically. Power–function relationships appear to represent a fundamental organizational principle by which the nervous system estimates magnitude across different sensory stimuli.[79] An exponent of 1 suggests that changes in mental representations remain proportionate to changes in physical stimuli.

Exponents less than 1, as occur in normal judgments of luminance magnitudes, suggest that mental representations are compressed in relation to the range of the physical stimulus.

The power functions derived from neglect patients' judgments of stimuli across various tasks have exponents that are diminished compared to functions derived from such judgments by normal subjects. Thus, while patients remain sensitive to changes in sensory magnitudes, their awareness of the magnitude of these changes is blunted.[74] For example, the exponent for normal judgments of linear extension is very close to 1. By contrast, neglect patients have diminished exponents suggesting that they, unlike normal subjects, experience horizontal lines of increasing lengths as increasing less than proportionately.[51,77] These observations also mean that magnitude transformations of sensations to mental representations occur nonlinearly within the central nervous system and not simply at sensory receptors, as implied by some psychophysicists.[80]

Representational Instability

Halligan and Marshall[81,82] discovered that patients with neglect tended to bisect short lines to the left of the objective midpoint and seemed to demonstrate ipsilesional neglect of these stimuli. This crossover behavior is found in most patients with neglect[51] and is not explained easily by most neglect theories. In fact, Bisiach referred to it as "a repressed pain in the neck for neglect theorists."[83] Using performance on single-word reading tasks, Chatterjee[78] showed that neglect patients sometimes confabulate letters to the left side of short words and thus read short words as longer than their objective length. He argued that this crossover behavior represented a contralesional release of mental representations—an idea found plausible in a formal computational model.[84]

The crossover in line bisection is influenced by the context in which these lines are seen. Thus, patients are more likely to cross over and bisect to the left of a true midpoint if these bisections are preceded by a longer line.[85,86] A phenomenon like crossover also occurs with weight judgments.[14,87] Patients with left neglect are likely to judge right-sided weights as heavier than left-sided weights. However, with lighter-weight pairs, this bias may reverse to where they judge the left side to be heavier than the right. Crossover seems to be a general perceptual phenomenon not restricted to vision. It also suggests that patients with left neglect are more susceptible to contextual biases when apprehending stimuli on the left than on the right.

SPATIAL REFERENCE FRAMES

Humans have the intuition and experience of a coherent sense of space in which we perceive and act on objects.[88] However, this coherent sense of space harbors different representations anchored to distinct reference frames.[89] These reference frames may be centered on the viewer, the object, or the environment. For example, we can locate a chair in a room in each of these frames. A viewer-centered frame would locate the chair to the left or right of the viewer. An object-centered frame refers to the intrinsic spatial coordinates of the object itself, its top or bottom or right and left. The object-centered reference frames is not altered by changes in the position of the viewer. The top of the chair remains its top regardless of where the viewer is located. An environment-centered reference frame refers to the location of the object in relation to its surroundings, also independent of the location of the viewer. The chair would be coded with respect to other objects in the room and its relation to gravitational coordinates.

Viewer-centered reference frames can be divided further into retinal, head-centered or body-centered coordinates. For example, Nadeau and Heilman[90] described a patient with a "gaze-dependent hemianopia." This patient seemed to have a left visual field defect when his eyes gazed straight ahead but not when he gazed 30 degrees to his right. His neglect of left-sided stimuli was determined by "left" with respect to his head or trunk and not his eyes. Others have described dissociations of neglect within different viewer-centered reference frames.[91] Karnath[92,93] showed that, in many patients, neglect is determined by the trunk or body-centered coordinates.

In object-centered neglect, patients are unaware of parts of objects in ways that cannot be explained by viewer-centered reference frames (although for some descriptions of object-centered neglect, this claim is disputed[94,95]). Low-level mechanisms by which objects are perceptually distinguished, such as figure-ground segmentation or principal axes, can influence which parts of a stimulus are neglected.[96,97] Forms of object-centered neglect have been demonstrated when patients draw pictures,[58] take photographs,[98] perceive rotated objects,[99] and read single words.[100] In one striking case,[101] a well-known sculptor sculpted a head that was grossly deformed on the left side despite the fact that the sculpture was done on a turntable and could be rotated!

Environment-centered coordinates may influence neglect in two ways. First, gravitational influences and the vestibular system help to anchor this reference frame.[67] Some patients' performance on search tasks and line-bisection tasks is influenced by changes in the patients' body position, which alter vestibular input and can disentangle the environmental axis from viewer and object axes. The lateralized biases in some patients are modulated by these changes in body position.[67,68,102–104] Second, environmental coordinates are also established by appreciating stable spatial relationships between objects that exist independent of the viewer's position. When searching for hidden objects, some patients are insensitive to cues provided by other objects in the environment.[105]

CROSS-MODAL AND SENSORIMOTOR INTEGRATION

Different sensory and motor systems interact to give rise to our sense of space. Cross-modal links between interoceptive sensations (vestibular and proprioceptive) with exteroceptive sensations (vision, audition, and touch) modulate neglect. Rubens and colleagues,[106] following an early observation by Silberfennig,[107] demonstrated that left-sided vestibular input with cold water caloric stimulation improves left-neglect. Such vestibular stimulation can also improve contralesional somatosensory awareness[108] and may transiently improve anosognosia.[109] The deployment of spatial attention may also be influenced by changes in posture, which are presumably mediated by otolith vestibular inputs.[67,68] Proprioceptive input from neck muscles can also modify neglect.[92,110]

Recent studies have also focused on cross-modal links between exteroceptive sensory modalities such as links between vision and touch. Visual input close to the location of tactile stimulation may improve contralesional tactile awareness.[111-113]

Movement may also modulate sensory awareness in these patients. Patients with tactile extinction are more likely to be aware of contralesional tactile stimuli when they actively move their limbs than when they apprehend these stimuli passively.[113] The fact that patients with neglect can have personal neglect and deficits of contralesional body representations[46,114] raises the question of how personal space is integrated with extrapersonal space. Tactile sensations are experienced as being produced by objects on the body, the surface of personal space. Visual sensations are experienced as being produced by objects at a distance from the body, in extrapersonal space. The integration of these two sources of information may contribute to bringing personal and peripersonal space into register.[115]

The manipulation of sensorimotor links may be helpful in rehabilitating patients with neglect. Reaching or pointing to objects involves coordinating vision and movement. This visuomotor mapping can be altered if a subject wears prisms that displace stimuli to the left or right of his or her field of view. Recent work suggests that forcing patients to remap ballistic movements leftward by having them wear prisms that displace visual stimuli to their right can improve neglect.[116] These preliminary data suggest that the improvement persists for some time even after the prisms are removed.

LEVELS OF PROCESSING

Processing without Attention

Visual information is processed in stages.[117] First, simple visual elements such as color and movement are extracted from the visual scene. This level of processing is followed by preattentive processing in that the figure is initially segmented from the background and the visual elements are grouped together. Thus, preattentive processing parses the visual scene into regions and possible objects, which are then subject to detailed scrutiny. Preattentive processing is generally automatic and operates in parallel across different locations. Brain damage can produce selective deficits at

the preattentive level with relatively preserved visual-spatial attention.[118,119] These patients view the world in a piecemeal fashion, since visual elements are not grouped together automatically.

If neglect is an attentional disorder, then preattentive processing might still be preserved. Neglect patients are able to segment figure from ground even when the relevant aspect of the object to be segmented is on the left.[120,121] They also perform better on extinction and bisection tasks when left-sided stimuli can be grouped with right-sided stimuli than when they are not so linked.[122,123] Finally, neglect patients are susceptible to various visual illusions, such as the Müller-Lyer and Oppel-Kundt illusions,[124-127] which are presumed to be processed preattentively. Together, these observations support the idea that preattentive processing of contralesional stimuli is often preserved in neglect patients.

Processing without Awareness

Are stimuli that are neglected processed at all? Volpe and colleagues[128] found that patients with visual extinction had some awareness of stimuli that were extinguished. They were able to judge if two pictures were the same or different more accurately than would be expected by chance, even though they claimed to be unaware that there was even a left-sided stimulus present. Marshall and Halligan[129] reported, curiously enough, a patient who could not distinguish between two pictures of a house in which one had flames emanating out a window on the left. However, when asked which house she would live in, she consistently chose the house without the flames. The implication was that she processed "neglected" stimuli sufficiently to make logical judgments despite not seeming to be aware of the basis for making these judgments. The interpretation of these findings has been questioned by Bisiach and colleagues,[130] who find that although patients may have consistent biases in the pictures they choose, their choices do not always make sense. Other reports confirm that some patients process neglected stimuli to quite high levels. For example, neglected pictures on the left can facilitate processing of words centrally located (and not neglected) if the pictures and words belong to the same semantic category, such as animals.[131] Similarly, when patients with neglect are asked to decide if a string of letters on the right form a real word, they perform better if the neglected contralesional string is a word that is associated with the target word.[132]

CONCLUSION

The syndrome of unilateral neglect has contributed greatly to our understanding of the general organizational principles of spatial attention, intention, and representation. However, neglect is also quite heterogeneous. Despite broad similarity of symptoms, the specific details vary considerably across patients.[35,133] Some theorists wonder if it is meaningful to consider neglect a coherent entity.[134] However, rather than a cause for alarm, this heterogeneity itself has been critical to investigations of the organization of spatial attention and representation. Widely distributed neural networks mediate spatial attention, intention, and representation. Damage to parts of these networks can produce subtle differences in deficits of these complex functions. These differences themselves offer insight into how space is organized into different regions and reference frames, how different sensory modalities and perceptual motor systems interact, and how information processing, attention, and awareness are related.

REFERENCES

1. Desimone R, Duncan J: Neural mechanisms of selective visual attention. *Annu Rev Neurosci* 18:193–222, 1995.
2. Kinsbourne M: A model for the mechanisms of unilateral neglect of space. *Trans Am Neurol Assoc* 95:143–147, 1970.
3. Kinsbourne M: Mechanisms of unilateral neglect, in Jeannerod M (ed): *Neurophysiological and Neuropsychological Aspects of Spatial Neglect.* New York: North Holland, 1987, pp 69–86.
4. Heilman KM: Neglect and related disorders, in Heilman KM, Valenstein E (eds): *Clinical Neuropsychology.* New York: Oxford University Press, 1979, pp 268–307.
5. Heilman KM, Van Den Abell T: Right hemisphere dominance for attention: the mechanisms underlying hemispheric asymmetries of inattention (neglect). *Neurology* 30:327–330, 1980.
6. Mesulam M-M: A cortical network for directed attention and unilateral neglect. *Ann Neurol* 10:309–325, 1981.
7. Mesulam M-M: Large-scale neurocognitive networks and distributed processing for attention, language and memory. *Ann Neurol* 28:597–613, 1990.
8. Heilman KM, Schwartz HD, Watson RT: Hypoarousal in patients with the neglect syndrome and emotional indifference. *Neurology* 28:229–232, 1978.
9. Coslett H, Bowers D, Heilman K: Reduction in cognitive activation after right hemisphere stroke. *Neurology* 37:957–962, 1987.
10. Duncan J, Olson A, Humphreys G, et al: Systematic analysis of deficits in visual attention. *J Exp Psychol Gen* 128:450–478, 1999.
11. Posner M, Walker J, Friedrich F, et al: Effects of parietal injury on covert orienting of attention. *J Neurosci* 4:1863–1874, 1984.
12. Bender MB, Furlow CT: Phenomenon of visual extinction and homonomous fields and psychological principles involved. *Arch Neurol Psychiatry* 53:29–33, 945.
13. Heilman KM, Pandya DN, Geschwind N: Trimodal inattention following parietal lobe ablations. *Trans Am Neurol Assoc* 95:259–261, 1970.
14. Chatterjee A, Thompson KA: Weigh(t)ing for awareness. *Brain Cogn* 37:477–490, 1998.
15. Rapcsak SZ, Watson RT, Heilman KM: Hemispace-visual field interactions in visual extinction. *J Neurol Neurosurg Psychiatry* 50:1117–1124, 1987.
16. Feinberg T, Haber L, Stacy C: Ipsilateral extinction in the hemineglect syndrome. *Arch Neurol* 47:802–804, 1990.
17. Rizzolatti G, Berti A: Neural mechanisms in spatial neglect, in Robertson IH Marshall JC (eds): *Unilateral Neglect: Clinical and Experimental Studies.* Hillsdale, NJ: Erlbaum, 1993, pp 87–105.
18. Milner A, Goodale M: *The Visual Brain in Action.* New York: Oxford University Press, 1995.
19. Watson RT, Valenstein E, Heilman KM: Nonsensory neglect. *Ann Neurol* 3:505–508, 1978.
20. Heilman K, Bowers D, Coslett H, et al: Directional hypokinesia: prolonged reaction times for leftward movements in patients with right hemisphere lesions and neglect. *Neurology* 35:855–859, 1985.
21. Rizzolatti G, Matelli M, Pavesi G: Deficits in attention and movement following the removal of postarcuate (area 6) and prearcuate (area 8) cortex in macaque monkeys. *Brain* 106:655–673, 1983.
22. Coslett HB, Bowers D, Fitzpatrick E, et al: Directional hypokinesia and hemispatial inattention in neglect. *Brain* 113:475–486, 1990.

23. Bisiach E, Geminiani G, Berti A, et al: Perceptual and premotor factors of unilateral neglect. *Neurology* 40:1278–1281, 1990.

24. Bisiach E, Tegnér R, Làdavas E, et al : Dissociation of ophthalmokinetic and melokinetic attention in unilateral neglect. *Cereb Cortex* 5:439–447, 1995.

25. Milner AD, Harvey M, Roberts RC, et al: Line bisection error in visual neglect: Misguided action or size distortion? *Neuropsychologia* 31:39–49, 1993.

26. Tegner R, Levander M: Through the looking glass. A new technique to demonstrate directional hypokinesia in unilateral neglect. *Brain* 114:1943–1951, 1991.

27. Na DL, Adair JD, Williamson DJG, et al: Dissociation of sensory-attentional from motor-intentional neglect. *J Neurol Neurosurg Psychiatry* 64:331–338, 1998.

28. Bisiach E, Ricci R, Lualdi M, et al: Perceptual and response bias in unilateral neglect: Two modified versions of the Milner landmark task. *Brain Cogn* 37:369–386, 1998.

29. Milner AD, Harvey M: Distortion of size perception in visuospatial neglect. *Curr Biol* 5:85–89, 1995.

30. Binder J, Marshall R, Lazar R, et al: Distinct syndromes of hemineglect. *Arch Neurol* 49:1187–1194, 1992.

31. Triggs WJ, Gold M, Gerstle G, et al: Motor neglect associated with a discrete parietal lesion. *Neurology* 44:1164–1166, 1994.

32. Mattingley JB, Bradshaw JL, Phillips JG: Impairments of movement initiation and execution in unilateral neglect. *Brain* 115:1849–1874, 1992.

33. Mattingley J, Husain M, Rorden C, et al: Motor role of the human inferior parietal lobe in unilateral neglect patients. *Nature* 392:179–182, 1998.

34. Adair JC, Na DL, Schwartz RL, et al: Analysis of primary and secondary influences on spatial neglect. *Brain Cogn* 37:419–440, 1998.

35. Chatterjee A: Motor minds and mental models in neglect. *Brain Cogn* 37:339–349, 1998.

36. Colby CL: Action oriented spatial reference frames in cortex. *Neuron* 20:15–24, 1998.

37. Graziano MSA, Gross CG: The representation of extrapersonal space: a possible role for biomodal, visual-tactile neurons, in Gazzaniga MS (ed): *The Cognitive Neurosciences*. Cambridge, MA: MIT Press, 1995, pp 1021–1034.

38. Bisiach E: Mental representation in unilateral neglect and related disorders: The twentieth Bartlett Memorial lecture. *Q J Exp Psychol* 46A:435–461, 1993.

39. Bisiach E, Luzzatti C: Unilateral neglect of representational space. *Cortex* 14:129–133, 1978.

40. Bisiach E, Luzzatti C, Perani D: Unilateral neglect, representational schema and consciousness. *Brain* 102:609–618, 1979.

41. Doricchi F, Guariglia C, Paolucci S, et al: Disturbance of the rapid eye movements (REM) of REM sleep in patients with unilateral attentional neglect: Clue for the understanding of the functional meaning of REMs. *Electroencephalogr Clin Neurophysiol* 87:105–116, 1993.

42. Anderson B: Spared awareness for the left side of internal visual images in patients with left-sided extrapersonal neglect. *Neurology* 43:213–216, 1993.

43. Coslett HB: Neglect in vision and visual imagery: A double dissociation. *Brain* 120:1163–1171, 1997.

44. Brain WR: Visual disorientation with special reference to lesions of the right hemisphere. *Brain* 64:224–272, 1941.

45. Previc FH: The neuropsychology of 3–D space. *Psychol Bull* 124:123–163, 1998.

46. Bisiach E, Perani D, Vallar G, et al: Unilateral neglect: Personal and extrapersonal. *Neuropsychologia* 24:759–767, 1986.

47. Halligan PW, Marshall JC: Left neglect for near but not for far space in man. *Nature* 350:498–500, 1991.

48. Beschin N, Robertson IH: Personal versus extrapersonal neglect: a group study of their dissociation using a reliable clinical test. *Cortex* 33:379–384, 1997.

49. Chatterjee A, Mennemeier M: Anosognosia for hemiplegia: Patient retrospections. *Cogn Neuropsychiatry*, 1:221–237, 1996.

50. Schenkenberg T, Bradford DC, Ajax ET: Line bisection and unilateral visual neglect in patients with neurologic impairment. *Neurology* 30:509–517, 1980.

51. Chatterjee A, Dajani BM, Gage RJ: Psychophysical constraints on behavior in unilateral spatial neglect. *Neuropsychiatr Neuropsychol Behav Neurol* 7:267–274, 1994.

52. Heilman KM, Valenstein E: Mechanisms underlying hemispatial neglect. *Ann Neurol* 5:166–170, 1979.

53. Chatterjee A, Mennemeier M, Heilman KM: Search patterns and neglect: A case study. *Neuropsychologia* 30(7):657–672, 1992.

54. Albert ML: A simple test of visual neglect. *Neurology* 23:658–664, 1973.

55. Chatterjee A, Mennemeier M, Heilman KM: A stimulus-response relationship in unilateral neglect: The power function. *Neuropsychologia* 30:1101–1108, 1992.

56. Chatterjee A, Thompson KA, Ricci R: Quantitative analysis of cancellation tasks in neglect. *Cortex* 35:253–262, 1999.

57. Rapcsak S, Verfaellie M, Fleet W, et al: Selective attention in hemispatial neglect. *Arch Neurol* 46:172–178, 1989.

58. Marshall JC, Halligan PW: Visuo-spatial neglect: A new copying test to assess perceptual parsing. *J Neurol* 240:37–40, 1993.

59. Seki K, Ishiai S: Diverse patterns of performance in copying and severity of unilateral spatial neglect. *J Neurol* 243:1–8, 1996.

60. Cowey A, Small M, Ellis S: Left visuo-spatial neglect can be worse in far than in near space. *Neuropsychologia* 32:1059–1066, 1994.

61. Vuilleumier P, Valenza N, Mayer E, et al: Near and far visual space in unilateral neglect. *Ann Neurol* 43:406–410, 1998.

62. Mark VW, Heilman KM: Diagonal neglect on cancellation. *Neuropsychologia* 35:1425–1436, 1997.

63. Rapcsak SZ, Fleet WS, Verfaellie M, et al: Altitudinal neglect. *Neurology* 38:277–281, 1988.

64. Butter CM, Evans J, Kirsch N, et al: Altitudinal neglect following traumatic brain injury. *Cortex* 25:135–146, 1989.

65. Shelton PA, Bowers D, Heilman KM: Peripersonal and vertical neglect. *Brain* 113:191–205, 1990.

66. Mennemeier M, Wertman E, Heilman KM: Neglect of near peripersonal space: Evidence for multidirectional attentional systems in humans. *Brain* 115:37–50, 1992.

67. Mennemeier M, Chatterjee A, Heilman KM: A comparison of the influences of body and environment centred references on neglect. *Brain* 117:1013–1021, 1994.

68. Pizzamiglio L, Vallar G, Doricchi F: Gravitational inputs modulate visuospatial neglect. *Exp Brain Res* 117:341–345, 1997.

69. Werth R, Poppel E: Compression and lateral shift of mental coordinate systems in a line bisection task. *Neuropsychologia* 26:741–745, 1988.

70. Anderson B: A mathematical model of line bisection behaviour in neglect. *Brain* 119:841–850, 1996.

71. Karnath H-O, Ferber S: Is space representation distorted in neglect? *Neuropsychologia* 37:7–15, 1999.

72. Bisiach E, Ricci R, Modona MN: Visual awareness and anisometry of space representation in unilateral neglect: A panoramic investigation by means of a line extension task. *Consc Cogn* 7:327–355, 1998.

73. Mennemeier M, Rapcsak SZ, Dillon M, et al: A search for the optimal stimulus. *Brain Cogn* 37:439–459, 1998.

74. Chatterjee A: Spatial anisometry and representational release in neglect, in Karnath H-O, Milner D, Vallar G (eds): *The Cognitive and Neural Bases of Spatial Neglect*. Oxford, England: Oxford University Press, In press.

75. Bisiach E, Bulgarelli C, Sterzi R, et al: Line bisection and cognitive plasticity of unilateral neglect of space. *Brain Cogn* 2:32–38, 1983.

76. Marshall JC, Halligan PW: Line bisection in a case of visual neglect: psychophysical studies with implications for theory. *Cogn Neuropsychol* 7(2):107–130, 1990.

77. Chatterjee A, Mennemeier M, Heilman KM: The psychophysical power law and unilateral spatial neglect. *Brain Cogn* 25:92–107, 1994.

78. Chatterjee A: Cross over, completion and confabulation in unilateral spatial neglect. *Brain* 118:455–465, 1995.

79. Stevens SS: Neural events and the psychophysical power law. *Science* 170(3962):1043–1050, 1970.

80. Stevens SS: A neural quantum in sensory discrimination. *Science* 177(4051):749–762, 1972.

81. Halligan PW, Marshall JC: How long is a piece of string? A study of line bisection in a case of visual neglect. *Cortex* 24:321–328, 1988.

82. Marshall JC, Halligan PW: When right goes left: An investigation of line bisection in a case of visual neglect. *Cortex* 25:503–515, 1989.

83. Bisiach E, Rusconi ML, Peretti VA, et al: Challenging current accounts of unilateral neglect. *Neuropsychologia* 32:1431–1434, 1994.

84. Monaghan P, Shillcock R: The cross-over effect in unilateral neglect. Modelling detailed data in the line-bisection task. *Brain* 121:907–921, 1998.

85. Marshall RS, Lazar RM, Krakauer JW, et al: Stimulus context in hemineglect. *Brain* 121:2003–2010, 1998.

86. Ricci R, Chatterjee A: Context and crossover in unilateral neglect. *Neuropsychologia* 39:1138–1143, 2001.

87. Chatterjee A, Ricci R, Calhoun J: Weighing the evidence for cross over in neglect. *Neuropsychologia* 38(10):1390–1397, 2000.

88. Driver J, Spence C: Cross-modal links in spatial attention. *Philos Trans R Soc Lond B* 353:1319–1331, 1998.

89. Feldman JA: Four frames suffice: a provisional model of vision and space. *Behav Brain Sci* 8:265–289, 1985.

90. Nadeau SE, Heilman KM: Gaze-dependent hemianopia without hemispatial neglect. *Neurology* 41:1244–1250, 1991.

91. Hillis AE, Rapp B, Benzing L, et al: Dissociable coordinate frames of unilateral spatial neglect: "Viewer-centered" neglect. *Brain Cogn* 37:491–526, 1998.

92. Karnath HO, Schenkel P, Fischer B: Trunk orientation as the determining factor of the "contralateral" deficit in the neglect syndrome and as the physical anchor of the internal representation of body orientation in space. *Brain* 114:1997–2014, 1991.

93. Karnath HO, Christ K, Hartje W: Decrease of contralateral neglect by neck muscle vibration and spatial orientation of trunk midline. *Brain* 116:383–396, 1993.

94. Buxbaum L, Coslett H, Montgomery M, et al: Mental rotation may underlie apparent object-based neglect. *Neuropsychologia* 34:113–126, 1996.

95. Mozer M: Explaining deficits in unilateral neglect with object-based frames of reference. *Prog Brain Res* 121:99–119, 1999.

96. Driver J, Halligan PW: Can visual neglect operate in object-centered coordinates? An affirmative single-case study. *Cogn Neuropsychol* 8:475–496, 1991.

97. Driver J: Object segmentation and visual neglect. *Behav Brain Res* 71:135–146, 1995.

98. Chatterjee A: Picturing unilateral spatial neglect: Viewer versus object centred reference frames. *J Neurol Neurosurg Psychiatry* 57:1236–1240, 1994.

99. Behrmann M, Moscovitch M, Black SE, et al: Object-centered neglect in patients with unilateral neglect: Effects of left-right coordinates of objects. *J Cogn Neurosci* 6:1–16, 1994.

100. Caramazza A, Hillis AE: Levels of representation, coordinate frames, and unilateral neglect. *Cogn Neuropsychol* 7:391–445, 1990.

101. Halligan PW, Marshall JC: The art of visual neglect. *Lancet* 350:139–140, 1997.

102. Calvanio R, Petrone PN, Levine DN: Left visual spatial neglect is both environment-centered and body-centered. *Neurology* 37:1179–1183, 1987.

103. Farah MJ, Brun JL, Wong AB, et al: Frames of reference for allocating attention to space: Evidence from the neglect syndrome. *Neuropsychologia* 28(4):335–347, 1990.

104. Ladavas E: Is the hemispatial damage produced by right parietal lobe damage associated with retinal or gravitational coordinates. *Brain* 110:167–180, 1987.

105. Pizzamiglio L, Guariglia C, Cosentino T: Evidence for seperate allocentric and egocentric space processing in neglect patients. *Cortex* 34:719–730, 1998.

106. Rubens A: Caloric stimulation and unilateral neglect. *Neurology* 35:1019–1024, 1985.

107. Silberfennig J: Contributions to the problem of eye movements. III. Disturbances of ocular movements with pseudohemianopsia in frontal lobe tumors. *Confin Neurol* 4:1–13, 1941.

108. Vallar G, Bottini G, Rusconi ML, et al: Exploring somatosensory hemineglect by vestibular stimulation. *Brain* 116:71–86, 1993.

109. Cappa S, Sterzi R, Guiseppe V, et al: Remission of hemineglect and anosagnosia during vestibular stimulation. *Neuropsychologia* 25:775–782, 1987.

110. Karnath H-O, Sievering D, Fetter M: The interactive contribution of neck muscle proprioception and vestibular stimulation to subjective "straight ahead" orientation in man. *Brain Res* 101:140–146, 1994.

111. di Pellegrino G, Basso G, Frassinetti F: Visual extinction as a spatio-temporal disorder of selective attention. *Neuroreport* 9:835–839, 1998.

112. Ladavas E, Di Pellegrino G, Farne A, et al: Neuropsychological evidence of an integrated visuotactile representation of peripersonal space in humans. *J Cogn Neurosci* 10:581–589, 1998.

113. Vaishnavi S, Calhoun J, Chatterjee A: Crossmodal and sensorimotor integration in tactile awareness. *Neurology* 53:1596–1598, 1999.

114. Coslett HB: Evidence for a disturbance of the body schema in neglect. *Brain Cogn* 37:529–544, 1998.

115. Vaishnavi S, Calhoun J, Chatterjee A: Binding personal and peripersonal space: Evidence from tactile extinction. *J Cogn Neurosci* 13(2):181–189, 2001.

116. Rossetti Y, GR, Pisella L, et al.: Prism adaptation to a rightward optical deviation rehabilitates left spatial neglect. *Nature* 395:166–169, 1998.

117. Farah M: *The Cognitive Neuroscience of Vision.* Malden, MA: Blackwell, 2000.

118. Vecera S, Behrmann M: Spatial attention does not require preattentive grouping. *Neuropsychology* 11:30–43, 1997.

119. Ricci R, Vaishnavi S, Chatterjee A: A deficit of preattentive vision: experimental observations and theoretical implications. *Neurocase* 5(1):1–12, 1999.

120. Driver J, Baylis G, Rafal R: Preserved figure-ground segregation and symmetry perception in visual neglect. *Nature* 360:73–75, 1992.

121. Marshall JC, Halligan PW: The yin and the yang of visuo-spatial neglect: A case study. *Neuropsychologia* 32:1037–1057, 1994.

122. Mattingley JB, Davis G, Driver J: Preattentive filling-in of visual surfaces in parietal extinction. *Science* 275:671–674, 1997.

123. Vuilleumier P, Landis T: Illusory contours and spatial neglect. *Neuroreport* 9:2481–2484, 1998.

124. Mattingley J, Bradshaw J, Bradshaw J: The effect of unilateral visuospatial neglect on perception of Muller-Lyer illusory figures. *Perception* 24:415–433, 1995.

125. Ricci R, Calhoun J, Chatterjee A: Orientation bias in unilateral neglect: Representational contributions. *Cortex* 36:671–677, 2000.

126. Ro T, Rafal R: Perception of geometric illusions in hemispatial neglect. *Neuropsychologia* 34:973–978, 1995.

127. Vallar G, Daini R, Antonucci G: Processing of illusion of length in spatial hemineglect: A study of line bisection. *Neuropsychologia* 38:1087–1097, 2000.

128. Volpe BT, Ledoux JE, Gazzaniga MS: Information processing of visual stimuli in an "extinguished" field. *Nature* 282:722–724, 1979.

129. Marshall JC, Halligan PW: Blindsight and insight in visuospatial neglect. *Nature* 336:766–767, 1988.

130. Bisiach E, Rusconi ML: Breakdown of perceptual awareness in unilateral neglect. *Cortex* 26:643–649, 1990.

131. McGlinchey-Berroth R, Milberg WP, Verfaellie M, et al: Semantic processing in the neglected visual field: evidence from a lexical decision task. *Cogn Neuropsychol* 10:79–108, 1993.

132. Ladavas E, Paladini R, Cubelli R: Implicit associative priming in a patient with left visual neglect. *Neuropsychologia* 31:1307–1320, 1993.

133. Halligan PW, Marshall JC: Visuo-spatial neglect: The ultimate deconstruction. *Brain Cogn* 37:419–438, 1998.

134. Halligan PW, Marshall JC: Left visuo-spatial neglect: a meaningless entity? *Cortex* 28:525–535, 1992.

135. Chatterjee A: Neglect, in D'Esposito M (ed): *Neurological Foundations of Cognitive Neuroscience*. Cambridge, MA: MIT Press. In press.

Part III

LANGUAGE

Chapter 16

APHASIA I: CLINICAL AND ANATOMICAL ISSUES

Michael P. Alexander

The clinical study of aphasia began in 1861 with the observations of Paul Broca.[1] Within 40 or 50 years, all of the basic clinical phenomena reviewed here had been described and many of the major flash points of clinical and theoretical disagreement had been identified. In the past 20 years, fresh interest has come to clinical aphasia research from two directions: modern neuroimaging and cognitive neurosciences. Together, they have additionally provided tools to carry out aphasia-related language experiments in normals. Furthermore, old questions such as cerebral laterality, the influence of handedness, the effects of gender and bilingualism on aphasia, and the mechanisms of recovery have been re-explored. Much of this chapter–which reviews the basic clinical features of aphasia–could have been written 20, 50, or even 100 years ago. In 2002, it is possible to consider this material with greater appreciation of the variability found in the basic syndromes, of their anatomic complexities, of the natural history of recovery, and (although here only briefly) of the cognitive and linguistic deficits that fundamentally underlie the classic syndromes. The chapters on neuroimaging (Chaps. 2–5) and on cognitive analysis of aphasia (Chap. 17) should be read along with this chapter.

CLINICAL SYNDROMES

The description of syndromes of aphasia arose out of much the same motivation as the identification of other clinical neurologic syndromes: the need to identify clinically useful associations between specific clusters of signs and the likely anatomy of the lesion producing them. The most clinically transparent signs of aphasia have generally been taken to be independent signs of brain damage. Thus, syndromes have been constructed out of reduced language output as well as impaired comprehension, repetition, and naming. Disorders of

written language have been divided into additional syndromes only as reading and writing have been impaired beyond spoken language impairments. The use of three independent signs generates eight syndromes, assuming naming to be impaired in all aphasic patients.

Although these syndromes have reasonable clinical validity, there are numerous limitations to this type of syndrome construction. First, the syndromes depend on a sign being normal or not, much as a hemiparesis is present or absent; but the complexity of impairments in comprehension and language production are less amenable to simple dichotomous judgments. Thus, distinctions come to depend on the statistical properties and structural assumptions of the test. Second, there is no certainty that signs all have the same pathophysiologic mechanism in all patients. For comprehension at the sentence level, in particular, there may be several independent pathways to impairment.[2] Third, the syndromes are not stable even when the anatomy is. A patient with a temporoparietal stroke may have an initial Wernicke's aphasia, but, over weeks, language improves to reach the clinical diagnosis of conduction aphasia.[3] Does one conclude that the behavioral-anatomic correlations are with Wernicke's or conduction aphasia? Can one be certain that there are two distinct syndromes if they blur into each other? Should one conclude that only the early-phase correlations hold, that all correlations have built in corollaries about recovery, or that both are true? Fourth, most syndromes are polytypic–that is, they are defined by several criteria.[4] What do we conclude if only some of the criteria are met? Would this be a less severe syndrome? A subsyndrome? A different syndrome altogether?

Despite these limitations, the classic syndromes do have utility. They serve as a type of shorthand for clinical communications. If told that a patient has a particular aphasic syndrome 2 weeks after a stroke, one would know approximately what to expect of language examinations, what the range of possible brain lesions would be, what the prognosis should be, and what some reasonable treatments might be. And although the clinical-anatomic correlations are imperfect, certainly nothing as robust as the brainstem syndromes, they are a good first fit.[5] Any alleged scientific account of aphasia must be compatible with the syndrome-lesion correlations. If so inclined, one could suggest directly from the classic syndrome which interesting cognitive neuroscience issues the patient might illuminate.

Broca's Aphasia

In Broca's aphasia, language output is nonfluent–that is, it is reduced in phrase length and grammatical complexity. This reduction can range from no recognizable output or repeated meaningless utterances to short, truncated phrases using only the most meaning-laden words (substantives). When truncated, the sentence structure is poor; articles, modifiers, complex verb forms, etc., are missing, and the overall structure of sentences is simplified. This is referred to as *agrammatism* when it is dominated by simplifications, elisions, and omissions. *Paragrammatism* is incorrect grammar, such as incorrect pronoun use, wrong verb tense, number disagreement, etc. Few patients with severe Broca's aphasia produce enough language to be paragrammatic. Numerous theories have been proposed to account for agrammatism; none is universally accepted. It is also possible that agrammatism/paragrammatism in these patients represents the loss of schematic procedural knowledge for the implementation of grammar and syntax. Kolk has demonstrated substantial similarities in the grammatical capacities of patients with chronic agrammatic aphasia and normal young children who have the lexical capacity to produce complex sentences but not the practiced ("proceduralized") subroutines of producing complexity.[6]

There is also usually considerable hesitation and delay in production. Speech quality is impaired. Articulation is poor (dysarthria). Melodic line is disrupted (dysprosody), partly due to dysarthria but often more than just secondary to it. Volume is usually reduced at first (hypophonia). With time, speech takes on hyperkinetic (dystonic and spastic) qualities. Language comprehension is adequate although rarely normal. Response to word-recognition tasks, simple commands,

and routine conversation is generally good. Response to multistep commands and complex syntactic requests is generally poor. Repetition is poor, although often better than speech. Relational words (functors–articles, conjunctions, modifiers, etc.) may be produced in repetition, but they are exceedingly uncommon in spontaneous speech. Written language parallels spoken, although some patients, while never regaining useful speech, develop writing that is telegraphic. Oral reading is usually agrammatic; so-called deep dyslexia (see Chap. 20) may emerge with this.[7] Naming is usually poor, but it may be surprisingly good in chronic patients. All types of errors can occur, although semantic errors are most typical for substantive words.[8] Objects are frequently named better than are actions.[9]

Broca's aphasia is commonly accompanied by right hemiparesis, buccofacial apraxia, and ideomotor apraxia of the left arm (or both arms in the nonparetic case). Right-sided sensory loss and right visual field impairments (extinction and/or lower-quadrant deficit) are less frequent. Depression, frequently major, develops in approximately 40 percent of patients with Broca's aphasia.[10]

Many patients have fractional syndromes of Broca's aphasia. Because all of these fractional disorders are still taxonomically closer to Broca's aphasia than to any of the other seven classic diagnoses, many aphasia systems will classify them all as Broca's aphasia.[11] In analyzing reports of Broca's aphasia, it is crucial to understand the taxonomic rules of the report's assessment tool. If all fractional cases are considered Broca's aphasia, the clinicoanatomic correlations will seem imprecise. This is an example of the difficulty inherent in building syndromes with polytypic qualities. Analysis of the clinicoanatomic relationships within these fractional cases may be much more informative than lumping them all together on the basis of some overlap with the full syndrome.

Chronic Broca's Aphasia   This syndrome, as described above, often emerges out of global aphasia.[12] Damage can vary in extent; there does not seem to be a necessary and sufficient lesion profile. The most common pattern is extensive dorsolateral frontal, opercular, rolandic, and anterolateral parietal cortical damage plus lateral striatal and extensive paraventricular white matter damage (Fig. 16-1).[13] Particularly critical to

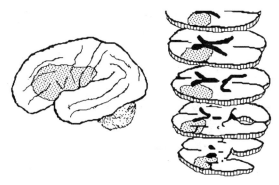

Figure 16-1

Typical lesion associated with severe chronic Broca's aphasia.

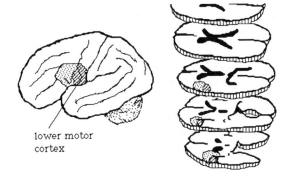

lower motor
cortex

Figure 16-2

Lesion distributions of incomplete forms of Broca's aphasia. The entire lesion would produce "acute" Broca's aphasia. The anterior component involved alone (stippled area) would typically evolve toward transcortical motor aphasia. The posterior component involved alone would typically evolve toward aphemia. In either case, the residual aphasia would be mild.

chronic Broca's aphasia is the subcortical extension of the lesion.[14] Long-lasting mutism can be seen after anterior deep lesions, undercutting supplementary motor area and cingulate-caudate projections.[15] Deep anterior periventricular white matter lesions disrupt dorsolateral frontal-caudate systems involved in ready access to complex output procedures.[16] They may also disrupt ascending anterior thalamic-frontal projections. Anterior supraventricular deep white matter lesions disrupt callosal frontal projections. Large periventricular and subcortical white matter lesions can disrupt all of the long, bidirectional parietotemporal-to-frontal projection pathways. All the distant corticocortical systems will be disrupted. A combination of these systems' disruptions seems to be the structural basis of persistent Broca's aphasia even with subcortical lesions only.

Acute Broca's Aphasia   Infarctions or trauma that produce acute Broca's aphasia often involve the frontal operculum, lower motor cortex, lateral striatum, and subcortical white matter (Fig. 16–2).[17] These patients recover over weeks to months, with variable mixtures of initiation delay, syntactic simplification, paraphasias, speech impairment, and usually with impaired repetition.

"Broca's Area" Lesion   Damage to the frontal operculum (areas 44 and 46) produces an acute aphasic disorder roughly compatible with Broca's aphasia (Fig. 16–2), but there is quite rapid improvement, usually to transcortical motor aphasia or even just mild

anomic aphasia.[11,17] Damage to the dorsolateral frontal cortex (areas 44, 46, 6, and 9) produces classic transcortical motor aphasia[15] (discussed in detail below). Damage to the subcortical frontal white matter or perhaps even to the dorsolateral caudate nuclei may produce the same deficit.[16,18] These observations suggest the existence of a "frontal-caudate" regional network required for construction of complex output procedures of language–syntax and narrative discourse at a minimum. Damage to this system is part of classic Broca's aphasia.

Lower Motor Cortex Lesion   Damage to the lower 50 percent of the prerolandic gyrus can acutely produce a deficit pattern roughly compatible with mild Broca's aphasia, but there is rapid recovery to a much more limited disorder of speech–predominantly of articulation and prosody–sometimes called aphemia (Fig. 16–2).[19] Damage to the subcortical outflow of lower motor cortex can produce the same speech deficit, suggesting the existence of a local (rolandic) network for articulation and some aspects of prosody that project to the brainstem. Some investigators consider this to be "apraxia of speech," a disruption in motor planning for speech movements.[20] This, too, is part of classic Broca's aphasia.

A rare variant of this restricted damage to motor systems of speech production is the foreign-accent syndrome.[21] A small number of cases have been described, usually emerging out of mild Broca's aphasia. In these patients, the predominant deficit is in speech prosody, but the quality of the prosodic deficit sounds to the listener like a foreign accent, not pathologic prosody. The reported lesions have all been in some component of the motor system for speech, either lower motor cortex[19] or putamen or deep connections between lower motor cortex and basal ganglia.[22,23] The precise speech impairment has not been consistent, and the foreign-accent syndrome probably represents a heterogeneous group with partial damage to the motor speech apparatus.

For all of these variants and fractional syndromes of Broca's aphasia, some improvement can be expected. The severe cases that often emerge from global aphasia typically have better recovery of comprehension than of speech; this recovery that may continue over a very long time.[3,24] Minimal recovery of spoken or written output from essentially none to classic telegraphic output is usually accompanied by lesion extent throughout the deep frontal white matter from the middle periventricular region to the region anterior and superior to the frontal horn.[14] The outcome of the milder cases is partly determined by lesion size,[11] but for these smaller lesions, precise lesion site seems to best account for evolution into the various fractional systems.[12,17,19] In both severe and milder cases, some patients may recover by reorganizing cerebral functions to allow some right-brain control of speech. Most current evidence comes from functional activation studies. Additional evidence comes from patients with serial frontal lesions[25] and from temporary inactivation of the right brain (Wada test) after left-brain stroke has produced severe nonfluent aphasia.[26] Recovery through increased compensatory regions in the right hemisphere is not uniformly present or definitively valuable. Some language tasks (semantic decision) may involve more distributed neural networks, and increased right opercular activity may compensate for left-sided damage.[27] Other functions (e.g., phonology) may be neurally restricted to a limited left hemisphere region, and right sided compensation cannot recreate the normal level of function. Only adjacent regions in the left hemisphere can compensate.

Wernicke's Aphasia

In this disorder, language output is fluent—that is, normal in mean phrase length, generally sentence-length, and using all grammatical elements available in the language. Content may be extremely paraphasic[8] or empty. Paraphasic speech conforms to the general rules of the language but contains substitutions at the phonemic level (phonemic paraphasias such as *smoon* for *spoon*), the word level (semantic paraphasias such as *cup* for *spoon*), or entirely novel but phonologically legal words (neologisms such as *snopel*). Empty speech may consist of either vague circumlocutions or single words (*thing, one, unit, it, going,* etc.). Lengthy, complex, phonologically rich output with varied neologisms is jargonaphasia. Although statements may be of sentence length, grammar may become quite imprecise, usually because of semantic ambiguity; this is paragrammatism.[2] Speech is normal. Language comprehension is poor at the levels of word recognition, simple commands, and simple conversation. Repetition is very poor. Written language is comparable to spoken. Naming is very poor. Errors are paraphasias, circumlocutions, and nonresponses.

Apraxia to command is common, but when the patient is given a model to imitate, performance can be extremely variable, from persistently severe apraxia to normal performance.[28] Deficits in the right visual field are common. In the acute phase, patients may be anosognosic; but with awareness of deficits, agitation and suspiciousness may emerge.

Fractional syndromes of Wernicke's aphasia are less common but can occur. Some patients have relatively better auditory comprehension (and usually repetition); others have relatively better reading comprehension. Severe limb apraxia (both ideomotor, even with imitation of gestures, and ideational) is sometimes seen.

The minimal lesion producing Wernicke's aphasia is damage to the superior temporal gyrus back to the end of the sylvian fissure (Fig. 16–3).[13] If damage includes additional adjacent structures, either the deep temporal white matter or the supramarginal gyrus or both, problems will be more persistent.[29–31] If damage includes middle and interior temporal gyri, initial deficits will be more severe, anomia will be more persistent, and reading comprehension will be poor even

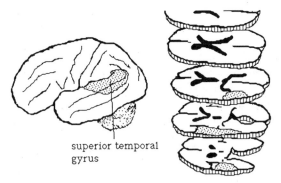

superior temporal
gyrus

Figure 16-3

Typical lesion producing Wernicke's aphasia. Persistence and severity would depend on lesion extent (see text).

if auditory comprehension improves. Patients with lesions restricted to the superior temporal gyrus may have predominantly auditory comprehension difficulties with relatively little anomia and much less reading impairment. The differential effects of lesion placement in the posterior temporal lobe certainly reflect variable damage to converging regional networks for several language processing systems. The auditory language system may be more specifically temporal, thus the relatively greater impairment of auditory comprehension. Visual language processing surely emerges out of the more posterior temporooccipitoparietal association cortex.[32] Cross-modal lexical and semantic knowledge emerges out of a broad range of regions in the posterior association cortex, but available evidence highlights the inferior temporal and middle temporal/angular gyrus transition as the particularly key regions for word retrieval.[33]

Severe and persistent Wernicke's aphasia seems to require damage to all of these regions or to their deep functional connections. The mechanisms of recovery are not completely known. As noted above, the brain regions involved in lexical-semantic function are broadly distributed in posterior association cortex. Size of lesion in these regions, extent of involvement of the superior temporal gyrus,[30,31] and extent of coincident damage to supramarginal and angular gyri[29] have all been implicated as factors in recovery of comprehension. Studies with positron emission tomography (PET) have demonstrated a variety of effects

related to recovery. Heiss and colleagues, studying subacute recovery in a mixed group of aphasic syndromes, demonstrated that recovery of comprehension was proportional to recovery of resting blood flow in the surviving left hemisphere, particularly the temporoparietal junction.[34] Weiller and coworkers demonstrated that recovery of Wernicke's aphasia is closely related to a shift in PET activation to semantic tasks from left temporal in normals to right temporal in patients with Wernicke's aphasia who recover.[35] Using a different paradigm with functional magnetic resonance imaging (fMRI), Cao et al. also demonstrated increased right-sided activation during lexical-semantic tasks in a mixed group of patients with aphasia, but the best recovery of comprehension was associated with the greatest activation of left-sided cortex adjacent to the lesion.[36] Heise et al. have reported identical results for comprehension, also in a mixed group of aphasic patients.[37] The precise meaning of these related studies is not known, but they all converge on the importance of posterior association cortex, either left or, if it is too damaged, right for recovery of comprehension.

Pure word deafness is sometimes considered a separate syndrome reflecting exclusive impairment to the auditory language processing system.[38] Most patients are only relatively "pure," emerging out of Wernicke's aphasia with relatively better recovery of reading comprehension for anatomically specific reasons proposed above. Some patients have had only small left temporal lesions[38]; others have had bilateral temporal lesions.[39] Depending upon the relative size and location of the bilateral lesions, these patients may be effectively deaf (cortical deafness: bilateral Heschl gyrus lesions) or have agnosia for the meaning of all sounds (machinery, animals, musical instruments, etc.), even though they hear them (auditory environmental agnosia: large right lesion, whatever the left lesion).[40] Also, depending on specific lesion sites, language output can be variably abnormal, although to be "pure," it should be normal. In this case, the implication is that underlying knowledge of word phonology is preserved because spontaneous production is normal. Depending on lesion site, patients with "relatively pure" Wernicke's aphasia may have considerable phonemic paraphasia or anomia.

The mechanism of pure word deafness is presumably damage to a system that converts the acoustic signal into a phonologically meaningful stimulus.[39] This is necessary but not sufficient for comprehension; for example, normals can repeat sentences in languages phonologically similar to their native one without understanding anything. There must still be a merger of the processed acoustic signal with a semantic system. In some patients with Wernicke's aphasia, the phonologic process seems very impaired; in others, the mapping to semantics; and in yet others, both are impaired.

Conduction Aphasia

In conduction aphasia, language output is fluent. Content is paraphasic, usually predominantly phonemic.[8] There may be frequent hesitations and attempts to correct ongoing phonemic errors (so-called *conduit d'approche*). Speech is normal. Language comprehension is good except for auditory span. Repetition is poor, not always worse than spontaneous output but dominated by phonemic paraphasias on substantive words, particularly phonologically complex target words (*happy hippopotamus*) or words embedded in phonologically complex sentences ("Dogs chase but rarely catch clever cats"). Written language is extremely variable in this syndrome. Writing is rarely better than speech, but it can be much more impaired. Oral reading is usually comparable to speech but can be better or worse. Reading comprehension is usually comparable to auditory but can be worse. Patients with the agraphia-with-alexia syndrome usually have conduction aphasia. Naming is also extremely variable, from extremely poor to nearly normal. Errors are paraphasias (phonemic especially).

Limb ideomotor apraxia is common initially but clears in most patients.[28] Right-sided sensory loss and visual field impairment (extinction and/or lower-quadrant deficit) are common.

Most patients with conduction aphasia have prominently reduced auditory verbal short-term memory (STM), tested as digit-span, word-span, or sentence-length effect in repetition. There is, however, little specificity of the STM problem, as many patients with perisylvian aphasias have a similar problem. The STM deficit also has little relevance to the language production problem, as similar output occurs in spontaneous output, oral reading and naming, and repetition. There is converging evidence that the inferior parietal

lobule, particularly the supramarginal gyrus, is critical for all aspects of phonologic processing. Thus, lesions there have been blamed for pure STM deficits,[41] phonologic agraphia,[42,43] and phonologic alexia, all of which commonly emerge from conduction aphasia.

Conduction aphasia is usually due to a lesion in the inferior parietal lobule, but lesions restricted to the posterosuperior temporal gyrus may also present with conduction aphasia.[44] As might be gathered from the discussion above of Wernicke's aphasia, involvement of the infrasylvian structures produces conduction aphasia with greater comprehension deficit than a purely suprasylvian one. Within the inferior parietal lobule, the classic lesion is in the supramarginal gyrus[45] (Fig. 16-4), involving the arcuate fasciculus, putatively connecting the temporal lobe to the frontal lobe.[46] Lesions in subcortical parietal white matter disrupt this fasciculus and may represent the classic correlation.[47] Lesions in white matter deep to sensory cortex or in the subinsular extreme capsule, as well as supramarginal cortex lesions, may also produce conduction aphasia.[48] These observations suggest that temporoparietal short association pathways (i.e., a regional network) may support the phonologic output structure of speech. This network is required for phonologic accuracy in spontaneous output, repetition, oral reading, and naming. If disturbed phonologic structure of output is the hallmark of conduction aphasia, this would be the criterion structural basis.

Figure 16-4

Typical lesion producing conduction aphasia. Smaller lesions within this region may also produce similar aphasia (see text).

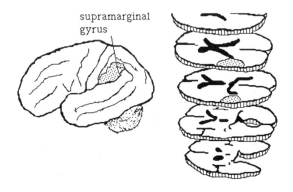

supramarginal
gyrus

Some patients have very extensive parietal lesions with more severe anomia, agraphia, and limb ideomotor apraxia. Partial involvement of the superior temporal gyrus can produce initial Wernicke's aphasia that evolves into conduction aphasia with very paraphasic output and severe anomia. Again, the overlap of syndromes should be evident. Patients whose perisylvian arterial architecture just happens to catch the superior temporal lobe in a predominantly parietal stroke will have elements of pure word deafness (decreased auditory comprehension) with conduction aphasia (phonemic paraphasias, anomia, and agraphia). That combination would be indistinguishable from Wernicke's aphasia; in fact, it probably is Wernicke's aphasia except that recovery of comprehension would be "surprisingly" good.

Most patients with acute conduction aphasia have good recovery over a few weeks, although residual writing impairments, mild anomia, and occasional phonemic errors can be observed. For the more severe cases with marked anomia and very paraphasic output, recovery is less complete. The combination of significant phonologic and semantic deficits despite good comprehension can be very long lasting. Over time, patients become less neologistic and more empty and circumlocutory, even if the basic deficits do not improve.[49]

Global Aphasia

In many ways global aphasia is the easiest syndrome to define. By definition, patients have significant impairments in all aspects of language. Language output is severely limited—there is no more than "yes," "no," and a recurring stereotypic utterance ("da, da," "no way, no way," etc.). In some patients with global aphasia (and Broca's aphasia) the recurring utterance may be repeated rapidly in a richly inflected manner that suggests fluent output if only it could be comprehended.[50] This is not jargonaphasia; it has none of the phonologic richness or preservation of grammatical infrastructure of jargonaphasia. The mechanism of this richly inflected stereotype is unknown, and it has no known prognostic significance.

Comprehension is very impaired. The Boston Diagnostic Aphasia Examination (BDAE) definition allows comprehension up to the 30th percentile for an aphasic population.[51] This is compatible with considerable single-word comprehension. The language comprehension tasks most likely to be preserved in global aphasia are pointing to a named location on a map,[52] pointing to personally highly familiar names from multiple choice or acknowledging them when they are presented auditorily, and a small subset of commands ("take off your glasses," "close your eyes," "stand up").[28] Some patients with global aphasia can do those tasks but little else. There is no repetition, naming, or writing.

Buccofacial and limb apraxia, to command and imitation, are nearly universal.[28] Right hemiplegia, hemisensory loss, and visual field impairments are all common but not invariable.

The most typical lesion involves or substantially undercuts the entire perisylvian region.[11,53] At least, this would require a combination of the Broca's and Wernicke's aphasia lesions, but much clinical variability is seen. Some patients with Broca's aphasia lesions present as having global aphasia without evident temporal lesions.[54] The mechanism of severe comprehension loss without a temporal lesion in a substantial fraction of patients with global aphasia is not known. The coincident frontal lesion may produce additional cognitive problems—such as inattention, underactivation, unconcern, poor problem solving (particularly relevant when the Token Test is the defining tool of comprehension), or perseveration—that interact with more modest phonologic/semantic deficits to produce more profound functional comprehension deficits.

A sufficiently great lesion of the deep temporal white matter might undercut connections to the temporal lobe.[55] Naeser and colleagues found these deep temporal lesions to be associated with poor comprehension in patient's with Wernicke's aphasia.[30] There was good recovery of comprehension in patients with deep temporal lesions but intact temporal cortex. As noted above, Heisse and coworkers have demonstrated a very high correlation between reduced temporoparietal blood flow in resting PET and poor comprehension, whatever the anatomic limits of the infarction.[34] Vignolo and associates[54] and DeRenzi and colleagues,[53] who have provided the most meticulous description of global aphasia without temporal lesions, have not found that temporal white matter lesions easily account for the deficits in comprehension. Conversely, some patients with very extensive posterior lesions that extend into subrolandic white matter present with global aphasia without any definite frontal or even anterior periventricular lesion.[11] The mechanism is not known.

Some patients with global aphasia have no hemiparesis. As a group, they are likely to have only a large frontal lesion or separate frontal and temporal lesions.[56] The purely frontal lesions are again presumably causing a "quasi"-comprehension deficit due to inattention, activation, perseveration, and so on. Many evolve into transcortical motor aphasia (see below).[57] These patients are also likely to have a better prognosis, but absence of hemiparesis is not a guarantee of a good outcome, as the absence of hemiparesis means only that a small portion of paraventricular white matter has been spared.[58]

When caused by infarction, global aphasia has a poor prognosis. Patients with smaller lesions (some without hemiparesis) will improve quickly. After infarction, patients still meeting taxonomic criteria for global aphasia at 1 month postonset have a very low probability of improving substantially.[3] Large hemorrhages may be associated with more late recovery, but by 2 months without improvement, the prognosis remains grim. Many patients show gradually improving comprehension over weeks and months and eventually reach taxonomic criteria for severe Broca's aphasia. Even with severe deficits in language comprehension, patients with global aphasia may have considerable retained capacity to understand the emotional intonation of speech.[59] Recognition of the gist or of the key words in an utterance, such as proper names, combined with accurate discrimination of emotional intent may be sufficient to power substantial social interaction. Many experienced clinicians have the impression that numerous patients with chronic global aphasia are even sensitive to the inflections of sarcasm.

Transcortical Motor Aphasia

In this syndrome, language output is commonly viewed as nonfluent because there is substantial initiation block, reduction in average phrase length, and simplification of grammatical form.[15] Many patients with transcortical motor aphasia (TCMA) are initially mute and may remain mute or nearly so for days or weeks. Note that if they are mute, repetition is obviously absent and, by strict taxonomic criteria, such patients would

initially be seen to have Broca's aphasia. Frank agrammatism is uncommon; responses are simply terse and delayed. Echolalia in various forms is frequently observed. Completely uninhibited echolalia is unusual, but fragmentary echoing, particularly of commands, may be observed. Incorporation echolalia is more common. The patient incorporates a portion of a question into the initial portion of his response. Speech quality is normal in the classic case. Repetition is, by definition, normal or at least vastly superior to spontaneous output. Recitation of even very complex overlearned material (e.g., the Lord's Prayer) may be flawless. Language comprehension is supposed to be normal, but, as observed above, the large frontal lesions most often associated with TCMA may produce substantial impairment of comprehension. Writing is usually similar to spoken output, but patients rarely write to dictation as well as they repeat. Reading comprehension parallels auditory. Oral reading may be quite normal if initial prompts are provided. Naming is quite variable. It may be quite normal. If not, errors are nonresponses, semantic paraphasias, or perseverations.

Transcortical motor aphasia may have any range of associated motor deficits, depending upon lesion site. The classic case has no motor deficit. Hemiparesis accompanies many cases of subcortical TCMA.[16] Inverted hemiparesis (leg worse than arm) and a contralateral grasp reflex accompany medial frontal TCMA.[15] Sensory loss and visual field deficits are not usually seen except in subcortical cases. Buccofacial apraxia may be seen, but limb ideomotor apraxia is less common.[28]

The classic patient has a large dorsolateral frontal lesion, typically extending into the deep frontal white matter (Fig. 16–5).[15] Identical cases have been reported with just a white matter lesion abutting the frontal horn of the lateral ventricle.[55] Very similar cases involve the capsulostriatal region, particularly the dorsolateral caudate and adjacent paraventricular white matter (Fig. 16–6).[16] The similarity of the aphasia associated with these disparate lesions is paralleled by the nearly identical reduction in blood flow seen on resting PET or single proton emission computed tomography (SPECT) in dorsolateral frontal cortex, whatever the lesion site.[60,61] The more posterior the lesion extends along the paraventricular white matter, the likelier the presence of dysarthria (see discussion of transcortical

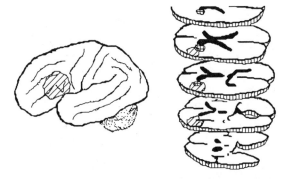

Figure 16-5
Typical lesions producing transcortical motor aphasia.
Note overlap with lesions in Broca's area (Fig. 16–2).

motor aphasia, above) and hemiparesis. Damage to the medial frontal lobe, particularly the supplementary motor area, produces TCMA-like disturbance.[62,63] Mutism may be more prolonged. When patients begin to speak, they rarely show any frankly aphasic qualities. They simply do not speak much.

Analysis of cortical and subcortical cases with TCMA suggests that one fundamental deficit is in generative language tasks.[16,64,65] The patients seem to have very limited capacity to generate complex syntax. They may reuse the syntax in a question they are asked (incorporation echolalia). They may produce short responses,

Figure 16-6
Large lenticulostriate lesion, which is often associated with transcortical motor aphasia, frequently accompanied by speech disturbance and hemiparesis. Smaller lesion (cross-hatched area) *may produce mild transcortical motor aphasia without motor deficits.*

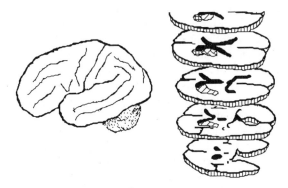

even short sentences, quite well. When asked an open-ended question, however, they do not have timely access to the range of syntax needed to answer. Patients with this profile—essentially normal responsive language but deeply limited open-ended language—have been said to have "dynamic aphasia." Several analyses of patients with this disorder point to disruption in the recruitment or deployment of schemas for complex language constructions, particularly when the utterance is not constrained in any way. That is, the speaker must generate an action plan for how the utterance will unfold, and this must happen over seconds.[66,67]

generative tasks—word-list generation, storytelling, or producing sentences using provided main verbs—will be impaired out of proportion to other language tasks. Patients with large dorsolateral frontal lesions may have little or no aphasia on standard tests but will still be unable to tell a story or recite a narrative in normal fashion. This level of language is called discourse.[68] In parallel with claims for utilization of learned schemas (procedures) for grammar and syntax, it has been claimed that discourse requires recruitment and utilization of a schema for unfolding a very complex utterance. All of these systems for utilizing language are embedded in related frontal structures.[69] Neither the functional nor anatomic boundaries are sharp between sentence structure and story structure. There is a series of interactive effector systems from conception and organization to rules of narrative to complex language to common grammar to speech. Their organization runs from prefrontal to lower motor cortex.

A second fundamental deficit in TCMA is reduction in activation to speak (or to write). Analysis of lesion site effects, particularly the profound mutism that occurs with medial frontal damage, suggests that reduced activation is due to loss of ascending dopaminergic pathways. The medial frontal regions are primary targets of the nonnigral dopaminergic system.[70] Bilateral damage to this system anywhere from the upper midbrain to the frontal cortex results in akinetic mutism,[71] evolving into less flagrant forms often called abulia.[72] Transcortical motor aphasia may represent a subsyndrome of akinetic mutism with more rapid clearing of mutism and less global akinesia because the lesion is only unilateral. The improvement in fluency and speech rate after administration of direct dopamine agonists supports this proposition.[73,74] Improvement with bromocriptine is almost uniquely seen in TCMA or in other nonfluent aphasias that also include significant speech and language initiation block[75,76]

Transcortical Sensory Aphasia

In transcortical sensory aphasia (TCSA), language output is fluent. Content is very empty, with semantic paraphasia predominating. All patients make abundant use of one-word circumlocutions and nonspecific filler words, such as *one, things, does,* etc. Phonemic paraphasias and neologistic jargon are less common, so that output is more accurately described as extended English jargon. Content is also often perseverative. Speech quality is normal. Repetition is, by definition, normal. Language comprehension is impaired. In particular, single-word comprehension may be quite poor. When accompanied by accurate repetition of the test words and even their incorporation in sentences ("A watch? I should know that. Is one of these a watch?"), the behavior has been called alienation of word meaning.[77] There may be category-specific comprehension impairments with particularly good performance at following commanded actions and very poor performance at pointing to named targets. Many patients will accept incorrect names or quibble over accuracy. ("You could call it a watch, but I don't think it is one.") Naming is poor, and again some category specificity may be observed. Some patients are worse at naming animals, insects, and other animate objects than tools and other inanimate objects.[78] There is no important discrepancy between naming performance to different sensory modalities. Many patients respond quickly to phonemic cues but will then reject or be uncertain about the correct response. This behavior has been called a two-way naming impairment.[79] Written output may be similar to spoken, but patients usually do not write extensively and are very perseverative. Reading aloud and reading comprehension are both abnormal. In many patients, reading comprehension is even worse than auditory comprehension.

Transcortical sensory aphasia has been described after lesions in middle and inferior temporal gyri (Fig. 16–7).[77] The temporal lesion may produce a right visual field defect if white matter extent reaches the geniculocalcarine pathways. Many cases of TCSA have unexpected lesion sites involving the entire perisyl-

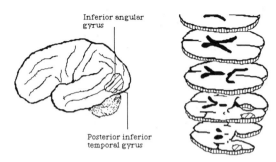

Inferior angular gyrus

Posterior inferior temporal gyrus

Figure 16-7
Typical lesion producing transcortical sensory aphasia. Lesions more medial and inferior, usually posterior cerebral artery infarctions, may produce similar aphasia (see text).

vian cortex, a lesion much likelier to produce global aphasia.[80] The mechanism for this is unknown, although some variant on bilateral language representation is usually recruited. Some cases with temporal lesions may also involve the inferior temporo-occipital region—for instance, after posterior cerebral artery infarction. These patients will certainly have very impaired reading.[32] Many have associative agnosia.[81] As reviewed in Chap. 9, not only can they not name an object or point to a named object but they cannot indicate its use or sort it into a correct functional category (i.e., put a pencil with chalk rather than with a knife). Thus, the deficit is not restricted to *lexical* semantic knowledge but involves actual semantic knowledge. This may be modality-specific, with visually presented tasks more impaired,[81] or it may affect all modalities equally.[81]

Transcortical sensory aphasia is almost monotypic in that it is fundamentally a disorder of semantic processing. Nevertheless, different aspects of semantic knowledge and access to such knowledge may be impaired in different cases. The inability of patients with TCSA to associate a name with an object is the result of a semantic disorder at the interface between language and semantic memory. When semantic memory is more globally affected, patients are unable to demonstrate recognition of objects by nonverbal means as well (see Chap. 27). This is most commonly seen in degenerative diseases with a predilection for temporal cortex, such as Alzheimer's disease or semantic dementia.[33,78,82–84]

Anomic Aphasia

Anomic aphasia is a much less homogeneous grouping than any of the other classic syndromes. By definition, language is fluent, comprehension good, and repetition good. The only deficit in spoken language is in word retrieval. Paraphasias are infrequent. Word-finding problems usually produce filler words[8] or circumlocutions. Other impairments vary with lesion site.

Anomic aphasia is the residual state of many aphasic disorders after time for improvement.[3] As a primary diagnosis, anomic aphasia usually accompanies lesions in the same regions as TCMA or TCSA or the anterior thalamus.

As noted, most patients with TCMA are or at least become basically fluent but with terse, unelaborated utterances. When it is accompanied by word-finding deficits, this condition would qualify as anomic aphasia. Anomic aphasia is also the mildest form of TCSA, representing a deficit only in lexical retrieval from semantic stores. Thus, when anomic aphasia is caused by a dorsolateral frontal lesion, there are no accompanying neurologic signs. When it is caused by a deep frontostriatal lesion, there may be dysarthria, hemiparesis, and buccofacial apraxia, depending upon lesion extent. When it is caused by a posterior association cortex lesion, there may be a visual field deficit and alexia, depending upon lesion extent. When anomic aphasia is the residual of partly recovered conduction or Broca's aphasia, the accompanying signs are as expected for those disorders.

Mixed Transcortical Aphasia

In mixed transcortical aphasia (MTA), language output is nonfluent. Comprehension is impaired. Naming is poor. Repetition is preserved. Echolalia and fragmentary sentence starters ("I don't . . . ," "Not with the . . .") are common. Speech quality is normal. Writing and reading are similarly reduced.

In the patient whose case report defined this syndrome, MTA was due to bilateral hypoxic neuronal loss in the arterial border zones,[85] but ischemic damage in the left border zones could presumably cause the same disorder. The implication is that MTA requires a combination of the lesions of TCMA and TCSA, with perisylvian structures allowing repetition preserved. Most cases are actually due to large frontal lesions in the region of TCMA lesions. The comprehension defect is probably due to a mixture of frontal impairments, exactly as described for restricted frontal lesions and global aphasia. Comprehension improves, and patients evolve toward TCMA. Associated lesions are as described for TCMA.

Large anterior thalamic lesions also produce MTA.[86–88] Most cases have involved the anterior, ventrolateral, and dorsomedian nuclei at a minimum. Damage to those three nuclei effectively deprives the frontal lobe of thalamic input and modulation. Patients are often mute initially. When they speak, the reduction in narrative and terseness of structure are similar to those of TCMA. The impairment in comprehension may be due to the speculative "frontal" mechanisms. The associated signs depend upon lesion extent out of the thalamus. Recovery of language is usually good.

CROSSED APHASIA AND APHASIA IN LEFT-HANDERS

The foregoing review is valid for most right-handers with lesions of the left hemisphere. For the 10 percent of the population that is left-handed and for the approximately 2 to 5 percent of the right-handed population that becomes aphasic after a right-brain lesion (crossed aphasia), some modifications of the clinical rules are required. For left-handers, the phenomenology of aphasia is complicated by the very issue of left-handedness. More than right-handers, all left-handers are not created equal; they vary greatly in degree and nature of hemispheric specialization for language. For both populations, the phenomenology is further complicated by irregularities in lateral dominance for other typically lateralized functions, such as praxis and some aspects of visuospatial function. Only a brief summary of these issues is possible here.

Crossed Aphasia

The incidence of crossed aphasia has been reported as anywhere from 1 to 13 percent.[89–91] The stroke population is least contaminated by possible bilateral lesions, but in all populations methodologic limitations (defining handedness and aphasia testing strategies) leave the actual incidence uncertain. A reasonable estimate is 2 to 5 percent.

Patients with crossed aphasia fall into two broad categories. About 70 percent have a standard aphasia syndrome associated with, at least approximately, the lesion site expected in the left hemisphere.[92] All types of aphasia profiles can occur with the expected lesions (albeit in the right hemisphere). The other 30 percent have striking anomalies in the aphasia-lesion relationship.[92] In this group, unexpectedly mild aphasia syndromes occur despite large lesions that would typically cause a more severe aphasia. Conduction aphasia or phonologic agraphia have been seen despite large perisylvian lesions.[92,93] In other patients with large perisylvian lesions, transcortical sensory aphasia or anomic aphasia has been described.[80,94] Alexander and Annett have suggested that these anomalous cases point to possible discrepant lateralizations of phonologic and semantic functions.[95] Patients with crossed aphasia, particularly if anomalous, may have a better capacity for recovery.

Lateralization of praxis and visuospatial functions in crossed aphasia has not been as definitely addressed as the language functions. Castro-Caldos and coworkers claim that these functions show anomalous lateralization less frequently than language, asserting that praxis remains in the left hemisphere contralateral to the preferred right hand and that visuospatial functions remain in the right hemisphere.[91] Others have disputed this, arguing from case reports that all functions show a high rate of anomalous lateralization.[94,96] Alexander and coworkers have reviewed the case reports of anomalous visuospatial lateralization to the left hemisphere in right-handers.[97] They have proposed that there is a subset of right-handers who have chance lateralization of all functions. These authors, among others, have even proposed that a genetic basis for the inheritance of handedness and laterality of cognitive functions, such as the right shift theory of Annett,[89,95] can account for the rates of all anomalies. The biological basis of crossed aphasia, however, remains unknown.

Aphasia in Left-Handers

Left-handers make up 10 percent of the population, but they are a much more heterogeneous group than right-handers. If a strict criterion for left-handedness is used, most of the left-handed population becomes relabeled as being mixed-handed.[89] Thus, some authorities simply refer to non-right-handers. The rate of cerebral lateralization of left-handers depends to some extent on the criteria used to define the group. Large studies of left-handed aphasics have been reasonably consistent, however, in finding that about 70 percent have left-brain lesions and 30 percent have right-brain lesions.[98] Hécaen computed that approximately 15 percent probably would be aphasic after a lesion of either hemisphere; that is, they have bilateral language representation. Whether aphasic after left or right brain lesions, the proportion of cases with anomalous aphasia-lesion relationships is higher than in right-handers.[99] It has been claimed that left-handers have better recovery than right-handers,[98] but, as with crossed aphasia, this question is muddied by the higher proportion of mild aphasics.[99] It is also unclear if better recovery means bilateral language capacity, so that all functions have higher potential for recovery, or divergent lateralization of functions, so that some are left uninvolved by any lateralized lesion.[90,95,100] Both factors are probably operative, but in different patients.

Lateralization of praxis and visuospatial function shows anomalies at a rate similar to those of crossed aphasia. Every possible arrangement of impaired and preserved functions has been reported after left or right lesions.[94] Since the biological basis of neither handedness nor the lateralization of cognitive functions has been established, it remains an open question how these anomalies occur in left-handers as well as right-handers.

EFFECT OF ETIOLOGY

Infarctions

Almost all of the foregoing is based on the literature accumulated from strokes. Infarcts have numerous advantages for clinicoanatomic correlations. They are sudden in onset, and there is therefore no accommodation and compensation prior to clinical presentation. Boundaries between damaged and nondamaged brain are fairly precise, so correlations are clearer. Nevertheless, the vascular system cannot provide every topographic variation of brain injury; therefore much of what has come to us as classic syndromes could easily be partially artifactual correlations produced by the limited independence of lesions sites from infarctions.

There are some aphasic syndromes that are commonly believed to be caused by emboli because the distribution of infarction seems most plausibly to be in the territory of a branch of the middle cerebral artery. The fractional Broca's aphasias, conduction aphasia, and Wernicke's aphasia all seem likely to have an embolic basis when due to infarction. Global aphasia and Broca's aphasia require more extensive damage in the territory of the middle cerebral artery. There is, however, no basis for presuming an infarction mechanism simply on the basis of these aphasia types.

Hemorrhages

All of the rules established for infarctions apply for hemorrhages if the hemorrhage happens to be in the same brain topography as an infarction pattern. Patients with hemorrhages may be much more impaired initially because of physiologic deficits not primarily related to aphasia–mass effects, intraventricular blood, and so on. Hemorrhages are not constrained by vascular patterns, so entirely novel arrangements of lesions can be seen. This may be exemplified most clearly with lesions of the lenticulostriate region. Infarctions tend to be partially or completely limited to the middle cerebral artery perforators, but hemorrhages can dissect out of that limited region. Much of the variability reported after lenticulostriate lesions[101] may be due to idiosyncratic extensions of hemorrhages.[102]

Trauma

Focal contusions can occur anywhere, depending upon the direction of the blow, skull fragments, and so forth. When the contusion is in a perisylvian region, the resulting aphasia will usually follow the rules established by infarctions. Conduction and Wernicke's aphasias may result from relatively superficial cortical lesions; thus traumatic contusions, which are also predominantly cortical, may produce typical profiles. Cortical contusions rarely cause injury deep enough to damage all of the required deep structures (see above) to produce lasting nonfluent aphasia. There is a strong tendency for traumatic contusions to arise from basal structures due to inertial effects. Focal contusions of the inferior temporal lobe will cause anomic aphasia. If the lesions are large and extend into lateral temporal lobe or hemorrhage dissects up into the deep temporal white matter, patients may present with Wernicke's aphasia or TCSA. Trauma can also cause large epidural or subdural hematomas that do not directly affect language zones. They cause cerebral herniation with entrapment of the posterior cerebral artery, causing occipitotemporal infarctions with alexia and anomia. This herniation-caused infarction can be superimposed on direct temporal contusion, resulting in a very severe fluent aphasia.

Tumors

The lesson for aphasia due to tumors is no different than that for any cognitive function. In general, large tumors produce relatively much less cognitive impairment than an infarction of the same size would produce, but tumors produce symptoms qualitatively appropriate for the region involved. Primary brain tumors tend to infiltrate and gradually disrupt function, allowing substantial compensation as the disorder progresses. The conformity with patterns established by infarctions will be correlated largely with the malignancy and speed of growth of the tumor.

Herpes Simplex Encephalitis

Although rare, herpes simplex encephalitis (HSE) has a predilection for the medial temporal lobes, basalmedial frontal lobes, and insular cortices. Survivors of HSE frequently have severe amnesia. Patients with extensive left-sided HSE lesions, including the inferotemporal lobe, commonly show category-specific semantic deficits.[78,103]

Dementia

The most common dementing illnesses—dementia of the Alzheimer's type (DAT) and multi-infarct dementia (MID)–both cause language impairments. DAT typically presents with memory and language disturbances.[83] The language problem begins as anomia and is often misidentified by families as memory impairment.

With time, the language disorder evolves toward TCSA, and the patient's semantic memory erodes.[104] The structure of this erosion is fairly predictable. Highly typical semantic associations survive longer than the semantic associations and attributes of low typicality.[104] For instance, the patients may still recognize the words and concepts behind cat but not the words and then even the concepts of leopard, fang, or litter. It has been proposed that this slow erosion of semantic knowledge—first words and then concepts—is the fundamental cognitive deficit of DAT.[105] Its presumed pathologic basis is the loss of neurons in posterior association cortex.

If one of the infarcts is in the language zone, MID may cause aphasia directly. The more typical pathology of MID is, however, numerous small infarcts in subcortical regions. These lesions may produce a variety of motor speech impairments such as articulatory problems, hypophonia, dysprosody, and rate disturbances. A recognizable aphasic syndrome does not occur, but patients may show cognitive deficits similar to those seen with frontal lobe lesions, including disturbances in all aspects of generative language: reduced word-list generation, terse or unelaborate utterances, and poor narrative ability. It has been suggested that a single small infarct in the genu of the left internal capsule is sufficient to disconnect frontothalamic circuitry and produce these deficits.[106]

A less common but hardly rare form of degenerative dementia, frontotemporal dementia, often presents with primary progressive aphasia. By definition, this disorder is characterized by a gradual decline that is essentially limited to language deficits.[107] The most common form is progressive loss of semantics and has therefore also been called semantic dementia (see Chap. 27). The presentation is usually similar to the language impairments of DAT–anomia initially progressing to TCSA and finally to loss of semantic concepts and knowledge. Unlike DAT, other cognitive functions remain are initially and often remain intact in these cases. Pathology is restricted to the anterior inferior temporal lobes. Two different "nonfluent" forms of primary progressive aphasia have also been described.[108–110] In one, the deficit is identical to dynamic aphasia described above, and imaging shows focal atrophy in the left prefrontal regions. In the other, the deficit is a progressive speech disorder, a mixture of articulation problems, stuttering, rate abnormalities, phonemic paraphasias, and facial apraxia. All forms are commonly associated with extrapyramidal disorders, either corticobasal degeneration or progressive supranuclear palsy.[111,112] In all forms of this disorder, the histopathology has been similar, although the distribution of the pathology has reflected the focal language profiles. Many patients would be labeled as having Pick's disease or a near variant.[113,114] A sizable minority is inherited, usually due to an abnormality on chromosome 17 in the gene for the tau protein, a critical element of axonal function.[111,115] For the neuroscientist, it should be fascinating to contemplate a single gene critical for language functions. What should be most interesting for students of aphasia is how closely the focal and multifocal degenerative disorders recapitulate the localization matrix created through the study of stroke.

REFERENCES

1. Broca P: Perte de la parole. Ramollissement chronique et destruction partielle du lobe anterieur gauche du cerveau. *Bull Soc Anthropol* 2:235, 1861.
2. Goodglass H: *Understanding Aphasia.* San Diego, CA: Academic Press, 1993.
3. Kertesz A, McCabe P: Recovery patterns and prognosis in aphasia. *Brain* 100:1–18, 1977.
4. Caramazza A: The logic of neuropsychological research and the problem of patient classification in aphasia. *Brain Lang* 21:9–20, 1984.
5. Kreisler A, Godefroy O, Delmaire C, et al: The anatomy of aphasia revisited. *Neurology* 54:1117–1123, 2000.
6. Kolk H: Does agrammatic speech constitute a regression to child language? A three-way comparison between agrammatic, child and normal ellipsis. *Brain Lang* 77:340–350, 2001.
7. Marshall JC, Newcombe F: Patterns of paralexia. *J Psycholinguist Res* 2:175–199, 1973.
8. Ardila A, Rosselli M: Language deviations in aphasia: A frequency analysis. *Brain Lang* 44:165–180, 1993.
9. Kohn SE: Verb finding in aphasia. *Cortex* 25:57–69, 1989.
10. Robinson RG, Kubos KL, Starr LB, et al: Mood disorders in stroke patients: Importance of location of lesion. *Brain* 107:81–93, 1984.

11. Mazzocchi F, Vignolo LA: Localisation of lesions in aphasia: Clinical–CT scan correlations in stroke patients. *Cortex* 15:627–654, 1979.

12. Mohr JP, Pessin MS, Finkelstein S, et al: Broca's aphasia: Pathologic and clinical. *Neurology* 28:311–324, 1978.

13. Naeser MA, Hayward RW: Lesion location in aphasia with cranial computed tomography and the Boston Diagnostic Aphasia Exam. *Neurology* 28:545–551, 1978.

14. Naeser MA, Palumbo CL, Helm-Estabrooks N, et al: Severe nonfluency in aphasia: Role of the medial subcallosal fasciculus and other white matter pathways in recovery of spontaneous speech. *Brain* 112:1–38, 1989.

15. Freedman M, Alexander MP, Naeser MA: Anatomic basis of transcortical motor aphasia. *Neurology* 34:409–417, 1984.

16. Mega MS, Alexander MP: Subcortical aphasia: The core profile of capsulostriatal infarction. *Neurology* 44:1824–1829, 1994.

17. Alexander MP, Naeser MA, Palumbo C: Broca's area aphasia. *Neurology* 40:353–362, 1990.

18. Nadeau S, Crosson B: Subcortical aphasia. *Brain Lang* 58:355–402, 1995.

19. Schiff HB, Alexander MP, Naeser MA, Galaburda AM: Aphemia: Clinical-anatomic correlation. *Arch Neurol* 40:720–772, 1983.

20. Fox RJ, Kasner SE, Chatterjee AC, Chalela JA: Aphemia: An isolated disorder of articulation. *Clin Neurol Neurosurg* 103:123–126, 2001.

21. Monrad-Krohn GH: Dysprosody or altered "melody of language." *Brain* 70:405–415, 1947.

22. Blumstein SE, Alexander MP, Ryalls JH: The nature of the foreign accent syndrome: A case study. *Brain Lang* 31:215–244, 1987.

23. Graff-Radford NR, Cooper WE, Colsher PL, Damasio AR: An unlearned foreign "accent" in a patient with aphasia. *Brain Lang* 28:86–94, 1986.

24. Prin RS, Snow E, Wagenaar E: Recovery from aphasia: Spontaneous speech versus language comprehension. *Brain Lang* 6:192–211, 1978.

25. Basso A, Gardelli M, Grassi MP, et al: The role of the right hemisphere in recovery from aphasia: Two case studies. *Cortex* 25:555–566, 1989.

26. Kinsbourne M: The minor hemisphere as a source of aphasic speech. *Trans Am Neurol Assoc* 96:141–145, 1971.

27. Calvert GA, Brammer MJ, Morris RG, et al: Using fMRI to study recovery from acquired dysphasia. *Brain Lang* 71:391–399, 2000.

28. Alexander MP, Baker E, Naeser MA, Kaplan E: Neuropsychological and neuroanatomical dimensions of ideomotor apraxia. *Brain* 118:87–107, 1992.

29. Kertesz A, Lau WK, Polk M: The structural determinants of recovery in Wernicke's aphasia. *Brain Lang* 44:153–164, 1993.

30. Naeser MA, Helm-Estabrooks N, Haas G, et al: Relationship between lesion extent in Wernicke's area on computed tomographic scan and predicting recovery of comprehension in Wernicke's aphasia. *Arch Neurol* 44:73–82, 1987.

31. Selnes OA, Knopman DS, Niccum N, et al: Computed tomographic scan correlates of auditory comprehension deficits in aphasia: A prospective recovery study. *Ann Neurol* 13:558–566, 1983.

32. Henderson VW, Friedman RB, Teng EL, Weiner JM: Left hemisphere pathways in reading: Inference from pure alexia without hemianopia. *Neurology* 35:962–968, 1985.

33. Damasio AR: Synchronous activation in multiple cortical regions: A mechanism for recall. *Semin Neurosci* 2:287–296, 1990.

34. Heiss W, Kessler J, Karbe H, et al: Cerebral glucose metabolism as a predictor of recovery from aphasia in ischemic stroke. *Arch Neurol* 50:958–964, 1993.

35. Weiller C, Isensee C, Rijintjes M, et al: Recovery from Wernicke's aphasia: A positron emission tomography study. *Ann Neurol* 37:723–732, 1995.

36. Cao Y, Vikingstad EM, George KP, et al: Cortical language activation in stroke patients recovering from aphasia with functional MRI. *Stroke* 30:2331–2340, 1999.

37. Heise WD, Karbe H, Weber-Luxenburger G, et al: Speech-induced cerebral metabolic activation reflects recovery from aphasia. *J Neurol Sci* 145:213–217, 1997.

38. Takahashi N, Kawamura M, Shinotou H, et al: Pure word deafness due to left hemisphere damage. *Cortex* 28:295–303, 1992.

39. Auerbach SH, Allard T, Naeser MA, et al: Pure word deafness: Analysis of a case with bilateral lesions and a defect at the prephonemic level. *Brain* 105:271–300, 1982.

40. Fujii T, Fukatsu, Watabe S, et al: Auditory sound agnosia without aphasia following a right temporal lobe lesion. *Cortex* 26:263–268, 1990.

41. Paulesu E, Frith CD, Frackowiack RSJ: The neural correlates of the verbal component of working memory. *Nature* 362:342–345, 1993.

42. Alexander MP, Friedman RB, Loverso F, Fischer RF: Lesion localization in phonological agraphia. *Brain Lang* 43:83–95, 1992.

43. Roeltgen DP, Sevush S, Heilman KM: Phonological agraphia: Writing by the lexical semantic route. *Neurology* 33:755–765, 1983.
44. Axer H, von Keyserlingk AG, Berks G, von Keyserlingk DG: Supra- and infrasylvian conduction aphasia. *Brain Lang* 76:317–331, 2001.
45. Palumbo CL, Alexander MP, Naeser MA: CT scan lesion sites associated with conduction aphasia, in Kohn S (ed): *Conduction Aphasia*. Hillsdale NJ: Erlbaum, 1992, pp 51–75.
46. Benson DF, Sheremata WA, Bouchard R, et al: Conduction aphasia: A clinicopathological study. *Arch Neurol* 28:339–346, 1973.
47. Mendez MF, Benson DF. Atypical conduction aphasia: A disconnection syndrome. *Arch Neurol* 42:886–891, 1985.
48. Damasio H, Damasio AR: The anatomical basis of conduction aphasia. *Brain* 103:337–350, 1980.
49. Kertesz A, Benson DF: Neologistic jargon: A clinicopathological study. *Cortex* 6:362–386, 1970.
50. Poeck K, de Bleser R, von Keyserlingk DG: Neurolinguistic status and localization of lesions in aphasic patients with exclusively consonant vowel recurring utterances. *Brain* 107:199–217, 1984.
51. Goodglass H, Kaplan E: *The Assessment of Aphasia and Related Disorders*. Philadelphia: Lea & Febiger, 1983.
52. Wapner W, Gardner H. A note on patterns of comprehension and recovery in global aphasia. *J Speech Hear Res* 29:765–771, 1979.
53. DeRenzi E, Colombo A, Scarpa M: The aphasic isolate. *Brain* 114:1719–1730,1991.
54. Vignolo LA, Boccardi E, Caverni L: Unexpected CT-scan finding in global aphasia. *Cortex* 22:55–69, 1986.
55. Alexander MP, Naeser MA, Palumbo CL: Correlations of subcortical CT lesion sites and aphasia profiles. *Brain* 110:961–991, 1987.
56. Tranel D, Biller J, Damasio H, Damasio AR: Global aphasia without hemiparesis. *Arch Neurol* 44:304–308, 1987.
57. Hanlon RE, Lux WE, Dromerick AW: Global aphasia without hemiparesis: Language profiles and lesion distribution. *J Neurol Neurosurg Psychiatry* 66:365–369, 1999.
58. Legatt AD, Rubin AJ, Kaplan LR, et al: Global aphasia without hemiparesis. *Neurology* 37:201–205, 1987.
59. Barrett AM, Crucian GP, Raymer AM, Heilman KM: Spared comprehension of emotional prosody in a patient with global aphasia. *Neuropsychiatry Neuropsychol Behav Neurosci* 12:117–120, 1999.
60. Alexander MP: Speech and language deficits after subcortical lesions of the left hemisphere: A clinical, CT, and PET study, in Vallar G CS, Wallesch C-W (eds): *Neuropsychological Disorders Associated with Subcortical Lesions*. Oxford: Oxford Science Publications, 1991, pp 454–477.
61. Démonet JF, Puel M: "Subcortical" aphasia: Some proposed pathophysiological mechanisms and their rCBF correlates revealed by SPECT. *J Neuroling* 6:319–344, 1991.
62. Alexander MP: Disturbances in language initiation: Mutism and its lesser forms, in Joseph AB, Young RR (eds): *Movement Disorders in Neurology and Psychiatry*. Boston: Blackwell, 1992, pp 389–396.
63. Rubens AB: Transcortical motor aphasia. *Stud Neuroling* 1:293–306, 1976.
64. Costello AL, Warrington EK: Dynamic aphasia. The selective impairment of verbal planning. *Cortex* 25:103–114, 1989.
65. Luria AR, Tsvetkova LS: Towards the mechanism of "dynamic aphasia." *Acta Neurol Psychiatr Belg* 67:1045–1067, 1967.
66. Robinson G, Blair J, Cipolotti L: Dynamic aphasia: An inability to select between competing verbal responses? *Brain* 121:77–89, 1998.
67. Thompson-Schill SL, Swick D, Farah MJ, et al: Verb generation in patients with focal frontal lesions: A neuropsychological test of neuroimaging findings. *Proc Natl Acad Sci U S A* 95:15855–15860, 1998.
68. Chapman SB, Culhane KA, Levin HS, et al: Narrative discourse after closed head injury in children and adolescents. *Brain Lang* 43:42–65, 1992.
69. Sirigu A, Cohen L, Zalla T, et al: Distinct frontal regions for processing sentence syntax and story grammar. *Cortex* 34:771–778, 1998.
70. Lindvall O, Bjorklund A, Moore RY, Stenevi U: Mesencephalic dopamine neurons projecting to neocortex. *Brain Res* 81:325–331, 1974.
71. Alexander MP: Chronic akinetic mutism after mesencephalic-diencephalic infarction: Remediated with dopaminergic medications. *Neurorehabil Neural Repair.* 15:151–156, 2001.
72. Fisher CM: Abulia minor vs agitated behavior. *Clin Neurosurg* 1985;31:9–31, 1985.
73. Albert ML, Bachman DL, Morgan A, Helm-Estabrooks N: Pharmacotherapy for aphasia. *Neurology* 38:877–879, 1988.
74. Saba L, Leiguarda R, Starkstein SE: An open-label trial of bromocriptine in nonfluent aphasia. *Neurology* 42:1637–1638, 1992.

75. Bragoni M, Altieri M, DiPiero V, Padovani A, et al: Bromocriptine and speech therapy in non-fluent chronic aphasia after stroke. *Neurol Sci* 21:19–22, 2000.

76. Gold M, VanDam D, Silliman ER: An open-label trial of bromocriptine in non-fluent aphasia: A qualitative analysis of word storage and retrieval. *Brain Lang* 74:141–156, 2000.

77. Alexander MP, Hiltbrunner B, Fischer RF: The distributed anatomy of transcortical sensory aphasia. *Arch Neurol* 46:885–892, 1989.

78. Warrington EK, Shallice T: Category-specific semantic impairment. *Brain* 107:829–854, 1984.

79. Benson DF: Neurologic correlates of anomia, in Whitaker HWH (ed): *Studies in Neurolinguistics*. New York: Academic Press, 1979, pp 293–328.

80. Berthier ML, Starkstein SE, Leiguarda R, et al: Transcortical aphasia. *Brain* 114:1409–1427, 1991.

81. Feinberg TE, Dyckes-Berke D, Miner CR, Roane DM: Knowledge, implicit knowledge and metaknowledge in visual agnosia and pure alexia. *Brain* 118:789–800, 1995.

82. Graff-Radford NR, Damasio AR, Hyman BT, et al: Progressive aphasia in a patient with Pick's disease. *Neurology* 40:620–626, 1990.

83. Price BH, Gurvit H, Weintraub S, et al: Neuropsychological patterns and language deficits in 20 consecutive cases of autopsy-confirmed Alzheimer's disease. *Arch Neurol* 50:931–937, 1993.

84. Riddoch MJ, Humphreys GW, Coltheart M, Funnell E: Semantic systems or system? Neuropsychological evidence re-examined. *Cogn Neuropsychol* 5:3–25, 1988.

85. Geschwind N, Quadfasel FA, Segarra JM: Isolation of the speech area. *Neuropsychologia* 6:327–340, 1968.

86. Cappa SF, Vignolo LA: "Transcortical" features of aphasia following left thalamic hemorrhage. *Cortex* 19:227–241, 1979.

87. Graff-Radford NR, Damasio H, Yamada T, et al: Nonhemorrhagic thalamic infarction. *Brain* 108:485–516, 1985.

88. McFarling D, Rothi LJ, Heilman KM: Transcortical aphasia from ischemic infarcts of the thalamus. *J Neurol Neurosurg Psychiatry* 45:107–112, 1982.

89. Annett M: *Left, Right, Hand and Brain: The Right Shift Theory*. Hillsdale, NJ: Erlbaum, 1985.

90. Bryden MP, Hécaen H, DeAgostini M: Patterns of cerebral organization. *Brain Lang* 20:249–262, 1983.

91. Castro-Caldas A, Confraria A, Poppe P: Nonverbal disturbances in crossed aphasia. *Aphasiology* 1:403–413, 1987.

92. Alexander MP, Fischette MR, Fischer RS: Crossed aphasia can be mirror image or anomalous. *Brain* 112:953–973, 1989.

93. Basso A, Capitani E, Laiacona M, Zanobio ME: Crossed aphasia: One or more syndromes? *Cortex* 25:25–45, 1985.

94. Alexander MP, Annett M: Crossed aphasia and related anomalies of cerebral organization: case reports and a genetic hypothesis. *Brain Lang* 55:213–239, 1996.

95. Annett M, Alexander MP: Atypical cerebral dominance: Predictions and tests of the RS theory. *Neuropsychologia* 34:1215–1227, 1996.

96. Trojano L, Balbi P, Russo G, Elefante R: Patterns of recovery in verbal and nonverbal function in a case of crossed aphasia. *Brain Lang* 46:637–661, 1994.

97. Fischer RS, Alexander MP, Gabriel C, Milione J: Reversed lateralization of cognitive functions in right handers. *Brain* 114:245–261, 1991.

98. Hécaen H, DeAgostini M, Monzon-Montes A: Cerebral organization in lefthander. *Brain Lang* 12:261–284, 1981.

99. Basso A, Farabola M, Grassi MP, et al: Aphasia in lefthanders. *Brain Lang* 38:233–252, 1990.

100. Naeser MA, Borod JC: Aphasia in lefthanders. *Neurology* 36:471–488, 1986.

101. Puel M, Démonet JF, Cardebat I, et al: Aphasies sous-corticales: Étude neurolinguistique avec scanner x de 25 cas. *Rev Neurol* 140:695–710, 1984.

102. D'Esposito M, Alexander MP: Subcortical aphasia: Distinct profiles following left putaminal hemorrhages. *Neurology* 45:33–37, 1995.

103. DeRenzi E, Lucchelli F: Are semantic systems separately represented in the brain? The case of living category impairment. *Cortex* 30:3–25, 1994.

104. Smith S, Faust M, Beeman M, et al: A property level analysis of lexical semantic representation in Alzheimer's disease. *Brain Lang* 49:263–279, 1995.

105. Hodges JR, Salmon DP, Butters N: Semantic memory impairment in Alzheimer's disease: Failure of access or degraded knowledge? *Neuropsychologia* 30:301–314, 1992.

106. Tatemichi TK, Desmond DW, Prohovnik I, et al: Confusion and memory loss from capsular genu infarction: A thalamocortical disconnection syndrome? *Neurology* 42:1966–1979, 1992.

107. Hodges JR, Patterson K, Oxbury S, Funnell E: Semantic dementia. *Brain* 115:1783–1806, 1992.

108. Mesulam M-M: Slowly progressive aphasia without generalized dementia. *Ann Neurol* 1982;11:592–598, 1982.

109. Mesulam M-M: Primary progressive aphasia. *Ann Neurol* 49:425–432, 2001.

110. Weintraub S, Rubin NP, Mesulam M-M: Primary progressive aphasia: Longitudinal course, neuropsychological profile and language features. *Arch Neurol* 47:1329–1335, 1990.

111. Foster NL, Wilhelmsen KC, Sima AAF, et al: Frontotemporal dementia and Parkinsonism linked to chromosome 17: A consensus conference. *Ann Neurol* 41:706–715, 1997.

112. Kertesz A, Martinez-Lage P, Davidson W, Munoz DG: The corticobasal degeneration syndrome overlaps progressive aphasia and frontotemporal dementia. *Neurology* 55(9):1368–1375, 2000.

113. Kertesz A, Davidson W, Munoz DG: Clinical and pathological overlap between frontotemporal dementia, primary progressive aphasia and corticobasal degeneration: The Pick complex. *Dement Geriatr Cogn Disord* 10 (Suppl 1):46–49, 1999.

114. Kertesz A, Hudson L, MacKenzie IRA, Munoz DG: The pathology and nosology of primary progressive aphasia. *Neurology* 44:2065–2072, 1994.

115. van Slegtenhorst M, Lewis J, Hutton M: The molecular genetics of the tauopathies. *Exp Gerontol* 35(4):461–471, 2000.

Chapter 17

APHASIA II: COGNITIVE ISSUES*

Eleanor M. Saffran

As is evident from the preceding chapter, much was known about aphasia prior to the emergence of cognitive neuropsychology in the 1970s. Symptoms had been described, diagnostic and treatment protocols developed, anatomic correlates established, and models proposed that interpreted aphasic phenomena within an anatomic theory based on aphasic data (see Ref. 1 for review). The cognitive neuropsychological approach represents a shift from clinical and anatomic concerns to an emphasis on functional architecture. One assumption that underlies this approach is that language breakdown patterns reflect the natural divisions of the language system and hence that the disorders reveal its componential structure. This school of neuropsychological research is closely tied to developments in cognitive psychology and psycholinguistics. Normative models guide the investigation of pathologic phenomena, which, in turn, provide fertile ground for testing and extending theories of language function.

The concern with functional architecture has implications not only for the types of questions that are addressed by aphasia research but also for methodology. Earlier investigators had relied extensively on the classic aphasia syndrome categories (e.g., Broca's aphasia, Wernicke's aphasia) as the basis for identifying and grouping subjects. While useful as behavioral descriptors and pointers to lesion site, the syndrome designations allow a considerable amount of variability.[2,3] Moreover, these fairly gross breakdown patterns did not map very neatly onto the models of normal language processing that psycholinguists were developing. The investigative focus therefore moved from what might be regarded as "typical" aphasic manifestations[†]—for example, the combination of receptive and expressive

symptoms that define Wernicke's aphasia—to deficits that were (1) of a more circumscribed nature and (2) had some clear relationship to models of language processing.[‡] An early statement of the assumptions underlying the approach was provided by Marin and colleagues[4]:

> . . . the behavior of the patient with organic brain disease largely reflects capacities which existed in the premorbid state. We should therefore be able to make some inferences about the organization of normal language function from patterns of functional preservation and impairment: if process X is intact where process Y is severely compromised or absent, and especially if the converse is found in other patients, there is reason to believe that X and Y reflect different underlying mechanisms in the normal state. At the very least, the resulting matrix of intact and impaired functions should yield a taxonomy of functional subsystems. It may not tell us how these subsystems interact—but it should identify and describe what distinct capacities are available (e.g., it might, to take a hypothetical instance, describe a semantic process that is distinct from a syntactic process). The method is, of course, limited by the functional topology of the brain. Because functions may overlap in their anatomical

---

[†] Although any experienced clinician would agree that many patients are not easily assigned to classic syndrome categories.

[‡] This is not to imply that the cognitive neuropsychology approach is without clinical relevance. The assumption is that analyses of disorders in terms of loci of disruption within processing models should provide the basis for developing treatment programs tailored to the underlying disturbance (e.g., Chap. 12 in Ref. 105).

---

* **ACKNOWLEDGMENT:** Preparation of this chapter was supported by grant DC00191 from the National Institutes of Health.

substrates, we cannot state with assurance that every functional system which could be observed will be observed. But positive evidence that functions are organized independently should be significant for a theory of the language process [pp. 869–870].

It follows from this emphasis on dissociations that, for investigative purposes, greater value is placed on the purity of the impairment than on its frequency of occurrence in the aphasic population. Since circumscribed deficits are relatively rare, studies of single patients are not only admissible but, in the view of some investigators (e.g., Ref. 5), constitute the only valid source of neuropsychological data for the purpose of testing models of cognitive function (see Chap. 10 in Ref. 6 for discussion). Many cognitive neuropsychologists do not subscribe to this position, and group studies that involve sets of patients identified as having a particular cognitive impairment (e.g., "asyntactic" comprehension; see below) are not uncommon. Moreover, although the case study approach clearly departs from the random sampling from a population that is standard for behavioral research, the data are nevertheless cumulative. Delineation of an impairment in a single case report often leads to the identification of other patients with similar impairments and ultimately to compilations of data from a number of cases whose deficits appear quite similar.[7,8]

The cognitive neuropsychological approach is clearly well suited to the investigation of cognitive systems with modular architectures, that is, systems with components that are discrete and isolable, both functionally and anatomically.[9] In a system so constituted, the effects of damage to a single component should be quite local; other components should continue to function much as they did before the damage was incurred.[6] According to this view, the behavioral deficit should directly reflect the nature of the underlying impairment; Caramazza[2] refers to this as the "transparency" assumption. We will return to this point again at the end of the chapter, after reviewing the major contri-

butions of cognitive neuropsychology to the study of aphasia.*

COMPONENTS OF LANGUAGE PROCESSING

Most psycholinguists would agree that a model of language processing should include the components identified in Fig. 17-1. The model distinguishes among three types of information—semantic, syntactic, and phonologic; it does not, however, specify the extent to which these forms of information are processed independently, a matter that is still much debated.[10–12] The model includes procedures for recognizing and producing spoken words and for recovering and generating syntactic structures; the extent to which components are shared by the comprehension and production streams is another open question.[13,14] Language breakdown patterns are germane to both of these issues.

Assuming that the model is correct and that the processes and components identified in Fig. 17-1 can be disrupted independently, it should be possible to find patients with deficits that reflect breakdown at particular loci in the model. We will examine evidence for such disorders in the sections that follow.

DISORDERS OF LANGUAGE PROCESSING

Processing of Single Words: Comprehension

Impairments in the comprehension of spoken words are common in aphasia, and it is evident from Fig. 17-1 that there are a number of ways in which comprehension might fail: faulty phonologic processing prior to lexical access; loss of or impaired access to the phonologic forms of words; and/or loss of or impaired access to word meanings. Disorders of the first type can be ruled out by tests of phoneme perception and the second by lexical decision tasks in which the patient is asked to determine whether a string of phonemes is or is not a word. If a semantic deficit is present, it should be manifest not only on tests of auditory word comprehension but on written word comprehension and

---

*Although the approach was first applied in the study of acquired dyslexia,[7] reading disorders are the subject of another chapter in this volume (Chap. 20) and are not discussed here.

SENTENCE COMPREHENSION AND PRODUCTION

A. COMPREHENSION

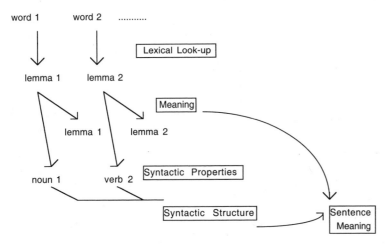

B. PRODUCTION

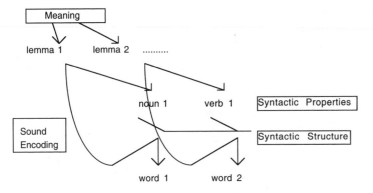

Figure 17-1
*Stages in language process-
ing. A. Processing of single
words. The lemma refers to a
processing level at which the
word is specified with respect
to meaning and grammatical
class but not encoded phonologically. B. Processing of sentences.*

production tasks as well. This follows from the widely
held assumption that comprehension and production
in both oral and written modalities rely on a common
conceptual base.[14]

Phonologic Processing

The task for the perceiver of spoken language is to
recover meaningful units (words) from the complex
and variable sound patterns produced by the human
vocal tract. Phonemes, such as *d*, *ow*, and *t*, which are
the basic building blocks of words, consist of several
distinct frequency bands (formants) that may differ in
their relative onset times as well as undergo transient
shifts in frequency. These acoustic properties can vary
depending on the context in which the phoneme occurs;
compare the *d* sound in the word *ride* with the *d* sound
in *rider*. A further complication is that the boundaries
between words are not systematically marked by gaps
in the acoustic stimulus, as they are in written text.
Thus the processing of speech input is a complicated
matter, which, it has been argued, requires specialized
mechanisms that are distinct from those used to process
other types of acoustic stimuli.[15]

The fact that the processing of speech sounds
can be selectively disrupted by brain damage supports
this view. Disorders that meet this description are labeled *pure word deafness*. They are the product of small

lesions, usually embolic in nature, that affect the superior temporal lobe on the left or, in other cases, that occur bilaterally. In its pure form, the disorder is relatively rare. In most cases the lesion is more extensive, resulting in the set of symptoms associated with Wernicke's aphasia, which may include features of word deafness.[16]

The hallmark of pure word deafness is that the patient has great difficulty comprehending and repeating what he or she hears but can read and speak virtually normally. The audiometric exam is essentially normal, and nonspeech sounds are interpreted without difficulty. Some patients have shown suppression of right-ear input under dichotic listening conditions, suggesting that auditory input is being processed in the right hemisphere[17,18] (but see Ref. 19). Auditory comprehension improves significantly when lip reading is allowed,[19] speech is slowed down,[17] and/or contextual constraints are provided. For example, Saffran and coworkers[18] described a patient whose ability to repeat words was better with semantically constrained than random word lists. These observations suggest that the auditory information available for word identification is in some way inadequate or degraded. Studies in which speech perception has been carefully examined have demonstrated deficits in the discrimination and identification of phonemes.[18-20] Vowels, made up of steady-state formants, tend to be better preserved than consonants, in which there are transient frequency shifts.[20] The processing of nonspeech sounds has not been examined as systematically. Although word-deaf patients are generally able to identify environmental stimuli such as the sounds of animals and musical instruments, they have seldom been called upon to make fine-grained judgments outside the speech domain, involving, for example, the temporal and waveform parameters that are manipulated in speech perception tasks. In the few studies that have included such investigations, deficits in the resolution of repetitive click stimuli have been identified.[17,19,21] This finding points to an impairment in auditory processes that are essential to phoneme perception but are not necessarily specific to speech. Auerbach and coworkers[19] have suggested that there may, in fact, be two forms of word deafness, one reflecting impairment of prephonetic auditory processing and the other specific to phonetic operations. This proposal requires further investigation.

Lexical Processing

Lexical access entails matching of the acoustic input to an entry in lexical memory that represents the word's phonologic form. Loss or degradation of lexical phonology is a possible cause of comprehension failure. Deciding whether a speech sound is a word or not (auditory lexical decision) should be impaired under these conditions, but it should still be possible to repeat words, treating them as one would normally treat nonwords. Lexical decision and comprehension of written words should be preserved. Deficits in word comprehension, with relatively preserved repetition, have been described under the label *word-meaning deafness*.[22-24] These patients are reported to have no comparable difficulty with written words and may resort to writing down spoken words in order to understand them. However, data on lexical decision have not been provided, and evidence for the critical phenomenon—failure to comprehend spoken words that can be understood in written form—are limited to a small number of examples.

The model outlined in Fig. 17-1 also suggests the possibility of preserved access to phonologic form with failure of access to word meaning. Franklin and associates[25] have recently reported a case that meets this description, at least for abstract words. This patient performed well on phonologic processing and auditory lexical decision tasks but was impaired in the auditory—but not written—comprehension of abstract words. He also had difficulty repeating abstract words as well as nonwords. Word meaning was clearly a significant factor in his repetition performance, as further indicated by a tendency to produce semantic errors in repeating single words. This pattern of repetition performance is termed *deep dysphasia* (for case reports, see Refs. 26 to 28). As shown below, this is but one of several disorders in which particular types of words are disproportionately affected.

Semantic Processing

Deficits that involve the loss of word meaning are frequently reported, although often in the context of other impairments (e.g., as in Wernicke's aphasia). Relatively pure cases have been described under the label *transcortical sensory aphasia,* a disorder in which repetition is spared relative to comprehension and spontaneous production.[29,30] Semantic disturbances are also found in cases of herpes encephalitis[31,32] and, in progressive form (*semantic dementia*), in association with degenerative brain disease[33,34]; these disorders involve damage to middle and inferior temporal lobe structures that lie outside the perisylvian zone usually associated with language function (see Chap. 27).

In some cases, the deficit is remarkably selective, affecting some categories of words more than others. The pattern that has been most frequently reported is a disproportionate loss of knowledge of biological kinds, such as animals, fruits, and vegetables; knowledge of artifacts, such as tools and furniture, is at least relatively preserved (see Ref. 35 for review). The semantic deficit is manifest on naming tasks as well as on a variety of measures of word comprehension. This "category-specific" disorder has most often been described in cases of herpes encephalitis but has also been found in one case of semantic dementia.[36] There have been attempts to account for this pattern in terms of confounding factors such as the greater visual complexity and lesser familiarity of animals relative to objects such as tools,[37,38] but the category differences have been shown to persist even when these factors are well controlled.[39] Moreover, the opposite pattern—better performance on living things—has been demonstrated in patients with frontoparietal lesions (see Ref. 35 for review). One possible account of this double dissociation is that biological kinds and artifacts depend in different degrees on different types of semantic information.[31,40] For example, animals are distinguished largely on the basis of perceptual characteristics such as shape and color (compare *lion* and *tiger*, for example), while artifacts are defined primarily by their function (namely, the diverse objects that qualify as radios).

These considerations are compatible with the view that semantic memory is distributed across subsystems specialized for different types of knowledge (but see Ref. 41). Figure 17-2, from Allport,[42] illustrates such a model: the shape of a telephone is stored in one subsystem, its sound in another, its function (not shown) in still another. Although represented in different subsystems, the properties of an object are linked in memory by virtue of the fact that they consistently occur together. When some features of an object (e.g., its shape) are accessed, properties that reside in other

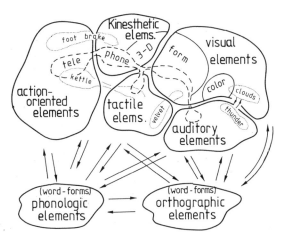

Figure 17-2

Schematic of a distributed model of conceptual representation. (From Allport,[42] with permission.)

subsystems (e.g., function) are automatically activated, instantiating the distributed activation pattern that corresponds to full knowledge of the object.

Semantic breakdown also occurs along the abstractness/concreteness dimension. Normal subjects show an advantage for concrete words,[43] and it would not be surprising if brain damage magnified this effect. This is, in fact, the result that is most frequently reported. For example, repetition of abstract words is disproportionately impaired in deep dysphasia,[26–28] a pattern that also holds for oral reading in deep dyslexia.[7] It is unlikely, however, that this effect simply reflects the greater difficulty of abstract words, as there are patients who show the reverse pattern, performing better on abstract than concrete words.[36,44,45] There is some evidence that abstract word superiority is associated with differential impairment within the class of concrete words, specifically, worse performance on words denoting living things than those denoting artifacts.[32,36] This would suggest that both patterns reflect disproportionate loss of perceptual components of meaning, which are irrelevant to abstract words and more salient for some categories of concrete words than others.

Processing of Single Words: Production

Psycholinguists conceive of production as a multistage process that begins with a concept and ends with movement of the articulators.[11,46,47] Here we concern ourselves only with the processes exemplified in Fig. 17-1, which involve selection of a lexical entry (lemma) that corresponds to the concept to be communicated, followed by access to the phonologic form of the word. The evidence that supports the two-stage retrieval process is not reviewed here (see Refs. 11, 46, and 47), but consideration of the tip-of-the-tongue phenomenon— knowing that one knows a word without being able to encode it phonologically—suggests that there is a stage of lexicalization that precedes access to phonology. The second stage, phonologic encoding, is a complex process involving retrieval of a set of phonemes, arranging them in the correct serial order, and specifying their stress pattern.[11]

Although there is general agreement that word retrieval is a two-step process, the nature of the relationship between the two stages is controversial. Some theorists maintain that lemma selection precedes and is entirely uninfluenced by phonologic encoding.[11] Others view lexical retrieval as an interactive process, involving feedback from phonology as well as activation in the forward direction, with the result that phonology can affect lemma selection.[10,48] Observations that favor the latter account include the fact that mixed errors that bear both a semantic and a phonologic relationship to the target word (e.g., *carrot, cabbage*) are more frequent than would be expected by chance.[49,50] This finding suggests that phonologic feedback interacts with feed-forward activation from semantics to promote the selection of alternatives that bear both a semantic and a phonologic relationship to the target.

Models of word production are based to a large extent on normal speech error patterns.[46,47] It should be possible to account for aphasic speech errors within the same theoretical framework. The errors produced by normal speakers include word substitutions that are semantically (e.g., *fork; spoon*) or phonologically related to the target (e.g., *index; insect*) as well as the mixed errors referred to above. Semantic errors are common in aphasics, and although the literature suggests that phonologically related word substitutions are rare (cf. Ref. 51), there are some patients who do produce high rates of these "formal paraphasias"[52,53] Perhaps the major difference between aphasic and normal speech errors (aside from the increase in overall rate of error production) is the frequency with which aphasic

patients generate errors that are not words; these are referred to as phonemic paraphasias, or neologisms. Some of these errors bear a clear phonologic relationship to the target (e.g., *scout; scut*); others, sometimes referred to as abstruse neologisms,[54] do not.

Although patients generally produce both semantic and phonologic errors, there are cases in which one type of error dominates. For example, Caramazza and Hillis[55] describe a patient who produced only semantic errors, while Caplan and coworkers[56] report a case in which errors were exclusively phonologic. In general, the error patterns of aphasics are consistent with the two-stage model, with indications that semantic and phonologic processes can, on occasion, be disrupted independently.

Recently, there have been efforts to bring aphasic data to bear on the question of independent stage versus interactive models of lexical retrieval. As noted earlier, the interactive model predicts that mixed (semantic + phonologic) errors should exceed levels expected by chance; this prediction should hold for aphasic individuals as well as for normals. Martin and coworkers[57] examined a corpus of errors elicited from aphasic patients in a picture-naming task and found that it does. Martin and colleagues[53] were also able to simulate error patterns of a patient who produced a high rate of form-based word substitutions by altering parameter settings on an implemented version of an interactive computational model.[10]

Grammatical class is another important variable in lexical retrieval. It is not unusual to find patients who show significant differences in their ability to retrieve nouns versus verbs.[58,59] Case studies include those of McCarthy and Warrington,[60] of a patient with a selective disturbance in verb production and comprehension, and Zingeser and Berndt,[61] whose patient showed preservation of action naming relative to object naming. Different lesion sites have been implicated in these selective impairments—specifically, a frontal locus for verbs and a temporal locus for nouns.[62] But the functional basis for these grammatical class effects is not entirely clear. As grammatical class reflects a conceptual distinction, one might expect this factor to be operative early in word retrieval; indeed, the lemma is assumed to specify grammatical class.[11] However, Caramazza and Hillis[63] have argued that phonologic output from the lexicon is also organized with respect to grammatical class. This proposal follows from their study of two patients who showed selective deficits for verbs in a single modality—oral production in one case and written production in the other. They interpret these patterns to reflect selective impairment for verbs at the level of orthographic or phonologic encoding.

Sentence-Level Processing: Comprehension

As inspection of the sentences below indicates, the meaning of a sentence is not solely a function of its lexical content. Failure to comprehend such sentences—interpreting sentence 1 to indicate that the cat was the chaser or that the dog was black—is not uncommon in aphasic individuals, even when they understand all of the individual words. In an influential study, Caramazza and Zurif[64] demonstrated such an impairment in patients with Broca's aphasia. Although their subjects had no difficulty understanding sentences like sentence 2, they performed at chance on sentences like sentence 1.

1. The cat that the dog chased was black.
2. The apple that the boy ate was red.

The difference between the two sentences, which have the same syntactic structure, is that the second one is semantically constrained (apples cannot eat boys), while the first is not. In order to interpret sentence 1 correctly, it is necessary to recover the syntax of the sentence and to use this information to assign the nouns to the thematic roles specified by the verb (i.e., *dog* to the role of agent, or chaser, and *cat* to the role of theme, or the entity being chased). Caramazza and Zurif's experiment showed that the aphasic subjects had difficulty utilizing syntactic information for this purpose, although they were clearly able to make use of semantic constraints. These authors showed, further, that performance was a function of syntactic complexity: although the patients did relatively well on simple active declarative sentences, their performance broke down on more complex structures, such as passives and object relatives (sentence 1, for example). Caramazza and Zurif interpreted this result to indicate that the patients were using heuristics such as "assign the preverbal noun the agent

role and the postverbal noun the role of theme." Reliance on heuristics, together with semantic constraints, would account for the fact that sentence comprehension appears relatively preserved in those with Broca's aphasia.

Difficulty in sentence production—the pattern known as "agrammatism"—is also part of the symptom complex in Broca's aphasia. The fact that syntactic impairments in comprehension and production occurred in the same patients gave rise to the hypothesis that the co-occurring deficits were due to a central syntactic deficit, characterized as a loss of grammatical knowledge.[65] Another influential view was that both disturbances reflect impairment to the closed class vocabulary, consisting of elements such as prepositions and tense markers, which convey syntactic information.[66] Both hypotheses were subsequently challenged by two sources of evidence: reports of cases in which production was agrammatic but comprehension was intact[67] and the demonstration that patients with agrammatic Broca's aphasia with the "asyntactic" comprehension pattern described by Caramazza and Zurif[64] were able to detect grammatical violations such as those in sentences 3a and 3b.[68,69]

3a. How many did you see birds in the park?
3b. John was finally kissed Louise.

These results, subsequently replicated in other laboratories,[70,71] present difficulty for both accounts of the agrammatic impairment. The ability to detect such violations requires knowledge of the grammar as well as sensitivity to the absence or presence and identity of the grammatical morphemes on which most of them depend.

What, then, is the basis for the "asyntactic" comprehension pattern? Linebarger and coworkers[68] suggested two possible accounts. The first of these is the limited capacity hypothesis. The patients have limited processing resources that will not suffice for parsing and interpretive operations; if they parse, they cannot interpret, and vice versa. Schwartz and coworkers[72] tested this hypothesis in a study in which patients judged the plausibility of sentences such as sentences 4a and 4b. The "padding" in sentence 4b should increase the difficulty of parsing relative to sentence 4a; on the limited capacity hypotheses, one might therefore expect worse performance on the padded sentences.

    4a.   The chicken killed the farmer.

    4b.   In the early part of the day, the chicken drank some water and then killed and ate the farmer.

    4c.   The farmer was killed by the chicken.

The results showed, however, that the effect of padding was negligible for the "asyntactic" comprehenders (though not for other aphasic patients); in contrast, the effect of the syntactic manipulation in sentence 4c, which involves movement of the nouns from their canonical (preverbal agent, postverbal theme) positions, was seriously detrimental. The second account is the mapping hypothesis. The patients are able to parse sentences but cannot carry out additional operations on the structures computed by the parser, such as mapping from a syntactic representation to thematic roles.

    Interpretation of the "asyntactic" comprehension pattern remains controversial. The mapping and limited capacity hypotheses are still debated, as are other interpretations motivated by recent developments in linguistic theory (see Ref. 69 for discussion). The mapping hypothesis has led to the development of treatment programs directed at the mapping operation (see Refs. 73 and 74 and Chap. 18, this volume), which have produced gains in some patients with chronic aphasia. The capacity limitation hypothesis has received support from studies conducted with normal subjects; it turns out that a variety of manipulations that might be expected to tax processing capacity (e.g., rapid serial visual presentation of the words in a sentence; divided attention; elimination of grammatical morphemes) result in comprehension patterns that mirror those of the aphasic individuals.[75–77] However, this evidence in itself is not compelling. Assuming that it is the recovery of syntactic information and/or the mapping from syntactic to semantic structures that are most vulnerable under these conditions, one would expect other factors that contribute to sentence interpretation to be more influential; these include a tendency to assign the preverbal noun the role of agent, which it often is in English sentences.[78] Other proposals have come from linguists, who have attempted to interpret the asyntactic comprehension pattern in terms of constructs in linguistic theory (see Ref. 69 and other papers in

that volume). To a large extent, these accounts emphasize the difficulty that these aphasic patients have in comprehending sentences with moved arguments; these structures are marked with "traces" (indicated by t) linked to the argument that has been moved, as in sentence 5:

    5.   The farmer was killed t by the chicken.

It is assumed that the necessity to link the moved argument (the farmer, in sentence 5) to the trace complicates sentence processing for those with aphasia. Often ignored by proponents of these views, however, is the fact that "asyntactic" patients frequently have difficulty with sentences that (at least according to most theories) lack traces, such as the simple active declarative[79,80] and locative[79,81] sentences exemplified by sentences 6a and 6b.

    6a.   The boy follows the girl.

    6b.   The paper is on the book.

Thus, while the basic phenomena are well established, there is as yet no generally accepted interpretation of the "asyntactic" comprehension pattern.

Short-Term Memory and Sentence Processing

Other studies of aphasia have focused on the role of short-term memory (STM) in sentence processing. Although most aphasic patients show some degree of short-term verbal memory impairment (see Ref. 82 for review), there are cases in which STM capacity, as measured by digit and word span, is markedly deficient in the context of relatively preserved language abilities.[83,84] The STM deficit appears to reflect impairment of a phonologic component of STM.[8] Most STM patients have difficulty with sentence comprehension, demonstrating the performance pattern characteristic of agrammatical aphasia that was described above.[85] It has proved difficult, however, to specify the relationship between these two impairments. One complicating factor is that the two are not perfectly correlated; there are instances in which reduced memory span is not accompanied by impairment in comprehension.[86,87] Studies of normal sentence processing indicate, moreover, that syntactic and semantic encoding occur on line,[88] so that there would seem to be no need to maintain the input in phonologic form. But while phonologic memory may not be necessary for first-pass encoding operations, it may serve as a backup store that allows the listener to revise interpretations in light of information that comes later in the sentence (for discussion, see Refs. 89 and 90).

Sentence-Level Processing: Production

A schema for sentence production is outlined in Fig. 17-1. Although not explicitly represented in the diagram, most psycholinguists assume that sentence production involves retrieval of a syntactic frame that stipulates word order (e.g., determiner-noun-auxiliary-verb. . .) and serves as a template into which phonologically specified words are later inserted (e.g., Refs. 47 and 48). While there are other aphasic patients who are impaired in some aspects of sentence production,[91] it is the deficits of agrammatical Broca's aphasia that have drawn most attention. The production of such patients is characterized by the limited use of syntactic structures and the omission of grammatical morphemes, such as tense markers (e.g., -ed), determiners (e.g., the), and prepositions (e.g., to). It seems likely that frame retrieval is seriously impaired in such patients, reflecting a reduction in the inventory of syntactic structures, their inaccessibility, or both.[92] The fact that patients occasionally produce utterances that are more complex than those constituting the bulk of their corpora suggests that inaccessibility of these structures is at least part of the problem.[93] In light of evidence from normals that use promotes further use,[94,95] it seems likely that a tendency to rely on a limited set of structures will render other structures progressively less accessible. There is some evidence that frame retrieval can be disrupted independently of access to grammatical morphology[67,96] and that bound (i.e., inflectional) and free-standing grammatical morphemes can be selectively affected.[97,98]

NEW DIRECTIONS

Cognitive neuropsychology adopted the box-and-arrow information processing models that were favored by cognitive psychologists in the 1970s. The boxes

stood for modules whose internal operations were largely unknown; the arrows symbolized the flow of information between them. More recently, cognitive theorists have turned to computer-implemented (neural network or "connectionist") models that specify more precisely how information is represented and processed (see Chap. 7). These models are networks of units that represent information; the informational significance of the units is either specified by the modeler (in "localist" models; e.g., Ref. 48) or acquired during learning trials [in parallel distributed processing (PDP) models; e.g., Refs. 40 and 99]. In the latter, inner layers of units are initially connected randomly to input and output layers in which units are specified for content. Thus, for example, models that learn to read aloud have input units that stand for individual letters or groups of letters and output units that stand for specific phonemes or groups of phonemes. Explorations of effects of "lesioning" these models (for example, by randomly eliminating units or altering the strength of connections between units) have revealed some interesting properties that have implications for fundamental assumptions in cognitive neuropsychology.

One major result of the simulation studies is that symptoms are not necessarily a direct reflection of the type of representation that is lesioned. For example, Shallice and colleagues[99,100] have developed a connectionist model of reading in which learning procedures are used to train graphemic units to activate units of meaning ("sememes" such as "brown," "has legs," etc.) that ultimately activate phoneme units. In other words, the model learns to pronounce written words by looking up their meanings. Lesioning of this model can result in semantic errors (e.g., reading *night* as *sleep*) of the sort that are produced by patients with deep dyslexia (see Chap. 20, this volume). These errors were generally thought to reflect impairment at the semantic level.[101] The simulations on this model demonstrate, however, that semantic errors can be generated by lesions elsewhere in the network. A related point is made by data from a study by Farah and McClelland,[40] who lesioned a semantic network to simulate the disorders involving living and nonliving things. The model included two semantic subsystems, one representing functional properties and the other visual properties, which predominated for living things. As a result of the connectivity patterns within the network, damage to the visual subsystem rendered the functional properties of living things inaccessible. The "symptoms" therefore reflected perturbations that extended well beyond the subsystem targeted by the lesion. The implication of these findings is that the relationship between symptom and deficit may not be as direct as it is often taken to be (cf. Ref. 102).

Other simulation studies demonstrate that performance patterns that appear selective can be generated by lesions that are widespread. Employing a localist model of word retrieval,[10] which allows activation to feed back from phonemes to lemma to semantic units as well as to proceed in the forward direction, our group has shown that shifts in the dominant error types can be produced by altering different parameters of the model.[53,103] The two parameters are connection strength, which affects the ease with which activation flows (in both directions) from one level to another, and decay rate, which affects the persistence of activation within representational levels. Different error patterns result from connection weight and decay rate lesions, both applied uniformly throughout the lexical system. A decrease in connection strength reduces the flow of activation to target-related units, resulting in an increase in nonword errors. Decay rate lesions have a different effect on the distribution of activation, shifting error production in the direction of semantic and formal substitutions. Lest it be thought that this is merely a formal exercise, manipulation of these two parameters closely simulated the individual error patterns of almost all (20 of 23) of the patients with fluent aphasia tested by us.

How seriously should we take these demonstrations of nonlocal effects of lesions, and do they in any way invalidate the 20-year research program in cognitive neuropsychology? Computational modeling in the language domain is relatively new, and it is too soon to determine how useful this approach will prove to be. However, recent psycholinguistic studies indicate that normal language processing is characterized by a good deal of interaction among processing components.[10,95,104] Interactive processing architectures complicate the task of inferring the locus of the deficit from a patient's performance. As Farah[102] has observed, the relationship between symptom and impaired process is no longer transparent; semantic errors, for example, need not necessarily reflect perturbation of a semantic process. But while it will be necessary to interpret new data more cautiously and, perhaps, to reexamine earlier conclusions, the effort to tie phenomena of language breakdown to models of normal language function remains useful and valid. Neuropsychological data extend the database and testing ground for normative models, and the models, in turn, provide a coherent framework for the investigation and interpretation of clinical phenomena.

REFERENCES

1. Goodglass H, Geschwind N: Language disorders (aphasia), in Carterette EC, Friedman MP (eds): *Handbook of Perception.* New York: Academic Press, 1976.
2. Caramazza A: The logic of neuropsychological research and the problem of patient classification in aphasia. *Brain Lang* 21:9–20, 1984.
3. Schwartz MF: What the classical aphasia categories can't do for us and why. *Cognit Neuropsychol* 21:3–8, 1984.
4. Marin OSM, Saffran EM, Schwartz MF: Dissociations of language in aphasia: Implications for normal function. *Ann NY Acad Sci* 280:868–884, 1976.
5. Caramazza A: On drawing inferences about the structure of normal cognitive systems from the analysis of patterns of impaired performance: the case for single-patient studies. *Brain Cogn* 5:41–66, 1986.
6. Shallice T: *From Neuropsychology to Mental Structure.* Cambridge, England: Cambridge University Press, 1988.
7. Coltheart M, Patterson KE, Marshall JC (eds): *Deep Dyslexia.* London: Routledge, 1980.
8. Vallar G, Shallice T (eds): *Neuropsychological Deficits in Short-Term Memory.* Cambridge, England: Cambridge University Press, 1990.
9. Fodor JA: *The Modularity of Mind.* Cambridge, MA: MIT Press, 1983.
10. Dell GS, O'Seaghdha PG: Mediated and convergent lexical priming in language production: A comment on Levelt et al. *Psychol Rev* 98:604–614, 1991.
11. Levelt WJM: Accessing words in speech production: Stages, processes and representations. *Cognition* 42:1–21, 1992.
12. Mitchell DC: Sentence parsing, in Gernsbacher MA (ed): *Handbook of Psycholinguistics.* San Diego, CA: Academic Press, 1994.
13. Allport DA: Speech production and comprehension: One lexicon or two? in Prinz W, Sanders AF (eds):

Cognition and Motor Processes. Berlin: Springer-Verlag, 1984.

14. Monsell S: On the relation between lexical input and output pathways for speech, in Allport A, MacKay D, Prinz W, Sheerer E (eds): *Language Perception and Production.* London: Academic Press, 1987.

15. Liberman AM, Studdert-Kennedy M: Phonetic perception, in Held R, Lebowitz H, Teuber H-L (eds): *The Handbook of Sensory Physiology: Perception.* Heidelberg: Springer-Verlag, 1978, vol 8, pp. 143–178.

16. Caramazza A, Berndt RS, Basili AG: The selective impairment of phonological processing: A case study. *Brain Lang* 18:128–174, 1983.

17. Albert ML, Bear D: Time to understand: A case study of word deafness with reference to the role of time in auditory comprehension. *Brain* 97:373–384, 1974.

18. Saffran EM, Marin OSM, Yeni-Komshian G: An analysis of speech perception in word deafness. *Brain Lang* 3:209–228, 1976.

19. Auerbach SH, Allard T, Naeser M, et al: Pure word deafness: Analysis of a case with bilateral lesions and defect at the prephonemic level. *Brain* 105:271–300, 1982.

20. Denes G, Semenza C: Auditory modality-specific anomie: Evidence from a case of pure word deafness. *Cortex* 14:41–49, 1975.

21. Tanaka Y, Yamadori A, Mori E: Pure word deafness following bilateral lesions. *Brain* 110:381–403, 1987.

22. Bramwell B: Illustrative cases of aphasia (case 11). *Lancet* 1:1256–1259, 1897. [Reprinted with an introduction by AW Ellis. *Cognit Neuropsychol* 1:245–258, 1984.]

23. Kohn SE, Friedman RB: Word-meaning deafness: A phonological semantic dissociation. *Cognit Neuropsychol* 3:291–308, 1986.

24. Schacter DL, McGlynn SM, Milberg WP, Church BA: Spared priming despite impaired comprehension: Implicit memory in a case of word-meaning deafness. *Neuropsychology* 7:107–118, 1993.

25. Franklin S, Howard D, Patterson K: Abstract word meaning deafness. *Cogn Neuropsychol* 11:1–34, 1994.

26. Howard D, Franklin S: *Missing the Meaning? A Cognitive Neuropsychological Study of Processing of Words by an Aphasic Patient.* Cambridge, MA: MIT Press, 1988.

27. Katz R, Goodglass H: Deep dysphasia: an analysis of a rare form of repetition disorder. *Brain Lang* 39:153–185, 1990.

28. Martin N, Saffran EM: A computational account of deep dysphasia: Evidence from a single case study. *Brain Lang* 43:240–274, 1992.

29. Berndt RS, Basili A, Caramazza A: Dissociation of functions in a case of transcortical sensory aphasia. *Cognit Neuropsychol* 4:79–101, 1987.

30. Martin N, Saffran EM: Factors underlying repetition and short-term memory in transcortical sensory aphasia. *Brain Lang* 37:440–479, 1990.

31. Warrington EK, Shallice T: Category-specific semantic impairments. *Brain* 107:829–854, 1984.

32. Sirigu A, Duhamel J-R, Poncet M: The role of sensorimotor experience in object recognition. *Brain* 114:2555–2573, 1991.

33. Snowden JS, Goulding PJ, Neary D: Semantic dementia: a form of circumscribed cerebral atrophy. *Behav Neurol* 2:167–182, 1989.

34. Hodges JR, Patterson K, Oxbury S, Funnell E: Semantic dementia: progressive fluent aphasia, with temporal lobe atrophy. *Brain* 115:1783–1806, 1992.

35. Saffran EM, Schwartz MF: Of cabbages and things: semantic memory from a neuropsychological perspective—a tutorial review, in Umilta C, Moscovitch M (eds): *Attention and Performance: XV. Conscious and Nonconscious Processes.* Cambridge, MA: MIT Press, 1994.

36. Breedin SD, Saffran EM, Coslett HB: Reversal of the concreteness effect in a patient with semantic dementia. *Cognit Neuropsychol* 11:617–660, 1994.

37. Funnell E, Sheridan J: Categories of knowledge? Unfamiliar aspects of living and non-living things. *Cognit Neuropsychol* 9:135–154, 1992.

38. Stewart F, Parkin AJ, Hunkin NM: Naming impairments following recovery from herpes simplex encephalitis: category specific? *Q J Exp Psychol* 44A:261–284, 1992.

39. Farah MJ, McMullen PA, Meyer MM: Can recognition of living things be selectively impaired? *Neuropsychologia* 29:185–193, 1991.

40. Farah MJ, McClelland JL: A computational model of semantic memory impairment: Modality specificity and emergent category. *J Exp Psychol (Gen)* 120:339–357, 1991.

41. Caramazza A, Hillis AE, Rapp B, Romani C: The multiple semantics hypothesis: Multiple confusion? *Cognit Neuropsychol* 7:161–189, 1990.

42. Allport DA: Distributed memory, modular subsystems and dysphasia, in Newman SK, Epstein R (eds): *Current Perspectives in Dysphasia.* Edinburgh: Churchill Livingstone, 1985, pp 32–60.

43. Paivio A: Dual coding theory: Retrospect and current status. *Can J Psychol* 45:255–258, 1991.

44. Warrington EK: The selective impairment of semantic memory. *Q J Exp Psychol* 27:635–657, 1975.

45. Cipolotti L, Warrington EK: Semantic memory and reading abilities: A case report. *J Int Neuropsychol Soc* 1:104–110, 1995.

46. Fromkin VA: The non-anomalous nature of anomalous utterances. *Language* 47:27–52, 1971.

47. Garrett MF: Levels of processing in sentence production, in Butterworth B (ed): *Language Production.* New York: Academic Press, 1980, vol 1.

48. Dell GS: A spreading activation theory of retrieval in language production. *Psychol Rev* 93:283–321, 1986.

49. Dell GS, Reich PA: Stages in sentence production: An analysis of speech error data. *J Verb Learn Verb Behav* 20:611–629, 1981.

50. Martin N, Weisberg R, Saffran EM: Variables influencing the occurrence of naming errors: Implications for models of lexical retrieval. *J Mem Lang* 28:462–485, 1989.

51. Ellis AW: The production of spoken words, in Ellis AW (ed): *Progress in the Psychology of Language.* London: Erlbaum, 1985, vol 2.

52. Blanken G: Formal paraphasias: A single case study. *Brain Lang* 38:534–554, 1990.

53. Martin N, Dell GS, Saffran EM, Schwartz MF: Origins of paraphasias in deep dysphasia: Testing the consequences of a decay impairment to an interactive spreading activation model of lexical retrieval. *Brain Lang* 47:609–660, 1994.

54. Schwartz MF, Saffran EM, Bloch DE, Dell GS: Disordered speech production in aphasic and normal speakers. *Brain Lang* 47:52–88, 1994.

55. Caramazza A, Hillis AE: Where do semantic errors come from? *Cortex* 26:95–122, 1990.

56. Caplan D, Vanier M, Baker C: A case study of reproduction conduction aphasia: I. Word production. *Cognit Neuropsychol* 3:99–128, 1986.

57. Martin N, Gagnon DA, Schwartz MF, et al: Phonological facilitation of semantic errors in normal and aphasic speakers. *Lang Cogn Process* 11:257–282, 1996.

58. Miceh G, Silveri MC, Romani C, Caramazza A: On the basis for the agrammatic's difficulty in producing main verbs. *Cortex* 20:207–220, 1984.

59. Kohn SE, Lorch MP, Pearson DM: Verb finding in aphasia. *Cortex* 25:57–69, 1989.

60. McCarthy R, Warrington EK: Category specificity in an agrammatic patient: The relative impairment of verb retrieval and comprehension. *Neuropsychologia* 23:709–727, 1985.

61. Zingeser LB, Berndt RS: Retrieval of nouns and verbs in agrammatism and anomia. *Brain Lang* 39:14–32, 1990.

62. Daniele A, Giustolisi L, Silveri MC, et al: Evidence for a possible neuroanatomical basis for lexical processing of nouns and verbs. *Neuropsychologia* 32:1325–1341, 1994.

63. Caramazza A, Hillis AE: Lexical organization of nouns and verbs in the brain. *Nature* 349:788–790, 1991.

64. Caramazza A, Zurif EB: Dissociations of algorithmic and heuristic processes in language comprehension: Evidence from aphasia. *Brain Lang* 3:572–582, 1976.

65. Caramazza A, Berndt RS: Semantic and syntactic processes in aphasia: A review of the literature. *Psychol Bull* 85:898–918, 1978.

66. Bradley DC, Garrett MF, Zurif EB: Syntactic deficits in Broca's aphasia, in Caplan D (ed): *Biological Studies of Mental Processes.* Cambridge, MA: MIT Press, 1980.

67. Miceli G, Mazzuchi A, Menn L, Goodglass H: Contrasting cases of Italian agrammatic aphasia without comprehension disorder. *Brain Lang* 19:65–97, 1983.

68. Linebarger MC, Schwartz MF, Saffran EM: Sensitivity to grammatical structure in so-called agrammatic aphasics. *Cognition* 13:641–662, 1983.

69. Linebarger MC: Agrammatism as evidence about grammar. *Brain Lang* 50:52–91, 1995.

70. Berndt RS, Salasoo A, Mitchum CC, Blumstein S: The role of intonation cues in aphasic patients' performance of the grammaticality judgment task. *Brain Lang* 34:65–97, 1988.

71. Shankweiler D, Crain S, Gorrell P, Tuller B: Reception of language in Broca's aphasia. *Lang Cogn Process* 4:1–33, 1989.

72. Schwartz MF, Linebarger M, Saffran EM, Pate DS: Syntactic transparency and sentence interpretation in aphasia. *Lang Cogn Process* 2:85–113, 1987.

73. Byng S: Sentence comprehension deficit: theoretical analysis and remediation. *Cognit Neuropsychol* 5:629–676, 1988.

74. Schwartz MF, Saffran EM, Fink RB, et al: Mapping therapy: A treatment program for agrammatism. *Aphasiology* 8:19–54, 1994.

75. Miyake A, Carpenter PA, Just MA: A capacity approach to syntactic comprehension disorders: Making normal adults perform like aphasics. *Cognit Neuropsychol* 11:671–717, 1994.

76. Blackwell A, Bates E: Inducing agrammatic profiles in normals: evidence for the selective vulnerability of morphology under cognitive resource limitation. *J Cogn Neurosci* 7:228–257, 1995.

77. Pulvermüller F: Agrammatism: Behavioral description and neurobiological explanation. *J Cogn Neurosci* 7:165–181, 1995.

78. Bever TG: The cognitive basis for linguistic structures, in Hayes JR (ed): *Cognition and the Development of Language.* New York: Wiley, 1970.

79. Schwartz MF, Saffran EM, Marin OSM: The word order problem in agrammatism: 1. Comprehension. *Brain Lang* 10:263–288, 1980.

80. Berndt RS, Mitchum CC, Haendiges AN: Comprehension of reversible sentences in "agrammatism." *Cognition.* In press.

81. Kolk H, Van Grunsven MJE: Agrammatism as a variable phenomenon. *Cogn Neuropsychol* 2:347–384, 1985.

82. Saffran EM: Short-term memory impairment and language processing, in Caramazza A (ed): *Advances in Cognitive Neuropsychology and Neurolinguistics.* Hillsdale, NJ: Erlbaum, 1990.

83. Saffran EM, Marin OSM: Immediate memory for word lists and sentences in a patient with deficient auditory short-term memory. *Brain Lang* 2:420–433, 1975.

84. Vallar G, Baddeley AD: Phonological short-term store, phonological processing and sentence comprehension: A neuropsychological case study. *Cognit Neuropsychol* 1:121–142, 1984.

85. Saffran EM, Martin N: Short-term memory impairment and sentence processing, in Vallar G, Shallice T (eds): *Neuropsychological Impairments of Short Term Memory.* Cambridge, England: Cambridge University Press, 1990.

86. Butterworth B, Campbell R, Howard D: The uses of short-term memory: A case study. *Q J Exp Psychol* 38:705–737, 1986.

87. Martin RC: Articulatory and phonological deficits in short-term memory and their relation to syntactic processing. *Brain Lang* 32:159–192, 1987.

88. Marslen-Wilson W, Tyler LK: The temporal structure of spoken language understanding. *Cognition* 8:1–71, 1980.

89. Caplan D: *Language: Structure, Processing and Disorders.* Cambridge, MA: MIT Press, 1992.

90. Gathercole SE, Baddeley AD: *Working Memory and Language.* Hillsdale, NJ: Erlbaum, 1993.

91. Butterworth B, Howard D: Paragrammatisms. *Cognition* 26:1–38, 1987.

92. LaPointe S, Dell GS: A synthesis of some recent work on sentence production, in Tanenhaus MK, Carlson G (eds): *Linguistic Structure in Language Processing.* Dordrecht: Kluwer, 1988.

93. Menn L, Obler LK (eds): *Agrammatic Aphasia: A Cross-Language Narrative Sourcebook.* Philadelphia: John Benjamins, 1990.

94. Bock JK: Syntactic persistence in language production. *Cognit Psychol* 18:355–387, 1986.

95. Bock JK: Structure in language: Creating form in talk. *Am Psychol* 45:1221–1236, 1990.

96. Saffran EM, Schwartz MF, Marin OSM: Evidence from aphasia: Isolating the components of a production model, in Butterworth B (ed): *Language Production.* London: Academic Press, 1980, pp 221–240.

97. Nespoulous J-L, Dordain M, Perron C, et al: Agrammatism in sentence production without comprehension deficits: reduced variability of syntactic structures and/or of grammatical morphemes? A case study. *Brain Lang* 33:273–295, 1988.

98. Saffran EM, Berndt RS, Schwartz MF: A scheme for the quantitative analysis of agrammatic production. *Brain Lang* 37:440–479, 1989.

99. Plaut D, Shallice T: Deep dyslexia: A case study of connectionist neuropsychology. *Cognit Neuropsychol* 10:377–500, 1993.

100. Hinton GE, Shallice T: Lesioning an attractor network: Investigations of acquired dyslexia. *Psychol Rev* 98:74–95, 1991.

101. Shallice T, Warrington EK: Single and multiple component central dyslexic syndromes, in Coltheart M, Patterson KE, Marshall JC (eds): *Deep Dyslexia.* London: Routledge, 1980, pp 119–145.

102. Farah MJ: Neuropsychological inference with an interactive brain: a critique of the "locality assumption." *Behav Brain Sci* 17:43–104, 1994.

103. Dell GS, Schwartz MF, Martin N, et al: Lesioning a connectionist model of lexical retrieval to simulate naming errors in aphasia. Presented at conference on Neural Modeling of Cognitive and Brain Disorders; June 9, 1995; College Park, MD.

104. MacDonald MC, Pearlmutter NJ, Seidenberg MS: Lexical nature of syntactic ambiguity resolution. *Psychol Rev* 101:676–703, 1994.

105. Howard D, Hatfield FM: *Aphasia Therapy: Historical and Contemporary Issues.* Hillsdale, NJ: Erlbaum, 1987.

106. Heilman KM, Scholes RJ: The nature of comprehension errors in Broca's conduction, and Wernicke's aphasics. *Cortex* 12:258–265, 1976.

107. Grodzinsky Y: The syntactic characterization of agrammatism. *Cognition* 16:99–120, 1984.

108. Kay J, Lesser R, Coltheart M: *Psycholinguistic Assessment of Language Processing in Aphasia (PALPA).* London: Erlbaum, 1992.

Chapter 18

APHASIA III: REHABILITATION*

Myrna F. Schwartz
Ruth B. Fink

It is widely accepted that the goal of aphasia rehabilitation is to maximize functional communication
skills. There is less agreement on the optimal route
to that goal. Speech-language pathologists are exposed
to a broad range of approaches and are expected to
make informed decisions about the best treatment for
an individual patient based on a number of factors
(e.g., etiology, severity, and type of aphasia). They
are trained to view aphasia as a complex cognitive/
linguistic/communication disorder requiring intervention that addresses the social, as well as the linguistic,
needs of the client,[1,2] and they work with patients in a
variety of settings (acute care hospitals, rehabilitation
units, home care, and outpatient facilities) throughout
the phases of recovery.

Differences aside, speech-language pathologists
typically perform three basic functions: assessment,
treatment, and outcome evaluation. The initial assessment is critical for establishing the diagnosis of aphasia
and differentiating it from other neuropathologies such
as dementia and dysarthria, communicating with other
professionals and the patient's family, and setting goals
and developing a treatment plan. Following a program
of treatment, an outcome evaluation is performed to determine how well the goals have been met. Each of these
three functions (assessment, treatment, and outcome
evaluation) is carried out at several levels of analysis.

LEVELS OF ANALYSIS: IMPAIRMENT, ACTIVITY LIMITATION, PARTICIPATION RESTRICTION

The World Health Organization (WHO)[3] has proposed
a useful framework which distinguishes three levels

at which functioning and disability may be described
and explained: *impairment, activity limitation,* and
participation restriction. These levels replace those
used in the 1980 *WHO International Classification of
Impairment, Disability and Handicap* (ICIDH)[4] and
reflect a revision in the classification system. The new
(ICIDH-2)[3] terminology extends the meanings to include descriptions of positive as well as negative experiences, as shown below.

ICIDH	ICIDH-2
Impairment	Body structure and function (impairment)
Disability	Activity (activity limitation)
Handicap	Participation (participation restriction)

Impairment refers to "problems in body function or structure such as significant deviation or loss"
(Ref. 3, p. 13). The classic taxonomy of aphasia
(Broca's aphasia, Wernicke's aphasia, conduction
aphasia, anomic aphasia) rests on a mix of anatomic-
psychological impairment symptoms [e.g., disruption
of auditory-phonologic images caused by lesions in the
left posterior temporal gyrus (Wernicke's area)]. The
contemporary cognitive neuropsychological approach,
which we focus on in later sections, derives its impairment categories from cognitive and psycholinguistic
theories of the normal language system.

Activity limitation (formerly *disability*) refers to
an individual's competence in executing a skill or activity. While the characterization of impairments is theory dependent, *activity limitation* refers to categories
of behavior that have strong face validity, such as producing and understanding speech, reading, or writing. When speech pathologists characterize an aphasic disturbance, they generally do so in terms of its
impact on skills like these. On the other hand, such

* **ACKNOWLEDGMENTS:** Preparation of this manuscript
was supported by NIH grants 1R01 DC01825 and
DC00191. Jessica Myers and Jennifer Bender provided invaluable assistance.

characterizations often also make reference to the units affected (e.g., word, phrase, sentence), in which case it becomes difficult to distinguish this level of description from the impairment level. In general, however, activity limitations are observable at the level of the person while the presence of an impairment is inferred from diagnostic tests that reflect on the functioning of a body organ or system.

Participation restriction (formerly *handicap*) refers to involvement in life situations or capacity to function in society. When communication is compromised by a speech/language disability (e.g., nonfluent speech) such that the individual can no longer function effectively in his or her role as parent, spouse, lawyer, etc., a participation restriction is present. The degree of restriction depends upon factors both within and external to the individual. These include the severity of the disability; the intactness of other avenues of communication, such as writing or gesturing; the readiness of others to shoulder the burden of communication; and the ability to use, and to afford, alternate communication systems like computers or communication boards. Participation restrictions are thus affected by social factors or barriers (structural or attitudinal) which limit fulfillment of roles or deny access to services and opportunities. They are observed at the interface of the individual and environment.

THE TRADITIONAL LANGUAGE-ORIENTED SCHOOL OF APHASIA THERAPY

In aphasia rehabilitation, any one of these three levels may be targeted for assessment, treatment, and outcome evaluation. The impairment-activity-participation matrix shown in Fig. 18-1 represents the various possibilities[5] and the shaded cells locate the endeavor we term the *traditional language-oriented school*. The majority of clinicians in the United States would probably identify themselves with this school, which is eclectic in its approach to assessment and treatment. Assessment draws upon standardized instruments that measure loss at both the activity and impairment level (e.g., Boston Diagnostic Aphasia Examination,[6] Western Aphasia Battery,[7] Minnesota

Test for Differential Diagnosis of Aphasia[8]). The assessment serves as a guide to treatment, which might target several impairments concurrently or bypass the impairment level altogether in favor of direct retraining or stimulation of the compromised language skill. Both the target of treatment and the treatment techniques are tailored to the needs of the individual patient. The clinician may chose from several approaches. For example, the "stimulation" approach advocated by Schuell and colleagues[9] uses intensive auditory or multimodality input to elicit language production through a variety of means (e.g., repetition, phonemic cueing, reading) and in a variety of contexts (linguistic and situational). Helm-Estabrooks developed a variant of this technique to facilitate sentence production. Helm's Elicited Language Program for Syntax Stimulation (HELPSS)[10] uses a combined delayed repetition/story elicitation procedure to stimulate production of specific syntactic structures (e.g., yes-no questions; passive voice constructions) in aphasics with grammatical disturbances. The rationale behind the stimulation approach is that aphasia represents reduced access or efficiency. An alternative view is that specific aspects of the language system are lost or disrupted. This view is represented in Shewan and Bandur's "language-oriented therapy,"[11] a comprehensive, psycholinguistically based treatment program that aims to strengthen the impaired function(s) using training methods derived from behavioral learning theory. The common thread among these different approaches is the focus on restoration of language skills as the route to improved functional communication.

The same language-oriented assessments used to evaluate the patient's initial status are generally used as well to measure the gains made in treatment. But this alone does not constitute outcome evaluation. Also required is an assessment of the extent to which the *functional goals* projected for the patient at the outset have been met.

Medicare guidelines[12] specifically require that a plan of treatment state functional goals and estimated rehabilitation potential: "Functional goals must be written by the speech and language pathologist to reflect the level of communicative independence the patient is expected to achieve, outside of the therapeutic environment. The long-term functional goals must

Figure 18-1

The impairment-activity-partic-ipation (ICIDH-2) matrix. Assessment, treatment, and outcome evaluation can be directed at any of the three levels. The traditional, language-oriented school of aphasia rehabilitation focuses primarily on the impairment and activity levels.

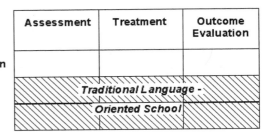

reflect the final level the patient is expected to achieve, be realistic, and have a positive effect on the quality of the patient's everyday functions."

To assess whether functional goals have been met, clinicians often rely on anecdotal reports from patients and family members. While formal assessments of functional communication are available (e.g., Functional Communication Profile,[13] Communicative Abilities in Daily Living,[14] Communicative Effectiveness Index,[15] ASHA's Functional Communication Scales for Adults[16]), many clinicians find that these instruments lack the requisite sensitivity or are too cumbersome to administer.[17] A new generation of functional assessments is being developed to better meet the needs of the clinic in documenting change associated with communication training. For example, conversational analysis[18,19] and discourse assessments (Assessment Profile of Pragmatic Language Skills,[20] Discourse Abilities Profile[21]) offer structured ways of assessing change in narrative and conversational discourse. Rating scales[15,22] and questionnaires[23] measure quality of life, ability to perform various communication tasks, and participation in social activities and social functioning.

That language-oriented therapy succeeds in enhancing the language skills of treated patients is demonstrated in a number of large-scale group studies,[24–28] as well as smaller, more focused studies.[29–33] There is less evidence that these gains translate into expanded participation and enhanced quality of life. Indeed, the general view is that language gains evident in the clinic do not generalize well to less constrained tasks or settings.[34] This is one problem with the traditional, language-oriented school of

aphasia therapy. A second is its weak theoretical base. Two newer schools have arisen in response to these perceived weaknesses: the functional/pragmatic/social school and the cognitive neuropsychological school.

THE FUNCTIONAL/PRAGMATIC/SOCIAL SCHOOL OF APHASIA THERAPY

If linguistic gains made in the clinic do not automatically translate into improved functional communication, then perhaps functional carryover should be programmed in as an integral part of the rehabilitation process. For adherents of the functional/pragmatic/social school, this means gearing therapy toward the enhancement of *communication,* nonverbal as well as verbal, in functional settings and/or with functional materials. Functional/pragmatic approaches typically capitalize on the patients' strengths and seek to train patients to use compensatory strategies when communicating. They may also involve use of behavioral methodology to achieve changes in pragmatic skills, as Doyle et al.[35] demonstrated in a study aimed at teaching patients with Broca's aphasia to make requests. The point of functional/pragmatic treatments is to develop communication skills that can be used in everyday life. The most widely known program of this type is Promoting Aphasics Communicative Effectiveness (PACE),[36] which fosters the communication of new information (the patient conveys a message unknown to the therapist, who must then figure it out) using whatever combination of strategies (verbal, written, gestural, graphic) achieves success. Another functional/pragmatic program, conversational coaching,[37]

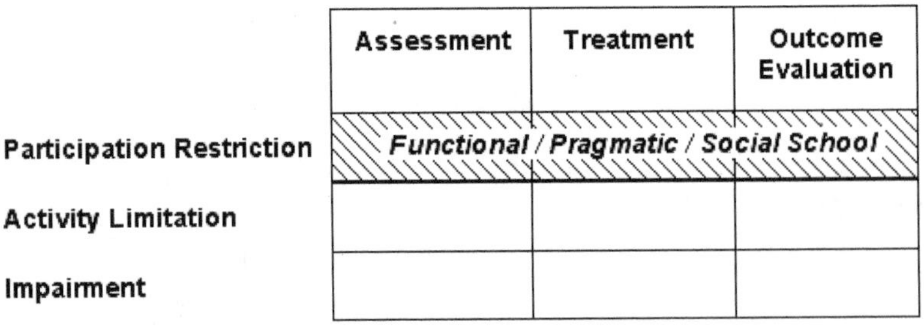

	Assessment	Treatment	Outcome Evaluation
Participation Restriction	*Functional / Pragmatic / Social School*		
Activity Limitation			
Impairment			

Figure 18-2
The functional/pragmatic/social school of aphasia rehabilitation focuses primarily on the level of participation restriction.

develops compensatory strategies in treatment sessions that simulate conversations that might take place outside the clinic. These include conversations with unfamiliar listeners to further extend generalization. Ultimately, the patient and his or her relatives are trained to use these strategies to communicate with maximum effectiveness.

Training aphasic patients to get their message across using compensatory strategies and multiple modalities is now a staple of most treatment programs. In recent years, however, there has been a growing movement toward "social" or "life participation" approaches to aphasia. These approaches have developed in response to the unmet needs and rights of those affected by aphasia and are in keeping with the disability movement and the revised WHO ICIDH-2 classification. The social approach, as we will call it, is a natural outgrowth of the functional/pragmatic school. It addresses activity and participation issues directly, by emphasizing the context in which communication occurs and involving family members and/or peers within the community. Treatment is not intended to make the person "talk" better. It is designed to improve the quality of interactions between individuals with aphasia and their communication partners. To this end, programs such as Communication Partners,[38] Supported Conversation for Adults with Aphasia (SCA),[39] family member training,[40,41] and Family Intervention in Chronic Aphasia (FICA)[42,43] train family members and other partners to take greater responsibility for facilitating and supporting the communicative exchanges. For example, in the FICA program, partners learn to identify facilitative and nonfacilitative behaviors, first in videotaped conversations, and then in actual conversations. (Nonfacilitative behavior includes such things as asking questions whose answers are already known;

interrupting and correcting the aphasic partner during a successful communication effort.) Subsequently, partners engage in "negative practice," wherein they deliberately employ nonfacilitative behaviors and explore the degree to which these behaviors impede the success of the interaction.

Preliminary research on the FICA program indicates that (1) education (e.g., disseminating and discussing information) alone is not sufficient for altering interaction patterns; (2) an increase in facilitative behaviors and decrease in nonfacilitatory behaviors occurs within 3 to 5 weeks of direct behavior training; and (3) changes in the quality of communicative interactions are recognized by uninvolved observers.[42,43]

In its pure form (depicted in Fig. 18-2), the functional/pragmatic/social school replaces the traditional emphasis on language impairment and disability with an emphasis on minimizing handicap through enhanced communication, activity, and participation. In actuality, however, even its strongest proponents advocate that pragmatic techniques be used in combination with language-based approaches.[37,44,45]

THE COGNITIVE NEUROPSYCHOLOGY (CN) SCHOOL

Cognitive neuropsychologists apply information-processing models of normal cognition to the analysis of disorders of higher cortical function, including language. Until recently, CN's major contribution to rehabilitation was the development of model-driven assessments for describing impairments. With increasing frequency, though, cognitive neuropsychologists are involving themselves in treatment. Speech-language pathologists have also begun to apply cognitive models

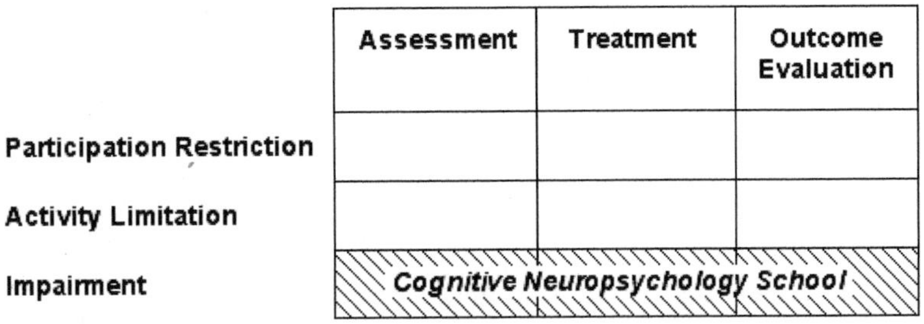

	Assessment	Treatment	Outcome Evaluation
Participation Restriction			
Activity Limitation			
Impairment	*Cognitive Neuropsychology School*		

Figure 18-3

The cognitive neuropsychology school of aphasia rehabilitation focuses primarily on the impairment level.

in the clinic. The basic idea is to pursue a more "rational" approach to treatment, in which the goals of the treatment program are informed by theory-based assessment of the patient's language capabilities.[46–48]*

CN assessments identify and measure impairments. It is not surprising, therefore, that impairments are also the focus of CN treatments and outcome evaluations. This restricted focus is in no way a necessary consequence of using cognitive theory to guide treatment, however. As noted by Caramazza,[49] the outcome of a cognitive assessment does not constrain the choice of therapeutic strategy; having characterized the patient's deficit at the level of impairment, one is perfectly free to target the level of activity or participation as the focus of treatment and/or outcome. Nevertheless, the bias in CN treatment research, if not in clinical practice, has been to target the impairment level as the focus for assessment, treatment, and outcome evaluation (Fig. 18-3).

Cognitive Neuropsychological Analysis Applied to Disorders of Word Retrieval (Anomia)

CN assessment begins where traditional assessment ends. For example, having identified a primary disorder of word retrieval, the CN-oriented clinician attempts to locate the deficit within the "functional architecture" of the language production system. The basic assumption is that one must probe for the explanation of a surface symptom like anomia; two patients with the same surface symptom may have very different underlying

deficits. Probing for underlying deficits proceeds with reference to an information processing model, using tests and procedures specifically developed with the model in mind.

Figure 18-4 presents a schematic version of a model that has been very influential in the analysis of word retrieval deficits and, in particular, deficits in picture naming.[50–52] The model subdivides word retrieval into two temporally distinct stages, each of which accomplishes a transcoding, or "mapping," from one type of representation to another. The first stage takes place within the "semantic lexicon"; here, the semantic code that defines the word's meaning is mapped into a phonologic address that provides key information about the word's pronunciation, for example, the initial sound in the word, the number of syllables it contains, and its stress pattern. The second stage takes place

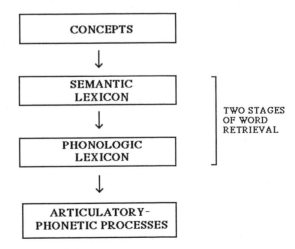

Figure 18-4

Schematic version of the two-stage model of word retrieval.

---

* The journal *Neuropsychological Rehabilitation* has devoted two special issues to the topic of cognitive neuropsychology and language rehabilitation: volume 5, issue 1/2 (March 1995) and volume 10, issue 3 (June 2000).

within the "phonologic lexicon." Here, the phonologic address for each known word is mapped onto an ordered string of phonemes specifying the full pronunciation, albeit still in a form more abstract than what the articulatory-motor system can take as input. The transcoding from a phonemic to articulatory-motor representation occurs at a subsequent step of word production. Disruption of this last step results in verbal "apraxia" of the sort we see in nonfluent (Broca's) aphasia. The types of word retrieval disorders that are of concern to us here are those that arise earlier in the process, at the first or second word-retrieval stage.

Various diagnostic tests are used to locate a picture naming deficit at one or the other of these stages (or both). Briefly, when we find that a patient's comprehension of pictures is unimpaired but he or she nevertheless makes semantic errors in naming (e.g., *horse* for *cow*), we immediately think of a problem in the semantic lexicon. If the patient makes semantic errors in comprehension as well as production, it is likely that the meaning representations in the semantic lexicon are degraded.[53] A patient studied by Howard and Orchard-Lisle[54] could not generate any names unless cued with the first phoneme of the target; when this patient was cued with the first phoneme of a semantically related word (e.g., shown a lion and cued with *t*), she showed a reliable tendency to produce the semantic substitution (*tiger*) and to accept that as the correct response. The implication of this "miscueing" effect is that degradation of semantic lexical entries resulted in the subthreshold activation of multiple entries in the semantic lexicon, and hence multiple phonologic addresses. Phonemic cues raised the activation value of corresponding addresses to threshold level; when the cue corresponded to the target, the correct name was produced; when it corresponded to a semantic coordinate, a semantic error was produced.

Many anomic patients can be cued phonemically to the correct target but do not show miscueing. Such patients are frequently able to provide partial information about the names they are unable to retrieve (e.g., that it is a long word or short word), and their errors, when they make them, bear a phonologic, rather than semantic, relation to the target.[55] These are indications that the problem arises in the retrieval of the full phonologic form, at the level of the phonologic lexicon.

Implications for Treatment of Word-Retrieval Deficits

The previous section illustrates the type of evidence that is used to locate a naming deficit within a functional model of the intact system. Reasoning about the treatment implications of such an analysis might proceed as follows: Patients whose deficits are centered in the semantic lexicon, i.e., in the semantic specification of words or the phonologic addressing mechanism, should benefit from interventions that encourage semantic processing of pictures in conjunction with phonologic processing of their names. A standard way of accomplishing this is to have the patient match pictures to written words, at least some of which bear a semantic relationship to the target name. The semantic component of such tasks should be less important for patients whose deficits are centered in the phonologic lexicon. These patients should benefit as much from purely phonologic techniques, such as oral reading, repeating the target name, or making a rhyme judgment.

A few studies have tested this model-driven prediction directly.[56-58] The conclusion at this point seems to be that patients with pure phonologic deficits do, as predicted, benefit from purely phonologic treatments. However, at least some patients with semantic involvement also benefit from phonologic techniques, which, if not pure, require only minimal semantic processing (e.g., responding to sentence-completion cues). It may be the key ingredient in phonologic techniques for patients with semantic or multilevel impairments is having some opportunity to strengthen the connections between corresponding entries in the semantic and phonologic lexicons.

Most CN treatment studies have not tested the model-based predictions directly. A number have assessed the short- and long-term effects of semantic and phonologic techniques in groups of subjects with undifferentiated naming deficits.[59,60] The results of these studies have generally favored semantic over phonologic techniques. Other studies have used the model-driven analysis to suggest the type of intervention called for (semantic or phonologic) in single cases or small homogeneous groups, but without examining whether the alternative approach would have been less successful. (Examples of these model-driven studies can be found in Refs. 56 to 58 and 61 to 71.)

Cumulatively, these CN-based studies provide conclusive evidence that anomia is amenable to treatment by a variety of semantic and phonologic techniques and that these benefits are maintained long after treatment ceases—as much as 1 year in the follow-up study reported by Pring and colleagues.[68] They also show that contrary to the findings of earlier single-exposure ("facilitation") studies[59,72] phonologic treatments have the potential to produce long-lasting effects and some degree of generalization. Further research is still needed to better understand who benefits

from what treatment and what constitutes the "active ingredient" in each treatment.

Cognitive Neuropsychological Analysis Applied to Agrammatism

The term *agrammatism* refers to the simplification and fractionation of morphosyntactic structure in the speech of patients with nonfluent Broca's aphasia (see Table 18-1). The traditional, language-oriented approach to treating agrammatism uses combinations of

Table 18-1

Examples of G.R.'s picture description performance at three points in time[a]

TARGET	**THE BOY IS SLEEPING IN THE BED.**
PRE M	Sleep . . . boy . . . bed . . .
POST M	The man is sleeping.
POST V	The boy is sleeping.
TARGET	**THE GIRL IS GIVING FLOWERS TO THE TEACHER.**
PRE M	Girl and woman . . . flowers . . .
POST M	The . . . girls is washing . . . daisies.
POST V	The girl is . . . giving the papsies [poppies] to the teacher.
TARGET	**THE ROCK IS FALLING ON THE BOY.**
PRE M	Rock . . .
POST M	The . . . the rock is small big . . . big . . .
POST V	The rock is . . . putting on the man.
TARGET	**THE BOY IS GIVING A VALENTINE TO THE GIRL.**
PRE M	Boy is . . . valentine . . . and . . . girl . . .
POST M	The man . . . valentine's day . . .
POST V	1. The boy is giving the girl to the no . . .
	2. The boy is holding the card to the girl . . . valentine.
	3. The boy is holding the valentine of the girl.
TARGET	**THE TRUCK IS TOWING THE CAR.**
PRE M	One grutch [truck] and one car . . .
POST M	The truck is . . . the car . . .
POST V	The truck is towing the car.
TARGET	**THE BOY IS WATCHING TELEVISION.**
PRE M	Television and man . . .
POST M	The man is TV opening the TV.
POST V	The boy is . . . putting on the TV.
TARGET	**THE BALL IS HITTING THE BOY IN THE HEAD.**
PRE M	Baseball hit . . .
POST M	The baseball is . . . ah no . . .
POST V	The . . . ball is striking the . . . boy.

Source: From Fink et al,[94] with permission.

[a] Pre-mapping therapy (Pre M), 1/20/90; post-mapping therapy (Post M), 5/11/90; post-verb studies (Post V), 12/7/90.

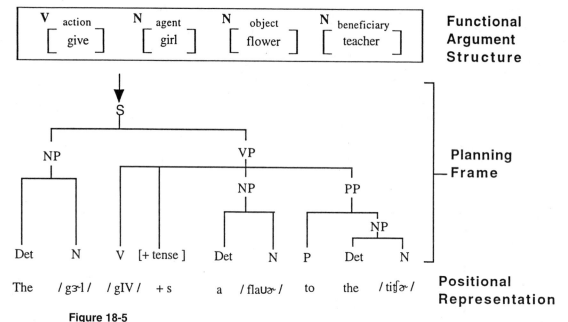

Figure 18-5

Schematic interpretation of Garrett's model of sentence production, applied to the sentence "The girl gives a flower to the teacher." The functional level contains content words only, and these are represented in the abstract format of the semantic lexicon. At the positional level, content words are represented in a phonologic format, while grammatical morphemes are represented more abstractly. S, sentence; NP, noun phrase; VP, verb phrase; PP, prepositional phrase; Det, determiner; N, noun; V, verb; P, preposition.

stimulation, repetition, and shaping techniques to facilitate production of affected structures. The CN approach aims deeper, at the underlying causes of the impaired production.

Psycholinguist Merrill Garrett[51,73] produced an account of sentence planning in normal speakers that has been very influential in the CN analyses of agrammatism. The model is illustrated in Fig. 18-5. The first stage involves formulation of the "functional argument structure" (alternatively, predicate- or verb-argument structure), which encodes the "who-is-doing-what-to-whom" information in the sentence. The "positional representation" encodes the surface form of the sentence, including the left-to-right order of the content words and the form as well as placement of the grammatical morphemes. Mapping from the functional to positional level is accomplished by means of "planning frames."

The diverse symptoms of agrammatism are associated with one or another stage of sentence planning. Problems in selecting or pronouncing grammatical morphemes are thought to arise at or after the creation of the positional level. Problems in retrieving verbs and their associated argument structures arise earlier, at the functional level, or in the mapping from the functional to the positional level. Schwartz and colleagues[74,75] have also identified faulty mapping between functional and positional representations as the basis for the syntactic comprehension disorder that often accompanies agrammatic speech.

The notion that a deficit in functional-positional level mapping is responsible for production and comprehension impairments in agrammatic aphasics motivated a number of treatment studies aimed at remediating the mapping deficit.[76–84] These "mapping treatments" represent a radical departure from traditional treatments for agrammatism. We illustrate the mapping-based approach with a 1986 case study by speech pathologist E. Jones.[80]

Jones's patient (B.B.) was a severely nonfluent agrammatic aphasic patient, who remained essentially at a single-word level 6 years after a left cerebrovascular accident despite many years of speech therapy. B.B.'s attempts at connected speech contained almost no verbs, but he was able to produce verbs on an action-naming test. Asked to describe pictures of simple transitive events, he had difficulty communicating the correct verb-argument structure. Even when supplied with the verb, he continued to have difficulty, for example, leaving out the subject (agent) or reversing the order of agent and object. Referring to the Garrett model, Jones interpreted these findings as evidence of a problem in the early stages of sentence planning, i.e., prior to the positional level.

In comprehension testing, B.B. was found to make errors in comprehending reversible sentences, ordering printed noun and verb constituents to convey the meaning of a picture, and rearranging printed phrases into sentences. Together with the production data, the findings are indicative of a deficit in mapping between sentence form (positional level) and sentence meaning (functional level).

To address this mapping deficit, Jones developed a highly structured treatment program using written sentences. B.B. was first trained to identify the verb in simple sentences, then to identify the arguments of the verb in response to probe questions: "Who (or what) is doing the action? To whom? Where?" After 3 months of this purely receptive treatment, B.B. demonstrated improved sentence comprehension for both written and spoken sentences. Moreover, his production improved as well, as indexed by increased use of correctly inflected verb phrases and increased use of prepositions, particles, and determiners. This improvement in production was noted in the home setting as well as on formal testing.

Jones's report was one of the first in a series of mapping therapy studies (see Refs. 76 to 79 and 81 to 84; for review, see Refs. 85 and 86). Most of these studies involved subjects with chronic aphasia who underwent detailed, model-driven assessments that yielded evidence consistent with a mapping deficit (e.g., impaired access to verbs and failure to comprehend se-

mantically reversible sentences). In each case a program was designed to remediate the mapping deficit. The specifics of the programs differed, but the strategy employed by most was to focus the patient's attention on the verb (or preposition, as in the case of locative sentences like "The pencil is *in* the sink.") and the roles it assigns to other constituents in the sentence (for an alternative approach, see Refs. 79 and 82). In most of the studies, production was not trained directly. Nevertheless, there were posttreatment gains in production, particularly those measures of production that reflect functional-level processes (i.e., production of verb, number of arguments produced, reduction in word-order errors).

That a treatment program involving no production training can nonetheless improve production is a striking finding. One possible explanation is that mapping therapy reeducates patients in mapping rules,[76] which can then be applied across tasks. However, since mapping rules are at least partly verb-specific, one would expect only limited generalization to untrained verbs, which is contrary to the findings of Jones's and other mapping therapy studies (e.g., Ref. 76, case 1; Ref. 84). A more plausible explanation is that the knowledge needed to map correctly is present prior to training, but not fully utilized. By drawing the patient's attention to the verb and the meaning it confers on sentence constituents, mapping therapy may shift or facilitate the allocation of processing resources to these aspects of sentence processing. Future studies should help resolve these issues. In any case, it is worth underscoring that the extent of the generalization to untrained materials and tasks that has been reported in some mapping therapy studies is substantially greater than what has been found with more traditional approaches that seek to train production directly.

The effect of mapping therapy on sentence comprehension is less impressive. While a number of subjects showed gains in syntactic comprehension of active reversible sentences, the gains and generalization patterns were variable within and across studies. Furthermore, half of the subjects studied did not show notable gains in syntactic comprehension in spite of their gains in production. This finding has both theoretical and practical implications regarding the underlying nature of the mapping disorder and how best to treat it (see Refs. 82, 84, and 87 for discussion).

Although the results of mapping therapy studies have been generally promising, a number of points are worth mentioning. First, the sentence query approach is not suitable for those with more complicated impairments, and it has yet to be shown that a standardized mapping protocol can benefit the wide range of agrammatic presentations that come through the clinic. Indeed, since agrammatism is a multifaceted condition, no single approach is likely to benefit all that carry this diagnosis. For example, depending on the nature of the verb retrieval problem, different approaches may be called for. Consequently, a complete program for agrammatism will likely require not one, but a series of targeted interventions. (We return to this point below, in the section on modular treatments.)

COGNITIVE NEUROPSYCHOLOGY AND APHASIA REHABILITATION: AN EVALUATION

While the CN approach has much to offer the rehabilitation enterprise, it is not a panacea. Cognitive models are of great value in specifying the locus of impairment in a particular patient, as well as the residual areas of strength, but it still falls to the clinician to use her or his judgment and experience to arrive at the optimal program of treatment, that is, whether to attempt to remediate the impaired process(es) and, if so, how. Rehabilitationists are being challenged to develop theories of how the damaged brain relearns and reorganizes itself,[88,89] and it is not clear whether and how cognitive models can contribute to this process (but see Ref. 90 for an encouraging step in this direction).

The length of CN assessments and the need to tailor such assessments to individual patients is poorly suited to the exigencies of the clinic. The development of model-driven language assessments that are standardized and normed [e.g., Psycholinguistic Assessment of Language Processing in Aphasia (PALPA)][91] has been of great help in this regard. Even so, the CN approach is probably not appropriate for all individuals with aphasia. Pinpointing the functional locus of a deficit rests on a fair degree of selectivity: the more global the deficit, the more problematic the endeavor.

CN interventions may be of greatest value when used as part of a more comprehensive treatment program that aims to achieve maximal carryover to real-world settings.[92] Toward this end, we advocate an approach that uses CN-motivated treatments as the building blocks or "modules" of a comprehensive treatment program.[93]

THE MODULAR-TREATMENTS APPROACH

In preceding sections we have enumerated a set of impairment symptoms that derive from contemporary models of spoken language production. At the level of the lexicon there are symptoms bearing on the representation and retrieval of meaning, and of phonology. At the sentence level there are symptoms having to do with the verb and its argument structure, the mapping between this and surface syntax, and the retrieval and/or phonologic realization of grammatical morphemes. In other domains, too—spoken language comprehension, written language production and comprehension—CN studies have elucidated a relatively small set of impairment symptoms that accounts for much of the variability in how disabilities in these domains are expressed.

Most aphasic patients display multiple impairments in more than one domain. The particular combination of impairment symptoms determines the patient's clinical classification. But most impairment symptoms are not restricted to a single clinical classification. For example, the lexical-semantic impairment that compromises word retrieval is found in patients with Broca's, Wernicke's, and anomic aphasia.

The goal of a CN assessment is to determine which impairment symptoms are present in the patient and which are amenable to treatment. For many patients, treatment will then aim to strengthen the impaired processes, one at a time or concurrently. To assist the therapist in this enterprise, we advocate the development of semistandardized treatment "modules," each of which targets a different impairment symptom. Such treatments should be designed to serve as broad a segment of the aphasia population as evinces the target symptom. This can be accomplished by graduating the demands of the treatment task and using multimodality treatment materials whenever possible. In Schwartz et al.,[93] we illustrated the requirements of treatment modules with experimental and clinical protocols already in use.

The basic idea behind this modular approach is that model-driven treatments that target specific impairments may produce narrow gains; however, the cumulative impact of multiple treatments can be substantial. Consider the case of G.R., a severely agrammatical patient who was 7 years postonset when he joined our mapping therapy study.[84] Comparison of his sentence production before and after mapping therapy revealed nontrivial gains on a 20-item picture description test: the percentage of words in sentences increased from 52 to 88; and the percentage of syntactically well-formed sentences increased from 30 to 44. He continued to experience difficulty retrieving verbs, however: the number of verbs produced was 10 before training and 11 after training (maximum 18). We therefore followed mapping therapy with a verb-treatment program designed to facilitate verb retrieval in the context of sentence production.[94] In this study, we compared the effects of two facilitation techniques: a repetition priming technique and a direct production technique that employs cueing and modeling in the context of mapping-type probe questions. The second technique proved more effective in facilitating acquisition of a small set of training verbs and carryover to untrained verbs.

At the end of the verb-treatment study, the number of verbs in G.R.'s picture description attempts increased from 11 to 18, and the number of appropriate verbs increased from 9 to 14. Examples of his picture description attempts at each stage of the treatment program are shown in Table 18-1. Although this was not designed as a test of the modular treatment approach, the results demonstrate the cumulative effects of treatments targeted at specific impairment symptoms.

CONCLUSION

The ICIDH-2 matrix serves as a reminder that the components of aphasia rehabilitation—assessment, treatment, and outcome evaluation—take place at multiple levels of analysis. The different schools of aphasia rehabilitation assign particular emphasis to one or another level, but, in reality, they are not as distinct from one another as Figs. 18-1 to 18-3 suggest. CN is really a branch of the language-oriented school that advocates using cognitive and psycholinguistic theory to direct rehabilitation activities. And as language-oriented therapists turn their attentions to the upper right-hand cell of the ICIDH-2 matrix, which insurance providers are increasingly requiring them to do, they are likely to draw on the theoretical and practical tools of the functional/pragmatic/social school.

What should be clear even from this brief discussion is that the future of aphasia rehabilitation will be shaped by interactions among clinicians and researchers with diverse perspectives and expertise. And there is much that we have not touched upon: research in neural plasticity is changing the way we think about the brain's capacity for recovery and reorganization after damage (e.g., Refs. 95 and 96); neural models that learn, and that relearn after "lesioning," provide a testing ground for theories of cognitive rehabilitation[90]; and advances in psychopharmacology[97–100] and computer technology[101–106] offer new avenues for treatment. Translating these promising trends into improved care for the individual with aphasia requires opportunities for clinicians, cognitive scientists, and neuroscientists to interact with one another and funding mechanisms to support and sustain such interdisciplinary collaborations.

REFERENCES

1. Chapey R: An introduction to language intervention strategies in adult aphasia, in Chapey R (ed): *Language Intervention Strategies in Adult Aphasia,* 2d ed. Baltimore: Williams & Wilkins, 1986, pp 2–11.
2. Wepman J: Aphasia therapy: Some "relative" comments and some purely personal prejudices, in Sarno M (ed): *Aphasia: Selected Readings.* New York: Appleton-Century-Crofts, 1972.
3. World Health Organization: *International Classification of Functioning, Disability and Health* (prefinal draft). Geneva: 2000.
4. World Health Organization: *International Classification of Impairments, Disabilities, and Handicaps: A Manual of Classification Relating to the Consequences of Diseases.* Geneva: World Health Organization, 1980.
5. Schwartz MF, Whyte J: *Methodological Issues in Aphasia Treatment Research: The Big Picture.* NIDCD Monograph, vol 2. Publication No. 93-3424:17–23. Bethesda, MD: National Institutes of Health, 1992.

6. Goodglass H, Kaplan E: *Assessment of Aphasia and Related Disorders*. Philadelphia: Lea & Febiger, 1983.

7. Kertesz A: *Western Aphasia Test Battery*. New York: The Psychological Corporation, 1982.

8. Schuell H: *Minnesota Test for Differential Diagnosis of Aphasia*. Minneapolis: University of Minnesota Press, 1965.

9. Schuell H, Jenkins JJ, Jimenez-Pabon E: *Aphasia in Adults: Diagnosis, Prognosis, and Treatment*. New York: Harper and Row, 1964.

10. Helm-Estabrooks NA: *Helm Elicited Language Program for Syntax Stimulation (HELPSS)*. Austin, TX: Exceptional Resources, 1981.

11. Shewan C, Bandur D: *Treatment of Aphasia: A Language-Oriented Approach*. Boston: College-Hill Press, 1986.

12. *Medicare Intermediary Manual, Billing Procedures for Part B Outpatient Speech and Language Services, 3905.3*. Washington, DC: US Government Printing Office.

13. Sarno MT: *Functional Communication Profile*. New York: Institute of Rehabilitation Medicine, 1969.

14. Holland AL, Frattali C, Fromm, D: *Communicative Abilities in Daily Living: Manual*. Austin, TX: Pro-Ed, 1999.

15. Lomas J, Pickard L, Bester S, et al: The communicative effectiveness index: Development and psychometric evaluation of a functional communication measure for adult aphasia. *J Speech Hear Disord* 54:113–124, 1989.

16. Frattali C, Thompson C, Holland A, et al: The FACS of Life. ASHA FACS: A functional outcome measure for adults. *ASHA* 37:40–46, 1995.

17. Frattali C, Thompson CK, Wohl CB: Trends in functional assessment. *Am Speech Lang Hear Assoc Newsl* 4:4–9, 1994.

18. Boles L, Bombard T: Conversational discourse analysis: Appropriate and useful sample sizes. *Aphasiology* 12:547–670, 1998.

19. Damico JS, Oelschlager M, Simmons-Mackie N: Qualitative methods in aphasia research: Conversational analysis. *Aphasiology* 13:667–679, 1999.

20. Gerber SK, Gerland GB: Applied pragmatics in the assessment of aphasia. *Semin Speech Lang* 10:14–25, 1989.

21. Terrell BY, Ripich DN: Discourse competence as a variable in intervention. *Semin Speech Lang* 10:282–297, 1989.

22. Sarno JE, Sarno MT, Levita E: The functional life scale. *Arch Phys Med Rehabil* 54:214–220, 1973.

23. Willer B, Rosenthal M, Kreutzer JS, et al: Assessment of community integration following rehabilitation for traumatic brain injury. *J Head Trauma Rehabil* 8:75–87, 1993.

24. Basso A, Capitani E, Vignolo LA: Influence of rehabilitation on language skills in aphasic patients: A controlled study. *Arch Neurol* 36:190–196, 1979.

25. Poeck K, Huber W, Williams K: Outcome of intensive language treatment in aphasia. *J Speech Hear Disord* 54:471–479, 1989.

26. Shewan CM, Kertesz A: Effects of speech and language treatment on recovery of aphasia. *Brain Lang* 23:272–299, 1984.

27. Wertz RT, Collins MJ, Weiss D, Kurtze JF, et al: Veterans administration cooperative study on aphasia: A comparison of individual and group treatment. *J Speech Hear Res* 24:580–594, 1981.

28. Wertz RT, Weiss DG, Aten JL, et al: Comparison of clinic, home, and deferred language treatment for aphasia. *Arch Neurol* 43:653–658, 1986.

29. Doyle PJ, Bourgeois MJ: The effect of syntax training on adequacy of communication in Broca's aphasia: A social validation study, in Brookshire RH (ed): *Clinical Aphasiology*. Minneapolis: BRK Publishers, 1986, vol 16, pp 123–132.

30. Doyle PJ, Goldstein H, Bourgeois M: Experimental analysis of syntax training in Broca's aphasia: A generalization and social validation study. *J Speech Hear Disord* 52:143–156, 1987.

31. Fink RB, Schwartz MF, Rochon E, et al: Syntax stimulation revisited: An analysis of generalization of treatment effects. *Am J Speech Lang Pathol* 4:99–104, 1995.

32. Helm-Estabrooks NA, Ramsberger G: Treatment of agrammatism in long-term Broca's aphasia. *Br J Disord Commun* 21:39–45, 1986.

33. Thompson CK, McReynolds LV: Wh-interrogative production in agrammatic aphasia: An experimental analysis of auditory-visual stimulation and direct-production treatment. *J Speech Hear Res* 29:193–206, 1986.

34. Thompson CK: Generalization research in aphasia: A review of the literature, in Prescott T (ed): *Clinical Aphasiology*. Boston: College-Hill Publications, 1989, vol 18, pp 195–222.

35. Doyle P, Goldstein H, Bourgeois M, Nakles K: Facilitating generalized requesting behavior in Broca's aphasia: a generalization and social validation study. *J Speech Hear Disord* 22:157–170, 1989.

36. Davis GA, Wilcox MJ: *Adult Aphasia Rehabilitation: Applied Pragmatics*. San Diego, CA: College Hill, 1985.

37. Holland AL: Pragmatic aspects of intervention in aphasia. *J Neuroling* 6:197–211, 1991.

38. Lyon JG, Cariski D, Keisler L, et al: Communication partners: enhancing participation in life and communication for adults with aphasia in natural settings. *Aphasiology* 11:693–708, 1997.

39. Kagen A: Supported conversation for adults with aphasia: Methods and resources for training conversation partners. *Aphasiology* 12:816–831, 1998.

40. Hinckley JJ, Packard MEW: Family education seminars and social functioning of adults with chronic aphasia. *J Commun Disord* 34:241–254, 2001.

41. Simmons N, Kearns K, Potechin G: Treatment of aphasia through family member training, in Prescott T (ed): *Clinical Aphasiology*. Austin, TX: Pro-Ed, 1987, vol 17, pp 106–116.

42. Rogers MA, Alarcon NB, Olswang LB: Aphasia management considered in the context of the World Health Organization model of disablements. *Phys Med Rehabil Clin North Am* 13:907–923, 1999.

43. Hickey E, Rogers MA, Alaron NB, et al: Social validity measures for family-based intervention for chronic aphasia (FICA): presentation. Clinical Aphasiology Conference. Asheville, NC, 1998.

44. Davis A: Pragmatics and treatment, in Chapey R (ed): *Language Intervention Strategies in Adult Aphasia,* 2d ed. Baltimore: Williams & Wilkins, 1986, pp 251–265.

45. Springer L, Glindemann R, Huber W, Williams K: How efficacious is PACE therapy when "language systematic training" is incorporated? *Aphasiology* 5:391–399, 1991.

46. Coltheart M: Editorial. *Cogn Neuropsychol* 1:1–8, 1984.

47. Mitchum CC, Berndt RS: Aphasia rehabilitation: An approach to diagnosis and treatment of disorders of language production, in Eisenbert MG (ed): *Advances in Clinical Rehabilitation*. New York: Springer-Verlag. 1989.

48. Seron X, Deloche G: Introduction, in Seron X, Deloche G (eds): *Cognitive Approaches in Neuropsychological Rehabilitation*. Hillsdale, NJ: Erlbaum, 1989, pp 1–16.

49. Caramazza A: Cognitive neuropsychology and rehabilitation: An unfulfilled promise? in Seron X, Deloche G (eds): *Cognitive Approaches in Neuropsychological Rehabilitation*. Hillsdale, NJ: Erlbaum, 1989, pp 383–398.

50. Butterworth B: Lexical access in speech production, in Marslen-Wilson W (ed): *Lexical Representation and Process*. Cambridge, MA: MIT Press, 1989, pp 108–135.

51. Garrett MF: Production of speech: observations from normal and pathological language use, in Ellis A (ed): *Normality and Pathology in Cognitive Functions*. London: Academic Press, 1982.

52. Levelt WJM: *Speaking: From Intention to Articulation*. Cambridge, MA: MIT Press, 1989.

53. Hillis A, Rapp B, Romani C, Carramazza A: *Selective Impairments of Semantics in Lexical Processing: Reports of the Cognitive Neuropsychology Laboratory*. Baltimore: Johns Hopkins University, 1989.

54. Howard D, Orchard-Lisle V: On the origin of semantic errors in naming: evidence from the case of a global aphasic. *Cogn Neuropsychol* 1:163–190, 1984.

55. Kay J, Ellis A: A cognitive neuropsychological case study of anomia. *Brain* 110:613–629, 1987.

56. Greenwald ML, Raymer AM, Richardson ME, Rothi LJG: Contrasting treatments for severe impairments of picture naming. *Neuropsychol Rehabil* 5:17–49, 1995.

57. Hillis AE, Caramazza A: Theories of lexical processing and rehabilitation of lexical deficits, in Riddoch MJ, Humphreys GW (eds): *Cognitive Neuropsychology and Cognitive Rehabilitation*. Hove, Sussex: Erlbaum: 1994, pp 449–484.

58. LeDorze G, Pitts C: A case study evaluation of the effects of different techniques for the treatment of anomia. *Neuropsychol Rehabil* 5:51–65, 1995.

59. Howard D, Patterson K, Franklin S, et al: The facilitation of picture naming in aphasia. *Cogn Neuropsychol* 2:48–80, 1985.

60. Howard D, Patterson K, Franklin S, et al: Treatment of word retrieval deficits in aphasia: A comparison of two therapy methods. *Brain* 108:817–829, 1985.

61. Fink RB, Brecher A, Schwartz MF: A computer implemented protocol for treatment of naming disorders: Evaluation of clinician-guided and partially self-guided instruction. *Aphasiology*. In press.

62. Hillis AE: Efficacy and generalization of treatment for aphasic naming errors. *Arch Phys Med Rehabil* 70:632–636, 1989.

63. Hillis AE: Effects of separate treatments for distinct impairments within the naming process, in Prescott T (ed): *Clinical Aphasiology*. Austin, TX: Pro-Ed, 1991, vol 19, pp 255–265.

64. Marshall J, Pound C, White-Thomson M, Pring T: The use of picture/word matching tasks to assist word retrieval in aphasic patients. *Aphasiology* 4:167–184, 1990.

65. Miceli G, Amitrano A, Capasso R, Caramazza A: The remediation of anomia resulting from output lexical damage: analysis of two cases. *Brain Lang* 52:150–174, 1996.

66. Nettleton J, Lesser R: Therapy for naming difficulties in aphasia: Application of a cognitive neuropsychological model. *J Neuroling* 6:139–154, 1991.

67. Nickels L, Best W: Therapy for naming disorders: Part 2. Specifics, surprises and suggestions. *Aphasiology* 10:109–136, 1996.

68. Pring T, White-Thomson M, Pound C, et al: Short report: picture/word matching tasks and word retrieval. Some follow-up data and second thoughts. *Aphasiology* 4:479–483, 1990.

69. Raymer AM, Thompson CK, Jacobs B, LeGrand HR: Phonological treatment of naming deficits in aphasia: model-based generalization analysis. *Aphasiology* 7:27–53, 1993.

70. Robson J, Marshall J, Pring T, Chiat S: Phonological naming therapy in jargon aphasia: positive but paradoxical effects. *J Int Neuropsychol Soc* 4:675–686, 1998.

71. Wambaugh J, Doyle P, Linebaugh C: Effects of deficit oriented treatments on lexical retrieval in a patient with semantic and phonological deficits. *Brain Lang* 69:446–450, 1999.

72. Patterson KE, Purell C, Morton J: Facilitation of word retrieval in aphasia, in Code C, Muller DJ (eds): *Aphasia Therapy*. London: Arnold, 1983, pp 76–87.

73. Garrett MF: Levels of processing in sentence production, in Butterworth B (ed): *Language Production*. New York: Academic Press, 1980, vol 1, pp 177–220.

74. Linebarger MC, Schwartz MF, Saffran EM: Sensitivity to grammatical structure in so-called agrammatic aphasics. *Cognition* 13:361–392, 1983.

75. Schwartz MF, Linebarger MC, Saffran EM: The status of the syntactic deficit theory of aggrammatism, in Kean MC (ed): *Agrammatism*. New York: Academic Press, 1985, pp 83–124.

76. Byng S: Sentence processing deficits: theory and therapy. *Cogn Neuropsychol* 1988; 5:629–676.

77. Byng S, Nickels L, Black M: Replicating therapy for mapping deficits in agrammatism: remapping the deficit. *Aphasiology* 8:315–341, 1994.

78. Fink RB, Schwartz MF, Myers, JL: Investigations of the sentence-query approach to mapping therapy. *Brain Lang* 65:203–207, 1998.

79. Haendiges AN, Berndt RS, Mitchum CC: Assessing the elements contributing to a "mapping deficit": A targeted treatment study. *Brain Lang* 52:276–302, 1996.

80. Jones EV: Building the foundations for sentence production in a non-fluent aphasic. *Br J Disord Commun* 21:63–82, 1986.

81. LeDorze G, Jacob A, Coderre L: Aphasia rehabilitation with a case of agrammatism: A partial replication. *Aphasiology* 5:63–85, 1991.

82. Mitchum, CC, Haendiges AN, Berndt RS: Treatment of thematic mapping in sentence comprehension: Implications for normal processing. *Cogn Neuropsychol* 12:503–547, 1995.

83. Nickels L, Byng S, Black M: Sentence processing deficits: A replication of therapy. *Br J Disord Commun* 26:175–199, 1991.

84. Schwartz MF, Saffran EM, Fink RB, et al: Mapping therapy: A treatment program for agrammatism. *Aphasiology* 8:19–54, 1994.

85. Fink RB: Mapping treatment: an approach to treating sentence level impairments in agrammatism. *Am Speech Lang Hear Assoc Newsl* 11:14–23, 2001.

86. Marshall J: The mapping hypothesis and aphasia therapy. *Aphasiology* 9:517–539, 1995.

87. Mitchum CC, Greenwald ML, Berndt RS: Cognitive treatments of sentence processing disorders: What have we learned? *Neuropsychol Rehabil* 10(3):311–336, 2000.

88. Byng S: A theory of the deficit: A prerequisite for a theory of therapy? *Clin Aphasiol* 22:265–273, 1994.

89. Holland AL: Cognitive neuropsychological theory and treatment for aphasia: Exploring the strengths and limitations. *Clin Aphasiol* 22:275–282, 1994.

90. Plaut DC: Relearning after damage in connectionist networks: Toward a theory of rehabilitation. *Brain Lang* 52:25–82, 1996.

91. Kay J, Lesser R, Coltheart M: *Psycholinguistic Assessment of Language Processing in Aphasia*. East Sussex, England: Erlbaum, 1992.

92. Lesser R, Algar L: Towards combining the cognitive neuropsychological and the pragmatic in aphasia therapy. *Neuropsychol Rehabil* 5:67–92, 1995.

93. Schwartz MF, Fink RB, Saffran EM: The modular treatment of agrammatism. *Neuropsychol Rehabil* 5:93–127, 1995.

94. Fink RB, Martin N, Schwartz MF, et al: Facilitation of verb retrieval skills in aphasia: A comparison of two approaches. *Clin Aphasiol* 21:263–275, 1992.

95. Thomas C, Altenmuller E, Marckmann G, et al: Language processing in aphasia: Changes in lateralization patterns during recovery reflect cerebral plasticity in adults. *Electroencephalogr Clin Neurophysiol* 102:86–97, 1997.

96. Thulborn KR, Carpenter PA, Just MA: Plasticity of language-related brain function during recovery from stroke. *Stroke* 30:749–754, 1999.

97. Bragoni M, Altieri M, DiPiero V, et al: Bromocriptine and speech therapy in non-fluent chronic aphasia after stroke. *Neuroscience* 21:10–22, 2000.

98. Gold M, VanDam D, Silliman ER: An open label trial of Bromocriptine in non-fluent aphasia: A qualitative analysis of word storage and retrieval. *Brain Lang* 74:141–156, 2000.

99. Kessler J, Thiel A, Karbe H, Heis WD: Piracetam improves activated blood flow and facilitates rehabilitation of post stroke aphasic patients. *Stroke* 31:2112–2116, 2000.

100. Walker-Batson D, Curtis S, Natarajan R, et al: A double blind placebo-controlled study of the use of amphetamine in the treatment of aphasia. *Stroke* 32:2093–2098, 2001.

101. Aftonomos LB, Steele R, Wertz R: Promoting recovery in chronic aphasia with an interactive technology. *Arch Phys Med Rehabil* 78:841–846, 1997.

102. Crerar M, Ellis A, Dean E: Remediation of sentence processing deficits in aphasia using a computer-based microworld. *Brain Lang* 52:229–275, 1996.

103. Katz RC, Wertz T: The efficacy of computer-provided reading treatment for chronic aphasic adults. *J Speech Lang Hear Res* 40:493–507, 1997.

104. Linebarger MC, Schwartz MF, Kohn SE: Computer-based training of language production: An exploratory study. *Neuropsychol Rehabil* 11(1):57–96, 2001.

105. Linebarger MC, Schwartz MF, Romania JR, et al: Grammatical encoding in aphasia: Evidence from a "processing prosthesis." *Brain Lang* 75:416–427, 2000.

106. Weinrich M, McCall D, Weber C, et al: Training on an iconic communication system for severe aphasia can improve natural language production. *Aphasiology* 9(4):343–364, 1995.

Chapter 19

APHASIA IV: ACQUIRED DISORDERS OF LANGUAGE IN CHILDREN*

Maureen Dennis

Childhood-acquired language disorder, or *childhood-acquired aphasia,* refers to language impairment that is evident after a period of normal language acquisition and that is precipitated by, or associated with, an identified form of brain insult. It differs from language acquisition disorders without clearly established brain pathology and from language deficits that emerge during or after initial language acquisition in children with neurodevelopmental brain disorders (see Chaps. 34 and 36).

In an earlier research era, acquired language disorders in children were referenced to adult aphasic syndromes. It was concluded that, compared to adults, children showed fewer aphasic symptoms (especially comprehension symptoms), more transient aphasic deficits, and fewer focal and lateralized precipitating brain insults.[1,2]

A more recent view of childhood-acquired aphasia has been shaped by the explosion of empirical studies; the publication of benchmarks, assessment instruments, and theoretical models of normal language development; and the availability of structural and functional imaging techniques to identify the brain correlates of aphasic disorders. It has also been shaped by developmental neuropsychological models of childhood brain disorders, which have proposed that functional outcome, including language, represents the effects of the biology of the brain injury, the age and development of the child, the time since onset of injury, and the available cognitive and psychosocial reserve.[3]

* **ACKNOWLEDGMENTS:** The author's research described in this paper was supported by project grants from the Ontario Mental Health Foundation and the Physicians' Services Incorporated Foundation and by NINDS Grant 2R01NS 21889-16, "Neurobehavioral Outcome of Head Injury in Children."

Any advantage for an earlier onset of acquired aphasia is short-lived and concerns the faster abatement of acute-stage aphasic symptoms. In the long term, children with acquired aphasia continue to exhibit language impairment. Age at aphasia-producing brain injury has proved to be less predictive of aphasic symptoms but more relevant to long-term language function than was previously thought. Given a similar brain injury, children and adults exhibit similar aphasic symptoms in the acute stage of acquired aphasia; however, while children show a faster resolution of aphasic symptoms than adults, their long-term language function may sometimes be poorer. These conclusions have emerged from studies conducted over the last 20 years, which have questioned many of the features once considered to define childhood-acquired aphasia—namely, fewer language symptoms, faster rate of recovery, less focal and lateralized lesions.

Nonfluent Characteristics of Childhood-Acquired Aphasia

Historically, childhood-acquired aphasia was characterized by nonfluent and impoverished spontaneous speech,[4-6] ranging in severity from mutism to articulatory difficulties, as well as by nonfluent language, often with simplified syntax, telegraphic speech, and word-finding difficulties (see Chap. 16 for a discussion of these aphasic signs). Dysfluency has been reported in both older[7-9] and more recent[10] studies of childhood-acquired aphasia.

Symptoms of adult fluent aphasia (logorrhea, verbal stereotypies, perseverations, neologisms, jargon, and paraphasias; see Chap. 16) would once have been thought to be rare in children with acquired language disorders.[8] More recently, studies have shown that children with acquired aphasia show fluent aphasia[11] that includes phonemic jargon, neologisms, and paraphasias[12] and also that aphasic symptoms in children are quite varied.[13] Moreover, a number of adult aphasic syndromes have been described in children: jargon aphasia[12,14]; Wernicke's aphasia and transcortical sensory aphasia[15]; conduction aphasia[16]; transcortical sensory aphasia[11,17]; anomic aphasia[18]; and alexia without agraphia.[19,20] In short, most adult aphasic syndromes can be observed in children, albeit with different base frequencies.[21]

From its first description in 1957, the Landau-Kleffner syndrome (LKS),[22] whose defining feature is a severe and long-lasting verbal auditory agnosia for words and for sounds, became the paradigm of childhood-acquired aphasia.[23] Comprehension deficits are features of the long-term language function in other childhood-acquired aphasic conditions and may even be more pronounced than in adults; for example, global aphasia from a childhood left middle cerebral artery infarct may resolve to a transcortical sensory aphasia characterized by poorer language comprehension than in comparable adult cases.[24]

Recent research has not supported the traditional view that comprehension, especially auditory comprehension, is preserved in childhood-acquired aphasia. Instead, it has shown comprehension deficits to be central to childhood-acquired aphasic disorders.

Transient Nature of Childhood-Acquired Aphasia

Recovery of aphasic symptoms in cases of childhood-acquired aphasia is often rapid,[25] although some 25 to 50 percent of cases still show residual aphasia 1 year later. Recent long-term follow-up studies, which have focused on recovery of language function rather than on abatement of aphasic symptoms, show that childhood-acquired aphasia is long-lasting, with effects that extend in time beyond the disappearance of aphasic symptoms.[23] Although clinical signs of aphasia somewhat similar to those in the adult occur in the acute phase of childhood-acquired aphasia, long-term language outcome may be poor even after aphasic symptoms have resolved,[26] especially for pragmatic language.[27,28]

Functional outcomes that require intact language skills, such as academic achievement, continue to be poor beyond the period of clinical aphasia recovery,[29–31] and problems in new academic learning[17] may even become exacerbated over time, perhaps because of the escalating demands of academic work in the higher grades.[32]

Nonfocal Brain Bases of Childhood-Acquired Aphasia

Early study groups of children with acquired aphasia had an overrepresentation of traumatic and infectious etiologies.[7] At that time, techniques for determining lesion lateralization involved principally clinical status, such as the presence of hemiplegia, which meant that actual lesions might have been bilateral or unilateral.[14] As a result of these limitations, the view arose that childhood-acquired aphasia involved nonfocal brain insult.

Child and adult aphasia–producing lesions may have different long-term effects on the brain. Some early lesions may leave little focal residual change,[33] with the result that the brain does not show characteristic gliotic changes but rather tissue shrinkage, so that even with an initially focal insult, brain lesions in childhood may involve decreased brain volume.[34]

Nonlateralized Brain Bases of Childhood-Acquired Aphasia

It was once assumed that the lateralization of language was incremental over the first decade of life, but the question then arose of a left hemisphere bias for language development (discussed in Refs. 21 and 35). Recent empirical studies have not only challenged the idea that aphasia after right-sided lesions is more common in children than in adults[14] but have shown that the risk of acquired aphasia after left hemisphere damage in right-handers is approximately the same in children and adults,[25,36,37] leading to the conclusion that, given a unilateral lesion to the dominant hemisphere, childhood aphasia is no more uncommon than adult aphasia.[38]

Even the characteristics of the aphasia are similar in children and adults. Left-sided lesions to the classic adult language areas in childhood produce a fluent aphasia with many neologisms and paraphasias.[39]

Recovery from childhood-acquired aphasia depends on the integrity of the left posterior language areas,[30] which suggests that a lateralized and focal language representation is well established by middle childhood and also that recovery from childhood-acquired aphasia may engage intact areas of the left hemisphere.[40]

Age-Related versus Etiologic Differences in Adult- and Childhood-Acquired Aphasia

In earlier studies, child and adult differences in outcome after acquired aphasia have been attributed to the younger age of the child (and to the putative plasticity of the brain for which the younger age was a marker). Early research selected study groups on the basis of aphasia and combined heterogeneous pathologies in assessing outcome.[7]

However, differences in age at aphasia onset are correlated with differences in etiology. Relative to an adult group, a child group studied because of aphasic symptoms will have an overrepresentation of traumatic and convulsive etiologies and an underrepresentation of vascular disorders. Because inferences about acquired aphasia are based on data from the etiology most frequently reported, views about adult-acquired aphasia have been shaped from parallels with arteritic stroke while those for childhood-acquired aphasia have been understood in terms of head injury and convulsive disorders.

Child and adult acquired aphasias typically differ in both age and etiology,[31] and recent studies have addressed the question of etiologic differences in childhood-acquired aphasia.[2,41] Recovery, both short- and long-term, varies with etiology.[26]

PRINCIPAL ETIOLOGIES OF CHILDHOOD-ACQUIRED APHASIA

This section reviews the characteristics of the principal etiologies of childhood-acquired aphasia. For each etiology, some general issues are discussed; where sufficient evidence is available, cross-etiology comparisons are facilitated by Tables 19-1 through 19-4.

Seizure and Seizure-Related Disorders: The Landau-Kleffner Syndrome (LKS)

Seizure disorders affect cognition and language,[42] and language symptoms have been observed both as part of clinical seizures and as part of ictal speech automatisms. Recurrent generalized seizures and medication may have diffuse effects that can confound the interpretation of otherwise focal lesions. The most fully studied aphasia-producing seizure disorder, however, is the LKS,[22] the characteristics of which are reviewed in Table 19-1.

Vascular Disorders

Vascular disorders involve interruptions to the blood supply within the brain as a result of occlusion (ischemic stroke) or rupture (hemorrhagic stroke). Most vascular diseases observed in the adult also occur in children, albeit with different base frequencies. Degenerative disorders like atherosclerosis are common in the middle-aged and elderly but rare in children, while vascular disorders associated with congenital heart disease occur more commonly in childhood[68] and may produce strokes by an embolism from the heart, from complications of heart surgery, or from hypoperfusion from prolonged hypotension. The characteristics of childhood-acquired aphasia from vascular diseases are reviewed in Table 19-2.

Traumatic Disorders

Traumatic head injury is a common cause of childhood-acquired aphasia. Children exhibit a range of aphasic symptoms and language disturbances after head injury.[76] The characteristics of childhood-acquired aphasia from traumatic disorders are reviewed in Table 19-3.

Brain Tumors

Brain tumors in children may be associated with language disturbances.[11,79,95] Language disturbances after tumors above the tentorium have been described, although studies are not numerous. Posterior fossa tumors occur with relatively high frequency in children,

Table 19-1
Childhood-acquired aphasia and the Landau-Kleffner syndrome

Definition

Landau-Kleffner syndrome (LKS) involves acquired aphasia with convulsive disorder[22] occurring in normal children who acutely or progressively lose previously acquired language ability.

A variety of typologies have been proposed.[43]

It was originally claimed that pregnancy, birth, and early development were normal in LKS,[44] and that, classically, LKS occurs after some period of normal language development. More recently, however, it has been found that a history of language pathology may precede the onset of language deterioration and loss,[45] with some 75 percent of patients exhibiting language disturbance before the aphasia.[46]

Loss of language is associated with either clinical seizures (generalized, partial, partial complex, or absence) or with an electroencephalogram (EEG) showing unilateral or paroxysmal activity, sometimes more prominent in slow-wave sleep.[47]

It has been argued that LKS overlaps with other epileptic conditions: rolandic epilepsy, electrical status epilepticus during sleep (ESES), and autistic regression and disintegrative disorder associated with unilateral or bilateral centrotemporal spike/spike-wave discharges.[21]

Core Features

A severe comprehension defect[48] occurs, characteristically with severe verbal auditory agnosia, which may involve both common sounds (such as a dog barking or a doorbell ringing) and words.[2,49]

Epileptic seizures occur in 70 to 75 percent of patients.[50]

Severe behavior disturbances occur in 75 percent of patients.[50] Long-term ($\geq$7 years) follow-up studies have reported mild behavior disturbance (hyperactivity, impulsivity, and oppositional behavior) that is chronologically linked with the language disturbances and follows their fluctuations.[51]

Oral expression is typically poorer than written expression,[52,53] although severe impairment of written language and mathematical skills has been reported.[48]

Neurologic examination is reported to be normal.[54]

Nonverbal intelligence appears to be well preserved.[55]

Half the published cases present first with comprehension disorder, the other half with seizures.[50]

Most LKS patients have a mild form of epilepsy that responds to drug therapy.[56]

There is a correlation between the aphasia and the seizure disorder, although both may fluctuate out of phase,[56] so that the relation is not obvious.[57]

Epidemiology, Demography, and Risk Factors

Some 200 cases have been reported from 1957 to 1995.[50]

The male:female ratio is 2:1.[50]

There are currently no epidemiologic data in regard to geography, infectious disease, toxins, nutrition, or environmental exposures.[58]

Age-Related Factors

Onset occurs from 3 to 8 years of age in 50 percent of cases.[50]

Onset is rare after 8 years of age, although several cases have been reported with loss of language after age 9. Later-onset cases are more likely to have a primarily expressive aphasia with dysfluency and word-finding difficulties.[59]

An age-prognosis relationship has been proposed, such that the younger the child, the poorer the recovery from the acquired aphasia—the reasoning being that newly acquired language skills are particularly vulnerable to bilateral brain pathology.[44] However, age-prognosis effects, such as the claim that recovery is worse with a diagnosis before age 5,[60] have not been replicated with more clearly defined case selection criteria.[51]

Table 19-1 (*Continued*)

<hr>

Time-Related Factors

<hr>

Language impairments in LKS persist for months or even years.[49]

Long-term language outcome is often poor. When studied 10 to 28 years after onset of acquired aphasia, more than half of an LKS sample continued to show language disorder.[47] In a long-term follow-up of at least 7 years—into the adolescent years—no individual with LKS fully recovered language.[51]

Typically, seizures remit before adulthood and the aphasia subsides, although not necessarily in parallel.[44]

The long-term outcome of the aphasia has been considered to be unpredictable with respect to medical history features,[47] despite the fact that both epilepsy and EEG abnormalities improve.[61] There is an unpredictable prognosis on an individual case basis, with a fluctuating course of remissions and exacerbations of both aphasia and EEG abnormalities.

In a long-term (2- to 15-year) follow-up of LKS cases, it was found that, even when the EEG normalized in the long term, few individuals achieved normal language, and, further, that no individual with persisting EEG abnormalities recovered normal or near normal language.[46] Thus, persisting EEG abnormalities appear to be a risk factor for continuing aphasia.

Neuropathologic Substrate

<hr>

Initially, it was unclear whether the language disturbances in LKS was functional or due to an identifiable brain lesion. Proposals for the brain basis of LKS have ranged widely.

It has been suggested that LKS might involve focal subclinical epileptogenic discharges involving the language areas. In this view, aphasic symptoms arise because persistent epileptic discharges cause functional ablation of the primary cortical language areas.[62]

Because the course of the aphasia in LKS may be linked to the appearance and disappearance of ESES,[61] LKS has been considered related to ESES. However, few children with ESES have specific language disorders, and the characteristic EEG of ESES is infrequently found in LKS.[56]

The mild to moderate elevation of cerebrospinal fluid proteins in some LKS cases[47,63] has been used to suggest a low-grade focal inflammation of the brain as the mechanism of LKS aphasia.[64]

Cortical biopsies in some LKS cases have shown changes indicative of a slow virus infection, implying that a subacute viral encephalitis might produce both aphasia and seizures, either from a low-grade selective encephalitis[55] or a subchronic viral encephalitis affecting both hemispheres.[44]

The finding of a positive autoimmune reaction to myelin during clinical deterioration of language in LKS patients has been used to suggest a disorder of myelin metabolism and to account for the positive effect of corticosteroids as immunosuppressive therapy.[65]

Computed tomography and structural magnetic resonance imaging are typically normal.[64]

Angiography has shown isolated arteritis of some branches of the carotid arteries, which implies that focal cerebral vasculitis may be involved in the pathogenesis of LKS.[64]

Positron emission tomography has shown abnormal glucose utilization during sleep, with lower metabolic rates in subcortical than in cortical areas.[66]

Treatment

<hr>

There is no convincing evidence of empirically effective therapy.[58]

Various drug treatments (antiepileptics, corticosteroids) have been tried, with success on an individual-case basis.

Based on the view that focal vasculitis is responsible for LKS, calcium channel blockers have been proposed as a possible therapy.[64]

Subpial resection has been proposed as therapy in some cases of LKS.

Speech and language therapy has long been used in the rehabilitation of individuals with LKS, but there has been controversy about whether therapy should involve enhancing the residue of oral language; intensive training in the visual domain (gestures, communication boards, signing, computers); brief training in the visual domain with rapid transfer to oral language; or a more pragmatic, multimodal approach. A recent review[67] suggests that no single therapy program will work, that LKS patients are not like deaf individuals, and that any therapy will likely take several years to be effective.

<hr>

Table 19-2

Language disturbances from vascular etiologies

Definition

Acquired aphasia may be precipitated by a vascular brain lesion occurring in children who acutely or progressively lose
previously acquired language skills.

Brain localization depends on the pathophysiology of the stroke. In children, most strokes are secondary to intracranial
occlusive disease and are localized in the basal ganglia;[69] however, cortical vascular lesions in the left temporoparietal
lobe that produce aphasia have been reported to occur from cerebral arteritis[39] and ruptured arteriovenous
malformations.[70]

Core Features

The type of aphasia depends on the localization of the lesion. Aphasia is fluent in form with lesions to the posterior left
hemisphere cortical language areas[71] but nonfluent with predominantly subcortical pathology.[72,73]

In the fluent form of aphasia, anomia, word-finding deficits, paraphasias, and circumlocutions occur.[39,70]

Reading and spelling may be relatively preserved with cortical lesions in the left hemispheric posterior language areas,
despite anomia,[39,70] which suggests poor phonologic representation of target words.

Reading and writing disorders are common in both the acute and chronic stages of subcortical vascular lesions.[73]

Epidemiology, Demography, and Risk Factors

Few cases have been reported.[71]

Age-Related Factors

Onset at any point throughout childhood.

Time-Related Factors

There is significant recovery from aphasic symptoms after vascular lesions,[73] although naming and word-finding problems
persist into the chronic stage of recovery.[39,70]

Neuropathologic Substrate

The laterality and localization of cortical lesions are similar to those of anomic aphasia in adults; damage occurs to the
posterior left hemisphere cortical language areas.[39,70]

Most subcortical vascular aphasias of childhood also appear to accord with the clinical-radiologic correlation observed in
adults with subcortical aphasias.[72,73]

Lesion laterality may be related to the pattern of impaired language comprehension. In a mixed group of brain-injured
children—many with acquired lesions from vascular etiologies—children with left-sided lesions were unable to integrate
pragmatic knowledge with syntactic constraints,[74] whereas those with right-sided lesions showed impairments in
lexical-semantic and pragmatic knowledge.[74,75]

Treatment

None specific.

Table 19-3
Language disturbances from head injury

Definition

Acquired aphasia may occur after a head injury, typically a closed head injury.

The aphasia is precipitated by injury to the brain, which includes both immediate-impact injury (contusions, diffuse axonal damage) and secondary brain damage involving intracranial events (hematomas, brain swelling, infections, subarachnoid hemorrhages, hydrocephalus) and extracranial factors (hypoxia, hypotension).

Focal brain contusions are common in the frontal and temporal lobes after head injury, whether or not the head has been struck in these particular regions.[77]

Core Features

Children with acquired aphasia from head injury show a variety of aphasic symptoms in the acute stage.[7,78,79]

Frank aphasia and adult-like aphasic syndromes occur infrequently.[76]

Mutism or reduced verbal output and anomia are common in the short term after head injury.[76,80,81]

Epidemiology, Demography, and Risk Factors

Head injury is the leading cause of childhood death in North America,[82] with an incidence of 200 per 10,000 per year.[83] Eighty percent of survivors of severe childhood head injury have learning difficulties, including problems in language-related skills.[84]

Age-Related Factors

Onset can occur at any point throughout childhood.

An earlier age at onset may be associated with more deficits in reading decoding and reading comprehension.[85]

Injury before age 7 versus injury at an older age is associated with more long-term difficulties in understanding the linguistic-symbolic nature of facial expressions, in metalinguistic awareness, and in comprehension monitoring.[86,87]

Time-Related Factors

Aphasic symptoms resolve over time in children with acquired aphasia from head injury.[7,78,79]

Anomia and reduced verbal fluency are consistent deficits after childhood head injury even 18 months postinjury.[37,88–90]

One group of persisting problems for children after head injury involve what have been termed *nonaphasic language disorders* with nonliteral language, discourse, and inferencing.[91] In the long term, head-injured children show a variety of discourse deficits, not so much in the gross aspects of communication[92,93] as in telling a story,[27] using and understanding idiomatic or ambiguous statements, making inferences, and producing speech acts appropriate to particular contexts.[28,94]

In the long term, children with head injury have difficulty in comprehension—monitoring tasks requiring them to evaluate statements that violate semantic selection rules, grammatical structures, or pragmatic constraints.[86]

In the long term, children who have had a head injury at a younger rather than an older age are poor at referential communication tasks requiring them to judge the relevance of an instruction, suggesting poor metacognitive function.[86]

Children with head injury have long-term difficulties in understanding how language is used to serve social-communicative goals that include emotional deception. These children have difficulty understanding the linguistic-symbolic nature of facial displays, such as those involved in the deceptive expression of emotion (e.g., they have difficulty selecting a neutral or happy expression when told that a story character is feeling sad but has a reason for hiding that feeling from another character).[87]

Academic abilities in language-related areas are poor in the long-term after childhood head injury.[80,81]

Vocabulary tests may deteriorate with increasing time, because head-injured children are unable to acquire new language-based knowledge at an age-appropriate rate.[29]

Table 19-3 (*Continued*)

Neuropathologic Substrate

The degree of residual language impairment appears to be related to the severity of the head injury,[5,81] and children with mild head injury recover functional language faster than do children with more severe injuries.[90]

The clinical-pathologic correlation of language disorders in childhood head injury is poorly understood, particularly as it concerns contusional damage to the frontal and temporal lobes. However, it is known that frontal contusions and left-sided contusions in children and adolescents with head injury are variously associated with problems in understanding the linguistic-symbolic nature of facial expressions, in metalinguistic awareness, and in oral comprehension monitoring.[86,87]

Early frontal lobe injury particularly affects nonaphasic discourse disorders in the long term after a childhood head injury,[86,87] which is consistent with the importance of an intact frontal lobe system for the development of social awareness and social cognition.

Treatment

None specific.

---

and studies of cerebellar medulloblastomas, astrocytomas, and ependymomas have provided the principal source of information about childhood brain tumors and language.[96] The features of childhood-acquired aphasia from posterior fossa tumors are reviewed in Table 19-4.

Cancer Treatments

Radiotherapy and chemotherapy are often part of the treatment for childhood cancers such as acute lymphoblastic leukemia. Central nervous system (CNS) prophylaxis is known to cause structural and functional damage to the brain.[108] Children treated for cancer show cognitive deficits[109] and a variety of impairments in speech and language,[110] including mutism, expressive aphasia, anomia, and problems with academic skills. These speech and language deficits are not fully understood with respect to the relations between degree of language impairment and prophylactic dose, the specificity of the language disorders within particular conditions, and the correlation between language function and neuropathology.

Infectious Conditions

Infectious diseases of the brain may involve viral, bacterial, spirochetal, and other microorganisms that infect the meninges (meningitis) and/or the brain (encephalitis). Infectious conditions, which have long-term cognitive effects,[111] are reported to produce childhood-acquired aphasia,[112] either as a primary effect of CNS involvement in conditions like herpes simplex encephalitis or as a secondary effect of sensorineural hearing loss in conditions such as bacterial meningitis or toxoplasmosis.

Studies of the effects of meningitis on language function have not provided clear information. While some studies have suggested that deficits in communication are an effect of meningitis, others have not.[112] Differences in research methods and assessment procedures for language may be responsible for the apparent inconsistency in results in studies of meningitis and language.

Aphasia is often part of the morbidity of herpes simplex encephalitis,[15,29,40,113] although antiviral medication in recent years has reduced the mortality associated with this condition. There is an acute-stage comprehension defect that is similar to that seen in global aphasia following an initial period of mutism and that involves a fluent aphasia with neologisms, semantic and phonemic paraphasias, stereotypies, and perseverations.[15,29] That a fluent form of aphasia is associated with herpes simplex encephalitis appears consistent with the fact that the herpesvirus has a tropism for the temporal lobes.[2]

Recovery from aphasia appears to be especially poor after herpes simplex encephalitis.[112] Children with aphasia from encephalitis exhibit long-term paraphasias, word-finding problems, and severe

Table 19-4
Language disturbances after posterior fossa brain tumors

Definition

Acquired aphasia occurs secondary to astrocytomas, medulloblastomas, and ependymomas of the cerebellum, fourth
    ventricle, and/or brainstem, occurring in children who acutely or progressively lose previously acquired language skills.

Core Features

Mutism occurs commonly in acute-stage cerebellar lesions of childhood.[97,98]

The mutism is not tumor-specific in that it involves various tumor pathologies.[97]

A syndrome of mutism and subsequent dysarthria (MSD) has been identified[99]; it is not obviously related to cerebellar ataxia
    but characterized by a complete but transient loss of speech resolving into dysarthria.

Analysis of the dysarthria of posterior fossa tumors in children suggests that it shares some of the features of adult
    dysarthria—namely, imprecise consonants, articulatory breakdowns, prolonged phonemes, prolonged intervals, slow rate
    of speech, lack of volume control, harsh voice, pitch breaks, variable pitch, and explosive onsets.[100–103]

There appears to be no adult-like pattern of fluent or nonfluent aphasia in children treated for posterior fossa tumors.
    However, children with treated posterior fossa tumors, including medulloblastomas, show mild language impairments in
    oral expression and auditory comprehension.[101]

Epidemiology, Demography, and Risk Factors

As of 1994, a total of 36 cases of MSD have been reported.[99]

In children with posterior fossa tumors, risk factors for the development of MSD are hydrocephalus at the time of tumor
    presentation, ventricular localization of the tumor, and postsurgical edema of the pontine tegmentum.[99]

Age-Related Factors

Some 90 percent of MSD patients are less than 10 years of age, and the condition has been described in children as young as
    age 2.[99]

Time-Related Factors

In cases of MSD, recovery of dysarthria to normal speech seems to be related to the recovery of complex movements of the
    mouth and tongue.[99]

A range of short- and long-term intellectual, neuropsychological, and academic difficulties have been identified in children
    with posterior fossa tumors,[95] including language-related difficulties. Academic failure occurs frequently in survivors of
    posterior fossa tumors; the rate is higher in survivors of medulloblastoma than in survivors of cerebellar
    astrocytomas.[104–106]

Neuropathologic Substrate

Mutism may occur with a midline location of the tumor combined with postoperative complications that involve destruction
    of the midline roof structures and penetration of the peduncles and/or lateral wall or ventricular floor parenchyma.[97]

Mutism occurs particularly with posterior fossa tumors located in the midline or vermis of the cerebellum and with tumors
    invading both cerebellar hemispheres or the deep nuclei of the cerebellum.[97,98]

Table 19-4 *(Continued)*

Isolated lesions in cerebellar structures are not sufficient to produce MSD. An additional ventricular location of the tumor and adherence to the dorsal brainstem are necessary—an idea supported by the frequent occurrence of pyramidal and eye-movement signs in children with MSD.[99]

Localization of the brainstem dysfunction in MSD appears to be rostral to the medulla oblongata and caudal to the mesencephalon.[99]

It has been proposed that the mutism of MSD is related to bilateral involvement of the dentate nuclei and that the subsequent dysarthric speech represents a recovering cerebellar mechanism.[105]

Treatment

None specific to the language disorders, only the appropriate course of tumor treatment.

comprehension deficits.[15,29] The poor outcome may be related to the bilateral effects of brain infections,[33] and also to the necrotic brain lesions and significant neurologic sequelae associated with herpesvirus infections.[114]

Hypoxic Disorders

Anoxia is a state in which the oxygen levels in the body fall below physiologic levels because of depleted oxygen supply. Anoxia can come about from various causes—including severe hypotension, cardiac arrest, carbon monoxide poisoning, near-drowning, and suffocation—that involve a drop in the level of cerebral blood flow or the oxygen content of the blood. In turn, this results in cerebral anoxia, a prolonged period of which will produce permanent brain damage or anoxic encephalopathy, which is associated with a range of neurologic disorders, including language deficits.[115]

Anoxic encephalopathy affects short- and long-term language function. An initial mutism resolves into a variety of forms of language disorder, ranging from dysarthria, increased speech rate, problems initiating speech movements, and anomia.[29,116] Children who suffer a near-drowning episode show speech and language disorders that appear to recover in the longer term,[117,118] although that subset of children who initially present as comatose after a near-drowning episode may continue to be at risk for language disorders.[115]

The neuropathology of cerebral anoxia is fairly well known, although there have been few research studies in children that correlate language status and patterns of anoxic brain damage. In one study, subcortical lesions resulting from anoxic encephalopathy in adolescence have been related to motor speech disorders involving a progression from mutism to dysarthria.[116]

Metabolic Disorders

Systemic metabolic disorders that result in the accumulation of metabolites in the bloodstream cause brain disruption and cognitive impairments[119] that may include speech and language deficits. Some of the inborn errors of metabolism that have been shown to affect speech and language include phenylketonuria (an absence of the liver enzyme phenylalanine), galactosemia (an inability to utilize the sugars galactose and lactose because of disordered carbohydrate metabolism), and Wilson's disease (a progressive degenerative disorder of the brain and liver resulting from inability to process dietary copper). Congenital hypothyroidism also affects intellectual functions, including language. Other hereditary metabolic diseases such as homocystinuria, a disorder of amino acid metabolism, may cause vascular occlusive disease when enzyme deficiencies damage blood vessels, leading to thrombosis and ischemic stroke.[68] The specificity of speech and language disorders and the relation between language and neuropathology are poorly understood in these various metabolic conditions.

CONCLUSIONS AND ONGOING DIRECTIONS

Recent studies of the acquired aphasias of childhood have provided the basis of more systematic knowledge about these conditions—specifically about language symptoms and type of aphasia, demographic and incidence, and the course of resolution of language symptoms.

Children show a wide range of acquired aphasic features. There is no single profile of language loss in the acquired aphasic conditions of childhood. Various profiles of language loss are associated with different etiologies of childhood-acquired aphasias, ranging from the mutism of cerebellar lesions through the impairments in pragmatic and social discourse commonly observed in the long term after childhood head injury.

The symptoms manifest in the acute phase of childhood-acquired aphasia often differ according to etiology, although some acquired aphasic symptoms are common to a range of etiologies while others occur in only a few conditions. For example, many types of childhood-acquired aphasia[120] resolve to anomic and word-finding deficits, while the severe auditory agnosia of LKS is distinctive.

Age-Related Issues: Similarities and Differences between Children of Different Ages and between Children and Adults

One age-related issue concerns the difference among children with acquired aphasia in relation to age at onset of language disorder. Language disturbances involving the use and understanding of mental states and social discourse are more common with an earlier rather than a later age at head injury.[86,87]

A second age-related issue concerns the consequences for language-related skills of the developmental timing of brain injury. If the onset of epilepsy coincides with beginning to read and write, it will impair the acquisition of written language.[42] The profile of reading outcome varies with the timing of childhood head injury with respect to phonologic skills.[85] Compared to later prophylaxis, earlier treatment for childhood acute lymphoblastic leukemia results in poorer phonemic awareness.[121] These data suggest that

actively developing but unconsolidated skills are highly vulnerable to disruption by brain damage.

Aphasic mutism is of interest under the above model of heightened vulnerability for skills that are in the course of acquisition but not yet automatized. Mutism occurs more commonly in children than in adults, variously from a range of etiologies that include the acute phase of vascular, epileptogenic, traumatic, tumorigenic, and infectious conditions. The ubiquity of aphasic mutism in childhood-acquired aphasia over the age range of childhood suggests that the initiation of speech is a volatile and imperfectly automatized language function during childhood.

An important age-related issue concerns similarities and differences between childhood- and adulthood-acquired aphasia. Children and adults show more similarities in aphasic patterns than was earlier recognized. This is not to argue, however, that the aphasic symptoms and patterns are identical in children and adults; for one reason, the base frequencies of symptoms like mutism are higher in children than in adults, whereas the base frequencies of symptoms like neologisms are lower in children than in adults.

The neuroanatomy of childhood-acquired aphasia is both similar to and different from that of adulthood-acquired aphasia.[17] When the same etiology is compared in childhood and in adulthood, a number of language deficits prove to be similar. In children as well as in adults, a lesion in the left hemispheric posterior cortical language areas produces a fluent aphasia and impaired comprehension[124]; specifically, the correlation between lesion site and aphasia in children duplicates the anatomic-clinical correlation in adults.[17] Further, age does not predict recovery from aphasic symptoms when etiology is constant.[30]

To be sure, aphasic symptoms are not identical in children and adults with the same brain damage. Unlike adults, for example, children do not suffer speech disturbances from damage to the superior paravermal cortical regions associated with posterior fossa tumors.[99] Differences in base rate and frequency of aphasic symptoms may be associated with different underlying neuropathologic substrates in children and adults.

The differences between acquired aphasia in children and in adults, once thought to concern short-term aphasic symptoms, now appear to relate more to long-term language function. With increasing time since aphasia, adult language improves, albeit at variable rates. Time does not always improve language function after childhood-acquired aphasia. Children with aphasia may show an increasing inability to accrue a new verbal knowledge base, which results in chronic problems in reading and vocabulary development.[29,73]

Time-Related Issues and Their Importance for Theoretical Accounts and Taxonomies of Childhood-Acquired Aphasia

The time course of aphasic symptoms and resolution of language seems to discriminate among different etiologies of childhood-acquired aphasia. Aphasic symptoms arising from head injury resolve more quickly than do symptoms from infectious and vascular etiologies. Granted that abatement of symptoms varies according to etiology,[26] a continuing task in understanding childhood-acquired aphasia is to specify the time course of symptoms within conditions.

A better understanding of the time course and pattern of preserved and disrupted language skills is essential to establishing a more theoretically grounded account of childhood-acquired aphasia. This is also relevant to the question of the taxonomy of these conditions.

At present, there are few plausible theories of the language disturbances underlying the principal forms of childhood-acquired aphasia. Certainly no single theory is likely to account for every manifestation of childhood aphasia. Even within a particular etiology, any theory must account for the vagaries of symptoms throughout the time course of the aphasia. For example, central receptive deficits have been proposed to be primary in LKS,[60] but a closer analysis of the time course in LKS patients with more slowly developing symptoms reveals a predominantly motor aphasia evident during a language deterioration phase,[45] which seems inconsistent with the idea of a core disorder that is exclusively receptive. By understanding patterns of language deficits that change over time, it will be possible to provide a theoretically motivated account of what distinguishes impaired from preserved language skills in childhood-acquired aphasia.

The neuroanatomy of symptom patterns over time is likely to provide important clues to the underlying mechanisms of language loss and hence to be part of any theory of acquired aphasia. It has been claimed that subcortical lesions in children may have long-term effects similar to those of cortical lesions; for example, one interpretation of the mutism from subcortical vascular lesions is that it arises from a transient frontal diaschisis secondary to subcortical damage. Correlations between language and neuroimaging to allow a detailed comparison of cortical and subcortical lesions producing acquired aphasia have not yet been reported.

It is likely that the same acquired aphasic symptom may be produced by more than one mechanism. In support of this, the time course of resolution of aphasic mutism appears to be different with supratentorial and subtentorial lesions. In the case of posterior fossa tumors, the mutism resolves to dysarthria; with vascular subcortical lesions, however, the resolution of the mutism does not appear to include dysarthric symptoms.[72] This is consistent with the developmental role of the cerebellum in a range of functions, including motor timing and speech production.[102,103,122]

Without a theory of language disruption grounded in the time course of symptoms and long-term language function, there can be no workable taxonomy for childhood-acquired aphasia and its symptom patterns. For the most part, the loose descriptive taxonomy that exists among etiologies is based simply on frequency of reporting and aphasic symptoms for particular etiologies, with a condition like LKS somewhat overrepresented in publications on childhood-acquired aphasia in relation to its frequency of occurrence.[2]

Neither the classic adult taxonomy of aphasia nor existing childhood language classification systems appear adequate to describe childhood-acquired aphasia. When such cases are coded according to a taxonomy of adult aphasia,[123] some 30 to 50 percent of cases cannot be classified.[124,125] Most children with acquired aphasia cannot be classified in either the adult taxonomy or a taxonomy devised for pediatric conditions.[126]

A productive approach to the issue of taxonomy would be one that used theory-driven paradigms of normal language development rather than a priori taxonomies. In recent reviews of childhood-acquired aphasia, there has been a more explicit awareness of the need for paradigms of normal language development.[54] At the same time, it has become apparent that any such paradigms must be complex and expressed as patterns of acquisition over very long time spans, because there are wide individual differences in the rate, strategy, and style of language acquisition in normally developing children, and brain damage affects language acquisition patterns in a number of different ways.[127]

Neuropathology of Language Disorders

One reason for the dearth of workable taxonomies of childhood-acquired aphasic conditions must be the limited number of clinical-pathologic correlations that would allow comparisons of patterns of neuropathology underlying language disorders. An important objective in studies of childhood-acquired aphasia has been to contrast the pathologic processes that produce acquired aphasia with those that do not.[33] Only noninvasive forms of neuroimaging make possible this endeavor; in recent years, structural and functional neuroimaging has provided information about the temporal and spatial extent of brain pathology and hence about the neuropathologic substrates of childhood-acquired aphasia. Of direct relevance are findings from functional neuroimaging studies suggesting what had long been suspected, that areas of brain dysfunction are much larger than the areas of structural lesion in some forms of aphasia-producing childhood vascular lesions.[128]

Studies that correlate language status with neuroimaging are able to identify the factors that produce poor recovery of language. Three such factors have been suggested: an infectious etiology, poor verbal comprehension, and involvement of Wernicke's area.[30] As a larger database of such studies is accrued, it will become easier to understand the mechanism of recovery in cases of childhood-acquired aphasia.[10]

Structural and functional neuroimaging studies have enormous value in shaping taxonomies of childhood-acquired aphasia. The correlation between language symptoms and brain pathology will inform any taxonomy of childhood-acquired aphasic conditions, which must also be grounded in developmental models of language.

REFERENCES

1. Collignon R, Hécaen H, Angelergues R: A propos de 12 cas d'aphasie acquise de l'enfant. *Acta Neurol Belg* 68:245–277, 1968.
2. Paquier P, Van Dongen HR: Current trends in acquired childhood aphasia: An introduction. *Aphasiology* 7:421–440, 1993.
3. Dennis M: Childhood medical disorders and cognitive impairment: Biological risk, time, development, and reserve, in Yeates KO, Ris MD, Taylor HG (eds): *Pediatric Neuropsychology: Research, Theory, and Practice.* New York: Guilford Press, 2000, pp 3–22.
4. Freud S: *Infantile Cerebral Paralysis* (1897). Russin LA (trans). Coral Gables, FL: University of Miami, 1968.
5. Assal G, Campiche R: Aphasie et troubles du langage chez l'enfant apres contusion cerebrale. *Neurochirurgie* 19(Suppl 4):399–406, 1973.
6. Byers RK, McLean WT: Etiology and course of certain hemiplegias with aphasia in childhood. *Pediatrics* 29:376–383, 1962.
7. Guttmann E: Aphasia in children. *Brain* 65:205–219, 1942.
8. Alajouanine TH, Lhermitte F: Acquired aphasia in children. *Brain* 88:653–662, 1965.
9. Hécaen H: Acquired aphasia in children and the ontogenesis of hemispheric functional specialization. *Brain Lang* 3:114–134, 1976.
10. Satz P: Symptom pattern and recovery outcome in childhood aphasia: A methodological and theoretical critique, in Martins IP, Castro-Caldas A, Van Dongen HR, Van Hout A (eds): *Acquired Aphasia in Children.* Dordrecht, The Netherlands: Kluwer, 1991, pp 95–114.
11. Van Dongen HR, Paquier P: Fluent aphasia in children, in Martins IP, Castro-Caldas A, Van Dongen HR, Van Hout A (eds): *Acquired Aphasia in Children.* Dordrecht, The Netherlands: Kluwer, 1991, pp 125–141.
12. Visch-Brink EG, Van de Sandt-Koenderman M: The occurrence of paraphasias in the spontaneous speech of children with an acquired aphasia. *Brain Lang* 23:258–271, 1984.
13. Van Hout A: Characteristics of language in acquired aphasia in children, in Martins IP, Castro-Caldas A, Van Dongen HR, Van Hout A (eds): *Acquired Aphasia in Children.* Dordrecht, The Netherlands: Kluwer, 1991, pp 117–124.
14. Woods BT, Teuber HL: Changing patterns of childhood aphasia. *Ann Neurol* 3:273–280, 1978.

15. Van Hout A, Evrard P, Lyon G: On the positive semiology of acquired aphasia in children. *Dev Med Child Neurol* 27:231–241, 1985.

16. Van Dongen HR, Loonen MCB, Van Dongen KJ: Anatomical basis for acquired fluent aphasia in children. *Ann Neurol* 17:306–309, 1985.

17. Cranberg LD, Filley CM, Hart EJ, Alexander MP: Acquired aphasia in childhood: Clinical and CT investigations. *Neurology* 37:1165–1172, 1987.

18. Dennis M: Dissociated naming and locating of body parts after left temporal lobe resection: An experimental case study. *Brain Lang* 3:147–163, 1976.

19. Makino A, Soga T, Obayashi M, et al: Cortical blindness caused by acute general cerebral swelling. *Surg Neurol* 29:393–400, 1988.

20. Paquier P, Saerens J, Parizel PM, et al: Acquired reading disorder similar to pure alexia in a child with ruptured arteriovenous malformation. *Aphasiology* 3:667–676, 1989.

21. Rapin I: Acquired aphasia in children. *J Child Neurol* 10:267–270, 1995.

22. Landau WM, Kleffner FR: Syndrome of acquired aphasia with convulsive disorder in children. *Neurology* 7:523–530, 1957.

23. Paquier P, Van Dongen HR: Acquired childhood aphasia: A rarity? *Aphasiology* 7(Suppl 5):417–419, 1993.

24. Ikeda M, Tanabe H, Yamada K, et al: A case of acquired childhood aphasia with evolution of global aphasia into transcortical sensory aphasia. *Aphasiology* 7 (Suppl 5):497–502, 1993.

25. Satz P, Bullard-Bates C: Acquired aphasia in children, in Sarno MT (ed): *Acquired Aphasia*. San Diego, CA: Academic Press, 1981, pp 399–426.

26. Loonen MCB, Van Dongen HR: Acquired childhood aphasia: Outcome one year after onset, in Martins IP, Castro-Caldas A, Van Dongen HR, Van Hout A (eds): *Acquired Aphasia in Children*. Dordrecht, The Netherlands: Kluwer, 1991, pp 185–200.

27. Chapman SB, Culhane KA, Levin HS, et al: Narrative discourse after closed head injury in children and adolescents. *Brain Lang* 43:42–65, 1992.

28. Dennis M, Barnes MA: Knowing the meaning, getting the point, bridging the gap, and carrying the message: Aspects of discourse following closed head injury in childhood and adolescence. *Brain Lang* 3:203–229, 1990.

29. Cooper JA, Flowers CR: Children with a history of acquired aphasia: Residual language and academic impairments. *J Speech Hear Disord* 52:251–262, 1987.

30. Martins IP, Ferro JM: Recovery of acquired aphasia in children. *Aphasiology* 6(Suppl 4):431–438, 1992.

31. Van Hout A: Outcome of acquired aphasia in childhood: Prognosis factors, in Martins IP, Castro-Caldas A, Van Dongen HR, Van Hout A (eds): *Acquired Aphasia in Children*. Dordrecht, The Netherlands: Kluwer, 1991, pp 163–169.

32. Cross JA, Ozanne AE: Acquired childhood aphasia: Assessment and treatment, in Murdoch BE (ed): *Acquired Neurological Speech/Language Disorders in Childhood*. London: Taylor & Francis, 1990, pp 66–123.

33. Woods BT: Patient selection in studies of aphasia acquired in childhood, in Martins IP, Castro-Caldas A, Van Dongen HR, Van Hout A (eds): *Acquired Aphasia in Children*. Dordrecht, The Netherlands: Kluwer, 1991, pp 27–34.

34. Taveras JM, Wood EH: *Diagnostic Neuroradiology*, 2d ed. Baltimore: Williams & Wilkins, 1976, vol 1.

35. Seron X: L'aphasie de l'enfant. *Enfance* 24:249–270, 1977.

36. Carter RL, Hohenegger MK, Satz P: Aphasia and speech organization in children. *Science* 218:797–799, 1982.

37. Hécaen H: Acquired aphasia in children: Revisited. *Neuropsychologia* 21:581–587, 1983.

38. Satz P, Lewis R: Acquired aphasia in children, in Blanken G, Dittmann J, Grimm H, et al. (eds): *Linguistic Disorders and Pathologies: An International Handbook*. Berlin: Walter de Gruyter, 1993, pp 646–659.

39. Dennis M: Strokes in childhood: I. Communicative intent, expression, and comprehension after left hemisphere arteriopathy in a right-handed nine-year-old, in Rieber R (ed): *Language Development and Aphasia in Children*. New York: Academic Press, 1980, pp 45–67.

40. Martins IP, Ferro JM: Recovery from aphasia and lesion size in the temporal lobe, in Martins IP, Castro-Caldas A, Van Dongen HR, Van Hout A (eds): *Acquired Aphasia in Children*. Dordrecht, The Netherlands: Kluwer, 1991, pp 171–184.

41. Murdoch BE: *Acquired Speech and Language Disorders: A Neuroanatomical and Functional Neurological Approach*. London: Chapman & Hall, 1990.

42. Williams J, Sharp GB: Epilepsy, in Yeates KO, Ris MD, Taylor HG (eds): *Pediatric Neuropsychology: Research, Theory, and Practice*. New York: Guilford Press, 2000, pp 47–73.

43. Deonna T, Beaumanoir A, Gaillard F, Assal G: Acquired aphasia in childhood with seizure disorder: A heterogeneous syndrome. *Neuropadiatrie* 8:263–273, 1977.

44. Lou HC, Brandt S, Bruhn P: Aphasia and epilepsy in childhood. *Acta Neurol Scand* 56:46–54, 1977.

45. Marien P, Saerens J, Verslegers W, et al: Some controversies about type and nature of aphasic symptomatology in Landau-Kleffner's syndrome: A case study. *Acta Neurol Belg* 93:183–203, 1993.

46. Soprano AM, Garcia EF, Caraballo R, Fejerman N: Acquired epileptic aphasia: Neuropsychologic follow-up of 12 patients. *Pediatr Neurol* (Suppl 3):230–235, 1994.

47. Mantovani JF, Landau WM: Acquired aphasia with convulsive disorder. *Neurology* 30:524–529, 1980.

48. Papagno C, Basso A: Impairment of written language and mathematical skills in a case of Landau-Kleffner syndrome. *Aphasiology* 7:451–461, 1993.

49. Cooper JA, Ferry PC: Acquired auditory verbal agnosia and seizures in childhood. *J Speech Hear Disord* 43:176–184, 1978.

50. Appleton RE: The Landau-Kleffner syndrome. *Arch Dis Child* 72:386–387, 1995.

51. Dugas M, Gerard CL, Franc S, Sagar D: Natural history, course and prognosis of the Landau and Kleffner syndrome, in Martins IP, Castro-Caldas A, Van Dongen HR, Van Hout A (eds): *Acquired Aphasia in Children.* Dordrecht, The Netherlands: Kluwer, 1991, pp 263–277.

52. Aicardi J: Syndrome of acquired aphasia with seizure disorder: Epileptic aphasia, Landau-Kleffner syndrome, and verbal auditory agnosia with convulsive disorder, in Aicardi J (ed): *Epilepsy in Children.* New York: Raven Press, 1986, pp 176–182.

53. Dugas M, Masson M, Le Heuzey MF, Regnier N: Aphasie "acquise" de l'enfant avec epilepsie (syndrome de Landau et Kleffner): Douze observations personnelles. *Rev Neurol* 138:755–780, 1982.

54. Martins IP: Introduction, in Martins IP, Castro-Caldas A, Van Dongen HR, Van Hout A (eds): *Acquired Aphasia in Children.* Dordrecht, The Netherlands: Kluwer, 1991, pp 3–12.

55. Worster-Drought C: An unusual form of acquired aphasia in children. *Dev Med Child Neurol* 13:563–571, 1971.

56. Genton P, Guerrini R: The Landau-Kleffner syndrome or acquired aphasia with convulsive disorder. *Arch Neurol* 50:1009, 1993.

57. Van Dongen HR, De Wijngaert E, Wennekes MJ: The Landau-Kleffner syndrome: Diagnostic considerations, in Martins IP, Castro-Caldas A, Van Dongen HR, Van Hout A (eds): *Acquired Aphasia in Children.* Dordrecht, The Netherlands: Kluwer, 1991, pp 253–261.

58. Landau WM: Landau-Kleffner syndrome. *Arch Neurol* 49:353, 1992.

59. Gerard C-L, Dugas M, Valdois S, et al: Landau-Kleffner syndrome diagnosed after 9 years of age: Another

Landau-Kleffner syndrome? *Aphasiology* 7:463–473, 1993.

60. Bishop DVM: Age of onset and outcome in "acquired aphasia with convulsive disorder." *Dev Med Child Neurol* 27:705–712, 1985.

61. Paquier PF, Van Dongen HR, Loonen CB: The Landau-Kleffner syndrome or "acquired aphasia with convulsive disorder." *Arch Neurol* 49:354–359, 1992.

62. Shoumaker RD, Bennett DR, Bray PF, Curless RG: Clinical and EEG manifestations of an unusual aphasic syndrome in children. *Neurology* 24:10–16, 1974.

63. McKinney W, McGreal DA: An aphasic syndrome in children. *Can Med Assoc J* 110:637–639, 1974.

64. Pascual-Castroviejo I, Lopez Martin VL, Martinez Bermejo AM, Perez Higueras AP: Is cerebral arteritis the cause of the Landau-Kleffner syndrome? Four cases in childhood with angiographic study. *Can J Neurol Sci* 19:46–52, 1992.

65. Nevsimalova S, Tauberova A, Doutlik S, et al: A role of autoimmunity in the etiopathogenesis of Landau-Kleffner syndrome? *Brain Dev* 14:342–345, 1992.

66. Maquet P, Hirsch E, Dive D, et al: Cerebral glucose utilization during sleep in Landau-Kleffner syndrome: A PET study. *Epilepsia* 31:778–783, 1990.

67. De Wijngaert E, Gommers K: Language rehabilitation in the Landau-Kleffner syndrome: Considerations and approaches. *Aphasiology* 7(Suppl 5):475–480, 1993.

68. Ozanne AE, Murdoch BE: Acquired childhood aphasia: Neuropathology, linguistic characteristics and prognosis, in Murdoch BE (ed): *Acquired Neurological Speech/Language Disorders in Childhood.* London: Taylor & Francis, 1990, pp 1–65.

69. Zimmerman RA, Bilaniuk LT, Packer RJ, et al: Computed tomographic-arteriographic correlates in acute basal ganglionic infarction in childhood. *Neuroradiology* 24:241–248, 1983.

70. Hynd GW, Leathem J, Semrud-Clikeman M, et al: Anomic aphasia in childhood. *J Child Neurol* 10:189–293, 1995.

71. Klein SK, Masur D, Farber K, et al: Fluent aphasia in children: Definition and natural history. *J Child Neurol* 7:50–59, 1992.

72. Aram DM, Rose DF, Rekate HI, Whitaker HA: Acquired capsular/striatal aphasia in childhood. *Arch Neurol* 40:614–617, 1983.

73. Martins IP, Ferro JM: Acquired childhood aphasia: A clinicoradiological study of 11 stroke patients. *Aphasiology* 7(Suppl 5):489–495, 1993.

74. Eisele JA: Selective deficits in language comprehension following early left and right hemisphere damage, in Martins IP, Castro-Caldas A, Van Dongen HR, Van Hout

A (eds): *Acquired Aphasia in Children*. Dordrecht, The Netherlands: Kluwer, 1991, pp 225–238.

75. Eisele JA, Aram DM: Differential effects of early hemisphere damage on lexical comprehension and production. *Aphasiology* 7:513–523, 1993.

76. Jordan FM: Speech and language disorders following childhood closed head injury, in Murdoch BE (ed): *Acquired Neurological Speech/Language Disorders in Childhood*. London: Taylor & Francis, 1990, pp 124–147.

77. Gennarelli TA, Graham DI: Neuropathology of the head injuries. *Semin Clin Neuropsychiatry* 3:160–175, 1998.

78. Van Dongen HR, Loonen MCB: Factors related to prognosis of acquired aphasia in children. *Cortex* 13:131–136, 1977.

79. Loonen MCB, Van Dongen HR: Acquired childhood aphasia: Outcome one year after onset. *Arch Neurol* 47:1324–1328, 1990.

80. Ewing-Cobbs L, Brookshire B, Scott MA, Fletcher JM: Children's narratives following traumatic brain injury: Linguistic structure, cohesion, and thematic recall. *Brain Lang* 61:395–419, 1998.

81. Ewing-Cobbs L, Fletcher JM, Levin HS, Eisenberg HM: Language functions following closed head injury in children and adolescents. *J Clin Exp Neuropsychol* 5:575–592, 1987.

82. Adelson PD, Kochanek PM: Head injury in children. *J Child Neurol* 13:2–15, 1998.

83. Kraus JF: Epidemiological features of brain injury in children: Occurrence, children at risk, causes and manner of injury, severity, and outcomes, in Broman SH, Michel ME (eds): *Traumatic Head Injury in Children*. New York: Oxford University Press, 1995, pp 22–39.

84. Ewing-Cobbs L, Fletcher JM, Levin HS, et al: Academic achievement and academic placement following traumatic brain injury in children and adolescents: A two-year longitudinal study. *J Clin Exp Neuropsychol* 20:769–781, 1998.

85. Barnes MA, Dennis M, Wilkinson M: Reading after closed head injury in childhood: Effects on accuracy, fluency, and comprehension. *Dev Neuropsychol* 15:1–24, 1999.

86. Dennis M, Barnes MA, Donnelly RE, et al: Appraising and managing knowledge: Metacognitive skills after childhood head injury. *Dev Neuropsychol* 12:77–103, 1996.

87. Dennis M, Barnes MA, Wilkinson M, Humphreys RP: How children with head injury represent real and deceptive emotion in short narratives. *Brain Lang* 61:450–483, 1996.

88. Jordan FM, Ozanne AE, Murdoch BE: Long-term speech and language disorders subsequent to closed head injury in children. *Brain Inj* 2:179–185, 1988.

89. Jordan FM, Ozanne AE, Murdoch BE: Performance of closed head injury children on a naming task. *Brain Inj* 4:27–32, 1990.

90. Jordan FM, Murdoch BE: A prospective study of the linguistic skills of children with closed-head injuries. *Aphasiology* 7:503–512, 1993.

91. Dennis M, Barnes MA: Speech acts after mild or severe childhood head injury. *Aphasiology* 14:391–405, 2000.

92. Dennis M, Purvis K, Barnes MA, Wilkinson M: Understanding of literal truth, ironic criticism, and deceptive praise following childhood head injury. *Brain Lang* 78:1–16, 2001.

93. Dennis M, Barnes MA: Comparison of literal, inferential, and intentional text comprehension in children with mild or severe closed head injury. *J Head Trauma Rehab* 16:456–468, 2001.

94. Barnes MA, Dennis M: Knowledge-based inferencing after childhood head injury. *Brain Lang* 76:253–265, 2001.

95. Dennis M, Spiegler B, Riva D, MacGregor DL: Neurocognitive outcomes after treatment for childhood brain tumors, in Walker D, Perilongo G, Punt J, Taylor R (eds): *Brain and Spinal Tumors of Childhood*. London: Arnold, 2002.

96. Hudson LJ: Speech and language disorders in childhood brain tumours, in Murdoch BE (ed): *Acquired Neurological Speech/Language Disorders in Childhood*. London: Taylor & Francis, 1990, pp 245–268.

97. Humphreys RP: Mutism after posterior fossa tumor surgery. *Concepts Pediatr Neurosurg* 9:57–64, 1989.

98. Rekate HL, Grubb RL, Aram DL, et al: Muteness of cerebellar origin. *Arch Neurol* 42:697–698, 1985.

99. Van Dongen HR, Catsman-Berrevoets CE, Van Mourik M: The syndrome of "cerebellar" mutism and subsequent dysarthria. *Neurology* 44:2040–2046, 1994.

100. Hudson LJ, Murdoch BE, Ozanne AE: Posterior fossa tumours in childhood: Associated speech and language disorders post-surgery. *Aphasiology* 3:1–18, 1989.

101. Hudson LJ, Murdoch BE: Language recovery following surgery and CNS prophylaxis for the treatment of childhood medulloblastoma: A prospective study of three cases. *Aphasiology* 6:17–28, 1992.

102. Huber-Okrainec J, Dennis M, Bradley K, Spiegler BJ: Motor speech deficits in long-term survivors of childhood cerebellar tumors: Effects of tumor type, radiation, age at diagnosis, and survival years (abstr). *Neurooncology* 3:371, 2001.

103. Huber-Okrainec J, Dennis M, Bradley K, Spiegler BJ: *Cerebellar tumor resection in childhood followed by transient cerebellar mutism: An investigation of residual speech deficits in long-term survivors.* (Retrieved January 7, 2002 from http://cnshome.org/abstracts/search.html.)

104. Dennis M, Spiegler BJ, Hetherington CR, Greenberg ML: Neuropsychological sequelae of the treatment of children with medulloblastoma. *J Neurooncol* 29:91–101, 1996.

105. Hirsch JF, Reiner D, Czernichow P, et al: Medulloblastoma in childhood: Survival and functional results. *Acta Neurochir* 48:1–15, 1979.

106. Johnson DL, McCabe MA, Nicholson HS, et al: Quality of long-term survival in young children with medulloblastoma. *J Neurosurg* 80:1004–1010, 1994.

107. Ammirati M, Mirzai S, Samii M: Transient mutism following removal of a cerebellar tumour: A case report and review of the literature. *Childs Nerv Syst* 5:12–14, 1989.

108. Withers HR: Biological basis of radiation therapy for cancer. *Lancet* 339:156–159, 1992.

109. Dropcho EJ: Central nervous system injury by therapeutic irradiation. *Neurol Clin* 9:969–988, 1991.

110. Hudson LJ, Buttsworth DL, Murdoch BE: Effect of CNS prophylaxis on speech and language function in children, in Murdoch BE (ed): *Acquired Neurological Speech/Language Disorders in Childhood.* London: Taylor & Francis, 1990, pp 269–307.

111. Smyth V, Ozanne AE, Woodhouse LM: Communicative disorders in childhood infectious diseases, in Murdoch BE (ed): *Acquired Neurological Speech/Language Disorders in Childhood.* London: Taylor & Francis, 1990, pp 148–176.

112. Paquier P, Van Dongen HR: Two contrasting cases of fluent aphasia in children. *Aphasiology* 5:235–245, 1991.

113. Van Hout A, Lyon G: Wernicke's aphasia in a 10-year-old boy. *Brain Lang* 29:268–285, 1986.

114. Kleiman MB, Carver DH: Central nervous system infections, in Black P (ed): *Brain Dysfunction in Children: Etiology, Diagnosis, and Management.* New York: Raven Press, 1981, pp 79–107.

115. Murdoch BE, Ozanne AE: Linguistic status following acute cerebral anoxia in children, in Murdoch BE (ed): *Acquired Neurological Speech/Language Disorders in Childhood.* London: Taylor & Francis, 1990, pp 177–198.

116. Murdoch BE, Chenery HJ, Kennedy M: Aphemia associated with bilateral striato-capsular lesions subsequent to cerebral anoxia. *Brain Inj* 3:41–49, 1989.

117. Pearn JM, DeBuse P, Mohay M, Golden M: Sequential intellectual recovery after near-drowning. *Med J Aust* 1:463–464, 1979.

118. Reilly K, Ozanne AE, Murdoch BE, Pitt WR: Linguistic status subsequent to childhood immersion injury. *Med J Aust* 149:225–228, 1988.

119. Ozanne AE, Murdoch BE, Krimmer HL: Linguistic problems associated with childhood metabolic disorders, in Murdoch BE (ed): *Acquired Neurological Speech/Language Disorders in Childhood.* London: Taylor & Francis, 1990, pp 199–215.

120. Dennis M: Word finding after brain-injury in children and adolescents. *Top Lang Disord* 13:66–82, 1992.

121. Kleinman SN, Waber DP: Neurodevelopmental bases of spelling acquisition in children treated for acute lymphoblastic leukemia. *Cogn Neuropsychol* 9:403–425, 1992.

122. Schmahmann JD: An emerging concept: The cerebellar contribution to higher function. *Arch Neurol* 48:1178–1186, 1991.

123. Goodglass H, Kaplan E: *The Assessment of Aphasia and Related Disorders.* Philadelphia: Lea & Febiger, 1972.

124. Marshall JC: The description and interpretation of aphasic language disorder. *Neuropsychologia* 24:5–24, 1986.

125. Martins IP, Ferro JM: Acquired conduction aphasia in a child. *Dev Med Child Neurol* 29:529–540, 1987.

126. Lees JA: Differentiating language disorder subtypes in acquired childhood aphasia. *Aphasiology* 7(Suppl 5):481–488, 1993.

127. Bates E, Thal D, Janowsky JS: Early language development and its neural correlates, in Boller F, Grafman J (eds): *Handbook of Neuropsychology.* Amsterdam: Elsevier, 1992, vol 7, pp 69–110.

128. Shahar E, Gilday DL, Hwang PA, et al: Pediatric cerebrovascular disease: Alterations of regional cerebral blood flow detected by TC 99m–HMPAO SPECT. *Arch Neurol* 47:578–584, 1990.

Chapter 20

ACQUIRED DISORDERS OF READING

H. Branch Coslett

The study of acquired dyslexia or disorders of reading dates at least to the contributions of Déjerine, who, in 1891 and 1892, described two patients with quite different patterns of reading impairment. Déjerine's first patient[1] developed an impairment in reading and writing subsequent to an infarction involving the left parietal lobe. Déjerine termed this disorder "alexia with agraphia" and attributed the disturbance to a disruption of the "optical image for words," which he thought to be supported by the left angular gyrus. In an account that in some respects presages contemporary psychological accounts, Déjerine concluded that reading and writing required the activation of these "optical images" and that the loss of the images resulted in an inability to recognize or write familiar words.

Déjerine's second patient[2] was quite different. This patient was unable to read aloud or for comprehension but could write, a disorder that Déjerine designated "alexia without agraphia" (also known as agnosic alexia and pure alexia). The patient had a right homonymous hemianopia from a left occipital lesion, which included the fibers carrying visual information from the right to the left hemisphere. Déjerine explained alexia without agraphia in terms of a "disconnection" between visual information confined to the right hemisphere and the left angular gyrus, which he assumed to be critical for the recognition of words.

After the seminal contributions of Déjerine, the study of acquired dyslexia languished for decades, during which the relatively few investigations that were reported focused primarily on the anatomic underpinnings of the disorders. The study of acquired dyslexia was revitalized, however, by the elegant and detailed investigation by Marshall and Newcombe,[3] demonstrating that by virtue of a careful investigation of the pattern of reading deficits exhibited by dyslexic subjects, distinctly different and reproducible types of reading deficits could be elucidated. These investigators described a patient (GR) who read approximately 50 per-

cent of concrete nouns but was severely impaired in the reading of abstract nouns and all other parts of speech. The most striking aspect of GR's performance, however, was his tendency to produce errors that appeared to be semantically related to the target word (e.g., *speak* read as "talk"). Marshall and Newcombe[3] designated this disorder "deep dyslexia." These investigators also described two patients whose primary deficit appeared to be an inability to derive the pronunciation of irregularly spelled words, such as "yacht." This disorder was designated "surface dyslexia."

On the basis of these data, Marshall and Newcombe[3] concluded that the meaning of written words could be accessed by two separate and distinct procedures. The first was a lexical (whole-word) procedure whereby familiar words activated the appropriate stored representation (or visual word form), which, in turn, activated meaning; reading in deep dyslexia was assumed to involve this procedure, labeled A in Fig. 20-1.

The second procedure was assumed to be a phonologically based process in which "grapheme-to-phoneme" (hereafter termed "print-to-sound") correspondences were employed to derive the appropriate phonology (that is, "sound out" the word); the reading of surface dyslexics was assumed to be mediated by this nonlexical procedure, labeled B in Fig. 20-1. Although a number of Marshall and Newcombe's specific hypotheses have been criticized, their argument that reading may be mediated by two distinct procedures has received considerable empirical support. Indeed, although it has occasionally been questioned,[4,5] the dual-route model of reading has provided the conceptual framework that has motivated most subsequent studies of acquired dyslexias and animates the present discussion.

In this chapter we briefly summarize the clinical features and conceptual basis of the major types of acquired dyslexia. Additionally, the possible role of

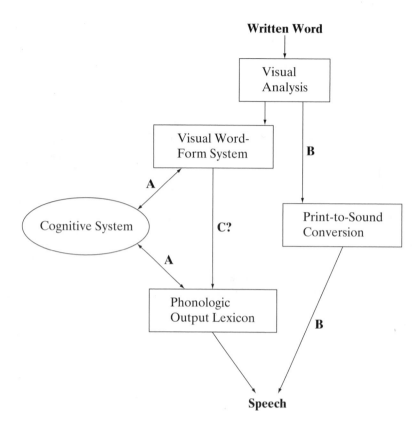

Written Word

Visual Analysis

Visual Word-Form System

B

Cognitive System

C?

Print-to-Sound Conversion

A

A

Phonologic Output Lexicon

B

Speech

Figure 20-1
A diagram of an information-processing model of reading incorporating three procedures for oral reading.

the right hemisphere in reading is briefly discussed. Finally, recent efforts to develop computational models of normal reading and acquired dyslexia are briefly described.

PERIPHERAL DYSLEXIAS

A useful starting point in the discussion of the dyslexias is the distinction offered by Shallice and Warrington[6] between "peripheral" and "central" dyslexias. The former are conditions characterized by a deficit in the processing of visual aspects of the stimulus that interferes with matching the familiar word to its stored orthographic representation or "visual word form."[6] Central dyslexias, in contrast, are attributable to an impairment of "deeper" or "higher" reading mechanisms by means of which visual word forms gain access to meaning or speech production mechanisms. The major types of peripheral dyslexia are briefly described below.

Alexia without Agraphia (Pure Alexia)

The classic syndrome of alexia without agraphia or pure alexia is perhaps the prototypical peripheral dyslexia. As noted above, the traditional account[2,7] of this disorder attributes the syndrome to a "disconnection" of visual information, which is restricted to the right hemisphere, from the left-hemispheric word-recognition system.

Though these patients do not appear to be able to read in the sense of fast, automatic word recognition, many are able to use a compensatory strategy that involves naming the letters of the word in serial fashion; they read, in effect, letter by letter. Using the slow and inefficient letter-by-letter procedure, pure alexics typically exhibit significant effects of word length, requiring more time to read long as compared to short words. In contrast to the central dyslexias, performance is typically not influenced by linguistic factors such as parts of speech (e.g., noun versus functor), the extent to which the referent of the word is concrete (e.g., *table*) or abstract (e.g., *destiny*), or whether the word is orthographically regular (that is, can be "sounded out").

A number of alternative accounts of the processing deficit in pure alexia have been proposed. Thus, some investigators have proposed that the impairment is attributable to a limitation in the transmission of letter identity information to the visual word system,[8] an inability to directly encode visual letters as abstract orthographic types,[9,10] or an inability to encode multiple visual shapes of any sort in rapid succession.[11,12] Other investigators have argued that the disorder is attributable to a disruption of the visual word-form system itself.[13,14]

Although most reports of pure alexia have emphasized the profound nature of the reading deficit, often stating that patients were utterly incapable of reading without recourse to a letter-by-letter strategy,[7,8] a number of investigators have reported data demonstrating that at least some pure alexic patients are able to comprehend words that they are unable to explicitly identify.[15–17] This capacity has been attributed by some investigators (e.g., Ref. 17) to the operation of a reading procedure based in the right hemisphere.

The anatomic basis of pure alexia has been extensively investigated. Although on rare occasions associated with lesions that "undercut" or disconnect the posterior perisylvian cortex on the left,[18] the disorder is typically associated with a lesion in the posterior portion of the dominant hemisphere, which compromises visual pathways in the dominant hemisphere and disrupts white matter tracts (such as the splenium of the corpus callosum or forceps major) critical for the interhemispheric transmission of visual information.[19,20]

Neglect Dyslexia

Neglect dyslexia, which is most commonly encountered in patients with left-sided neglect, is characterized by a failure to explicitly identify the initial portion of a letter string. Interestingly, the performance of patients with neglect dyslexia is often influenced by the nature of the letter string; thus, patients with this disorder may fail to report the initial letters in nonwords (e.g., the "ti-" in a nonword such as "tiggle") but read real words (e.g., "giggle") correctly (Ref. 21; see also Refs. 22 and 23). The fact that performance is affected by the lexical status of the stimulus has been taken to suggest that neglect dyslexia is not attributable to a failure to register letter information but reflects an attentional impairment at a higher level of representation (see also Chap. 7).

Although neglect dyslexia is generally seen in the context of the neglect syndrome (see Chaps. 14 and 15), it has occasionally been observed in isolation or even in the context of neglect of the opposite side of space.[24]

Attentional Dyslexia

Perhaps the least studied of the acquired dyslexias, attentional dyslexia is characterized by the relative preservation of single-word reading in the context of a gross disruption of reading when words are presented in text or in the presence of other words or letters.[25–28] Patients with this disorder may also exhibit difficulties identifying letters within words, even though the words themselves are read correctly,[25] and be impaired in identifying words flanked by extraneous letters (e.g., "Iboat"). We[28] have recently investigated a patient with attentional dyslexia secondary to autopsy-proven Alzheimer disease who produced frequent "blend" errors in which letters from one word of a two-word display intruded into the other word (e.g., "take lime" read as "tame"). Although several accounts for this disorder have been proposed, the disorder has been attributed by several investigators to an impairment in visual attention or a loss of location information. As visual attention may be critical to mapping the location of visually presented objects, these accounts are not clearly distinguishable.

CENTRAL DYSLEXIAS

In this section we briefly describe the clinical features and conceptual basis of the major types of central dyslexia including "deep," "phonologic," and "surface" dyslexia. Additionally, the phenomenon of "reading without meaning" is discussed.

Deep Dyslexia

Deep dyslexia, the most extensively investigated central dyslexia (see, for example, Coltheart and colleagues[29]) is in many respects the most compelling. The allure of deep dyslexia is due in large part to the intrinsically interesting hallmark of the syndrome, *semantic errors.* When shown the word *castle,* a deep dyslexic may respond "knight"; similarly, these interesting patients may read *bird* as "canary." At least for some deep dyslexics, it is clear that these errors are not circumlocutions and that the patients are not even aware that they have erred.

While semantic errors are typically regarded as essential for the diagnosis of deep dyslexia, the frequency with which deep dyslexics produce them is quite variable; for some patients, semantic errors may represent the most frequent error type, whereas for others they constitute a small proportion of reading errors. These patients also produce a variety of other types of reading errors, including "visual" errors in which the response bears a clear visual similarity to the target (e.g., *skate* read as "scale") and "morphologic" errors, in which a prefix or suffix is added, deleted, or substituted (e.g., *scolded* read as "scolds"; *governor* read as "government").

Additional hallmarks of the syndrome include a greater success in reading words of high as compared to low imageability. Thus, words such as *table, chair, ceiling,* and *buttercup,* the referents of which are concrete or imageable, are read more successfully by deep dyslexics than words such as *fate, destiny, wish,* and *universal,* the referents of which are abstract.

Also characteristic of the syndrome is part-of-speech effect, such that nouns are read more reliably than modifiers (adjectives and adverbs), which are, in turn, read more accurately than verbs. Deep dyslexics manifest particular difficulty in the reading of functors (a class of words that includes pronouns, prepositions, conjunctions, and interrogatives such as *that, which, they, because, under,* etc.). The striking nature of the part-of-speech effect is illustrated by the patient reported by Saffran and Marin[30] who correctly read the word *chrysanthemum* but was unable to read the *the*! Many errors to functors involve the substitution of a different functor (*that* read as *which*) rather than the production of words of a different class, such as nouns or verbs.

As functors are, in general, less imageable than nouns, verbs, or adjectives, some investigators have claimed that the apparent effect of part of speech is

in reality a manifestation of the pervasive imageability effect described above.[31] We have reported a patient,[32] however, whose performance suggests that the part-of-speech effect is not simply a reflection of a more general deficit in the processing of low-imageability words, as the difference remained after functors and content words were matched for imageability.

Finally, all deep dyslexics exhibit a substantial impairment in the reading of nonwords; when confronted with letter strings such as *flig* or *churt,* deep dyslexics are typically unable to employ print-to-sound correspondences to derive phonology; nonwords frequently elicit "lexicalization" errors (e.g., *flig* read as "flag"), perhaps reflecting a reliance on lexical reading in the absence of access to reliable print-to-sound correspondences.

How can deep dyslexia be accommodated by the model of reading depicted in Fig. 20-1? Several alternative explanations have been proposed. Most investigators agree that multiple processing deficits must be hypothesized to account for the full range of symptoms found in deep dyslexia. First, the strikingly impaired performance in reading nonwords and other tasks assessing phonologic function suggests that the print-to-sound conversion procedure is disrupted. Second, the presence of semantic errors and the effects of imageability (a variable usually thought to influence processing at the level of semantics) have been interpreted by many investigators as evidence that these patients also suffer from a semantic impairment; it should be noted in this context, however, that some deep dyslexic patients perform well on tests of comprehension with words they are unable to read aloud. Semantic errors in these patients have been attributed to a deficit in or access to representations in the output phonologic lexicon (Ref. 33; see also Ref. 6). Last, the production of visual errors has been interpreted by some to suggest that these patients suffer from an impairment in the visual word-form system. Other investigators (e.g., Coltheart,[34] Saffran and coworkers[35]) have argued that deep dyslexics' reading is mediated by a system not normally used in reading—that is, the right hemisphere. We will return to the issue of reading with the right hemisphere below.

Although deep dyslexia has occasionally been associated with posterior lesions, this disorder is typically encountered in association with large perisylvian lesions extending into the frontal lobe. As might be expected given the lesion data, deep dyslexia is usually associated with global or Broca's aphasia but may rarely be encountered in patients with fluent aphasia.

Phonological Dyslexia: Reading without Print-to-Sound Conversion

First described in 1979 by Derouesne and Beauvois,[36] phonological dyslexia is, perhaps, the "purest" of the central dyslexias in that the syndrome appears to be attributable to a selective deficit at some stage in the procedure mediating the translation from print to sound. Thus, although in many respects less arresting than deep dyslexia, phonological dyslexia is of considerable theoretical import. It is of interest to note that the existence of this syndrome was *predicted* by dual-route accounts of reading similar to that proposed by Marshall and Newcombe[3] and subsequently identified when dyslexic patients were assessed with theoretically motivated tasks. It has since become the subject of intensive study by cognitive neuropsychologists interested in the organization of reading in the brain.[37]

Phonological dyslexia is a relatively mild disorder in which reading of real words may be only slightly impaired. Many patients with this disorder, for example, correctly read 85 to 95 percent of real words (e.g., Refs. 32, 36, 38). Some patients with this disorder read all different types of words with equal facility,[38–40] whereas other patients are relatively impaired in the reading of functors.[41,42] Unlike patients with surface dyslexia, described below, the regularity of print-to-sound correspondences is not relevant to the performance of phonological dyslexics; thus, these patients typically pronounce orthographically irregular words such as *colonel* and words with standard print-to-sound correspondences such as *administer* with equal facility. Most errors in response to real words appear to have a visual basis, often involving the substitution of visually similar real words (e.g., *topple* read as "table").

The striking and theoretically relevant aspect of the performance of phonological dyslexics is a substantial impairment in the oral reading of nonword letter strings. A number of investigators have described patients with this disorder, for example, who read more than 90 percent of real words of all types yet correctly pronounce only about 10 percent of nonwords.[32,36]

Most errors in nonword reading involve the substitution of a visually similar real word (e.g., *phope* read as "phone") or the incorrect application of print-to-sound correspondences (e.g., *stime* read as "stim," rhyming with "him").

Within the context of the reading model depicted in Fig. 20-1, the account for this disorder is relatively straightforward. The patients' good performance with real words suggests that the processes involved in normal "lexical" reading—that is, visual analysis, the visual word-form system, semantics, and the phonological output lexicon—are at least relatively preserved. The impairment in nonword reading suggests that the print-to-sound translation procedure is disrupted.

A final point of interest is that a number of phonological dyslexics exhibit substantial deficits in processing morphologically complex words—that is, words with prefixes and suffixes.[38,42] The explanation for this association is not clear.

Phonological dyslexia has been observed in association with lesions in a number of sites in the dominant perisylvian cortex and, on occasion, with lesions of the right hemisphere (e.g., Ref. 42). Damage to the superior temporal lobe and angular and supramarginal gyri in particular is found in most but not all patients with this disorder. Although quantitative data are lacking, the lesions associated with phonological dyslexia appear to be smaller on average than those associated with deep dyslexia.

Just as there is variability with respect to the lesion site associated with phonological dyslexia, there is variability with respect to the type and severity of aphasia observed in these patients. A phonological dyslexic reported by Derouesne and Beauvois,[36] for example, did not exhibit a significant aphasia, whereas Funnell's patient W.B.[38] appears to have had a severe nonfluent aphasia.

Surface Dyslexia

Surface dyslexia is a disorder characterized by the inability to read words with "irregular" or exceptional print-to-sound correspondences. Patients with surface dyslexia are thus unable to read aloud words such as *colonel, yacht, island, have,* and *borough,* the pronunciation of which cannot be derived by phonological or "sounding out" strategies. In contrast, these patients read words containing regular correspondences (e.g., *state, hand, mint, abdominal*) as well as nonwords (e.g., *blape*) quite well.

As noted above, normal subjects may read familiar words by matching the letter string to a stored representation of the word and retrieving the pronunciation by means of a mechanism linked to semantics (or, as discussed below, by means of a nonsemantic "direct" route). As this procedure involves the activation of stored representations, the pronunciation of the word is not computed by rules but is retrieved; consequently, the regularity of print-to-sound correspondences would not be expected to play a major role in performance.

In the context of a dual-route model of reading, the sensitivity to the regularity of the print-to-sound correspondences provides prima facie evidence that the impairment in surface dyslexia is in the mechanism(s) mediating lexical reading. Similarly, the preserved ability to read regular words and nonwords provides compelling support for the claim that the procedures by which pronunciations are computed by the application of print-to-sound correspondences are at least relatively preserved.

Noting that there is substantial variability in the performance of surface dyslexics with respect to leading latencies as well as accuracy, Shallice and McCarthy[43] suggested that the syndrome of surface dyslexia be fractionated. Type 1 surface dyslexia, they suggested, is characterized by effortless and accurate reading of nonwords and regular words with poor performance with irregular words only. Type 2 surface dyslexia, in contrast, is characterized by slow, effortful reading; although these patients read irregular words less well than regular words and nonwords, they make errors with all types of stimuli. More recently, Shallice[44] suggested that at least for patients with type 2 surface dyslexia, the syndrome may reflect an attempt to compensate for damage to early stages of the reading process.

Other investigators have suggested that the syndrome may be fractionated even more. Thus, for example, surface dyslexia may be associated with disruption of the visual word-form system,[3] with a disruption of semantics (in conjunction with deficit in the "direct" route),[45,46] or with a lesion involving the phonological output lexicon.[47] Indeed, Coltheart and Funnell[48] pro-

posed that within the context of a multiroute model of reading, surface dyslexia might be associated with as many as seven distinct types of impairment.

Finally, if as suggested above, patients with surface dyslexia are unable to access semantics by means of a direct lexical procedure, one might ask how these patients derive word meaning. At least for some surface dyslexics, access to a word's meaning appears to occur only after the phonological form of the word has been derived. Thus, when presented the word *listen,* a patient described by Marshall and Newcombe[3] responded "Liston" and added "that's the boxer."

The anatomic correlate of surface dyslexia has not been well established. Indeed, in recent years the syndrome has been reported most frequently in the context of dementia.[46,49–54] Accordingly, surface dyslexia in demented patients is sometimes termed "semantic dyslexia." Many of these patients have exhibited brain atrophy most prominent in the temporal lobes (e.g., Refs. 50 and 53).

Reading without Meaning

In 1979, Schwartz and coworkers[45] reported a patient (WLP) who exhibited a profound loss of semantics in the context of dementia. Her performance was of particular interest because, unlike patients with surface dyslexia, she correctly read aloud both regular and irregular words that she was unable to comprehend. Thus, for example, when asked to sort written words into their appropriate semantic categories, she correctly classified only 7 of 20 animal names; critically, WLP correctly read aloud 18 of these animal names, including such orthographically ambiguous or irregular words as *hyena* and *leopard.* The same basic phenomenon—that is, the ability to read aloud regular and irregular words that the patient does not understand—has subsequently been reported by a number of investigators (see Refs. 55 and 56).

The pattern of performance exhibited by WLP and similar patients is of considerable theoretical interest. Recall that to this point, two procedures have been described by which written words may be pronounced. The first (labeled A in Fig. 20-1) involves the activation of an entry in the visual word-form system, access to semantic information, and ultimately activation of an entry in the phonological output lexicon. The second (B in Fig. 20-1) involves the nonlexical print-to-sound translation process. Reading without semantics is of interest precisely because it cannot readily be accommodated by such an account. The fact that these patients do not comprehend the words they correctly pronounce indicates that their oral reading is not mediated by the semantically based reading procedure. Additionally, the fact that these patients can read irregular words suggests that they are not relying on a sublexical print-to-sound conversion procedure.

How, then, do these patients read aloud? Several explanations have been proposed. One response was to suggest that oral reading may be mediated by a third mechanism or route (e.g., Ref. 57). This mechanism was assumed to be lexically based, involving the activation of an entry in the visual word-form system and the "direct" activation of an entry in the phonological output lexicon (C in Fig. 20-1); note that this procedure differs from the lexical procedure described above in that there is no intervening activation of semantic information. Based on the analysis of a phonological dyslexic's performance across a variety of reading, writing, and repetition tasks, we[32] have reported data providing additional support for the existence of a lexical but nonsemantic reading procedure. An alternative hypothesis was proposed by Shallice and colleagues (Refs. 44 and 46; see also Ref. 58). These investigators attempted to explain reading without semantics within the context of a dual-route model by proposing that the phonological reading procedure employs not only grapheme-to-phoneme correspondences but also correspondences based on larger units including syllables and even morphemes. Thus, on this account, WLP and similar patients are assumed to compute the pronunciation of irregular words they cannot understand by relying on the multiple levels of print-to-sound correspondences available in the phonological system. Finally, Hillis and Caramazza[59] have suggested that the apparent ability to read without meaning is attributable to the fact that, while the patient is impaired, the semantic and phonological reading procedures provide partial information that constrains the subject's responses. Thus, on this account, neither the semantic nor phonological procedure is assumed to be capable of generating the correct response, but the combination of partial phono-

logical and incomplete semantic information is often sufficient to identify the stimulus.

READING AND THE RIGHT HEMISPHERE

One important and controversial issue regarding reading concerns the putative reading capacity of the right hemisphere. For many years investigators argued that the right hemisphere was "word blind."[2,6,7] In recent years, however, several lines of evidence have suggested that the right hemisphere may possess the capacity to read. One seemingly incontrovertible line of evidence comes from the performance of a patient who underwent a left hemispherectomy at age 15 for treatment of seizures caused by Rasmussen's encephalitis;[60] after the hemispherectomy, the patient was able to read approximately 30 percent of single words and exhibited an effect of part of speech; she was also utterly unable to use a print-to-sound conversion process. Thus, in many respects this patient's performance was similar to that of a person with deep dyslexia, a pattern of reading impairment that has been hypothesized to reflect the performance of the right hemisphere.[34,35]

The performance of some split-brain patients is also consistent with the claim that the right hemisphere is literate. These patients may, for example, be able to match printed words presented to the right hemisphere with an appropriate object.[61,62] Interestingly, the patients are apparently unable to derive sound from the words presented to the right hemisphere; thus, they are unable to determine if a word presented to the right hemisphere rhymes with an auditorially presented word.

Another line of evidence supporting the claim that the right hemisphere is literate comes from evaluation of the reading of patients with pure alexia and optic aphasia.[17,63] We reported data, for example, from four patients with pure alexia who performed well above chance on a number of lexical decision and semantic categorization tasks with briefly presented words that they could not explicitly identify. Three of the patients who regained the ability to identify rapidly presented words explicitly exhibited a pattern of performance consistent with the right-hemisphere reading hypothesis. These patients read nouns better than functors and words of high (e.g., *chair*) better than words of low (e.g., *destiny*) imageability. Additionally, both patients for whom data were available demonstrated a deficit in the reading of suffixed (e.g., *flowed*) as opposed to pseudo-suffixed (e.g., *flower*) words. These data are consistent with a version of the right-hemisphere reading hypothesis postulating that the right-hemisphere lexical-semantic system primarily represents high imageability nouns. On this account, functors, affixed words, and low imageability words are not adequately represented in the right hemisphere.

Finally, we reported data from an investigation with a patient with pure alexia in which transcranial magnetic stimulation (TMS) was employed to directly test the hypothesis that the right hemisphere mediates the reading of at least some patients with acquired dyslexia.[64] We reasoned that if the right hemisphere provides the neural substrate for reading, the transient, localized disruption of cortical processing caused by TMS of the right hemisphere would interfere with reading. An extensively investigated patient with pure alexia who exhibited the reading pattern described above was asked to read aloud briefly presented words, half of which were presented in association with TMS. Consistent with the hypothesis that his reading was mediated by the right hemisphere, stimulation of the right hemisphere interfered with oral reading, whereas left-hemisphere stimulation had no significant effect.

Although a consensus has not yet been achieved, there is mounting evidence that, at least for some people, the right hemisphere is not word-blind but may support the reading of some types of words. The full extent of this reading capacity and whether it is relevant to normal reading, however, remain unclear.

COMPUTATIONAL MODELS OF THE DYSLEXIAS

To this point, the discussion of acquired reading disorders has been motivated by a widely though not universally (see Refs. 4 and 5) accepted multiroute information processing model of reading. In recent years, however, computer-implemented parallel distributed processing (PDP) models of cognitive processing have made important contributions in many domains of cognitive science, including reading (see Chap. 7). These models, which differ from traditional information processing models in that they offer (and in fact require) greater specification of the manner in which information is represented and processed, have called into question the necessity of hypothesizing two routes to account for the syndromes reviewed here. Although a detailed discussion of these models is beyond the scope of this chapter, several PDP accounts of reading are briefly summarized below.

Seidenberg and McClelland[65] have reported a PDP model of single-word reading in which the procedure for computing pronunciation directly from orthography (that is, without semantic mediation) is assumed to be mediated by a single network in which orthographic patterns are linked to phonological representations by means of an intermediate "hidden layer."[65] In contrast to the information processing accounts described above, this model does not postulate a discrete "lexical" or word-representation procedure or distinct lexical and sublexical procedures for the computation of phonology. Of particular relevance in the present context is the fact that investigators have attempted to simulate the performance of dyslexic patients by modifying or "lesioning" this PDP model. Patterson and colleagues,[66] for example, have attempted to model the performance of surface dyslexics by eliminating a proportion of the connections or units at different "lesion" sites. Although the simulations do not appear to capture all of the characteristic features of the performance of surface dyslexics, the lesioned models generate data that are in many interesting and important respects similar to those of patients. More recently, Plaut and Shallice[67] have reported a series of simulations of different PDP architectures in an attempt to model the performance of patients with deep dyslexia.

Finally, Seidenberg and Joanisse have recently extended their computational approach to reading to an issue of considerable theoretical importance: the reading of prefixed and suffixed (that is, "multimorphemic") words.[68] On the basis of empiric studies with normals as well as data from a computational model, Gonnerman et al.[69,70] argue that morphologic structure is an "emergent, interlevel representation that mediates computations between form and meaning" rather than an explicit level of representation.

An alternative computational account of reading has been developed by several investigators. Reggia and coworkers[71] developed a model that incorporates both lexical and nonlexical procedures for the computation of phonology. This model, which employs a competitive distribution of activation to govern interaction between competing concepts, simulates many aspects of normal reading performance. In a series of elegant investigations, Coltheart and colleagues[72,73] have described a computationally instantiated version of dual-route theory similar to that presented in Fig. 20-1, the "dual-route cascaded" model. This account incorporates a "lexical" route (similar to C in Fig. 20.1) as well as a "nonlexical" route by which the pronunciation of graphemes is computed on the basis of position-specific correspondence rules. Like the PDP models described above, the dual-route cascaded model accommodates a wide range of findings from the literature on normal reading. And as with the PDP models, "lesioning" the dual-route cascaded model produces disorders that are, at least in many respects, similar to acquired dyslexias described earlier in this chapter.[74]

A full discussion of the relative merits of these models as well as other approaches to the understanding of reading and acquired dyslexia (e.g., Ref. 75) is beyond the scope of this chapter. It would appear likely, however, that investigations of acquired dyslexia will help to adjudicate between competing accounts of reading and that these models will continue to offer critical insights into the interpretation of data from brain-injured subjects.

REFERENCES

1. Déjerine J: Sur un cas de cécité verbale avec agraphie, suivi d'autopsie. *C R Séances Soc Biol* 3:197–201, 1891.
2. Déjerine J: Contribution à l'étude anatomo-pathologique et clinique des différentes variétés de cécité verbale. *C R Séances Soc Biol* 4:61–90, 1892.
3. Marshall JC, Newcombe F: Patterns of paralexia: A psycholinguistic approach. *J Psycholinguist Res* 2:175–199, 1973.
4. Marcel AJ: Surface dyslexia and beginning reading: A revised hypothesis of the pronunciation of print and its impairments, in Coltheart M, Patterson KE, Marshall JC (eds): *Deep Dyslexia*. London: Routledge, 1980.
5. Van Orden GC, Pennington BF, Stone GO: Word identification in reading and the promise of subsymbolic psycholinguistics. *Psychol Rev* 97:488–522, 1990.
6. Shallice T, Warrington EK: Single and multiple component central dyslexic syndromes, in Coltheart M, Patterson K, Marshall JC (eds): *Deep Dyslexia*. London: Routledge, 1980.
7. Geschwind N: Disconnection syndromes in animals and man. *Brain* 88:237–294, 585–644, 1965.
8. Patterson K, Kay J: Letter-by-letter reading: Psychological descriptions of a neurological syndrome. *Q J Exp Psychol* 34A:411–441, 1982.
9. Arguin M, Bub DN: Pure alexia: Attempted rehabilitation and its implications for interpretation of the deficit. *Brain Lang* 47:233–268, 1994.
10. Arguin M, Bub DN: Single-character processing in a case of pure alexia. *Neuropsychologia* 31:435–458, 1993.
11. Kinsbourne M, Warrington EK: A disorder of simultaneous form perception. *Brain* 85:461–486, 1962.
12. Farah MJ, Wallace MA: Pure alexia as a visual impairment: A reconsideration. *Cognit Neuropsychol* 8:313–334, 1991.
13. Warrington EK, Shallice T: Word-form dyslexia. *Brain* 103:99–112, 1980.
14. Warrington EK, Langdon D: Spelling dyslexia: A deficit of the visual word-form. *J Neurol Neurosurg Psychiatry* 57:211–216, 1994.
15. Landis T, Regard M, Serrat A: Iconic reading in a case of alexia without agraphia caused by a brain tumor: A tachistoscopic study. *Brain Lang* 11:45–53, 1980.
16. Shallice T, Saffran EM: Lexical processing in the absence of explicit word identification: Evidence from a letter-by-letter reader. *Cognit Neuropsychol* 3:429–458, 1986.
17. Coslett HB, Saffran EM: Evidence for preserved reading in pure alexia. *Brain* 112:327–329, 1989.
18. Greenblatt SH: Subangular alexia without agraphia or hemianopia. *Brain Lang* 3:229–245, 1976.
19. Binder JR, Mohr JP: The topography of callosal reading pathways: A case-control analysis. *Brain* 115:1807–1826, 1992.
20. Damasio AR, Damasio H: The anatomic basis of pure alexia. *Neurology* 33:1573–1583, 1983.
21. Sieroff E, Pollatsek A, Posner MI: Recognition of visual letter strings following injury to the posterior visual spatial attention system. *Cognit Neuropsychol* 5:427–449, 1988.
22. Behrman M, Moscovitch M, Black SE, Mozer M: Perceptual and conceptual mechanisms in neglect dyslexia. *Brain* 113:1163–1183, 1990.

23. Berti A, Frassinetti F, Umilta C: Nonconscious reading? Evidence from neglect dyslexia. *Cortex* 30:181–197, 1994.

24. Costello AD, Warrington EK: The dissociation of visual neglect and neglect dyslexia. *J Neurol Neurosurg Psychiatry* 50:110–116, 1987.

25. Shallice T, Warrington EK: The possible role of selective attention in acquired dyslexia, *Neuropsychologia* 15:31–41, 1977.

26. Price CJ, Humphreys GW: Attentional dyslexia: The effects of co-occurring deficits. *Cognit Neuropsychol* 6:569-592, 1993.

27. Warrington EK, Cipolotti L, McNeil J: Attentional dyslexia: A single case study. *Neuropsychologia* 31:871–886, 1993.

28. Saffran EM, Coslett HB: "Attentional dyslexia" in Alzheimer's disease: A case study. *Cognit Neuropsychol.* In press.

29. Coltheart M, Patterson K, Marshall JC (eds): *Deep Dyslexia.* London: Routledge, 1980.

30. Saffran EM, Marin OSM: Reading without phonology: Evidence from aphasia. *Q J Exp Psychol* 29:515–525, 1977.

31. Allport DA, Funnell E: Components of the mental lexicon. *Phil Trans R Soc Lond B* 295:397–410, 1981.

32. Coslett HB: Read but not write "idea": Evidence for a third reading mechanism. *Brain Lang* 40:425–443, 1991.

33. Caramazza A, Hillis AE: Where do semantic errors come from? *Cortex* 26:95–122, 1990.

34. Coltheart M: Deep dyslexia: A right hemisphere hypothesis, in Coltheart M, Patterson K, Marshall JC (eds): *Deep Dyslexia.* London: Routledge, 1980.

35. Saffran EM, Bogyo LC, Schwartz MF, Marin OSM: Does deep dyslexia reflect right-hemisphere reading? in Coltheart M, Patterson K, Marshall JC (eds): *Deep Dyslexia.* London: Routledge, 1980.

36. Derouesne J, Beauvois M-F: Phonological processing in reading: Data from alexia. *J Neurol Neurosurg Psychiatry* 42:1125–1132, 1979.

37. Coltheart M (ed): *Special Issue on Phonological Dyslexia, Cognit Neuropsychol,* 13, 1996.

38. Funnell E: Phonological processes in reading: New evidence from acquired dyslexia. *Br J Psychol* 74:159–180, 1983.

39. Bub D, Black SE, Howell J, Kertesz A: Speech output processes and reading, in Coltheart M, Sartori G, Job R (eds): *Cognitive Neuropsychology of Language.* Hillsdale, NJ: Erlbaum, 1987.

40. Friedman RB, Kohn SE: Impaired activation of the phonological lexicon: Effects upon oral reading. *Brain Lang* 38:278–297, 1990.

41. Glosser G, Friedman RB: The continuum of deep/ phonological dyslexia. *Cortex* 26:343–359, 1990.

42. Patterson KE: The relation between reading and psychological coding: Further neuropsychological observations, in AW Ellis (ed): *Normality and Pathology in Cognitive Functions.* London: Academic Press, 1982.

43. Shallice T, McCarthy R: Phonological reading: From patterns of impairment to possible procedures, in Patterson KE, Coltheart M, Marshall JC (eds): *Surface Dyslexia.* London: Erlbaum, 1985.

44. Shallice T: *From Neuropsychology to Mental Structure.* Cambridge, England: Cambridge University Press, 1987.

45. Schwartz MF, Saffran EM, Marin OSM: Dissociation of language function in dementia: A case study. *Brain Lang* 7:277–306, 1979.

46. Shallice T, Warrington EK, McCarthy R: Reading without semantics. *Q J Exp Psychol* 35A:111–138, 1983.

47. Howard D, Franklin S: Three ways for understanding written words, and their use in two contrasting cases of surface dyslexia (together with an odd routine for making "orthographic" errors in oral word production), in Allport A, Mackay D, Prinz W, Scheerer E (eds): *Language Perception and Production.* New York: Academic Press, 1987.

48. Coltheart M, Funnell E: Reading writing: One lexicon or two? in Allport DA, MacKay DG, Printz W, Scheerer E (eds): *Language Perception and Production: Shared Mechanisms in Listening, Speaking, Reading and Writing.* London: Academic Press, 1987.

49. Warrington EK: The selective impairment of semantic memory. *Q J Exp Psychol* 27:635–657, 1975.

50. Hodges JR, Patterson K, Oxbury S, Funnell E: Semantic dementia: Progressive fluent aphasia with temporal lobe atrophy. *Brain* 115:1783–1806, 1992.

51. Patterson K, Hodges J: Deterioration of word meaning: Implications for reading. *Neuropsychologia* 30:1025–1040, 1992.

52. Graham KS, Hodges JR, Patterson K: The relationship between comprehension and oral reading in progressive fluent aphasia. *Neuropsychologia* 32:299–316, 1994.

53. Breedin SD, Saffran EM, Coslett HB: Reversal of the concreteness effect in a patient with semantic dementia. *Cognit Neuropsychol* 11:617–660, 1994.

54. Cipolotti L, Warrington EK: Semantic memory and reading abilities: A case report. *J Int Neuropsychol Soc* 1:104–110, 1994.

55. Friedman RB, Ferguson S, Robinson S, Sunderland T: Dissociation of mechanisms of reading in Alzheimer's disease. *Brain Lang* 43:400-413, 1992.

56. Raymer AM, Berndt RS: Models of word reading: Evidence from Alzheimer's disease. *Brain Lang* 47:479–482, 1994.

57. Morton J, Patterson KE: A new attempt at an interpretation, or an attempt at a new interpretation, in Coltheart M, Patterson K, Marshall JC (eds): *Deep Dyslexia*. London: Routledge, 1980.

58. McCarthy RA, Warrington EK: Phonological reading: Phenomena and paradoxes. *Cortex* 22:359–380, 1986.

59. Hillis AE, Caramazza A: Mechanisms for accessing lexical representations for output: Evidence from a category-specific semantic deficit. *Brain Lang* 40:106–144, 1991.

60. Patterson K, Vargha-Khadem F, Polkey CF: Reading with one hemisphere. *Brain* 112:39–63, 1989.

61. Zaidel E: Lexical organization in the right hemisphere, in Buser P, Rougeul-Buser A(eds): *Cerebral Correlates of Conscious Experience*. Amsterdam: Elsevier, 1978.

62. Zaidel E, Peters AM: Phonological encoding and ideographic reading by the disconnected right hemisphere: Two case studies. *Brain Lang* 14:205–234, 1981.

63. Coslett HB, Saffran EM: Preserved object recognition and reading comprehension in optic aphasia. *Brain* 12:1091–1110, 1989.

64. Coslett HB, Monsul N: Reading and the right hemisphere: Evidence from transcranial magnetic stimulation. *Brain Lang* 46:198–211, 1994.

65. Seidenberg MS, McClelland JL: A distributed, developmental model of word recognition and naming. *Psychol Rev* 96:522–568, 1989.

66. Patterson KE, Seidenberg MS, McClelland JL: Connections and disconnections: Acquired dyslexia in a computational model of reading processes, in Morris RGM (ed): *Parallel Distributed Processing: Implications for Psychology and Neurobiology*. Oxford, England: Oxford University Press, 1989.

67. Plaut D, Shallice T: Deep dyslexia: A case study of connectionist neuropsychology. *Cognit Neuropsychol* 10:377–500, 1993.

68. Joanisse MF, Seidenberg MS: Impairments in verb morphology after brain injury: A connectionist model. *Proc Natl Acad Sci U S A* 96:7592–7597, 1999.

69. Plaut DC, Gonnerman LM: Are non-semantic morphological effects incompatible with a distributed connectionist approach to lexical processing? *Lang Cogn Proc* 15:445–485, 2000.

70. Gonnerman M, Devlin JT, Andersen ES, Seidenberg MS: Derivational morphology as an emergent interlevel representation (personal communication, 2002).

71. Reggia J, Marsland P, Berndt R: Competitive dynamics in a dual-route connectionist model of print-to-sound transformation. *Complex Systems* 2:509–547, 1988.

72. Rastle K, Coltheart, M: Serial and strategic effects in reading aloud. *J Exp Psychol Hum Percept Perform* 25:482–503, 1999.

73. Coltheart M, Rastle, K, Perry C, et al: DRC: A dual route cascaded model of visual word recognition and reading aloud. *Psychol Rev* 108:204–256, 2001.

74. Coltheart M, Langdon R, Haller M: Simulations of acquired dyslexias by the DRC model, a computational model of visual word recognition and reading aloud, in Proceedings of the 1995 Workshop on Neural Modeling of Cognitive and Brain Disorders, College Park, MD: University of Maryland, June 8–10, 1995.

75. Van Orden GC, Jansen op de Haar MA, Bosman AM: Complex dynamic systems also predict dissociations but they do not reduce to autonomous components. *Cognit Neuropsychol* 14:131–165, 1997.

Chapter 21

THE APROSODIAS*

Elliott D. Ross

Communication is a multifaceted behavior whereby organisms exchange information through various mediums and sensory systems, such as olfaction, vocalization, and posturing. In lower animals, much of the communication takes place through species-specific displays that are relatively hard-wired and organized, at the lowest level, by the mesencephalic periaqueductal gray, with higher-order control furnished by the hypothalamus and limbic system.[1-4] In humans and to a far lesser degree in higher-order primates, communication in the form of language is organized predominantly by the neocortex and is no longer constrained by the innate and nonflexible demands of species-specific displays. This has allowed language to evolve as a graded, infinitely variable behavior.

The fundamental discoveries of Broca[5] and Wernicke[6] that focal lesions in the left hemisphere cause spectacular deficits in many aspects of language have led to the widely held belief that human language is a dominant and highly lateralized function of the left hemisphere, with the right hemisphere being relegated to a "minor" or "nondominant" role in language, communication, and overall control of behavior.[7,8] Over the last two and a half decades, however, considerable evidence has accrued to support the thesis that communication functions are distributed between the hemispheres.[9-37]

The left hemisphere is primarily concerned with lexical and syntactic processing and related functions such as pantomime, pragmatics, denotation, and the linguistic and dialectal aspects of prosody. The right hemisphere is primarily concerned with affective prosody, gestures, and certain related functions such as connotation, thematic inference, and comprehension of nonliteral phrases and complex linguistic relations. Numerous functional neuroimaging studies have established an active role for the right hemisphere in language.[11,38-40] The most intensively analyzed right hemisphere function has been affective prosody and gestures.

ELEMENTS OF LANGUAGE AND COMMUNICATION

Language and communication are characterized by four major constituents: the lexicon (vocabulary), syntax (grammar), prosody, and kinesics. The segment is the smallest articulated feature of a language which, in nontechnical terms, is most closely allied with the syllable.[41,42] Segments, therefore, are the primary building blocks for creating words which form the lexicon. Words, in turn, are concatenated into grammatical relationships to form phrases, sentences, and discourse. It is the segmentally related or verbal-propositional features of language that are primarily disrupted by focal left brain injury that cause aphasic syndromes.

Prosody is a nonverbal or suprasegmental feature of language that conveys various levels of information to the listener, including linguistic, affective (attitudinal and emotional), dialectal, and idiosyncratic data.[31,42-45] The acoustic features underlying prosody include pitch, intonation, melody, cadence, loudness, timbre, tempo, stress, accent, and pauses. Although the preeminence of the propositional aspects of language is well accepted, developmental studies have established that the earliest building blocks of language are prosodic-intonational rather than verbal-segmental features.[46-50] As children acquire the verbal-segmental features of language, prosodic phenomena eventually become embedded and carried by the articulatory line.

Kinesics refers to the limb, body, and facial movements associated with language and communication.[51] Movements that are used for semiotic purposes,

* ACKNOWLEDGMENT: This work was supported in part by grants from the Merit Review Board, Medical Research Service, Department of Veterans Affairs, Washington, DC, and OCAST, Oklahoma City, Oklahoma, to Dr. Ross.

such as the "V for victory" sign, are classified as pantomime, since they convey specific semantic information; whereas movements used to color, emphasize, and embellish speech are classified as gestures.[51,52] Most spontaneous kinesic activity associated with discourse usually blends gestures and pantomime into a single movement.

Neurology of Prosody

The first in-depth inquiry into the neurology of prosody was initiated by Monrad-Krohn.[44,53] During World War II he cared for a native Norwegian woman who sustained a shrapnel wound to the left frontal area, causing an acute Broca's aphasia. The woman made an excellent recovery except for a lingering accent, which caused her great emotional distress during the Nazi occupation, since she was consistently mistaken for being German and was, consequently, socially ostracized. Her speech was reported to have preserved melody, as evidenced by her ability to sing, intone, and emote. The acquired foreign accent was due to inappropriate application of stresses and pauses to the articulatory line.

On the basis of this patient and others, Monrad-Krohn[44] divided prosody into three major components as indicated by the italicized words. *Intrinsic* (linguistic) prosody provides the means for using nonverbal features to enhance the linguistic functions of a language; for example, raising the intonation at the end of a statement to indicate a question, changing the stress and timing on certain segments of a phrase to clarify meaning [e.g., "the Redcoats are coming" (British regulars) versus "the red coats are coming" (red-colored coats)], or changing the stress on certain words and altering the pause structure to clarify potentially ambiguous syntax [e.g., "The man . . . and woman dressed in black . . . came to visit" (only the woman was dressed in black) versus "The man and woman dressed in black . . . came to visit" (both were dressed in black)].[31,43,45] Dialectal and idiosyncratic prosody are also to some degree subsumed by the term *intrinsic prosody* and refer to regional and individual differences in speech quality. *Intellectual* prosody imparts attitudinal information to discourse that may drastically alter meaning. For example, if the sentence "He is clever" is emphatically stressed on *is,* it becomes a resounding acknowledgment of the person's ability; whereas if the emphatic stress resides on *clever,* with a terminal rise

in intonation, sarcasm becomes apparent. *Emotional* prosody injects primary types of emotions into speech, such as happiness, sadness, fear, and anger. The term *affective prosody* refers to the combination of attitudinal and emotional prosody. *Inarticulate* prosody is the use of certain paralinguistic nonverbal elements, such as grunts and sighs, to embellish discourse.

Monrad-Krohn[44] also described various clinical disorders of prosody. *Dysprosody* is a change in voice quality that gives rise to a foreign accent syndrome. Since it is encountered primarily in patients with fairly good recovery from motor types of aphasia, it is associated with left hemisphere lesions that alter the patient's dialectal and idiosyncratic aspects of prosody. *Aprosody* is the general lack of prosody encountered in Parkinson's disease as part of the akinesia, masked facies, and soft monotone voice. *Hyperprosody* refers to the excessive use of prosody observed in mania or in patients with Broca's aphasia who have very few words at their disposal but use them to their utmost to convey attitudes and emotions. Although Monrad-Krohn did not describe prosodic disorders from focal right brain damage, he did predict that disorders of prosodic comprehension should also be encountered in brain-damaged patients.

Recent clinical studies have shown that focal right brain damage may seriously impair, in various combinations, the production, comprehension, and repetition of the affective-prosodic elements of language without disrupting its propositional elements (see below).[8–10,12,13,16,17,19,22–25,27–30,35,37] These affective-prosodic components, when coupled with gestures, impart vitality to discourse and, in many instances, are far more important than the verbal-linguistic message. Various studies have shown that if a statement contains an affective-prosodic message that is at variance with its verbal-linguistic meaning, the prosodic message normally takes precedence in adults and to a lesser degree in children.[12,54–57] For example, if the sentence "I had a really great day" is spoken using irony it will be understood as communicating a meaning that is actually opposite to its linguistic content.

Neurology of Kinesics

Disturbances in the production and comprehension of pantomimal kinesics have been firmly linked to left brain damage.[57,58] Goodglass and Kaplan[59] proposed that pantomimal disorders in aphasics with significant comprehension deficits can be attributed to their general inability to comprehend symbols, whereas pantomimal disorders in aphasics without significant comprehension deficits can be attributed to ideomotor apraxia. Other investigators, however, have not shown such tight correlation of a specific pantomimal disturbance with a specific linguistic disturbance,[60–62] although all studies to date have found that disorders of pantomime are almost always the result of left hemisphere damage resulting in aphasic disturbances.[59–63]

Gestural kinesics, on the other hand, has not been well studied neurologically, although occasionally clinical researchers have mentioned that gestural activity is often preserved in aphasic patients.[51,52] The first paper to specifically address the possible relationship of gestures to right brain damage and loss of affective prosody was published in 1979 by Ross and Mesulam.[8] They observed that lesions of the right frontal operculum may cause complete loss of spontaneous gestural activity in the nonparalyzed right face and limbs without any disturbance in praxis. The suggestion was made, therefore, that gestural behavior as opposed to pantomime was a dominant function of the right hemisphere. Since then a number of studies have lent further support to this hypothesis by showing that the right hemisphere is not only specialized for producing gestures but also for comprehending their meaning.[9,22,27,64–67]

THE APROSODIAS

Although Hughlings-Jackson[52] suggested almost a hundred years ago that the right hemisphere may have a dominant role in emotional communication, the first clinical study of affective prosody was published in 1975 by Heilman et al.[24] They assessed the ability of patients with right and left hemisphere strokes in the posterior sylvian distribution to recognize the affective content of verbally neutral statements that were spoken with various emotional intonations. Patients with right brain damage were markedly impaired on the task when compared to normals and (mildly) aphasic patients with left brain damage. In a follow-up study, Tucker et al.[30] found that patients with right but not left brain damage also had great difficulty in inserting affective variation into verbally neutral sentences on request and on a repetition task.

In 1979, Ross and Mesulam[8] described two patients with infarctions of the right anterior suprasylvian region verified by computed tomography (CT). Neither patient was aphasic or apraxic, but both complained bitterly of their almost total inability to insert affective variation into their speech and gestural behavior. Both patients seemed to have no difficulty perceiving affective displays in others and both insisted that they could feel and experience emotions inwardly. Based on these patients and the previous publications by Heilman and associates,[24,30] it was hypothesized that (1) the right hemisphere was dominant for organizing the affective-prosodic components of language and gestural behavior and (2) the functional/anatomic organization of affective language in the right hemisphere was analogous to the organization of propositional language in the left hemisphere. An issue not resolved in the paper, however, was whether the prosodic deficits from right brain damage also involved the linguistic aspects of prosody. Subsequent studies by Weintraub et al.,[35] Heilman et al.,[23] and Danly et al.[68,69] have looked more carefully at this issue in both right and left brain–damaged patients. The composite data indicate that the linguistic features of prosody may be impaired by either right or left brain damage but that the affective components seem to be disrupted exclusively by right brain damage.

In 1981, Ross[27] approached the issue of whether the anatomic organization of affective language in the right hemisphere was, in fact, similar to the organization of propositional language in the left hemisphere. Ten patients with focal right brain damage, localized by CT, underwent a bedside assessment of their ability to modulate affective prosody and gestures in a manner similar to methods utilized for propositional language. Thus, the patients were examined qualitatively for (1) spontaneous use of affective prosody and gesturing during conversation, (2) ability to repeat verbally neutral sentences with affective variation, (3) ability to auditorily comprehend affective prosody, and (4) ability to visually comprehend gestures. All patients who had lesions bordering the right sylvian fissure had some disorder of affective language. Because specific combinations of affective-prosodic deficits occurred following circumscribed lesions in the right hemisphere, which were analogous to the functional-anatomic clustering of aphasic deficits observed after focal left brain damage,[7] these particular syndromes were called

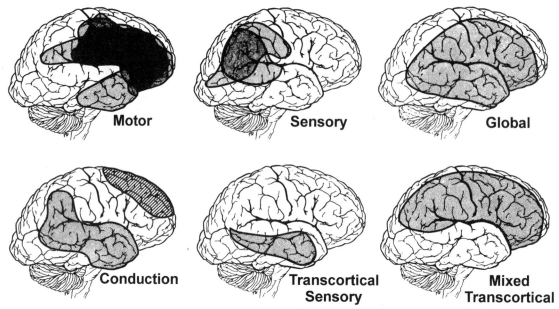

Figure 21-1

Composite cortical distribution of published CT scan lesions associated with various aprosodias[22,27] projected onto a lateral template of the right hemisphere. Stippled areas represent ischemic infarctions except for the patient with transcortical sensory aprosodia, who had a discrete hemorrhage without edema. Although the stippled lesion causing conduction aprosodia should have produced a sensory aprosodia, an analogous lesion in the left hemisphere may occasionally cause conduction rather than Wernicke's (sensory) aphasia[7,108,109]; the patient represented by the hatchmarked lesion in the lower left panel had a mild conduction aprosodia that evolved from an initial motor-type aprosodia.[27]

aprosodias and the same modifiers were applied for classification purposes as those used in the aphasias (Fig. 21-1, Table 21-1).[27] In a follow-up study, using blinded evaluations of affective language, Gorelick and Ross[22] corroborated that patients with focal right brain lesions display various deficits in affective language that corresponded with the aprosodic classifications and localizations published previously. They also reported that the prevalence of aprosodia following right brain damage was equal to the prevalence of aphasia following left brain damage, thus underscoring that the aprosodias are common rather than esoteric syndromes.

Although quantitative acoustic and neuropsychological testing paradigms exist for assessing affective prosody and communication,[26,28,29] clinicians can, with some practice and familiarization, readily incorporate an assessment of aprosodia into their bedside

neurologic examination much as one assesses patients for aphasia.

Spontaneous Affective Prosody and Gesturing During the interview, observations are made as to whether the patient gestures and imparts affect into his or her spontaneous conversation, especially when asked emotionally loaded questions about current illness or about past emotional experiences. Overall, loudness or softness of speech should be ignored, with attention paid to intonational variation in voice and gesturing to determine if emotional information appropriate to the situation under discussion is incorporated into the patient's discourse.

Repetition of Affective Prosody A declarative sentence, void of emotional words, is used to test

Table 21-1

The aprosodias

Type of aprosodia	Spontaneous affective prosody and gesturing	Affective prosodic repetition	Affective prosodic comprehension	Gestural comprehension
Motor*	poor	poor	good	good
Sensory*	good	poor	poor	poor
Conduction	good	poor	good	good
Global*	poor	poor	poor	poor
Transcortical motor	poor	good	good	good
Transcortical sensory*	good	good	poor	poor
Agesic†	good	good	good	poor
Mixed transcortical	poor	good	poor	poor

*Indicates aprosodias having anatomic correlations to right hemisphere lesions that are analogous to left hemisphere lesions resulting in similar types of aphasia (see Fig. 21-1).

†Agesic aprosodia is analogous to anomic aphasia,[7] initially described by Bowers and Heilman.[107]

affective repetition. After producing a token sentence using, for example, a happy, sad, tearful, disinterested, angry, or surprised tone of voice, the examiner immediately asks the patient to repeat the sentence. Repetition should be judged on how well the patient imitates the affective prosody of the examiner; raising or lowering the overall loudness of voice, slightly raising the voice at the end of a statement to indicate a question rather than surprise, or producing an incorrect emotion should not be considered a correct response.

Comprehension of Affective Prosody A declarative statement, void of emotional words, is used. The examiner injects the sentence with different affects and asks the patient to either verbally identify the emotion or choose the correct answer from a verbal list of five choices. Standing behind the patient during this assessment avoids giving the patient visual clues through gestural behaviors.

Comprehension of Gestures This is accomplished by standing in front of the patient and conveying a particular affective state using only gestural activity involving the face and limbs. As with affective-prosodic comprehension, the patient is asked to either identify the emotion verbally or, if necessary, choose the correct answer from a verbal list of five choices.

Using the bedside evaluation outlined above, aprosodias may be identified and subtyped as shown in Table 21-1. CT correlates of aprosodias involving a predominantly cortical-subcortical distribution are presented in Fig. 21-1. For detailed clinical descriptions of the aprosodias, the indicated references should be consulted.[22,27,37]

To date, aprosodias resulting from predominantly cortical lesions, assessed early poststroke (2 to 8 weeks), before long-term recovery of deficits occurs, appear to have a functional-anatomic organization in the right hemisphere analogous to aphasias caused by left hemisphere injury (see Figs. 21-1 and 21-2).[16,17,22,25,27,70,71] Other researchers, however, have not confirmed this observation. Some, such as Baum and Pell,[72,73] have studied patients approximately 1 to 4 years poststroke, which probably confounds their data because of long-term recovery mechanisms, much like what has been reported in the aphasia literature.[74] Others, such as Bradvik et al.,[75] have studied patients with predominantly lacunar-type infarctions that were assessed many months poststroke (mean of 13.5 months). In addition, some of the recovery patterns observed in patients with aprosodia[27] are similar to those described with aphasias,[7,76] and subcortical lesions in the right hemisphere may produce aprosodias,[22,27,37,77] just as subcortical lesions in the left hemisphere may produce aphasias.[78–80] There have also been case reports of crossed aprosodia, in which a strongly right-handed patient becomes aprosodic but not aphasic following a left hemisphere stroke, similar to cases of crossed aphasia in which a strongly right-handed patient becomes aphasic following a

Affective Prosody

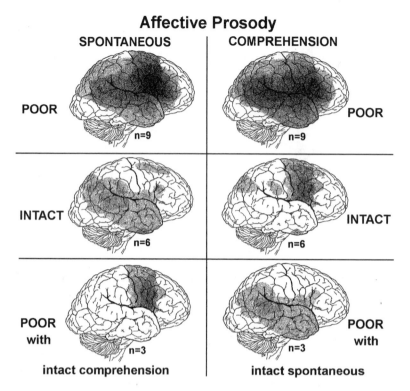

POOR
n=9

POOR
n=9

INTACT
n=6

INTACT
n=6

POOR
with
n=3

POOR
with
n=3

intact comprehension | intact spontaneous

Figure 21-2
Cortical distributions of ischemic strokes observed on MRI scan in 22 patients with right unilateral brain damage[71] classified by affective-prosodic performance on the Aprosodia Battery[96] based on spontaneous affective prosody and affective-prosodic comprehension. As in the case of aphasic deficits from left hemisphere lesions,[7] injury to the right inferior frontal region causes loss of spontaneous affective prosody in speech (analogous to aphasic nonfluency), whereas injury to the posterosuperior temporal lobe causes loss of affective-prosodic comprehension (analogous to aphasic loss of comprehension).

right hemisphere stroke.[81] Last, acquired aprosodias in children[82] and developmental disorders of affective prosody associated with aberrant psychosocial development resulting from early right brain damage[83-85] have been published that are comparable to the syndromes of acquired aphasia in children and with developmental dyslexia.

Hemispheric Lateralization of Affective Prosody

The terms *dominant* and *lateralized* are used interchangeably in the literature to describe brain function, even though they have overlapping but somewhat different neurologic implications. A brain function is considered dominant if a unilateral lesion produces a behavioral deficit that subtends both sides of space,[86,87] a criterion easily met by the various aphasic and aprosodic syndromes. For a function to be strongly lateralized, however, it must also be shown that the behavioral deficit does not occur following lesions of the opposite hemisphere. In this regard, it is of historic interest that, soon after his initial discovery that

damage to the foot of the left third frontal convolution caused loss of articulate speech,[5] Broca[88] reported that right hemisphere lesions did not result in the loss of articulate speech, thus establishing that articulation was both a dominant and highly lateralized function of the left hemisphere.[89] Unlike the aphasias, however, the degree of lateralization of affective prosody has not been established, since various publications have documented affective-prosodic disturbances in aphasic patients with left hemisphere strokes. In some instances authors have assumed incorrectly that all prosodic systems—intrinsic, affective, idiolectal, and dialectal, rather than just affective prosody—are modulated by the right hemisphere.[90,91] Nevertheless, certain publications[92-94,95] have reported considerable disturbances in the production and comprehension of affective prosody in left brain–damaged patients with severe aphasias, suggesting that affective prosody may not be strongly lateralized to the right hemisphere even though it appears to be a dominant function of that hemisphere.

De Bleser and Poeck[92] examined prosodic intonation in severe global aphasics whose speech output was restricted to one or two recurring syllables. Their intonations tended to be very stereotypic, bringing into question the original observations by Hughlings-Jackson[52] that severely aphasic patients are able to communicate through emotional channels. Schlanger et al.[93] reported affective-prosodic comprehension deficits in aphasics in opposition to the original studies by Heilman et al.[24] On reviewing the data published by both groups, it would appear that the discrepancy is most likely attributable to the distribution and severity of aphasic deficits; Heilman et al.[24] used patients with relatively preserved comprehension, whereas Schlanger et al.[93] used patients with significant deficits in verbal comprehension. More importantly, however, when Schlanger et al.[93] sorted their patients into "low-verbal" and "high-verbal" groups, the low-verbal aphasics were significantly more impaired on the emotional comprehension task than the high-verbal aphasics. Similarly, Seron et al.[94] also reported a significant positive correlation between scores of affective performance and verbal comprehension in

aphasic patients. This would suggest, therefore, that verbal impairments per se rather than a primary defect in affective processing underlie deficient performances on affective comprehension tasks in aphasic patients.

To further address this issue, Ross and colleagues[96] developed an Aprosodia Battery to assess affective prosody in a series of right and left brain–damaged (RBD, LBD) patients using a quantitative testing paradigm in which the verbal-articulatory demands were progressively reduced by using token sentences in which various emotions are carried by words, a repeated monosyllable ("ba ba ba ba ba ba"), and an asyllabic articulation ("aaaaaahhhhhhh"). In the LBD patients, reducing the verbal-articulatory load caused statistically robust improvement in their ability to comprehend affective prosody and to produce affective prosody on a repetition task, whereas no improvement occurred in the RBD patients (Fig. 21-3). Interestingly, the performance of LBD patients was not correlated with the presence, severity, or type of aphasic deficit(s).

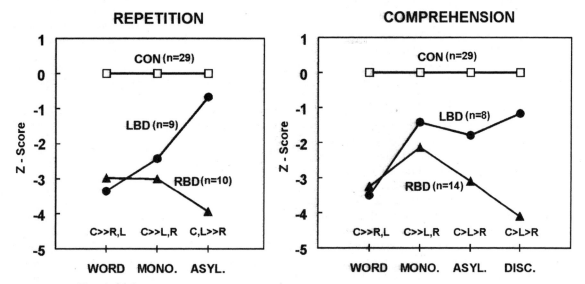

Figure 21-3

Patterns of deficits found on the Aprosodia Battery[96] in 22 RBD and 21 LBD patients with unilateral ischemic strokes compared to 29 controls.[71] Only LBD and RBD patients who had Z-scores of < −1.64, compared to controls on any repetition subtask or any comprehension subtask were included in the figure to focus attention on abnormal performance. Mono. = monosyllabic; Asyl. = asyllabic; Disc. = discrimination subtasks; C = Controls; R = RBD; and L = LBD with post hoc statistical relations for each subtask (alpha = 0.01) shown just above the abscissa. (See text and Ross et al.[96] for details about construction of the Aprosodia Battery and reasons for testing subjects under reduced verbal-articulatory demands.)

Based on functional-anatomic correlations for both spontaneous affective prosody and affective-prosodic repetition, deep white matter lesions located below the supplementary motor area that disrupt interhemispheric connections coursing through the midrostral corpus callosum seem to contribute to affective-prosodic deficits that are both additive and independent of any aphasic deficits. These findings, therefore, sustain the hypothesis that affective prosody is both a dominant and a lateralized function of the right hemisphere and lend strong support to research by Blonder et al.[10] and Bowers et al.[12,13] suggesting that RBD causes loss of affective-communicative representations as the theoretical basis for the aprosodias, similar to LBD causing the loss of verbal-syntactic representations as the theoretical basis for the aphasias.[96]

Neurology of Emotions

The aprosodias represent disturbances of graded emotional behavior encompassing both affective prosody and gestures. These behaviors are organized predominantly at the level of the neocortex as part of the language-related systems of communication. Since the experiential and display aspects of emotions are available to patients with aprosodia,[27,97,98] seemingly paradoxical behaviors may occur during clinical and social interactions. The most dramatic examples reported to date are patients with motor-types of aprosodia who are also experiencing severe depression. Because of their aprosodia, they exhibit a flat affective demeanor even when discussing highly emotional issues, such as suicide.[97,98] Consequently, their verbal reports of emotional distress can easily be discounted by both clinicians and family. Other patients may verbally deny depression but have vegetative indicators of melancholia that respond readily to antidepressant treatment. Current evidence has implicated the temporal limbic system, in particular the amygdala, as the nodal point of a neuroanatomic network for experiencing emotions and related phenomena.[99–103] Patients with motor or global aprosodia may also be observed to display extremes of emotions during very sad, happy, or angry situations despite their otherwise affectively flat demeanor.[22,27,97,98] These displays tend to be all or none, uncontrollable, and socially embarrassing, giving them the quality of pathologic regulation of affect, similar to behaviors encountered in patients with pseudobulbar palsy.[7,104,105]

Thus, the organization of emotional displays must also be modulated by areas outside the right neocortical motor system. The critical areas seem to reside in the temporal limbic system and basal forebrain, which have descending connections to alpha motor neurons through hypothalamus, periaqueductal gray, locus ceruleus, subceruleus, and the median raphe,[98,106] since lesions and epileptic discharges in these regions are known to induce sham emotional displays that usually take the form of pathologic regulation of affect.[104] For a more complete review of the neurology of emotions, the reader is referred to a recent article by Ross et al.[102] addressing the differential hemispheric lateralization of emotions and related behaviors based on the concept that emotions may be classified as having either primary or social properties.

REFERENCES

1. Bandler R, Keay KA: Columnar organization in the midbrain periaqueductal gray and the integration of emotional expression. *Prog Brain Res* 107:285–300, 1996.
2. Jurgens U, Zwirner P: The role of the periaqueductal grey in limbic and neocortical vocal fold control. *Neuroreport* 7:2921–2923, 1996.
3. Davis PJ, Zhang SP, Winkworth A, Bandler RJ: Neural control of vocalization: Respiratory and emotional influences. *J Voice* 10:23–38, 1996.
4. Jurgens U: Neural pathways underlying vocal control. *Neurosci Biobehav Rev* 26:235–258, 2002.
5. Broca P: Remarques sur le siege de la faculte du langage articule, suives d'une observation d'aphemie. *Bull Soc Anthropol Paris* 6:330–337, 1861. (Translated in von Bonin G: *The Cerebral Cortex.* Springfield, IL: Charles C Thomas, 1960.)
6. Wernicke C: *Der Aphasische Symptomencomplex. Eine Psychologische Studie auf Anatomischer Basis.* Breslau: Cohn & Weigert, 1874. (Translated in Eggert GH: *Wernicke's Works on Aphasia: Sourcebook and Review.* The Hague: Mouton, 1977.)
7. Benson DF: *Aphasia, Alexia and Agraphia.* Edinburgh: Churchill Livingstone, 1979.
8. Ross ED, Mesulam MM: Dominant language functions of the right hemisphere? Prosody and emotional gesturing. *Arch Neurol* 36:144–148, 1979.
9. Benowitz LI, Bear DM, Rosenthal R, et al: Hemispheric specialization in nonverbal communication. *Cortex* 19:5–14, 1983.

10. Blonder LX, Bowers D, Heilman KM: The role of the right hemisphere in emotional communication. *Brain* 114:1115–1127, 1991.

11. Bottini G, Corcoran R, Sterzi R, et al: The role of the right hemisphere in the interpretation of figurative aspects of language: A positron emission tomography activation study. *Brain* 117:1241–1253, 1994.

12. Bowers D, Coslett HB, Bauer RM, et al: Comprehension of emotional prosody following unilateral hemispheric lesions: Processing defect versus distraction defect. *Neuropsychologia* 25:317–328, 1987.

13. Bowers D, Bauer RM, Heilman KM: The nonverbal affect lexicon: Theoretical perspectives from neuropsychological studies of affect perception. *Neuropsychology* 7:433–444, 1993.

14. Brownell HH, Potter HH, Bihrle A: Inference deficits in right brain-damaged patients. *Brain Lang* 29:310–321, 1986.

15. Brownell HH, Potter HH, Michelow D, Gardner H: Sensitivity to lexical denotation and connotation in brain-damaged patients: A double dissociation? *Brain Lang* 22:253–265, 1984.

16. Darby DG: Sensory aprosodia: A clinical clue to lesions of the inferior division of the right middle cerebral artery? *Neurology* 34:567–572, 1993.

17. Denes G, Caldognetto EM, Semenza C, et al: Discrimination and identification of emotions in human voice by brain damaged subjects. *Acta Neurol Scand* 69:154–162, 1984.

18. Edmondson JA, Ross ED, Chan JL, Seibert GB: The effect of right-brain damage on acoustical measures of affective prosody in Taiwanese patients. *J Phonet* 15:219–233, 1987.

19. Ehlers L, Dalby M: Appreciation of emotional expressions in the visual and auditory modality in normal and brain-damaged patients. *Acta Neurol Scand* 76:251–256, 1987.

20. Emmorey K: The neurologic substrates for the prosodic aspects of speech. *Brain Lang* 30:305–320, 1987.

21. Foldi NC: Appreciation of pragmatic interpretations of indirect commands: Comparison of right and left brain-damaged patients. *Brain Lang* 31:88–108, 1987.

22. Gorelick PB, Ross ED: The aprosodias: Further functional-anatomic evidence for the organization of affective language in the right hemisphere. *J Neurol Neurosurg Psychiatry* 50:553–560, 1987.

23. Heilman KM, Bowers D, Speedie L, Coslett HB: Comprehension of affective and nonaffective speech. *Neurology* 34:917–921, 1984.

24. Heilman KM, Scholes R, Watson RT: Auditory affective agnosia: Disturbed comprehension of affective speech. *J Neurol Neurosurg Psychiatry* 38:69–72, 1975.

25. Hughes CP, Chan JL, Su MS: Aprosodia in Chinese patients with right cerebral hemisphere lesions. *Arch Neurol* 40:732–736, 1983.

26. Kent RD, Rosenbeck JC: Prosodic disturbances and neurologic lesion. *Brain Lang* 15:259–291, 1982.

27. Ross ED: The aprosodias: Functional-anatomic organization of the affective components of language in the right hemisphere. *Arch Neurol* 38:561–569, 1981.

28. Ross ED, Edmondson JA, Seibert GB, Homan RW: Acoustic analysis of affective prosody during right-sided Wada test: A within-subjects verification of the right hemisphere's role in language. *Brain Lang* 33:128–145, 1987.

29. Shapiro B, Danly M: The role of the right hemisphere in the control of speech prosody in propositional and affective contexts. *Brain Lang* 25:19–36, 1985.

30. Tucker DM, Watson RT, Heilman KM: Discrimination and evocation of affectively intoned speech in patients with right parietal disease. *Neurology* 27:947–950, 1977.

31. Van Lancker D: Cerebral lateralization of pitch cues in the linguistic signal. *Int J Hum Commun* 1980; 13:201–277.

32. Van Lancker D: The neurology of proverbs. *Behav Neurol* 3:169–187, 1990.

33. Van Lancker D, Kempler D: Comprehension of familiar phrases by left- but not right-hemisphere damaged patients. *Brain Lang* 32:256–277, 1987.

34. Wapner W, Hamby S, Gardner H: The role of the right hemisphere in the apprehension of complex linguistic materials. *Brain Lang* 14:15–33, 1981.

35. Weintraub S, Mesulam MM, Kramer L: Disturbances in prosody. *Arch Neurol* 38:742–744, 1981.

36. Winner E, Gardner H: The comprehension of metaphor in brain-damaged patients. *Brain* 100:717–729, 1977.

37. Wolfe GI, Ross ED: Sensory aprosodia with left hemiparesis from subcortical infarction. Right hemisphere analogue of sensory-type aphasia with right hemiparesis? *Arch Neurol* 44:661–671, 1987.

38. Meyer M, Alter K, Friederici AD, et al: fMRI reveals brain regions mediating slow prosodic modulations in spoken sentences. *Hum Brain* 17:73–88, 2002.

39. Ferstl E, von Cramon D: The role of coherence and cohesion in text comprehension: An event-related fMRI study. *Cogn Brain Res* 11:325–340, 2001.

40. Bookheimer S: Functional MRI of language. *Ann Rev Neurosci* 25:151–188, 2002.

41. Ladefoged P: *A Course in Phonetics*. New York: Harcourt Brace Jovanich, 1975.

42. Kent RD, Read C: *The Acoustic Analysis of Speech*. San Diego, CA: Singular Publishing Group, 1992.

43. Crystal D: *The English Tone of Voice.* New York: St Martin's Press, 1975.

44. Monrad-Krohn GH: The third element of speech: Prosody and its disorders, in Halpern L (ed): *Problems in Dynamic Neurology.* Jerusalem: Hebrew University Press, 1963, pp 101–118.

45. Van Lancker D, Canter GJ, Terbeek D: Disambiguation of ditropic sentences: Acoustic and phonetic cues. *J Speech Hear Res* 24:330–335, 1981.

46. Crystal D: Non-segmental phonology in language acquisition: Review of the issues. *Lingua* 32:1–45, 1973.

47. Lewis A: *Infant Speech: A Study of the Beginnings of Language.* New York: Harcourt Brace, 1936.

48. Werker JF, Tees RC: Cross-language speech perception: Evidence for perceptual reorganization during the first year of life. *Infant Behav Devel* 7:49–63, 1984.

49. Moon C, Cooper RP, Fifer WP: Two-day-old infants prefer their native language. *Infant Behav Dev* 16:495–500, 1993.

50. Dehaene-Lambbertz G, Houston G: Faster orientation latencies toward native language in two-month-old infants. *Lang Speech* 41:21–43, 1998.

51. Critchley M: *The Language of Gesture.* London: Edward Arnold, 1939.

52. Hughlings-Jackson J: On affectations of speech from diseases of the brain. *Brain* 38:106–174, 1915.

53. Monrad-Krohn GH: Dysprosody or altered "melody of language." *Brain* 70:405–415, 1948.

54. Ackerman BP: Form and function in children's understanding of ironic utterances. *J Exp Child Psychol* 35:487–508, 1983.

55. Bolinger D (ed): *Intonation.* Hardmondsworth: Penguin Press, 1972.

56. De Groot A: Structural linguistics and syntactic laws. *Word* 5:1–12, 1949.

57. De Renzi E, Motti F, Nichelli P: Imitating gestures: A quantitative approach to ideomotor apraxia. *Arch Neurol* 37:6–10, 1980.

58. Gainotti G, Lemmo M: Comprehension of symbolic gestures in aphasia. *Brain Lang* 3:451–460, 1976.

59. Goodglass H, Kaplan E: Disturbance of gesture and pantomime in aphasia. *Brain* 86:703–720, 1963.

60. Cicone M, Wapner W, Foldi N, et al: The relationship between gesture and language in aphasic communication. *Brain Lang* 8:324–349, 1979.

61. Delis D, Foldi NS, Hambe S, et al: A note on temporal relations between language and gestures. *Brain Lang* 8:350–354, 1979.

62. Feyereisen P, Seron X: Nonverbal communication and aphasia: A review (in 2 parts; I. Comprehension, II. Expression). *Brain Lang* 16:191–212, 213–236, 1982.

63. Seron X, Van der Kaa MA, Remitz A, Van der Linden M: Pantomime interpretation and aphasia. *Neuropsychologia* 17:661–668, 1979.

64. Borod JC, Koff E, Lorch MP, Nicholas M: Channels of emotional communication in patients with unilateral brain damage. *Arch Neurol* 42:345–348, 1985.

65. Borod JC, Koff E, Perlman M, et al: The expression and perception of facial emotion on focal lesion patients. *Neuropsychologia* 24:169–180, 1986.

66. Cicone M, Wapner W, Gardner H: Sensitivity to emotional expressions and situations in organic patients. *Cortex* 16:145–158, 1980.

67. DeKosky ST, Heilman KM, Bowers D, Valenstein E: Recognition and discrimination of emotional faces and pictures. *Brain Lang* 9:206–214, 1980.

68. Danly M, Cooper WE, Shapiro B: Fundamental frequency, language processing, and linguistic structure in Wernicke's aphasia. *Brain Lang* 19:1–24, 1983.

69. Danly M, Shapiro B: Speech prosody in Broca's aphasia. *Brain Lang* 16:171–190, 1982.

70. Starkstein SE, Federoff JP, Price TR, et al: Neuropsychological and neuroradiologic correlates of emotional prosody comprehension. *Neurology* 44:515–522, 1994.

71. Ross ED, Orbelo DM, Burgard M, Hansel S: Functional-anatomic correlates of aprosodic deficits in patients with right brain damage. *Neurology* 50(suppl 4):A363, 1998.

72. Baum SR, Pell MD: Production of affective and linguistic prosody by brain-damaged patients. *Aphasiology* 11:177–198, 1997.

73. Pell MD, Baum SR: The ability to perceive and comprehend intonation in linguistic and affective contexts by brain-damaged patients. *Brain Lang* 57:80–99, 1997.

74. Goodglass HG: *Understanding Aphasia.* New York: Academic Press, 1993, chap. 3.

75. Bradvik B, Dravins C, Holtas S, et al: Disturbances of speech prosody following right hemisphere infarcts. *Acta Neurol Scand* 84:114–126, 1991.

76. Kertesz A: *Aphasia and Associated Disorders.* New York: Grune & Stratton, 1979.

77. Ross ED, Harney JH, de Lacoste C, Purdy P: How the brain integrates affective and propositional language into a unified brain function. Hypotheses based on clinicopathological correlations. *Arch Neurol* 38:745–748, 1981.

78. Alexander MP, LoVerme SR: Aphasia after left hemispheric intracerebral hemorrhage. *Neurology* 30:1193–1202, 1980.

79. Damasio AR, Damasio H, Rizzo M, et al: Aphasia with nonhemorrhagic lesions in the basal ganglia and internal capsule. *Arch Neurol* 39:15–20, 1982.

80. Naeser MA, Alexander MP, Helm-Estabrooks N, et al: Aphasia with predominantly subcortical lesion sites: Description of three capsular/putaminal aphasia syndromes. *Arch Neurol* 39:2–14, 1982.

81. Ross ED, Anderson B, Morgan-Fisher A: Crossed aprosodia in strongly dextral patients. *Arch Neurol* 46: 206–209, 1989.

82. Bell WL, Davis DL, Morgan-Fisher A, Ross ED: Acquired aprosodias in children. *J Child Neurol* 5:19–26, 1989.

83. Weintraub S, Mesulam MM: Developmental learning disabilities of the right hemisphere: Emotional, interpersonal, and cognitive components. *Arch Neurol* 40:463–468, 1983.

84. Manaoch DS, Sandson TA, Weintraub S: The developmental social-emotional processing disorder is associated with right hemisphere abnormalities. *Neuropsychiatr Neuropsychol Behav Neurol* 8:99–105, 1995.

85. Voeller KKS: Right hemisphere deficit syndrome in children. *Amer J Psychol* 143:1004–1009, 1986.

86. Denny-Brown D, Banker BQ: Amorphosynthesis from left parietal lesion. *Arch Neurol Psychiatry* 71:302–313, 1954.

87. Denny-Brown D, Meyer JS, Horenstein S: The significance of perceptual rivalry resulting from parietal lesion. *Brain* 75:433–471, 1952.

88. Broca P: Du siege de la faculte du langage articule. *Bull Soc Anthropol Paris* 6:337–393, 1865.

89. Lecours AR, Lhermitte F: Historical review: From Franz Gall to Pierre Marie, in Lecours AR, Lhermitte F, Bryans B (eds): *Aphasiology*. London: Baillière Tindall, 1983, pp 12–14.

90. Ryalls J: Concerning right-hemisphere dominance for affective language. *Arch Neurol* 45:337–338, 1988.

91. Ross ED: Prosody and brain lateralization: Fact vs fancy or is it all just semantics? *Arch Neurol* 45:338–339, 1988.

92. de Bleser R, Poeck K: Analysis of prosody in the spontaneous speech of patients with CV-recurring utterances. *Cortex* 21:405–416, 1985.

93. Schlanger BB, Schlanger P, Gerstmann LJ: The perception of emotionally toned sentences by right hemisphere-damaged and aphasic subjects. *Brain Lang* 3:396–403, 1976.

94. Seron X, van der Kaa MA, van der Linden M, et al: Decoding paralinguistic signals: Effect of semantic and prosodic cues on aphasic comprehension. *J Commun Disord* 15:223–231, 1982.

95. Cancelliere AEB, Kertesz A: Lesion localization in acquired deficits of emotional expression and comprehension. *Brain Lang* 13:133–147, 1990.

96. Ross ED, Stark RD, Yenkosky JP: Lateralization of affective prosody in brain and the callosal integration of hemispheric language functions. *Brain Lang* 56:27–54, 1997.

97. Ross ED, Rush AJ: Diagnosis and neuroanatomical correlates of depression in brain-damaged patients: Implications for a neurology of depression. *Arch Gen Psychiatry* 38:1344–1354, 1981.

98. Ross ED, Stewart R: Pathological display of affect in patients with depression and right focal brain damage: An alternative mechanism. *J Nerv Ment Dis* 175:165–172, 1978.

99. Gloor P: Experiential phenomena of temporal lobe epilepsy: Facts and hypothesis. *Brain* 113:1673–1694, 1990.

100. Gloor P, Olivier A, Quesney LF, et al: The role of the limbic system in experiential phenomena of temporal lobe epilepsy. *Ann Neurol* 12:129–144, 1982.

101. LeDoux JE: Emotion and the amygdala, in Aggleton JP (ed): *The Amygdala: Neurobiological Aspects of Emotion, Memory, and Mental Dysfunction*. New York: Wiley-Liss, 1992, pp 339–351.

102. Ross ED, Homan RW, Buck R: Differential hemispheric lateralization of primary and social emotions: Implications for developing a comprehensive neurology for emotion, repression, and the subconscious. *Neuropsychiatr Neuropsychol Behav Neurol* 7:1–19, 1994.

103. Zola-Morgan S, Squire LR, Alvarez-Royo P, Clower RP: Independence of memory functions and emotional behavior: Separate contributions of the hippocampal formation and the amygdala. *Hippocampus* 1:207–220, 1991.

104. Poeck K: Pathophysiology of emotional disorders associated with brain damage, in Vinken PJ, Bruyn GW (eds): *Handbook of Clinical Neurology*. Amsterdam: North-Holland, 1969, vol 3, pp 343–367.

105. Wilson SAK: Some problems in neurology: II. Pathological laughing and crying. *J Neurol Psychopathol* 4:299–333, 1924.

106. Kuypers HGJM: A new look at the organization of the motor system. *Prog Brain Res* 57:381–403, 1982.

107. Bowers D, Heilman KM: Dissociation between the processing of affective and nonaffective faces: A case study. *J Clin Neuropsychol* 6:367–379, 1984.

108. Benson DF, Sheremata WA, Bouchard R, et al: Conduction aphasia: A clinicopathologic study. *Arch Neurol* 28:339–346, 1973.

109. Damasio H, Damasio AR: The anatomical basis of conduction aphasia. *Brain* 103:337–350, 1980.

Part IV

EXECUTIVE FUNCTION,
MEMORY, AND OTHER
COGNITIVE PROCESSES

Chapter 22

FRONTAL LOBES I: CLINICAL AND ANATOMICAL ISSUES

Bruce L. Miller
D. Frank Benson
Julene K. Johnson

For over a century, the frontal lobes have been an enigma to brain scientists. Significant progress has been made in the past several decades, but many anatomic and functional aspects remain mysterious. The frontal lobes, particularly in humans, are massive in relation to other, better-understood cortical areas, and it was long considered that the frontal lobes were the seat of human intelligence. This proved overly simple, at least as intelligence is defined by psychometric testing. A better generalization is that prefrontal cortex is concerned with the regulation of mental activities[1] and thus stands in a superordinate relation to the activities of posterior cortical areas.[2] As this chapter and the next will attest, our understanding the functions of the frontal lobes in human behavior is still at an early stage.

Classic neuroanatomy divides the cortical surface of the frontal lobes into three major segments: (1) motor–the narrow strip of cortical tissue located just anterior to the rolandic fissure; (2) premotor–the larger area of frontal tissue anterior to the motor strip that acts as a motor association cortex (Brodmann areas 6 and 8); and (3) prefrontal–the vast amount of frontal cortex anterior to the premotor cortex, including a significant amount of the anterior/lateral cortex, most of the medial frontal cortex, and the entire orbital frontal cortex. In the classification suggested by Luria, the motor and premotor areas of the frontal lobes would be included in the sensorimotor division and the prefrontal cortex would carry out the regulatory activities. The motor functions of the frontal lobes are adequately reviewed in many neuroanatomy texts. The prefrontal regulatory functions are important for psychology and are the topic of this chapter.

Of considerable significance in discussion of the neural basis of prefrontal psychological functions are the connections of frontal cortex with other brain areas.

The prefrontal cortex receives direct or indirect input from most ipsilateral cortical areas and from the opposite hemisphere via callosal connections. In addition, prefrontal cortex receives strong input from a number of significant subcortical sources: (1) the limbic system, (2) the reticular system, (3) the hypothalamus, and (4) neurotransmitter systems. Prefrontal cortex is the only cortical area that receives strong sensorimotor, limbic, and reticular input. Additional input of hypothalamic and autonomic information and the effects of the cholinergic, serotoninergic, noradrenergic, and glutamatergic neurotransmitter systems arriving from subcortical regions place prefrontal cortex in a strong position to monitor both intrinsic and extrinsic stimuli and to exert regulatory control of brain functions.

PREFRONTAL FUNCTION: INSIGHTS FROM THE CLINIC

The precise contribution of prefrontal cortex to behavior has proven difficult to delineate. To date, most information has been derived from the study of behavioral aberrations that develop following frontal brain damage. In the past several decades some psychological tests aimed directly at the assessment of prefrontal function have been devised (see Chap. 33), and more recently psychological testing has been combined with functional brain imaging techniques to provide valuable insights into the dynamic functions of prefrontal cortex. In general, however, psychological tests of prefrontal function demand inferences from data obtained through primary sensorimotor functions, which themselves may be impaired.[3]

A second problem in studying prefrontal function is a lack of cleanly delineated clinical/neuropathologic correlations. Frontal brain tumors tend to become massive, affecting both posterior ipsilateral tissues and tissues in the opposite frontal lobe, before diagnosis can be made. The only vascular lesion confined to prefrontal cortex involves the anterior cerebral artery, a vessel with considerable collaterals; consistent vascular lesions are rare. Prefrontal leukotomies provided clean, relatively precise prefrontal lesions but were performed only in individuals with significant behavioral abnormality prior to the operation; postsurgical testing was often frustrated by the inherent mental disorder. Finally, degenerative disorders, particularly frontotemporal dementia, offer insights into the functions of the frontal lobes, but patients tend to be recognized by physicians only after massive loss of function has occurred.

Perhaps because of these problems, the underlying impairment in frontally damaged patients has yet to be satisfactorily established. A review of current attempts at characterizing prefrontal function and its impairment is presented in the following chapter. Here we note some of the more common effects of prefrontal damage in terms of their clinical manifestations.

Personality changes following frontal lobe lesions are of two main types. One type could be called pseudoretarded or pseudodepressed, and is characterized by apathy, lethargy, little spontaneity of behavior, unconcern, reduced sexual interest, little overt emotion, and reduced ability to plan ahead. Although such patients appear retarded, their IQs may be normal or near normal. The other type could be called pseudopsychopathic and is characterized by inappropriate social behavior, lack of concern for others, increased motor activity, sexual disinhibition, and "Witzelsucht," an inappropriately puerile, jocular attitude. There is some suggestion of differential localization for these two types of personality change, the former being associated with dorsolateral lesions and the latter with orbitofrontal lesions. However, because of the nonfocal effects of many frontal lesions, mentioned above, patients will frequently manifest an almost paradoxical mixture of both personality types.

The right and left frontal lobes have differing contributions to behavior. Injury to the right frontal lobe is more likely to cause gross social impairment than is injury to the left side. Loss of insight, verbal and behavioral disinhibition, loss of respect for the interpersonal space of others, and changes in personality are common features of patients with asymmetric injury to the right frontal injury.

The cognitive impairments of patients with prefrontal damage are apparent in a variety of tasks, some of which are reviewed in the following chapter. The domains affected include complex motor behavior (see also Chap. 16), planning and sequencing, attention, memory, and language (see discussions of Broca's aphasia and transcortical motor aphasia in Chap. 11). Often patients can perform well on standard tests of intelligence but fail miserably in less constrained real-life situations calling for planning and flexibility.

MAJOR ETIOLOGIES OF PREFRONTAL DYSFUNCTION

Vascular

Ischemic Infarction   The vascular territory for the frontal lobes comes from the anterior cerebral artery (ACA) and middle cerebral artery (MCA), both of which are branches of the internal carotid artery.[4] The anterior and medial portions of the frontal lobes are supplied by the ACA, while the anterior branch of the MCA supplies most of the lateral dorsal frontal cortex. With ACA infarctions (see Fig. 22-1), the eyes tend to deviate toward the injured hemisphere. This conjugate eye deviation occurs following injury to the frontal eye fields in Brodmann area 8 and is accompanied by frontal neglect. Conjugate deviation following injury to area 8 tends to disappear after a few days, while the frontal neglect often persists. Neglect from frontal injury is not always easily differentiated from neglect due to parietal injury but is characterized motor akinesia rather than visual or sensory neglect on formal testing. Because the medial portion of the motor strip of the frontal cortex contains fibers for the leg, weakness and sensory loss associated with these infarctions is greatest in the leg, with relative sparing of motor and sensory function in the arm and face. Involvement of the supplementary motor area leads to a forced grasp of the contralateral hand. Transcortical motor aphasia is the most common aphasia syndrome seen with ACA occlusion of the dominant hemisphere.[5] Following ACA infarcts, common behavioral abnormalities include profound apathy and loss of executive control. A manic

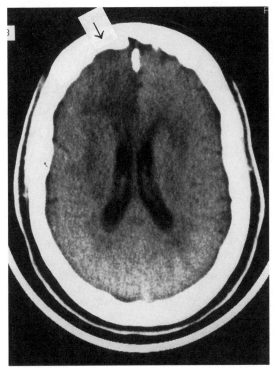

Figure 22-1
Computed tomography scan showing findings of a large anterior cerebral artery infarction involving the medial frontal cortex.

syndrome sometimes follows acute injury, particularly when the infarction involves the right hemisphere. Depression can occur with injury to either side. Rarely, a single ACA supplies both medial frontal lobes; ACA occlusion can produce bifrontal infarction leading to an akinetic mute state.

Strokes of the dominant MCA lead to paralysis of the face and arm on the contralateral side, with the eyes deviated toward the side of infarction (away from the paralysis). When the stroke is restricted to the anterior MCA branch of the dominant hemisphere, Broca's aphasia occurs; in contrast, complete MCA strokes lead to global aphasia. Loss of sequencing ability and disturbed executive control may be persistent problems. Forced grasp is not a feature of MCA stroke. Neglect occurs following either right- or left-sided MCA occlusion, but denial of illness is more common with right-sided lesions.

Other Vascular Lesions   Other types of vascular injury can also produce frontal dysfunction. A common site for aneurysms is the ACA; following rupture, ischemia or infarction within the territory of the ACA often occurs. The sagittal sinus lies adjacent to the medial portions of the frontal lobes, and thrombus formation in this sinus can produce variations on anterior artery syndromes, although seizures and alterations in consciousness are more common with sinus thrombosis than with simple arterial infarction. This disease is often idiopathic, although hypercoagulable states such as pregnancy, dehydration, and sickle cell anemia are known to cause this disorder.[6]

Trauma

The poles of the frontal lobes lie adjacent to frontal bone, while the basal (orbital) frontal regions sit on the skull's cribriform plate. The frontal lobe's intimate association with bone makes this area particularly prone to injury following trauma (see Fig. 22-2). Patients often recover from the motor and sensory deficits that follow a head injury only to be left with profound behavioral abnormalities such as disinhibition, apathy, and loss of executive control. Disinhibition associated with head trauma is often associated with injury of frontal orbitobasal regions. Loss of executive control is a sequela of injury involving dorsolateral cortex.[3] Neuropsychological tests of executive function can help to identify a frontal injury. When the injury affects orbitofrontal regions, test results may be normal, even when there is profound behavioral disinhibition.[7] In these patients, careful questioning and recording of the insights of the family, along with systematic observations by the physician, help delineate the presence and severity of the frontal syndrome.

Documentation of the severity of frontal dysfunction associated with head injury is important, as therapy for these patients is difficult. A rigidly structured environment can help patients with frontal injury cope with routine daily activities. Unfortunately, current therapies and management of apathy and loss of executive control have only limited efficacy. Antidepressant medications may help to relieve the depressions that follow frontal injury; divalproex sodium (Depakote) and atypical antipsychotics have some efficacy for disinhibition, violence, and irritability.

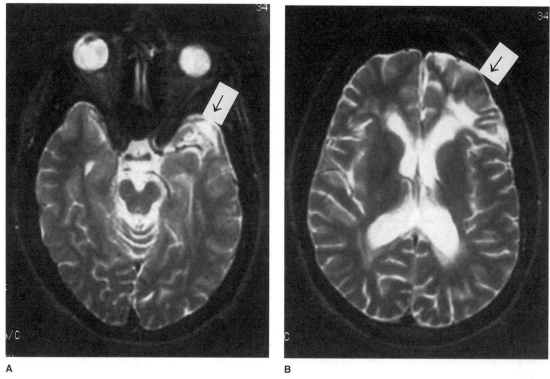

Figure 22-2
These T2-weighted MRI scans from the anterior temporal (A) and anterior frontal (B) lobes demonstrate loss of tissue secondary to trauma. The patient was a sexually and verbally disinhibited male with profound frontal systems deficits on neuropsychological testing.

Tumors

Tumors—either intrinsic or extrinsic to the frontal lobes—can produce frontal lobe symptomatology. The most common extrinsic tumors are meningiomas, which typically compress the frontal lobes in either the parasagittal (see Fig. 22-3) or cribriform plate regions.[8] Parasagittal meningiomas affect the medial aspects of the frontal lobes, so that bilateral leg weakness is a common finding. Once these tumors become sufficiently large, apathy, loss of executive control, or disinhibition can occur. Loss of the sense of smell is a common finding because of the close association of midline frontal tumors to the olfactory nerves. Cribriform plate meningiomas affect the basofrontal lobes, and behavioral disinhibition is common.

Primary brain tumors (gliomas, oligodendrogliomas, etc.) and metastases that involve the frontal lobes also alter frontal function. In current practice, these lesions are easily detected with computed tomography (CT) or magnetic resonance imaging (MRI), and effective surgical and medical therapies can be administered. However, diagnosis is often preceded by vague behavioral alterations that, in retrospect, are found to have been caused by frontal dysfunction.

Hydrocephalus

Abnormal absorption of cerebrospinal fluid (CSF) via the arachnoid granulation can cause "normal-pressure hydrocephalus" (NPH). The classic triad of hydrocephalus includes memory disturbance, urinary

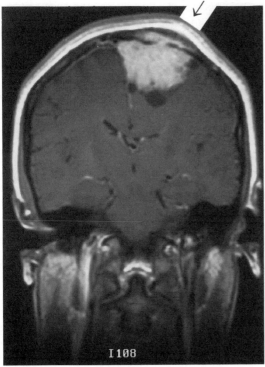

Figure 22-3
This T1-weighted gadolinium-enhanced MRI scan demonstrates a large parasagittal frontal meningioma.

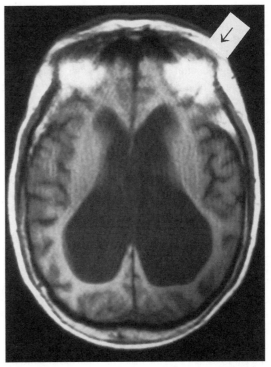

Figure 22-4
A T1-weighted MRI scan demonstrating hydrocephalus with enlarged frontal and posterior ventricles. There is no periventricular extravasation of fluid.

incontinence, and gait apraxia. Other common findings are profound apathy and even akinetic states.[9] MRI typically shows the panventricular dilatation (see Fig. 22-4) as well as extravasated periventricular fluid. The treatment of obstructive hydrocephalus (including NPH) is shunting CSF from the ventricles to a distant area for absorption. Unfortunately, this therapy is effective in only a minority of cases, and complications of shunt therapy can be troublesome.

Infections

Many infectious processes can involve frontal cerebral tissues. Bacterial, tuberculous, fungal, cysticercal, and toxoplasmal abscesses can selectively penetrate the frontal regions. Tertiary syphilis, or "general paresis of the insane" (GPI), now rare, showed a predilection to involve the frontal regions.[10] One of the

clinical syndromes associated with GPI was characterized by disinhibition and grandiose manic syndromes. Another was characterized by disinterest and slowed cognitive processing. An apathetic frontal lobe syndrome is the most typical clinical feature of dementia due to human immunodeficiency virus (HIV). This is probably based on involvement of both subcortical and frontal structures.[11] Often, HIV dementia responds at least transiently to antiviral therapy. Creutzfeldt-Jakob disease can begin in the frontal lobes.

Degenerative Dementias

Frontotemporal Dementia As reviewed in greater detail in Chap. 32, frontotemporal dementia (FTD) is a neurodegenerative disorder that involves progressive degeneration of the frontal and/or temporal lobes. It is probably the second most common pre-senile neurodegenerative disorder, ranking second only to early-onset Alzheimer's disease. Onset of FTD typically occurs in the fifth and sixth decade.[12] Neurodegeneration in FTD can be either symmetrical or asymmetrical, involving one or both frontal or temporal lobes. The clinical presentation of FTD, therefore, can be heterogeneous and reflects the relative pathologic involvement of the frontal and/or temporal cortices.[13]

The initial symptoms of FTD most commonly involve behavioral abnormalities and/or language impairments. Disinhibition, apathy, social withdrawal, loss of insight and social awareness, emotional blunting, and compulsive behaviors are common manifestations of FTD and relate to alterations in the frontal lobes. Additional impairments in executive functioning—such as planning, organizing, and shifting attention—are also common on neuropsychological testing.[14] Language is also affected by FTD. In a variant of FTD known as "primary progressive aphasia," there is a progressive nonfluent language presentation, with difficulties with speech output, grammar, and paraphasias (e.g., incorrect substitution of words or phonemes). Other individuals can present with a fluent-type aphasia and exhibit a progressive loss of semantic knowledge known as "semantic dementia," resulting in empty speech (e.g., "Show me the thing. I went to that place.").[15] Those symptoms are secondary to temporal, not frontal involvement (see also Chap. 39). The striking frontal and language impairments in FTD often contrast with a preservation of visuospatial abilities (e.g., copying designs, navigating around a neighborhood) and calculations, thereby reflecting the relative preservation of the parietal cortex. Memory abilities are also often preserved. This constellation of impaired and preserved symptoms in FTD and its variants contrasts with Alzheimer's disease, in which memory and word-finding impairments are most commonly the prominent early symptoms.

Focal presentations of FTD occur; patients with predominantly left-sided degeneration usually show progressive aphasia, while those with right-sided degeneration exhibit profound alterations of social skills. FTD invariably progresses; in the later stages, parkinsonian features and eye-movement abnormalities are common, reflecting degeneration in the basal ganglia.

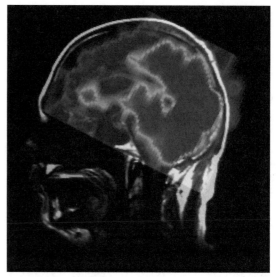

Figure 22-5

This is a xenon-133–corrected HMPAO SPECT coregistered upon a T2-weighted MRI scan from a patient with frontotemporal dementia. There is profound frontal hypoperfusion.

Eventually, profound apathy supervenes and most subjects enter a mute, akinetic state.[16] Recently, an international group of investigators proposed consensus criteria for three clinical subgroups of frontotemporal lobar degeneration: (1) frontotemporal dementia (FTD proper), (2) progressive nonfluent aphasia, and (3) semantic dementia.[17] Clinical misdiagnosis of FTD is common, but recent studies suggest that the combination of clinical data, behavioral questionnaires, and neuroimaging tools can yield a more accurate diagnosis. In most FTD patients, MRI shows atrophy of the frontal lobe and anterior temporal lobes (see Fig. 22-5), but generalized atrophy or even normal MRIs may be seen. Functional studies [e.g., single photon emission tomography (SPECT) or positron emission tomography (PET)] invariably show focal frontal or temporal deficits.

Histopathologic studies of FTD reveal severe neuronal loss and gliosis that is most prominent in the frontal and anterior temporal regions. In approximately 20 percent of FTD patients, cellular inclusions called Pick bodies are also found. Gliosis in the thalamus and basal ganglia can also be evident. Severe deficiencies in serotonin may correlate with clinical findings of weight gain and compulsions. Mutations in the tau gene on chromosome 17 have been linked to some kindreds with FTD and are associated with tau-positive neuronal or glial inclusions.[18]

Other Degenerative Dementias   Most of the degenerative dementias eventually involve the frontal lobes, even though primary pathology is elsewhere. A few disorders appear to have a selective influence upon frontal lobe function.

Alzheimer's Disease   Alzheimer's disease typically begins in the medial temporal cortex; frontal deficits rarely herald this dementia. However, a frontal variant of Alzheimer's disease has been described, and in these patients the syndrome is characterized by apathy, behavioral disorder, and loss of executive function. Their pathology is localized to frontal cortex.

Progressive Supranuclear Palsy   In this degenerative disorder the primary pathology is located in the midbrain. Extensive frontal connections with midbrain may explain the combination of midbrain and frontal lobe findings. Primary frontal degeneration occurs in some of these patients. The classic clinical findings in progressive supranuclear palsy (PSP) include frequent falls, axial rigidity, pseudobulbar palsy, apathy, and loss of both executive function, and vertical gaze. On functional imaging, dorsolateral and mediofrontal hypoperfusion is seen.[19]

Metachromatic Leukodystrophy   This degenerative disorder selectively injures white matter underlying the frontal cortex. A progressive frontal dementia occurs; diagnosis is made by demonstration of an enzymatic abnormality in arylsulfatase A. Although most cases occur in childhood and early adolescence, late-life onset can occur.[20]

Alcohol   Many toxins can affect cerebral cortex, but the symptom picture most often suggests diffuse (toxic) rather than focal abnormalities. The concept of alcohol-induced dementia remains somewhat controversial; in some individuals, chronic alcohol abuse appears to be associated with selective dysfunction of the frontal lobes (apathy and cognitive slowing).

In some instances, the frontal symptoms disappear or are considerably improved following abstinence from alcohol; in other cases, permanent dementia seems to develop.[21] The pathology of this dementia is poorly understood, but the presence of frontal symptoms is consistent.

REFERENCES

1. Luria AR: *The Working Brain: An Introduction to Neuropsychology.* Haig B, trans. New York: Basic Books, 1973.
2. Albert ML: Subcortical dementia, in Katzman R, Terry RD, Bick KI (eds): *Alzheimer's Disease, Senile Dementia and Related Disorders.* New York: Raven Press, 1978, pp 173–180.
3. Stuss DT, Benson DF: *The Frontal Lobes.* New York: Raven Press, 1986.
4. Gauthier JC, Mohr JP: Intracranial internal carotid artery disease, in Barnett HJM, Mohr JP, Stein BM, Yatsu FM (eds): *Stroke.* New York: Churchill Livingstone, 1986, pp 337–350.
5. Benson DF: *Aphasia, Alexia, and Agraphia.* New York: Churchill Livingstone, 1979.
6. Tsai FY, Higashida RT, Matovich V, Alrieri K: Acute thrombosis of the intracranial dural sinus: Direct thrombolytic treatment. *Am J Neuroradiol* 13:1137–1141, 1992.
7. Damasio AR: The frontal lobes, in Heilman KM, Valenstein E (eds): *Clinical Neuropsychology.* New York: Oxford University Press, 1979, pp 360–412.
8. Adams RD, Victor M: *Principles of Neurology,* 5th ed. New York: McGraw-Hill, 1993.
9. Hakim S: Biomechanics of hydrocephalus, in Harbert JC (ed): *Cisternography and Hydrocephalus.* Springfield, IL: Charles C Thomas, 1972, pp 22–25.
10. Cummings JL, Benson DF: *Dementia: A Clinical Approach.* Boston: Butterworth-Heinemann, 1992.
11. Price RW, Brew B, Sidtis J, et al: The brain in AIDS: Central nervous system HIV-1 infection and AIDS dementia complex. *Science* 239:286–292, 1988.
12. Brun A: Frontal lobe degeneration of non-Alzheimer type: I. Neuropathology. *Arch Gerontol Geriatr* 6:193–208, 1987.
13. Neary D, Snowden JS, Northen B, Goulding PJ: Dementia of frontal lobe type. *J Neurol Neurosurg Psychiatry* 51:353–361, 1988.
14. Miller BL, Cummings JL, Villanueva-Meyer J, et al: Frontal lobe degeneration: Clinical, neuropsychological

and SPECT characteristics. *Neurology* 41:1374–1382, 1991.

15. Hodges JR, Patterson K: Nonfluent progressive aphasia and semantic dementia: A comparative neuropsychological study. *J Int Neuropsychol Soc* 1996;6:511–524.

16. Miller BL, Chang L, Mena I, et al: Progressive right frontotemporal degeneration: clinical, neuropsychological and SPECT characteristics. *Dementia* 4:204–213, 1993.

17. Neary D, Snowden JS, Gustafson L, et al: Frontotemporal lobar degeneration: A consensus on clinical diagnostic criteria. *Neurology* 51:1546–1552, 1998.

18. Hutton M, Lendon C, Rizzu P, et al. Association of missense and 5'splicesite mutations in tau with the inherited dementia FTDP-17. *Nature* 393:702–705, 1998.

19. Johnson KA, Sperling RA, Holman BL, et al: Cerebral perfusion in progressive supranuclear palsy. *J Nucl Med* 33:704–709, 1992.

20. Austin J, Armstrong D, Fouch S, et al: Metachromatic leukodystrophy (MLD). *Arch Neurol* 18:225–240, 1968.

21. Lishman WA: Cerebral disorder in alcoholism: syndromes of impairment. *Brain* 104:1–20, 1981.

Chapter 23

FRONTAL LOBES II: COGNITIVE ISSUES

Martha J. Farah

Behavioral neurology has long recognized the crucial importance of prefrontal cortex in human behavior; the previous chapter summarizes much of what has been learned clinically about the effects of damage to this part of the brain from disease or injury. The goal of the present chapter is to review the current state of scientific understanding of prefrontal function. The emphasis is on those scientific findings and theories that help illuminate the role of prefrontal cortex (PFC) in normal human behavior and the underlying cognitive changes responsible for changes in behavior following PFC damage.

EFFECTS OF PREFRONTAL DAMAGE IN CLINICAL AND LABORATORY TASKS

The previous chapter described some of the behavioral changes seen following damage to PFC, which are typically observed (with concern) by family members, medical staff, and sometimes the patients themselves. These changes involve cognitive, social, and emotional functioning in patients' everyday lives. A complementary approach to characterizing the effects of PFC lesions is with relatively simple tasks that are either standardized relative to the performance of other people or designed to isolate specific cognitive abilities underlying task performance. Countless such tasks have been administered to PFC-damaged patients in the context of systematic research programs. The tasks and results described here are a small but representative sample.

Sequencing Tasks

A variety of clinical tests assess the ability to sequence items, from simple hand motions to strategic games such as the Towers of Hanoi. Penfield and Evans (1935) describe the difficulty that Penfield's sister had in preparing a meal after surgery to remove a frontal brain tumor. She could perform all the individual actions necessary to cook dinner but could not actually prepare the meal without someone to tell her the order in which to do things. Most clinical tests of sequencing involve simple gestures or stimuli; it is typically found that PFC-damaged patients are the most impaired (e.g., Kimura, 1982). Although the well-known tendency of PFC-damaged patients to perseverate would be expected to interfere with sequencing tasks, the errors made by such patients include nonperseverative errors. However, even more abstract sequencing tasks, such as the classic Towers of Hanoi game, reveal impairments in PFC-damaged patients (Morris et al., 1997; Shallice, 1982).

Fluency Tasks

"Fluency" tasks might be better named *generation* or *continuous generation* tasks. They require patients to generate as many exemplars of a category as possible within a time limit. Commonly used clinical tests of verbal fluency include *category fluency* tasks, in which a semantic category is used, for example naming as many animals as possible in 60 s, and *letter fluency* tasks, in which words beginning with a particular letter must be generated. Such tasks are particularly dependent on left PFC. *Design fluency,* which is most often compromised after right PFC damage, requires patients to draw a series of unique nonsense shapes to a certain specification, such as all having three sides (Jones-Gotman and Milner, 1977). As with sequencing performance, fluency is somewhat compromised by the occurrence of perseveration, but patients' output is generally impoverished beyond the "crowding out" of new items by perseverative responses.

Tests of Response Inhibition

Although important differences exist among the tasks used to assess response inhibition, they all share the following property: there are stimuli to which the subject must respond, certain stimulus-response pairings are "stronger" than others, and the tasks require that subjects override these stronger pairings in producing a correct response. Perhaps the best-known such task is the Stroop task (Stroop, 1935), in which subjects must name the ink color in which words are written, but the words themselves are color names (e.g., the word "red" written in blue ink). A lifetime of reading has automatized the process enough that effort is required to suppress the incorrect word-reading response and produce the correct color-naming response. A number of researchers report that left PFC–damaged patients have difficulty in so doing and are prone to frequent word-reading intrusion errors (Perret, 1974; Stuss and Benson, 1984).

The Go-No-Go task also taxes the testee's ability to restrain a strongly established response. There are many versions of this task, in which one stimulus-response pairing is strengthened by practice (e.g., "always tap twice when I tap once," or "always push the button when you see a letter") and then becomes the incorrect response (e.g., "now don't tap when I tap once," or "keep pushing for all the letters except for M"). Go-No-Go performance has long been recognized to depend on PFC (Drewe, 1975). Yet another test of inhibitory control is the Anti-Saccade Task, in which subjects strengthen the already potent tendency to look toward a sudden salient stimulus by performing a number of such saccades toward such stimuli but must then carry out the opposite action: saccading away from the sudden salient stimulus. This ability depends crucially on PFC (Roberts et al., 1994).

The Wisconsin Card Sorting Test (WCST) is often used as a test of prefrontal function and does require the inhibition of a recently rewarded response, although it also requires other abilities, some with nonfrontal localizations (e.g., Stuss et al., 2000; Monchi et al., 2001). The patient's task is to sort cards—on which are sets of geometric shapes that can vary in their color, shape, and numerosity—into piles according to one of these variables (e.g., blue cards together, red cards together, etc.). The task begins with the patient being given one card at a time and discovering the correct sorting rule by placing each card on a pile and being told "right" or "wrong." At some point after the patient has discovered the rule, the rule is changed (e.g., from sorting on the basis of color to sorting on the basis of shape). Thus the patient is required to shift his or her responding away from the recently used successful sorting rule. It is at this stage of the task, rather than the initial rule discovery, that PFC-damaged patients fail (e.g., Milner, 1963; Nelson, 1976).

Delayed Response and Span Tasks

Although not usually classified together under a single heading, both Delayed Response and Span tasks test the ability to maintain information in working memory. The Delayed Response task was first used in the animal literature many decades ago (Jacobsen, 1936) and has been adapted for humans more recently (Freedman and Oscar-Berman, 1986). In a typical simple version of the task, a stimulus object is shown and then hidden in one of a small number of locations. A delay interval of some number of seconds ensues, during which the subject cannot see the locations (to prevent simply fixating the correct location for the duration of the delay). The locations are then revealed and the subject must locate the hidden object, providing a measure of how accurately the location was maintained in spatial working memory. Both the animal and human lesion literature indicates prefrontal involvement in Delayed Response tasks (D'Esposito and Postle, 1999; Freedman and Oscar-Berman, 1986).

Whereas the limiting factor on performance in Delayed Response is the length of time over which information must be maintained, in Span tasks the limiting factor is the number of items. In a typical Span task, multiple items are presented to the subject, who must retain them in working memory just long enough to repeat or reproduce them. The most familiar version of this task is the forward Digit Span task, although spatial span is also frequently assessed by clinicians. In their literature review on Span-lesion correlations, D'Esposito and Postle (1999) found a weak trend toward decreased span in patients with focal damage to the lateral PFC.

Decision-Making Tasks

One of the most noticeable effects of PFC damage is personality change. The social-emotional dysfunction and poor judgment in such cases have recently become topics of study in cognitive neuropsychology. A number of researchers have attempted to capture these changes in relatively simple and controlled laboratory tasks, which can be grouped under the general rubric of Decision-Making tasks. The best known of these, the Iowa Gambling task (Bechara et al., 1997), requires patients to choose cards from among decks with different likelihoods and magnitudes of wins and losses. Patients with ventromedial PFC damage tend to persist in choosing from decks with large rewards, ignoring the intermittent losses from those decks, which more than wipe out their gains. Rogers and colleagues (Mavaddat et al., 2000; Rogers et al., 1999) developed a simpler type of gambling task that enables various aspects of decision making to be assessed and thus allows a more specific characterization of ventromedial PFC-damaged patients' impairment. In an even simpler decision-making task, choosing among alternative stimuli to obtain rewards, Rolls and colleagues (1994) demonstrated that socially dysfunctional PFC-damaged patients have difficulty avoiding a punishment-associated stimulus if that stimulus was once rewarding for them.

PFC-Damaged Patients in the Cognitive Neuropsychology Lab: Diversity and Commonality

The abilities tested by these tasks have a certain "family resemblance," which hints at underlying commonalities. For example, one could view perseveration on the WCST as the result of inadequate inhibition of previously successful sorting responses. Sequencing a set of pictures to tell a story requires an adequate working memory span, because the sequential position of each picture can be assessed only by comparing its temporal and causal relations with those of all the other pictures. Verbal fluency performance depends in part on a strategic search through alternative candidate words, not unlike the search through alternative candidate sorting criteria in the WCST. And most of the decision-making tasks involve the integration of positive and negative feedback over multiple trials, requiring working memory over delays.

In view of these interrelations among many of the PFC tasks, it is not surprising that patients may display impairments on many or all of the tasks described above. Yet dissociations are also frequently observed, implying that the different processing systems may in fact underlie this network of similarities and calling into question the concept of a "frontal syndrome." Patients may have normal working memory spans but profound impairments in decision making (Bechara et al., 1998) or normal fluency but severely impaired problem solving (Goldstein et al., 1993). The recent burgeoning of functional neuroimaging studies of PFC function have also highlighted the likely multiplicity of underlying cognitive systems within PFC. Well-designed experiments with normal subjects can isolate systems whose anatomic boundaries would likely be crossed by naturally occurring lesions.

CURRENT THEORIES OF PREFRONTAL FUNCTION

Given the range of impairments found after PFC damage and their dissociability, is it foolish to seek "a theory of prefrontal function"? Is this as ill conceived as, for example, a search for "a theory of temporal lobe function," when we already know that the temporal lobe subserves such diverse abilities as vision, hearing, and memory? The answer is no, and the reason highlights a difference between the organization of prefrontal and temporal cortex. Whereas vision, hearing, and memory are sufficiently independent systems that they can operate normally without one another, the function of PFC is highly integrated. For example, damage to auditory parts of temporal cortex has no effect on the function of visual parts or on a patient's visual ability. In contrast, even though the subsystems of PFC have distinct functions, these functions normally dovetail. The major functional distinctions and their interrelations are summarized here.

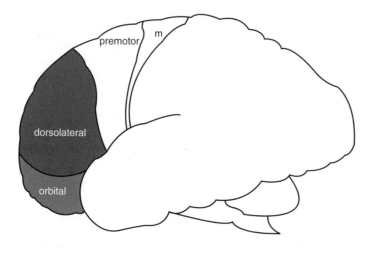

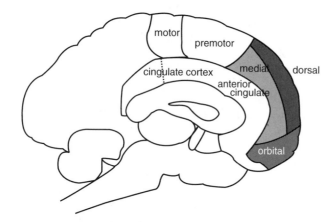

Figure 23-1
Areas of prefrontal cortex and neighboring brain regions.

The clinical observation, described in the previous chapter, of different behaviors following dorsolateral and orbital PFC damage, combined with laboratory tasks used with patients and in neuroimaging studies, leads to the following generalization about the organization PFC function. Lateral regions of PFC are essential for working memory and hence for a multitude of cognitive tasks that depend on working memory, including working memory for task instructions that run counter to prepotent response tendencies (e.g., in the Stroop task). Ventral and medial regions, including orbital cortex, play an important role in reward-related cognition and hence in tasks that require learning about, or making decisions about, reward- and punishment-related stimuli. In addition, the anterior cingulate cortex, which is not strictly speaking part of PFC but is closely related both spatially and functionally, is an integral part of this system. Its function has been characterized as "conflict monitoring"—in other words assessing the degree to which one's actual or planned response conflicts with the desired outcome (Botvinick et al., 2001). Figure 23-1 shows the locations of these areas.

These simple generalizations have been elaborated in various ways by different scientists, some of whom focus their interest on one particular component

Table 23-1
Representative current theories of prefrontal function

Theory: specific to a region	Representative reference
Somatic marker hypothesis (ventromedial PFC)	Damasio (1995)
Reversal learning (ventromedial PFC)	Rolls (2000)
Domain-specific working memory (lateral PFC)	Smith and Jonides (1999)
Process-specific working memory (lateral PFC)	Owen (1997)
Working memory and inhibition combined (dorsolateral PFC)	Diamond (1989)
Selection (inferolateral PFC)	Thompson-Schill (1997)
Theory: Unified	
Supervisory attentional system	Shallice and Burgess (1991)
Working memory	Kimberg and Farah (2000)
Adaptive coding	Duncan (2001)

of PFC and others of whom attempt a unification. Table 23-1 lists a number of these theories. A well-known theory of relatively narrow scope is Damasio's (1994) *somatic marker hypothesis,* which assigns ventromedial PFC a role in mediating intuitive "hunches" based on (literally) gut and other bodily reactions. An alternative conception of this area is offered by Rolls (2000), who emphasizes the importance of this area in the updating of *reversal of stimulus-reward associations.* There are also different theories of the organization of working memory within lateral PFC, with some authors suggesting a stimulus domain or *modality-specific organization* (e.g., Smith and Jonides, 1999) or alternatively a *process-specific organization,* whereby the nature of the processing to be performed on working memory governs the functional anatomy (e.g., Owen, 1997). Diamond (1989) has hypothesized that dorsolateral PFC is essential only for the *joint use of working memory and inhibitory control.* The *selection hypothesis* of Thompson-Schill (1997) concerns the role of inferior lateral PFC in memory and language tasks; she suggests that this region of PFC is needed when task-relevant information must be selected from competing irrelevant information. Finally, the *conflict-monitoring*

hypothesis of anterior cingulate function (Botvinick et al., 2001) asserts that this region measures conflict between task goals and performance in order to control attentional allocation.

Unified theories of PFC function are less common now than in previous decades. This may be the result of our increasing awareness of dissociations among "PFC tasks," thanks to a shift in neuropsychology research from large group studies of patients' performance on one task to single case studies of patients' performance on many tasks, which can reveal dissociations (see Chap. 1), as well as the proliferation of functional imaging studies capable of isolating small foci of activation. Some of the unified theories described in the previous edition of this book are now of more historical than scientific interest. Three unified theories with some currency are summarized here.

Supervisory Attentional System

This theory is based on an information processing model developed by Norman and Shallice (1986), which distinguishes between routine, automatic actions, and more novel actions requiring attentional control. Shallice and Burgess (1991) have proposed that the supervisory attentional system (SAS) is implemented in PFC, and argue that a wide variety of behavioral impairments following PFC damage can be attributed to the weakening or loss of this system. The sensitivity of PFC-damaged patients' performance to the familiarity of the task and the degree of constraint provided by the task, as well as the tendency of routinized actions to intrude when inappropriate (e.g., word-reading in the Stroop task), are among the characteristics consistent with an impaired SAS.

Working Memory

Although only a subset of the laboratory tasks described earlier are considered tests of working memory per se, cognitive psychologists have long hypothesized that working memory plays a crucial role in the performance of a wide variety of verbal and visuospatial tasks (Miyake and Shah, 1999). On the basis of extensive single-cell recording and lesion data linking PFC to working memory (e.g., Goldman-Rakic, 1987), Kimberg and Farah (1993, 2000) used computer simulation to determine whether the wider array of cognitive impairments following PFC damage could result from an underlying impairment in working memory. The simulations demonstrated that the weakening of working memory associations was in itself sufficient to evoke perseveration in the WCST, word-reading intrusions in the Stroop task, perseverative and nonperseverative errors in a sequencing task, and disinhibited responses in the antisaccade task, among other signs of PFC damage. The possibility that different domains of working memory might have different anatomic loci makes it possible for this hypothesis to account for dissociations among tasks. The extension of this idea to the domain of emotional or reward-related working memory (see Davidson and Sutton, 1995) suggests its applicability to even those tasks associated with orbital cortex.

Adaptive Coding

A related proposal concerning prefrontal function explains many aspects of patient behavior after PFC damage, as well as the results of neuroimaging experiments, in terms of the flexible response properties of PFC neurons. Drawing on the results of single cell recording in monkeys, John Duncan (2001) notes that many PFC neurons represent different information in different task contexts. This must be so, he points out, given the large proportion of neurons found to be responsive to the particular stimuli used in any given task. For example, in a dog-cat discrimination task 20 percent of neurons are selective for pictures of dogs versus cats. This seems more likely to be the result of adaptive coding in response to task demands than a reflection of the permanent response properties of these neurons prior to the task, particularly when one considers that the sum of just a few such experiments' responsive neurons exceeds 100 percent! According to Duncan, PFC neurons have the capacity to respond selectively to a wide range of input information, thanks to the extensive connectivity of PFC and posterior cortices and within the PFC itself. The dynamic reassignment of PFC representations functions as a kind of working memory, which is used to guide processing, as described in the previous section.

The more recent hypotheses concerning PFC function make contact, to varying degrees, with our growing knowledge of individual neuron behavior and of the computational properties of ensembles of neurons. Such evidence entered to a degree in the formulation of Kimberg and Farah's (1993, 2000) working memory hypothesis, and it plays a central role in Duncan's (2001) adaptive coding hypothesis. Future development in this field will undoubtedly continue to integrate evidence from animal studies, including neurochemical studies of many cortical-cortical and cortical-subcortical circuits through which PFC function influences behavior. (Robbins, 2000).

REFERENCES

Bechara A, Damasio H, Tranel D, Damasio AR: Deciding advantageously before knowing the advantageous strategy. *Science* 275:1293–1295, 1997.

Bechara A, Damasio H, Tranel D, Anderson SW: Dissociation of working memory from decision making within the human prefrontal cortex. *J Neurosci* 18:428–437, 1998.

Botvinick M, Braver TS, Barch DM, et al: Conflict monitoring and cognitive control. *Psychol Rev* 108:624–652, 2001.

Cohen JD, Servan-Schreiber D: Context, cortex, and dopamine: A connectionist approach to behavior and biology in schizophrenia. *Psychol Rev* 99:45–77, 1992.

Damasio AR: *Descartes' Error*. New York: Grosset, Putnam, 1994.

Diamond A: Developmental progression in human infants and infant monkeys, and the neural bases of inhibitory control of reaching, in Diamond A (ed): The *Development and Neural Bases of Higher Cognitive Functions*. New York: New York Academy of Science Press, 1989.

Drewe EA: The effect of type and area of brain lesion on Wisconsin Card Sorting Test performance. *Cortex,* 10:159–170, 1974.

Drewe EA: Go-no go learning after frontal lobe lesions in humans. *Cortex* 11:8–16, 1975.

Freedman M, Oscar-Berman M: Bilateral frontal lobe disease and selective delayed response deficits in humans. *Behav Neurosci* 100:337–342, 1986.

Goldman-Rakic PS: Circuitry of primate prefrontal cortex and regulation of behavior by representational memory, in Plum F, Mountcastle V (eds): *Handbook of Physiology, The Nervous System V.* Bethesda, MD: American Physiological Society, 1987.

Jacobsen CF: Studies of cerebral functions in primates. I. The function of the frontal association areas in monkeys. *Comp Psychol Monogr* 13:1–60, 1936.

Jones-Gotman M, Milner B: Design fluency: The invention of nonsense drawings after focal cortical lesions. *Neuropsychologia* 15:653–674, 1977.

Kimberg DY, Farah MJ: A unified account of cognitive impairments following frontal lobe damage: The role of working memory in complex, organized behavior. *J Exp Psychol Gen* 122:411–428, 1993.

Kimberg DY, Farah MJ: Is there an inhibitory module in prefrontal cortex? Working memory and the mechanisms of cognitive control, in Monsell S, Driver J (eds): *Control of Cognitive Processes: Attention and Performance XVIII.* Cambridge, MA: MIT Press, 2000.

Kimura D: Left-hemisphere control of oral and brachial movements and their relation to communication. *Philos Trans R Soc Lond B* 298:135–149, 1982.

Mavaddat N, Kirkpatrick PJ, Rogers RD, Sahakian BJ: Deficits in decision-making in patients with aneurysms of the anterior communicating artery. *Brain* 123:2109–2117, 2000.

Milner B: Effects of different brain lesions on card sorting. *Arch Neurol* 9:90–100, 1963.

Miyake A, Shah P (eds). *Models of Working Memory: Mechanisms of Maintenance and Executive Control.* New York: Cambridge University Press, 1999.

Nelson HE: A modified card sorting test sensitive to frontal lobe defects. *Cortex* 12:313–324, 1976.

Owen AM: Memory: Dissociating multiple memory processes. *Curr Biol* 8:850–852, 1998.

Penfield W, Evans J: The frontal lobe in man: a clinical study of maximum removals. *Brain* 58:115–133, 1935.

Perret E: The left frontal lobe of man and the suppression of habitual responses in verbal categorical behavior. *Neuropsychologia* 12:323–330, 1914.

Roberts RJ, Hager LD, Heron C: Prefrontal cognitive processes: Working memory and inhibition in the antisaccade task. *J Exp Psychol Gen* 123:374–393, 1994.

Robbins TW: Chemical modulation of frontal-executive functions in humans and other animals. *Exp Brain Res* 133:130–138, 2000.

Rogers RD, Owen AM, Middleton HC, et al: Choosing between small, likely rewards and large, unlikely rewards activates inferior and orbital prefrontal cortex. *J Neurosci* 20:9029–9038, 1999.

Rolls ET: The orbitofrontal cortex and reward. *Cereb Cortex* 10:284–294, 2000.

Rolls ET, Hornak J, Wade D, McGrath J: Emotion-related learning in patients with social and emotional changes associated with frontal lobe damage. *J Neurol Neurosurg Psychiatry* 57:1518–1524, 1994.

Shallice T: Specific impairments of planning. *Philos Trans R Soc Lond B* 298:199–209, 1982.

Shallice T, Burgess P: Higher-order cognitive impairments and frontal lobe lesions in man, in Levin HS, Eisenberg HM, Benton AL (eds): *Frontal Lobe Function and Dysfunction.* New York: Oxford University Press, 1991.

Smith EE, Jonides J: Storage and executive processes in the frontal lobes. *Science* 283:1657–1661, 1999.

Stroop JR: Studies of interference in serial verbal reactions. *J Exp Psychol* 18:643–662, 1935.

Stuss DT, Benson DF: Neuropsychological studies of the frontal lobes. *Psychol Bull* 95:3–28, 1984.

Thompson-Schill S, D'Esposito M, Aguirre GK, Farah MJ: The role of left prefrontal cortex in semantic retrieval: A re-evaluation. *Proc Natl Acad Sci U S A* 94:14792–14797, 1997.

Chapter 24

AMNESIA I: CLINICAL AND ANATOMICAL ISSUES

Matthias Brand
Hans J. Markowitsch

Memory is one of the most important and complex human brain functions and disturbances of memory processes can result in disastrous restrictions of life quality. Amnesic syndromes can occur as a consequence of widespread brain damage, as in Alzheimer's disease, as well as following tiny lesions of specific structures (e.g., in amnesics with diencephalic or mediotemporal lobe damage), or functional alterations of the brain (e.g., in psychogenic amnesia). Our knowledge of brain and memory interactions has increased greatly in recent years. The expansion of various methods to study brain-behavior interactions—primarily modern static and functional neuroimaging methods but also refined techniques in studying brain-lesioned animals—has substantiated our knowledge of interactions between different brain structures, neural nets, and specific memory processes. Detailed descriptions and neuropsychological examinations of brain-damaged patients complete the multifarious spectrum of methods used in neuroscientific reasearch and have considerably advanced our theoretical framework with respect to brain-memory relations.

CLASSIFICATION OF MEMORY

Memory can be subdivided along the dimensions of time (e.g., short- and long-term memory)[1] and content (e.g., episodic and semantic memory). Along the content-based distinction of memory, the division of four long-term memory systems—originally postulated by Tulving[2]—is widely accepted: episodic memory, semantic memory, procedural memory, and priming[3] (see also Chap. 25). The *episodic memory* system represents episodes of a person's life with respect to time and locus (e.g. "my first trip to New York in summer 1990"). The *semantic memory* system,

discussed in Chap. 27, comprises facts without a personal reference (e.g., arithmetical rules, world knowledge). *Procedural memory* comprises motor, sensory, and cognitive skills (e.g., knowing how to play cards), and *priming* describes the improved reproduction or recognition of information that has already been experienced. Retrieval of episodic memories occurs explicitly or intentionally, while retrieval of information of the other memory systems is implicit or incidental.[2]

Furthermore, memory can be classified according to the stages of information processing, whereby the *encoding* (initial entry into memory), *consolidation* (gradually increasing durability of the memory) as well as, *storage,* and *retrieval* of information are established. Regarding this subdivision, it is assumed that specific brain structures, so-called bottleneck structures (e.g., Refs. 4 and 5), are primarily involved in different memory processes (see Table 24-1).

Memory depends on a wide range of sensory, perceptual, attentive, emotional, and motivational processes and their neuroanatomic correlates. As discussed in Chap. 4, the role of a brain area cannot be understood either through isolated lesion studies or functional imaging studies in normal subjects. Specifically in the domain of memory, Chow[7] has pointed out that if a brain lesion does not affect a learning task, it cannot be concluded that this brain region is not involved in that function. And further, if the lesion influences the performance of a task, it does not unconditionally mean that it is the only structure engaged. The aim of ablation methods to clarify the functions of damaged brain structures is effectively never attainable, for it is based on observations in patients without the region of interest. It is important to take these statements into account in interpreting and integrating results from descriptions of brain-damaged patients as well as from neuroimaging studies.

Table 24-1

Structures relevant for the four long-term memory systems and the different memory processes

	Episodic memory	Semantic memory	Procedural memory	Priming
Encoding and consolidation	Limbic system, prefrontal cortex?*	Limbic system/ cerebral cortex	Basal ganglia, cerebellar structures	Cerebral cortex (uni- and polymodal areas)
Storage	Cerebral cortex (mainly association areas), limbic regions?*	Cerebral cortex (mainly association areas)	Basal ganglia, cerebellar structures	Cerebral cortex (uni- and polymodal areas)
Retrieval	Temporofrontal cortex (right)	Temporofrontal cortex (left)	Basal ganglia, cerebellar structures	Cerebral cortex (uni- and polymodal areas)

*No consistent evidence.
Source: Modified from Markowitsch.[6]

AMNESIC SYNDROMES

In describing patients' amnesic symptoms, the distinction between anterograde and retrograde amnesia is of crucial importance. Patients with anterograde amnesia are unable to form new memories, whereas patients with retrograde amnesia are impaired in retrieving "old" memories stored in the long-term memory system. Figure 24-1 shows relations between the point of a critical incident and possible amnesic states.

The term *amnesia* comprises various amnesic types, which differ in the severity and specificity of their symptoms as well as in their origins. The most extensive type is global amnesia, consisting of both anterograde and retrograde memory impairments. Global amnesia can occur following different etiologies with various lesion sites of brain damage. In Table 24-2, common etiologies of global amnesia and affected brain regions are listed. Examples of different amnesic states are given in Table 24-3.

The following sections contain examples of typical amnesic syndromes and their neuroanatomic and functional aspects.

H.M.: The Classic Case of Mediotemporal Lobe Amnesia

H.M. is probably the most extensively studied patient of this type and represents one of the milestones in the history of neuropsychological research. H.M., a 23-year-old right-handed man of average intelligence, was suffering from pharmacologically intractable epilepsy when his doctor decided to perform a bilateral resection of major portions of his mediotemporal lobes in order to reduce the frequency of H.M.'s attacks.[10] Magnetic resonance imaging (MRI), done several decades later, showed brain lesions comprising the amygdala, the parahippocampal-entorhinal cortex, and the anterior hippocampus bilaterally.[11] After surgery, H.M. became persistently anterograde amnesic. He lost his ability to store new information long-term, so that

Figure 24-1
Possible consequences of critical incidences or brain injury on the formation of new information and/or the retrieval of old memories. (Modified from Markowitsch).[9]

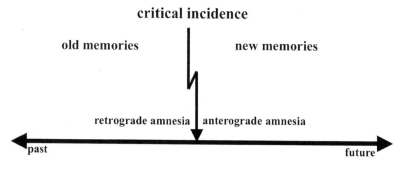

Table 24-2

Overview of patient groups in whom global amnesic syndromes may be prominent

Etiology	Most common lesion sites
Intracranial tumors	Limbic thalamus, medial temporal lobe, posterior cingulate gyrus, fornix, orbitofrontal cortex
Cerebral infarctions, ruptured aneurysms, aneurysm surgery	Limbic nuclei of the thalamus (paramedian, polar artery), orbitofrontal cortex and basal forebrain (anterior communicating artery)
Closed head injury	Orbitofrontal cortex, temporal pole
Viral infections (e.g., herpes simplex encephalitis)	Limbic and paralimbic cortex
Avitaminoses (e.g., B_1 deficiency)	Limbic thalamus, mammillary bodies (as in Korsakoff's syndrome)
Neurotoxin exposure	Hippocampus
Temporal lobe epilepsy	Temporal lobe
Degenerative diseases of the CNS (e.g., Alzheimer's or Pick's disease)	Entorhinal cortex, hippocampal formation, amygdala, prefrontal and inferotemporal cortex
Anoxia or hypoxia (e.g., after a heart attack or drowning)	Hippocampus (CA1 sector)
Drugs	Limbic system
Electroconvulsive therapy	Probably limbic system

Source: Modified from Markowitsch.[8]

time appeared to have stopped for him. Intellectual functions as well as emotional, behavioral, and social skills were not disturbed. Furthermore, impairments in short-term memory, working memory, and other cognitive abilities like reading, writing, and calculating were not observed. Recall of remote autobiographic memories was also unaffected. H.M. was extensively examined from 1955 to the present, and the reports on H.M. have pointed out the importance of the mediotemporal lobes for forming new memories.

The Korsakoff's Syndrome: A Classic Disease Related to Medial Diencephalic Lesions

Korsakoff's syndrome results from long-term alcohol addiction or abuse. Brain damage as well as neuro-

chemical dysfunctions in Korsakoff's patients are probably due to thiamine (vitamin B_1) deficiency and/or additional neurotoxic effects of ethanol. The damage presumably resulting in memory deficits in Korsakoff's syndrome comprises medial diencephalic structures such as the mammillary bodies, the mediodorsal and anterior thalamic nuclei, as well as nonspecific medial thalamic nuclei and the medial pulvinar.

Clinical symptoms of Korsakoff's patients consist of remarkable memory impairments, largely comparable to those after mediotemporal lobe damage, while intelligence may remain unchanged. Besides the mnestic deficits, disorientation and a tendency to confabulate are traditionally associated with Korsakoff's syndrome.[12]

The main symptom, the inability to store new information, includes both verbal and figural memory. Figure 24-2 shows an example for the deficient

Table 24-3

Examples of different types of amnesia and amnesic states

Amnesia type or state	Amnesic symptoms
Anterograde amnesia	The failure to store new memories long-term
Retrograde amnesia	The failure to retrieve (or ecphorize) old memories
Transient global amnesia	Anterograde (and possibly, although to a lesser degree, retrograde) amnesia for a time period of 1 day or less
Psychogenic amnesia	Retrograde (and in rare instances, also anterograde) amnesia without (obvious) brain damage, usually as a consequence of strong psychic pressure(s)
Functional amnesia	Retrograde (and in rare instances, also anterograde) amnesia of differing, but at least partly psychic, origin
Material- and modality-specific amnesias	Inability to retrieve specific material (e.g., common names) or to process within a specific modality (e.g., to remember or retrieve colors)
Reduplicative paramnesia	The phenomenon of being convinced that a person, place, or object exists twice

Source: Modified from Markowitsch.[9]

Figure 24-2

A. The nearly perfect copy of the Rey-Osterrieth complex figure (R-O-F) made by a 45-year-old male Korsakoff's patient.

B. Drawing of the R-O-F from memory after a 30-min delay by the same patient.

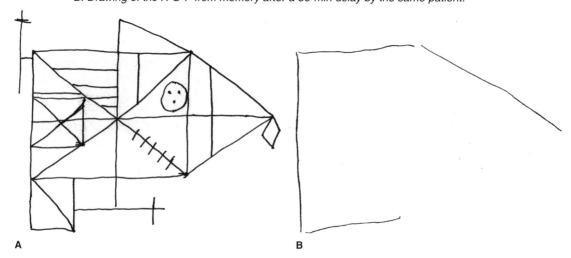

A   B

figural memory of a patient with Korsakoff's symptomatology.

Retrograde amnesia can also be observed in Korsakoff's patients, but to a more variable degree.[13-15] Furthermore, recent studies have revealed additional impairments of other cognitive domains in Korsakoff's patients, primarily of functions associated with the frontal lobes.[16]

The relevance of individual diencephalic structures for the memory deficits of Korsakoff's patients has been controversial. Mair et al.[17] described in detail neuropsychological changes and pathological alterations of the brain after postmortem analyses of two cases and concluded that the mammillary bodies and anterior and midline thalamic nuclei (e.g., the paratenial nuclei) are involved in the amnesic symptoms of Korsakoff's syndrome, whereas the medial dorsal nuclei play a minor role only. To work out structures involved in Korsakoff's syndrome, more recent reports differentiate between the Wernicke's encephalopathy, the first, transient phase of the Wernicke-Korsakoff syndrome, and the later and chronic Korsakoff's state. In this context, Harding et al.[18] revealed that the anterior thalamic nuclei are probably specifically affected in the Korsakoff's state but not in the Wernicke's phase and therefore might be relevant for the amnesic symptoms.

Although Korsakoff's syndrome is one of the most common etiologies for diencephalic amnesia, other causes for damage of diencephalic structures such as thalamic infarctions (e.g., Refs. 19 and 20) can also result in memory disturbances.

Given these examples of classic amnesic syndromes, we come back to the main subject of this chapter: the anatomic bases of memory and amnesia.

THE BRAIN SITES OF MEMORY PROCESSES AND THEIR DISTURBANCES

Encoding and Consolidation

The different memory systems described above are probably represented in specific agglomerates of brain regions. For the episodic memory system the medial temporal lobes, the medial diencephalon, and the basal forebrain as well as prefrontal regions act as so-called "bottleneck structures"[4,5] and their involvement in encoding and consolidation of (episodic and semantic) information is described consistently.[8] For encoding and consolidation of information, two interconnected but separable limbic circuits are proposed to act: the Papez circuit and the amygdaloid (basolateral limbic) circuit (Figs. 24-3 and 24-4).

Papez himself[21] viewed the circuit named after him as principally relevant for emotional analyses, but more recent studies have revealed a strong engagement of these structures and fiber connections in the

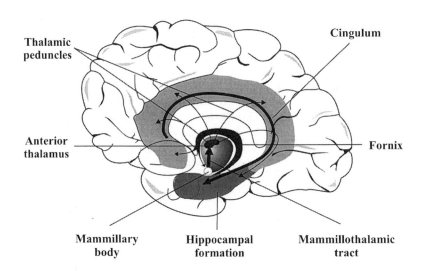

Thalamic peduncles

Cingulum

Anterior thalamus

Fornix

Mammillary body

Hippocampal formation

Mammillothalamic tract

Figure 24-3
The Papez circuit.

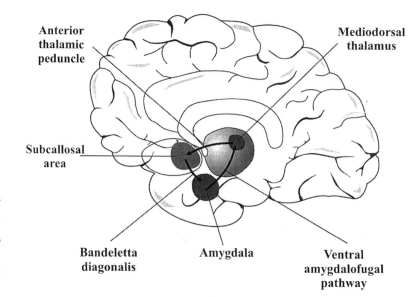

Figure 24-4
The basolateral limbic circuit comprising the amygdala, the mediodorsal nucleus of the thalamus, and portions of the basal forebrain as well as various interconnecting fibers such as the bandeletta diagonalis.

transfer of all kinds of information from short- to long-term memory.[22] The amygdaloid or basolateral limbic circuit, on the other hand, seems to be predominantly engaged in emotional processing and in encoding the emotional valence of experiences.

The hippocampal-entorhinal complex and the limbic thalamic nuclei, especially, are most closely related to the encoding and consolidation of information of the episodic memory system. Damage to these regions usually causes severe memory impairments. Vargha-Khadem and coworkers[23] have suggested that the hippocampus proper is of crucial importance for episodic memory encoding (for a discussion of their findings).[24]

Different cortical and subcortical limbic structures are involved in memory and emotional processes to a variable degree. The functional specificity of several limbic structures is shown in Table 24-4.

Various clinical observations suggest a dissociation between initial encoding and the subsequent and more stable consolidation of information. Furthermore, various case reports lead to the assumption that different brain structures are engaged at different periods of the memory process. For instance, Markowitsch et al.[26] described a 30-year-old female patient who became amnesic after a whiplash trauma. Neuroradiologic investigations revealed no specific brain damage, but she

had sustained hearing deficits and a tunnel view after her injury. She lost her ability to retrieve newly acquired information within 30 min to a few hours, whereas non-memory-related verbal and nonverbal functions remained unchanged and her intelligence was quite superior.

Another patient, reported by Kapur et al.,[27] suffering from temporal lobe epilepsy, showed remarkable impairments to remember information 40 days after learning, although he was able to encode and recall information for hours and days. O'Connor et al.[28] described a comparable patient with temporal lobe epilepsy and paraneoplastic limbic encephalitis who could retrieve information after hours and days but suffered an unusually high rate of forgetting thereafter. Case reports like these support the assumption of the involvement of different (limbic) structures and mechanisms in encoding and consolidation.

Evidence for the engagement of structures of the basal forebrain in memory processes (e.g., the septal nuclei, the nucleus accumbens, the nuclei of the diagonal band of Broca, as well as the nucleus basalis of Meynert) comes from patients with ruptured aneurysms of the anterior communicating artery (ACoA),[29] causing damage to the basal forebrain. The eventually resulting AcoA syndrome consists of amnesia, a tendency to confabulate, and personality changes. The memory

Table 24-4
Structures of the limbic system and their principal functional involvements

Structure	Functional implication(s)
Telencephalon, cortical	
Cingulate gyrus	Attention, drive, pain reception
Hippocampal formation	Memory, spatiotemporal integration
Entorhinal region	Memory
Telencephalon, subcortical	
Amygdala	Emotional evaluation, motivations, olfaction
Basal forebrain	Emotional evaluation, memory
Diencephalon	
Mammillary bodies	Memory, emotion?*
Anterior thalamic nucleus	Memory, emotion, attention
Mediodorsal thalamic nucleus	Memory, consciousness?*/sleep, emotion
Nonspecific thalamic nuclei	Consciousness?*
Associated regions ("paralimbic cortex"; expanded limbic system)	
Medial and orbitofrontal cortex	Emotional evaluation, social behavior, initiative (initiation of retrieval)
Insula	Sensory-motivational integration?*
Temporal pole (area 38)	Memory-related sensory integration, initiation of recall

*No consistent evidence.
Source: Modified from Markowitsch.[25]

impairments comprise both recall and recognition, with a disproportionate deficit in recall probably caused by additional frontal lobe lesions. Furthermore, septal lesions or damage of interconnecting fibers between the septum and hippocampal formation can lead to anterograde and retrograde amnesia.[30]

Storage

Long-term storage of information is presumed to involve widespread cortical regions— primarily association cortices—with alterations in synaptic conjunctions.[31] For binding information, limbic regions seem to play a critical role.[8]

The role of both cortical and limbic regions for long-term storage is shown, for instance, in patients with Alzheimer's disease. Alzheimer's patients are known to have persistent and severe memory impairments comprising episodic (e.g., Refs. 32 and 33) as well as semantic memory (e.g., Refs. 34 and 36). Furthermore, priming deficits and procedural mem-

ory impairments can occur.[37-39] Short-term and working memory functions may also be affected,[40,41] just like attention and executive functions.[42,43] Further possible symptoms of Alzheimer's disease are agnosia, apraxia, and aphasia. Though Alzheimer's disease is discussed as being a "cortical dementia," it must be mentioned that noncortical limbic and other subcortical structures are affected as well.[44] Therefore the various memory deficits observed in Alzheimer's patients may not be caused by damage of cortical and limbic structures alone. For instance, procedural memory deficits of Alzheimer's patients are found similarly as in patients with Huntington's or Parkinson's disease. As mentioned above, the third long-term memory system— procedural memory—depends significantly on basal ganglial structures. Therefore it is not unexpected that patients with damage of these regions are impaired in procedural memory.

Support for the major role of uni- and polymodal neocortical areas for priming—the fourth long-term memory system—came, for instance, from the study of Nielsen-Bohlman et al.[45] They found that patients with temporooccipital lesions are impaired in an implicit memory task (word-stem completion task). Though their patients suffered from lesions extending to mediotemporal lobe structures, these investigators argued that priming deficits are not typical in patients with mediotemporal lobe amnesia; they therefore concluded that the deficits of their patients were caused by the temporooccipital lesions (cf. also Refs. 46 and 47).

The important role of neocortical regions for the storage and retrieval of information can also be seen in material- and modality-restricted forms of amnesia (cf. Table 24-3); as an example, Reinkemeier et al.[48] reported the case of a patient who, following neocortical damage, was unable to remember names and faces.

Retrieval

For retrieval of information, a right-left distinction is assumed: the right hemisphere is viewed as to be primarily engaged in retrieval of episodic memories, while the left hemisphere seems to play a critical role in retrieval of semantic memories.[8,49] The brain region most strongly associated with retrieval is the prefrontal cortex of both hemispheres, following the content-based distinction (right-left) mentioned previously. Additionally, anterior temporal and limbic structures of the medial diencephalon and mediotemporal lobe regions support the retrieval especially of emotionally flavored information.[5]

The role of the hippocampal formation in episodic memory retrieval has been controversial. While Conway et al.[50] did not find substantial differences between hippocampal activation in recent and remote memory, Haist et al.[51] revealed a probable time-limited engagement of the hippocampal formation in human memory. They argued that the entorhinal cortex would be more involved than the hippocampus in remote memory functions. Similarly, Piefke et al.,[52] in a study with functional magnetic resonance imaging, demonstrated a time-limited engagement of the hippocampal formation for the retrieval of autobiographical events.

Lepage et al.[53] proposed that there is a distinction between different portions of the hippocampal formation and suggested that encoding is associated with activation of rostral portions of the hippocampal forma-

tion, whereas retrieval is related to activation of the caudal portions of this region. Dolan and Fletcher[54] confirmed this anterior-posterior functional segregation of the mediotemporal lobe (which had been questioned by Schacter and Wagner[55]).

Case reports of patients with more or less isolated retrograde amnesia support the involvement of mediotemporal regions in retrieval of memories.[56] In line with the mentioned right-left distinction of prefrontal activation in retrieval in healthy subjects, left-sided damage to the anterior temporal regions is related to semantic remote memory impairments,[57,58] whereas right-sided lesions tend to produce autobiographical memory disturbances.[59,60]

To summarize, the neural correlate of memory is not a single brain structure but a distributed network of structures and fiber connections. Figure 24-5 provides an overview of structures and circuits assumed to be centrally engaged in memory processes.

MEMORY AND EMOTION

The affective connotation of information is of crucial importance for its encoding and consolidation as well as for storage and retrieval. The most widely mentioned brain structure for an evaluation of the affective valence of information is the amygdala.[61] The amygdala, located in the anterior medial portion of the temporal lobe, consists of various nuclei and is connected with the hippocampal formation and further cortical and subcortical structures.[62] Various studies have revealed an amygdalar activity–dependent modulation of long-term memory storage and retrieval,[63] with an unequal participation of the two amygdalae.[64] Research on the functions of the amygdala in memory have revealed that gender is a major factor influencing the right-left distinction, with increased activity of the right amygdala in men related to emotion-induced improved recall of material and increased activity of the left amygdala in female subjects linked to better recall of emotional stimuli.[65] In addition to the amygdala, the septum plays an important role in emotional processing.[66]

The emotional valence of information can affect both increasing and decreasing storage. It has long been known that bilateral damage of the amygdaloid complex may lead to the Klüver-Bucy syndrome.[67]

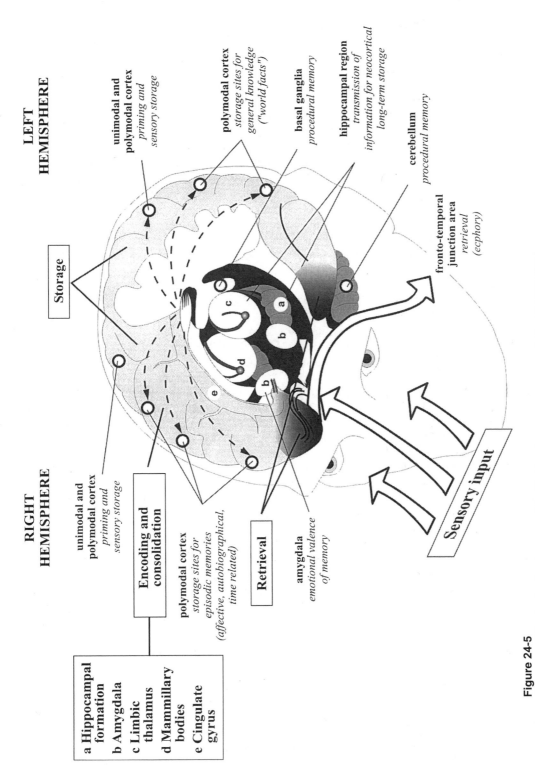

RIGHT HEMISPHERE

unimodal and polymodal cortex
priming and sensory storage

Encoding and consolidation

polymodal cortex
storage sites for episodic memories (affective, autobiographical, time related)

Retrieval

amygdala
emotional valence of memory

Storage

LEFT HEMISPHERE

unimodal and polymodal cortex
priming and sensory storage

polymodal cortex
storage sites for general knowledge ("world facts")

basal ganglia
procedural memory

hippocampal region
transmission of information for neocortical long-term storage

cerebellum
procedural memory

fronto-temporal junction area
retrieval (ecphory)

Sensory input

a Hippocampal formation
b Amygdala
c Limbic thalamus
d Mammillary bodies
e Cingulate gyrus

Figure 24-5
Overview of the brain structures engaged in long-term memory encoding and consolidation, storage, and retrieval. (Modified from Markowitsch.[8])

The Klüver-Bucy syndrome is composed of a complex symptomatology that includes (anterograde) amnesia and emotional disturbances as well as agnosia, hypersexuality, hyperorality, hyperphagia, tameness, and hypermetamorphosis. More recently, descriptions of patients with a selective mineralization of the amygdaloid complex due to Urbach-Wiethe disease (UWD)[68] have supported the assumption of the relevance of this limbic structure for the enhancement of memory for emotionally arousing information.[69,70]

Besides the reduced memory performance for emotional material because of brain damage (primarily damage to limbic regions), emotional overflow can also result in memory impairments. For instance, traumatic stress accompanied by improper coping strategies may lead to remarkable encoding and retrieval disturbances, probably due to increased release of stress-related hormones.[71] The intense release of such glucocorticoids may result in morphologic and functional alterations of limbic structures, especially in mediotemporal regions.[72,73] These can cause broad changes in neurotransmitter systems of the brain, such as of the cholinergic,[74] the serotoninergic,[75] the dopaminergic,[76] and the GABAergic systems.[77]

The relation between traumatic stress and functional brain alterations has been pointed out by recent descriptions of cases with so called "psychogenic amnesia." Markowitsch et al.[78] described a male patient (A.M.N.) who, at age 4, had seen a man burning to death. At the age of 23, A.M.N. experienced a fire in his house and became anterogradely amnesic immediately after that event. Additionally, he developed a retrograde amnesia concerning the period of the last 6 years of his life. Conventional neurologic and neuroradiologic (MRI) investigations failed to reveal clinically relevant morphologic changes. However, a positron emission tomography (PET) investigation showed functional alterations (decreased regional cerebral glucose metabolism) of the brain, particularly in memory-associated regions of the mediotemporal lobe and the medial diencephalon. In the case of A.M.N., these functional changes were temporary, and he returned to a normal level of functioning following pharmacologic and psychotherapeutic interventions. Similarly, his amnesic symptoms improved.

Another case of probable stress-related amnesia is that of F.A., also reported by Markowitsch et al.[79] F.A., a 46-year-old male patient, showed severe and persistent anterograde amnesia and short-term memory deficits with otherwise largely preserved intellectual capacities. He was diagnosed as being depressed, but different forms of drug treatment as well as psychotherapeutic interventions were ineffective. Exploration revealed a complicated, stressful life since childhood (e.g., severe conflicts with his authoritarian father). Neurologic investigations including static and dynamic neuroimaging did not reveal any pathologic brain alteration. The authors concluded that stress- or depression-related prolonged glucosteroid release can cause functional changes in memory-associated brain structures and introduced the term of *mnestic block syndrome* to describe memory impairments without clear organic or explicit psychogenic origin and including the various characteristics of functional amnesia.

CONCLUSION

As pointed out above, amnesia can be due to various etiologies and therefore by alterations to various and very divergent structures of the brain as well as by functional alterations of neuronal nets, induced by stress-hormone releases. Major mnestic disturbances can occur as a consequence of damage to a single brain structure, as has been seen in patients with focal mediotemporal lobe lesions, or they can be caused by neurodegenerative diseases affecting widespread cortical and subcortical regions. Psychic pressure and enduring or massive stress may also lead to severe memory impairments.

Amnesia also differs in quantitive and qualitative aspects of its appearance. While in some amnesic patients encoding and consolidation is more or less selectively disturbed, in others the retrieval of old episodic or semantic memories is impaired. Nevertheless, there are only very rare instances where the ability to encode and store information long-term as well as the recall of old memories is totally abolished. For instance, riding a bike or learning to avoid unpleasant stimuli in an implicit way is almost always preserved even in patients with persistent and severe amnesic syndromes such as in mediotemporal lobe amnesia.

Although our knowledge of the neuroanatomic bases and clinical features of amnesia has increased in recent years, mainly due to the expanded and refined methodologic repertoire of neuroscientic research, many questions remain unsettled. For example, the specific contribution of individual structures to specific memory processes is still a subject of controversy. In this context, for example, the specific engagement of the hippocampal formation in recent and/or remote memory and the importance of further limbic regions for storage and retrieval are still being debated. Likewise, the mechanisms of recovery from amnesic states, as in the case of patient A.M.N., described above, have not been unraveled in a satisfactory way. However, studies of such patients stress a dynamic view of the brain and suggest a potential for neural plasticity even in severely brain-damaged patients.

REFERENCES

1. Rosenzweig MR, Bennett EL, Colombo PJ, et al: Short-term, intermediate-term, and long-term memories. *Behav Brain Res* 57:193–198, 1993.
2. Tulving E: Organization of memory: Quo vadis? in Gazzaniga MS (ed): *The Cognitive Neurosciences*. Cambridge, MA: MIT Press, 1995, pp 839–847.
3. Markowitsch HJ: Anatomical basis of memory disorders, in Gazzaniga MS (ed): *The Cognitive Neurosciences*. Cambridge, MA: MIT Press, 1995, pp 947–967.
4. Brand M, Markowitsch HJ: The principle of bottleneck structures, in Kluwe RH, Lüer G, Rösler F (eds): *Principles of Learning and Memory*. Basel: Birkhäuser. In press.
5. Markowitsch HJ: Which brain regions are critically involved in the retrieval of old episodic memory? *Brain Res Rev* 21:117–127, 1995.
6. Markowitsch HJ: *Gedächtnisstörungen*. Stuttgart: Kohlhammer, 1999.
7. Chow KL: Effects of ablation, in Quarton GC, Melnechuk T, Schmitt FO (eds): *The Neurosciences*. New York: Rockefeller University Press, 1967, pp 705–713.
8. Markowitsch HJ: Memory and amnesia, in Mesulam M-M (ed): *Principles of Behavioral and Cognitive Neurology*. New York: Oxford University Press, 2000, pp 257–293.
9. Markowitsch HJ: The anatomical bases of memory, in Gazzaniga MS (ed): *The New Cognitive Neurosciences*. 2nd ed. Cambridge, MA: MIT Press, 2000, pp 781–795.
10. Scoville WB, Milner B: Loss of recent memory after bilateral hippocampal lesions. *J Neurol Neurosurg Psychiatry* 20:11–21, 1957.
11. Corkin S, Amaral DG, Gonzalez RG, et al: H.M.'s medial temporal lobe lesion: Findings from magnetic resonance imaging. *J Neurosci* 17:3964–3979, 1997.
12. Bonhoeffer K: Der Korsakowsche Symptomenkomplex in seinen Beziehungen zu den verschiedenen Krankheitsformen. *Allgem Zeitsch Psychiatrie* 61:744–752, 1904.
13. Kopelman MD, Stanhope N, Kingsley D: Retrograde amnesia in patients with diencephalic, temporal lobe or frontal lesions. *Neuropsychologia* 37:939–958, 1999.
14. Mayes AR, Daum I, Markowitsch HJ, et al: The relationship between retrograde and anterograde amnesia in patients with typical global amnesia. *Cortex* 33:197–217, 1997.
15. Shimamura A, Squire LR: Korsakoff's syndrome: A study of the relation between anterograde amnesia and remote memory impairment. *Behav Neurosci* 100:165–170, 1991.
16. Joyce EM, Robbins TW: Frontal lobe function in Korsakoff and non-Korsakoff alcoholics: Planning and spatial working memory. *Neuropsychologia* 29:709–723, 1991.
17. Mair WGP, Warrington EK, Weiskrantz L: Memory disorder in Korsakoff's psychosis. *Brain* 102:749–783, 1979.
18. Harding A, Halliday G, Caine D, et al: Degeneration of anterior thalamic nuclei differentiates alcoholics with amnesia. *Brain* 123:141–154, 2000.
19. Graff-Radford NR, Tranel D, Van Hoesen GW, et al: Diencephalic amnesia. *Brain* 113:1–25, 1990.
20. Markowitsch HJ, von Cramon DY, Schuri U: Mnestic performance profile of a bilateral diencephalic infarct patient with preserved intelligence and severe amnesic disturbances. *J Clin Exp Neuropsychol* 15:627–652, 1993.
21. Papez JW: A proposed mechanism of emotion. *Arch Neurol Psychiatry* 38:725–743, 1937.
22. Markowitsch HJ: The biological basis of memory, in Tröster AI (ed): *Memory in Neurodegenerative Disease: Biological, Cognitive and Clinical Perspective*. New York: Cambridge University Press, 1998, pp 140–153.
23. Vargha-Khadem F, Gadian DG, Watkins KE, et al: Differential effects of early hippocampal pathology on episodic and semantic memory. *Science* 277:376–380, 1997.
24. Tulving E, Markowitsch HJ: Episodic and declarative memory: Role of the hippocampus. *Hippocampus* 8:198–204, 1998.
25. Markowitsch HJ: Cognitive neuroscience of memory. *Neurocase* 4:429–435, 1998.
26. Markowitsch HJ, Kessler J, Kalbe E, et al: Functional amnesia and memory consolidation. A case of persistent anterograde amnesia with rapid forgetting following whiplash injury. *Neurocase* 5:189–200, 1999.

27. Kapur N, Millar J, Colbourn C, et al: Very long-term amnesia in association with temporal lobe epilepsy: Evidence for multiple-stage consolidation process. *Brain Cogn* 35:58–70, 1997.

28. O'Connor M, Sieggreen MA, Ahern G, et al: Accelerated forgetting in association with temporal lobe epilepsy and paraneoplastic encephalitis. *Brain Cogn* 35:71–84, 1997.

29. De Luca J, Diamond BJ: Aneurysm of the anterior communicating artery: A review of neuroanatomical and neuropsychological sequelae. *J Clin Exp Psychol* 17:100–121, 1995.

30. Von Cramon DY, Markowitsch HJ: The septum and human memory, in Numan R (ed): *The Behavioral Neuroscience of the Septal Region.* Berlin: Springer-Verlag, 2000, pp 380–413.

31. Baily CH, Kandel ER: Molecular and structural mechanisms underlying long-term memory, in Gazzaniga MS (ed): *The Cognitive Neurosciences.* Cambridge, MA: MIT Press, 1995, pp 19–36.

32. Beatty WW, Salmon DP, Butters N, et al: Retrograde amnesia in patients with Alzheimer's disease or Huntington's disease. *Neurobiol Aging* 8:181–186, 1988.

33. Bondi MW, Salmon DP, Butters N: Neuropsychological features of memory disorders in Alzheimer disease, in Terry RD, Katzman R, Bick KL (eds): *Alzheimer Disease.* New York: Raven Press, 1994, pp 41–63.

34. Hodges JR, Salmon DP, Butters N: Semantic memory impairment in Alzheimer's disease: Failure of access of degraded knowledge. *Neuropsychologia* 30:301–304, 1992.

35. Lambon Ralph MA, Patterson K, Hodges JR: The relationship between naming and semantic knowledge for different categories in dementia of Alzheimer's type. *Neuropsychologia* 35:1251–1260, 1997.

36. Nebes RD: Semantic memory in Alzheimer's disease. *Psychol Bull* 106:377–394, 1989.

37. Salmon DP, Shimamura AP, Butters N, et al: Lexical and semantic priming deficits in patients with Alzheimer's disease. *J Clin Exp Neuropsychol* 10:477–494, 1988.

38. Shimamura AP, Salmon DP, Squire LR, et al: Memory dysfunction and word priming in dementia and amnesia. *Behav Neurosci* 101:347–351, 1987.

39. Starkstein SE, Sabe L, Cuerva AG, et al.: Anosognosia and procedural learning in Alzheimer's disease. *Neuropsychiatry Neuropsychol Behav Neurol* 10:96–101, 1997.

40. Collette F, Van der Linden M, Bechet S, et al: Phonological loop and central executive functioning in Alzheimer's disease. *Neuropsychologia* 37:905–918, 1999.

41. White DA, Murphy CF: Working memory for nonverbal auditory information in dementia of the Alzheimer type. *Arch Clin Neuropsychol* 13:339–347, 1998.

42. Perry RJ, Hodges JR: Attention and executive deficits in Alzheimer's disease. A critical review. *Brain* 122:383–404, 1999.

43. Perry RJ, Watson P, Hodges JR: The nature and staging of attention dysfunction in early (minimal an mild) Alzheimer's disease: Relationship to episodic and semantic memory impairment. *Neuropsychologia* 38:252–271, 2000.

44. Braak H, Braak E: Frequency of stages of Alzheimer-related lesions in different age categories. *Neurobiol Aging* 18:351–357, 1997.

45. Nielsen-Bohlman L, Ciranni M, Shimamura AP, et al: Impaired word-stem priming in patients with temporal-occipital lesions. *Neuropsychologia* 35:1087–1092, 1997.

46. Schacter DL, Buckner RL: Priming and the brain. *Neuron* 20:185–195, 1998.

47. Buckner RL, Koutstaal W, Schacter DL, et al: Functional MRI evidence for a role of frontal and inferior temporal cortex in amodal components of priming. *Brain* 123:620–640, 2000.

48. Reinkemeier M, Markowitsch HJ, Rauch B, et al: Memory systems for people's names: A case study of a patient with deficits in recalling, but not learning people's names. *Neuropsychologia* 35:677–684, 1997.

49. Tulving E, Kapur S, Craik FIM, et al: Hemispheric encoding/retrieval asymmetry in episodic memory: Positron emission tomography findings. *Proc Natl Acad Sci U S A* 91:2016–2020, 1994.

50. Conway MA, Turk DJ, Miller SL, et al: A positron emission tomography (PET) study of autobiographical memory retrieval. *Memory* 7:679–702, 1999.

51. Haist F, Bowden Gore J, Mao H: Consolidation of human memory over decades revealed by functional magnetic resonance imaging. *Nature* 4:1139–1145, 2001.

52. Piefke M, Weiss PH, Zilles K, et al: Differential remoteness and emotional tone modulate the neural correlates of autobiographical memory. *Brain.* In press.

53. Lepage M, Habib R, Tulving E: Hippocampal PET activations of memory encoding and retrieval: The HIPER model. *Hippocampus* 8:313–322, 1998.

54. Dolan RJ, Fletcher PC: Encoding and retrieval in human medial temporal lobes: An empirical investigation using functional magnetic resonance imaging (MRI). *Hippocampus* 9:25–34, 1999.

55. Schacter DL, Wagner AD: Medial temporal lobe activations in fMRI and PET studies of episodic encoding and retrieval. *Hippocampus* 9:7–24, 1999.

56. Kopelman MD, Kapur N: The loss of episodic memories in retrograde amnesia: single case and group studies. *Philos Trans R Soc Lond Ser B: Biol Sci* 356:1409–1421, 2001.

57. De Renzi E, Liotti M, Nichelli P: Semantic amnesia with preservation of autobiographic memory. A case report. *Cortex* 23:575–597, 1987.

58. Markowitsch HJ, Calabrese P, Neufeld H, et al: Retrograde amnesia for famous events and faces after left fronto-temporal brain damage. *Cortex* 35:243–252, 1999.

59. O'Connor M, Butters N, Miliotis P, et al: The dissociation of anterograde and retrograde amnesia in a patient with herpes encephalitis. *J Clin Exp Neuropsychol* 14:159–178, 1992.

60. Kroll N, Markowitsch HJ, Knight R, et al: Retrieval of old memories—the temporo-frontal hypothesis. *Brain* 120:1377–1399, 1997.

61. LeDoux JE: The amygdala and emotion: a view through fear, in Aggleton JP (ed): *The Amygdala,* 2d ed. Oxford, UK: Oxford University Press, 2000, pp 289–310.

62. Sarter M, Markowitsch HJ: Involvement of the amygdala in learning and memory: A critical review, with emphasis on anatomical relations. *Behav Neurosci* 99:342–380, 1985.

63. Cahill L: Modulation of long-term memory storage in humans by emotional arousal: Adrenergic activation and the amygdala, in Aggleton JP (ed): *The Amygdala: A Functional Analysis.* Oxford, UK: Oxford University Press, 2000, pp 425–446.

64. Markowitsch HJ: Differential contribution of right and left amygdala to affective information processing. *Behavioural Neurology* 11:233–244, 1998/1999.

65. Cahill L, Haier RJ, White NS, et al: Sex-related differences in amygdala activity during emotionally influenced memory storage. *Neurobiol Learn Mem* 75:1–9, 2001.

66. Von Cramon DY, Markowitsch HJ, Schuri U: The possible contribution of the septal region to memory. *Neuropsychologia* 31:1159–1180, 1993.

67. Klüver H, Bucy PC: "Psychic blindness" and other symptoms following bilateral temporal lobectomy in rhesus monkeys. *Am J Physiol* 119:352–353, 1937.

68. Urbach E, Wiethe C: Lipoidosis cutis et mucosae. *Virchows Arch* 273:285–319, 1929.

69. Tranel D, Hyman BT: Neuropsychological correlates of bilateral amygdala damage. *Arch Neurol* 47:349–355, 1990.

70. Markowitsch HJ, Calabrese P, Würker M, et al: The amygdala's contribution to memory—a study on two patients with Urbach-Wiethe disease. *Neuroreport* 5:1349–1352, 1994.

71. Markowitsch HJ: Stress-related memory disorders, in Nilsson L-G, Markowitsch HJ (eds): *Cognitive Neuroscience of Memory.* Göttingen, Germany: Hogrefe, 1999, pp 193–211.

72. Sapolsky RM: Stress, glucocorticoids, and damage to the nervous system: The current state of confusion. *Stress* 1:1–19, 1996.

73. Lupien SJ, McEwen BS: The acute effects of corticosteroids on cognition: Intergration of animal and human model studies. *Brain Res Rev* 24:1–27, 1997.

74. Kaufer D, Friedman A, Seldman S, et al: Acute stress facilitates long-lasting changes in cholinergic gene expression. *Nature* 393:373–377, 1998.

75. Davis LL, Suris A, Lambert MT, et al: Post-traumatic stress disorder and serotonin: New directions for research and treatment. *J Psychiatry Neurosci* 22:318–326, 1997.

76. Arnsten AFT, Goldman-Rakic PS: Noise stress impairs prefrontal cortical cognitive function in monkeys. *Arch Gen Psychiatry* 55:362–368, 1998.

77. Rupprecht R: The neuropsychopharmacological potential of neuroactive steroids. *J Psychiatr Res* 31:297–314, 1997.

78. Markowitsch HJ, Kessler J, Van der Ven C, et al: Psychic trauma causing grossly reduced brain metabolism and cognitive deterioration. *Neuropsychologia* 36:77–82, 1998.

79. Markowitsch HJ, Kessler J, Russ MO, et al: Mnestic block syndrome. *Cortex* 35:219–230, 1999.

Chapter 25

AMNESIA II: COGNITIVE ISSUES*

Margaret M. Keane
Mieke Verfaellie

The hallmark of the amnesic syndrome is a severe deficit in new learning (anterograde amnesia) coupled with a variable impairment in the ability to retrieve memories formed prior to the onset of the amnesia (retrograde amnesia). As reviewed in the previous chapter, amnesia is typically associated with lesions of the hippocampus and/or related structures in the mediotemporal lobe and diencephalon[1] and can have a variety of etiologies including Korsakoff's disease, anoxia, herpes simplex encephalitis, and vascular accident.

Over the past several decades, studies of human amnesia have yielded crucial insights into the functional role of the hippocampus and related structures in human memory. In this chapter, we review three important behavioral phenomena in amnesia. We first review patterns of retrograde memory loss in amnesia and consider their implications for the role of the hippocampus in memory consolidation. We then turn to anterograde memory. First we consider the distinction between episodic and semantic memory and evaluate the role of the hippocampus in the acquisition of new semantic knowledge. Then we discuss the distinction between explicit and implicit memory and consider the differential role of the hippocampus in memory tasks that vary in terms of their underlying processing demands. Research within each of these domains has enhanced our understanding of the nature and neural bases of distinct memory processes.

* **ACKNOWLEDGMENTS:** Writing of this chapter was supported by NINDS Program Project Grant NS 26985 and NIMH Grant 57681 to Boston University and by the Medical Research Service of the VA Healthcare system.

RETROGRADE AMNESIA

An influential theory about the role of the mediotemporal lobe in memory function[2–4] came from the observation that the retrograde memory impairment in amnesia is typically temporally limited, such that very remote memories are spared. Clear examples of this pattern are provided by patients with documented damage to the hippocampal region. In one patient whose damage was limited to the CA1 field of the hippocampus, retrograde amnesia was limited to 1 or 2 years before the onset of amnesia.[5] In several other patients with more extensive damage, retrograde amnesia covered as much as 15 years but did not extend to earlier time periods.[6] In a patient with virtually complete damage to the hippocampus as well as extensive damage to adjacent structures, spatial memories acquired many years before the onset of amnesia were nonetheless preserved.[7]

These findings have been taken as evidence for the view that the hippocampus and related mediotemporal-lobe structures have a time-limited role in the *consolidation* (stabilization) of new memories, which are ultimately stored in neocortex. Anatomically, this process is enabled by the extensive and reciprocal connections that exist between the medial temporal lobe (particularly the hippocampus and related cortices) and distributed neocortical sites. During initial learning, such connections allow the hippocampus to bind together the various neocortical sites that represent the memorial event. Subsequently, when the memory is partially reactivated, the hippocampus serves as a "pointer," enabling activation of the full complement of neocortical sites associated with that memory. During consolidation, repeated (hippocampally mediated) coactivation of these neocortical components facilitates the establishment of corticocortical connections, which bind these components together directly. Thus, when consolidation is complete, the hippocampus is no longer necessary for memory retrieval.

By this view, retrograde amnesia reflects the disruption of memories that are in the process of consolidation (and thus still dependent on the hippocampus). The preservation of very remote memories is attributed to the fact that the consolidation process for those memories is complete, so that the hippocampus is no longer necessary for retrieval. Importantly, the theory postulates that the mediotemporal lobe has a similar role in the consolidation of episodic memory (memory for personally experienced events that occurred in a particular temporospatial context) and of semantic memory (i.e., memory for facts and general world knowledge).[8] Several computational models have been developed that successfully simulate the findings in amnesia and shed light on the reasons why such consolidation mechanisms might have evolved.[4,9,10]

Nadel and colleagues[11-13] have recently challenged consolidation theory, arguing instead that the hippocampal complex has a permanent role in the storage and retrieval of autobiographical (episodic) memories regardless of the age of those memories. This theory (known as "multiple memory trace" or MMT theory[11]) agrees with consolidation theory that memories are initially encoded by the hippocampus and stored as hippocampal-neocortical ensembles. According to MMT theory, each time a memory is retrieved, the hippocampus engages in a new encoding event, yielding a new (hippocampal-neocortical) memory trace, wherein the hippocampal component provides the spatial contextual framework for the memory.[14] Semantic memories (which are context-free) are believed to become stabilized over time in neocortex and thus ultimately independent of the hippocampus (a point on which MMT and consolidation theory agree). Episodic memories, by contrast, are thought to depend permanently on the hippocampus for the "spatial scaffold" that is essential to such memories.[14] By this view, in contrast to the consolidation view, extensive damage to the hippocampal complex should produce retrograde amnesia for episodes covering all time periods prior to the onset of the disorder.

Indeed, Nadel and Moscovitch[11,15] have challenged common notions about the nature of retrograde amnesia following damage to the mediotemporal lobe,

pointing to evidence that the retrograde memory loss is often extensive, sometimes covering an entire lifetime. MMT theory attributes the apparent sparing of very remote memories to the greater accumulation of memory traces associated with those memories compared to more recent memories.[16] Importantly, however, MMT theory predicts that even remote memories in individuals with hippocampal damage should differ in quality from remote memories retrieved by neurologically intact individuals, whose retrieval of such memories would benefit from the availability of the hippocampal storage system. By contrast, consolidation theory predicts that very remote memories should be qualitatively and quantitatively equivalent in individuals with and without hippocampal damage, because such memories are thought to be independent of the hippocampus.[2,3]

Thus, consolidation theory and MMT theory differ in how they characterize retrograde amnesia following damage to the hippocampal complex: as a temporally limited phenomenon, applying equally to episodic and semantic memory, with complete sparing of very remote memories, or as a temporally extensive phenomenon, applying primarily to episodic memory and covering very remote as well as more recent time periods. Empiric evidence from human and animal studies has been marshaled in support of each viewpoint (Refs. 3, 13, and 15 to 18), and the debate awaits resolution.

The distinction between episodic and semantic memory drawn by MMT theory, but not by consolidation theory, echoes a long-standing debate about the relative status of semantic and episodic memory in amnesia. In the next section, we consider this debate in the context of findings concerning the acquisition of new semantic memories following hippocampal damage.

SEMANTIC MEMORY IN AMNESIA

One of the early theoretical accounts of amnesia borrowed from a distinction between episodic and semantic memory that was first developed by Tulving[19,20] in the context of normal cognition. *Episodic memory* refers to memory for personally experienced events that occurred in a particular spatiotemporal context, whereas *semantic memory* refers to general knowledge of the world (including knowledge of words and their meanings), which is abstracted from the specific time and place in which the knowledge was acquired (see Chap. 27). The episodic/semantic distinction seemed to account well for the observation that amnesic individuals are severely impaired in remembering personally experienced events (including, for example, recalling or recognizing stimuli in a recently presented list) but nonetheless retain their fund of general world knowledge, including "the vocabulary and syntax of the language, the social amenities, or other much rehearsed skills."[21] (See also Refs. 20, 22, and 23.) As the basis for an episodic/semantic theory of impaired and intact memory in amnesia, however, such observations were flawed insofar as they confounded the type of memory (episodic or semantic) with the time period in which the memory was acquired (post- or premorbidly). Subsequent tests of the episodic/semantic account remedied this flaw by holding constant the time period of acquisition, either evaluating remote memory for both kinds of information or examining new (anterograde) learning for both kinds of information.

We focus below on studies that assessed new learning of episodic and semantic information in adult- and childhood-onset amnesia. It is noncontroversial that new episodic learning is impaired in amnesia, so the critical question addressed in these studies concerns the status of new semantic learning in amnesia.

Studies of new semantic learning in individuals with adult-onset amnesia vary markedly in the theoretical conclusions they elicit. Some researchers emphasize the fact that amnesic patients can acquire *some* semantic knowledge (a finding taken as support for the episodic/semantic account), while others highlight the fact that the amount of semantic knowledge acquired in amnesia is far below that of normal individuals (a finding taken as counterevidence to the episodic/semantic account). Thus, for example, several studies report that amnesic individuals can acquire some semantic information in the form of factual statements[24,25] or simple computer commands and vocabulary.[26,27] On the other hand, studies of new vocabulary learning have reported severe impairments in amnesia in the acquisition of knowledge about words new to the language since the onset of amnesia.[28,29]

In studies of childhood-onset amnesia, the status of new semantic learning is typically evaluated by examining the child's academic progress in school or performance on standardized tests that tap semantic knowledge. The assumption in these studies is that, prior to the onset of amnesia, a semantic knowledge base had not yet been well established. Thus, demonstrations of good semantic knowledge must be due to postmorbid acquisition (new learning). The evidence from two initial case studies was mixed, with one study demonstrating good academic progress in a child with amnesia secondary to encephalitis[30,31] and another demonstrating poor academic progress and impaired performance on several laboratory tests of semantic knowledge in a child with amnesia consequent to anoxia.[32]

More recently, Vargha-Khadem and coworkers[33–35] described as many as 11 cases of childhood-onset amnesia resulting from hypoxic-ischemic damage occurring at time points ranging from birth to 14 years. Magnetic resonance imaging data in these individuals revealed clear, bilateral damage to the hippocampus and apparent sparing of underlying cortices, including the entorhinal, perirhinal, and parahippocampal cortices. Across these cases, the investigators report a pattern of spared new semantic learning as measured by progress in school, performance on IQ tests, and/or performance on standardized tests of reading, spelling, and reading comprehension, coupled with marked impairments on standardized tests of episodic memory.

Thus, the behavioral evidence, from studies of both adult-onset amnesia and childhood-onset amnesia, is mixed, with some studies reporting marked semantic learning and others reporting little or no such learning in amnesic individuals. These findings have been interpreted in two different ways. On the one hand, Tulving and colleagues[25] have argued that these data favor an episodic/semantic memory account of amnesia insofar as they demonstrate that amnesic individuals can acquire an impressive amount of new semantic knowledge despite profound impairments in episodic memory. Such results are taken as evidence that semantic knowledge can be acquired independently of the mediotemporal-lobe structures that are damaged in amnesia. According to this view, that such knowledge is acquired quite slowly and does not reach normal levels is attributable to the fact that healthy individuals may draw on intact episodic memory abilities to enhance their semantic learning, putting amnesic individuals at a disadvantage.

On the other hand, Squire and colleagues[8,36,37] have argued that these results do not provide compelling evidence in support of an episodic/semantic account of amnesia because, in those instances in which semantic learning was significant, there was no evidence that such learning went beyond what would be expected on the basis of residual episodic memory. According to this view, episodic and semantic memory are similarly dependent on the mediotemporal-lobe structures that are damaged in amnesia. In support of this view, Hamann and Squire[37] directly compared memory for facts (semantic information) and events (episodic information) to which amnesic and control participants had been exposed during the course of an experiment. Although the amnesic group acquired some factual information, such knowledge was proportional to their level of episodic memory. More specifically, when the performance of the amnesic group was compared to that of a control group tested after a longer delay, the two groups showed similar levels of episodic memory performance and similar levels of semantic memory performance, indicating that semantic memory was not disproportionately spared in amnesia.

An alternative suggestion put forward by Vargha-Khadem and colleagues[33–35] offers a neuroanatomic account of spared semantic learning in their studies of childhood-onset amnesia and provides a possible way to reconcile conflicting results on this question across other studies. Specifically, based on their combined behavioral and neuroimaging findings (described above), Vargha-Khadem and colleagues have proposed that subhippocampal cortices (entorhinal, perirhinal, and parahippocampal) may be sufficient to support the acquisition of semantic memories, whereas the hippocampus may be additionally necessary for the acquisition of episodic memories. By this view, both forms of memory (episodic and semantic) depend on the integrity of the mediotemporal-lobe system, but each depends upon a distinct component of that system. Thus, the variable findings across studies concerning the status of new semantic learning in amnesia could be accounted for by the variable involvement of subhippocampal cortices in the amnesic individuals under study (for review, see Ref. 38).

This neuroanatomic hypothesis could be considered a neurally specified variation of Tulving's theory concerning the separability of episodic and semantic

memory in amnesia.[20,25] Both accounts stand in contrast to Squire and colleagues' view that episodic and semantic memory are equivalently impaired in amnesia and similarly dependent on all components of the mediotemporal/diencephalic system implicated in amnesia.[8,37] A clear resolution to this debate will require precise and detailed information about the nature and extent of the brain lesions in each amnesic individual under study as well as a consensus about what kind of evidence is necessary to demonstrate a disproportionate sparing of semantic memory in amnesia (see Ref. 8).

EXPLICIT AND IMPLICIT MEMORY

Whereas the distinction between episodic and semantic memory is based on the kind of information to be remembered (personally experienced episodes versus general world knowledge), the distinction between explicit and implicit memory (first introduced by Graf and Schacter[39]) is based upon the way in which memory is tested. In explicit memory tasks, subjects are asked to make deliberate (explicit) reference to a prior episode. In the laboratory, for example, subjects might be exposed to a list of words or pictures in a "study" phase and then asked to recall those stimuli in a subsequent "test" phase. By contrast, in implicit memory tasks, subjects are not required to make deliberate reference to a prior episode; memory for that episode is "implicit" in performance on a subsequent task. For example, subjects might be exposed to a list of stimuli in a study phase and, in a subsequent test phase, asked to perform a seemingly unrelated task, such as identifying stimuli flashed very briefly on a computer screen or generating exemplars from particular semantic categories. Half of the stimuli in the test phase correspond to stimuli from the prior study phase and half correspond to new, unstudied stimuli. (The unstudied items are included to provide a measure of baseline or "chance" performance.) Implicit memory for the study episode is reflected in subjects' enhanced performance in identifying or generating studied compared to unstudied stimuli (an effect known as *priming*). Thus, explicit memory tasks require conscious and deliberate reference to a prior experience, whereas implicit memory tasks measure the influence of prior experience without requiring conscious reference to it. In the following sections, we review some major theoretical issues regarding the status of explicit and implicit memory in amnesia.

Explicit Memory in Amnesia

Explicit memory is typically tested using either recall or recognition tasks. In free recall tasks, subjects are asked to remember and generate (without cues) previously encountered stimuli, whereas in recognition tasks, subjects are presented with a stimulus and asked to judge whether it was encountered previously. Dual-process models[40,41] have postulated that performance on such tasks is the product of two distinct processes: (1) recollection—an effortful process by which information from a prior experience is deliberately brought to mind, and (2) familiarity—a facility or fluency in stimulus processing that is attributed to prior experience with the stimulus. Free recall performance is thought to depend primarily on recollection, whereas recognition performance may be mediated both by recollection and by familiarity.

Amnesic individuals typically show impaired performance both on recall and on recognition tasks. There is debate, however, about the *relative* impairment of recall and recognition memory performance in amnesia, and this debate is closely linked to the question of whether recollection and familiarity are differentially affected in amnesia. Some studies demonstrate a disproportionate deficit in recall compared to recognition in amnesia,[42,43] and such results are taken as evidence that amnesia is associated with a greater impairment in recollection than in familiarity. Other studies demonstrate that recall and recognition are equivalently (proportionately) impaired in amnesia,[44-47] suggesting that recollection and familiarity are similarly affected.

Because the measurement scales in recall and recognition tasks are so different, most studies comparing the status of these two kinds of memory in amnesia do so by equating performance in amnesic and control subjects on a recognition task (either by providing additional study exposure to amnesic subjects or by delaying the memory test for control subjects) and then comparing the performance of the two groups on a recall task under the same experimental conditions. Equivalent performance in the two groups on the recall task suggests a proportionate recall deficit in amnesia, whereas impaired recall performance in the amnesic group suggests a disproportionate recall deficit in amnesia.

Giovanello and Verfaellie[48] suggested that the discrepancies in the literature concerning the relative status of recall and recognition in amnesia may be due to variability across studies in the method used to equate recognition performance in amnesic and control subjects. They tested this hypothesis by comparing two different methods within their own study: they equated recognition performance in amnesic and control groups in experiment 1 by administering six study presentations to the amnesic group and one to the control group and in experiment 2 by testing the amnesic group after a 1-min study-test delay and the control group after a 24-h delay. Their results showed that recall performance was impaired in the amnesic group in experiment 1 but not in experiment 2.

Giovanello and Verfaellie[48] suggested that these results could be understood in the context of two assumptions: (1) that familiarity is less impaired than is recollection in amnesia and forms the basis of explicit memory performance in amnesia and (2) that equating recognition memory performance in amnesic and control groups does not necessarily equate the processes underlying performance in the two groups. Thus, when recognition memory performance is equated by providing additional study exposures to the amnesic patients (experiment 1), performance in amnesia is nonetheless mediated solely by familiarity (albeit enhanced familiarity), whereas performance in control subjects is mediated both by familiarity and by recollection. Under these conditions, control subjects showed an advantage over amnesic subjects in recall performance because of their ability to use recollection. On the other hand, increasing the delay between study and test has been shown to have a larger detrimental effect on recollection than on familiarity.[49,50] Thus, when recognition performance in amnesic and control groups is equated by delaying the test for the control group, performance in both groups is likely mediated by familiarity. Under these conditions, recall performance is similar in amnesic and control subjects. In sum, Giovanello and Verfaellie[48] argue that the recall and recognition data from amnesic patients are consistent with the notion that the impairment in amnesia in recollection is more severe than the impairment in familiarity. Yonelinas[51] reached a similar conclusion in a comprehensive review of studies using a variety of techniques to assess the integrity of recollection and familiarity in amnesia.

Based on an extensive review of findings in animals as well as in humans, Aggleton and Brown[52,53] have recently suggested that recollection and familiarity are mediated by two distinct memory circuits, a hippocampal anterior thalamic system mediating recollection, and a perirhinal dorsal mediothalamic system mediating familiarity. Thus, the relative preservation of familiarity in amnesic patients may be accounted for by the fact that the hippocampus is typically more severely compromised than are the surrounding sub-hippocampal (i.e., entorhinal, perirhinal, and parahippocampal) cortices. This proposal can also account for the recent observation that recognition memory can be fully preserved in patients with lesions limited to the hippocampus proper.[33,54,55]

Arguing against the foregoing account, Squire and colleagues have demonstrated that recognition memory can be markedly impaired even when lesions are restricted to the hippocampus.[56,57] At present, the reason for the inconsistent results across studies is unclear, but such discrepancies highlight the importance of precise neuroanatomic characterization of the patients under study. Clearly, further work will be needed to reach firmer conclusions about the role of specific neuroanatomic structures in the mediation of different processes that contribute to explicit memory.

Implicit Memory in Amnesia

Perceptual and Conceptual Priming   Numerous studies have demonstrated that, despite impaired performance on explicit memory tasks, amnesic patients can show normal performance on implicit memory or priming tasks (for review, see Refs. 58 and 59). It is useful to draw a distinction between priming tasks that draw primarily on perceptual processes and those that draw primarily on conceptual processes.[60,61] In perceptual priming paradigms, the test-phase task requires subjects to identify a stimulus under speeded conditions, or given incomplete or degraded perceptual information (e.g., words or pictures presented very briefly or in fragmented form). In conceptual priming

paradigms, by contrast, subjects must retrieve a word that satisfies a particular semantic constraint (e.g., is a member of a specified semantic category or is semantically related to a cue word), or must evaluate a semantic property of a stimulus (e.g., decide whether it denotes an abstract or concrete concept). Operationally, perceptual and conceptual priming effects can be distinguished in terms of their sensitivity to various experimental manipulations. Manipulations of the surface similarity of stimuli in the study and test phases (e.g., study-test changes in sensory modality) influence the magnitude of perceptual priming effects[62-65] but not conceptual priming effects.[66,67] On the other hand, variations in the level of semantic processing of stimuli during the study phase have little effect on perceptual priming[63] but have a marked effect on conceptual priming.[66,68]

Amnesic patients have shown normal performance both on perceptual[69-72] and conceptual[73-76] priming tasks. These findings indicate that perceptual and conceptual priming effects do not depend upon the integrity of the mediotemporal-lobe and diencephalic brain structures that are damaged in amnesia. However, such findings fail to reveal which of the brain structures spared in amnesia support normal priming in this group and leave open the question of whether perceptual and conceptual priming depend on a unitary neural system or on dissociable neural systems.

Answers to such questions have been yielded by studies examining perceptual priming in individuals with brain lesions outside of the mediotemporal/diencephalic system. Important insights have come from studies of priming in patients with Alzheimer's disease (AD). AD resembles amnesia in that it is associated with lesions of the hippocampal formation,[77] but it differs from amnesia in that it is also associated with neocortical lesions of temporal, parietal, and frontal cortices.[78-80] Importantly for the present discussion, primary sensory cortices are relatively spared in AD.[80-82] The hippocampal lesions that are common to amnesia and AD account for the explicit memory deficits that are observed in AD patients.[83] However, because priming survives the hippocampal lesions in amnesia, we can infer that priming deficits observed in AD reflect pathology outside of that region.

A wide range of studies have shown that the status of priming in AD varies depending on the particular priming task. AD patients have shown normal priming in visual identification of briefly presented words,[84,85] auditory identification of words presented in white noise,[86] speeded lexical decision (deciding whether a string of letters constitutes a real word),[87,88] speeded picture identification,[89,90] and visual pattern completion.[91] In contrast, they have shown impaired priming in category exemplar production (generating exemplars in response to category cues)[90,92] and in word-association tasks (generating the first word that comes to mind in response to a word cue).[93–95] This pattern of results may be understood with reference to the distinction between perceptual and conceptual priming: AD patients appear to show normal priming on perceptual tasks but impaired priming on conceptual tasks. These findings suggest that conceptual priming is mediated by neocortical association areas that are compromised in AD, whereas perceptual priming may be mediated by sensory cortices that are relatively preserved in AD.

To address this neuroanatomic hypothesis, researchers have examined both forms of priming in individuals with focal occipital lobe lesions. Such individuals would be expected to exhibit impaired performance on visual perceptual priming tasks but normal performance on conceptual priming tasks. Consistent with this hypothesis, these patients have shown impaired priming on visual word identification but normal priming in category exemplar production.[67,96]

Converging evidence regarding the neural separability and localization of perceptual and conceptual priming comes from neuroimaging studies in healthy individuals. These studies have shown that priming is typically accompanied by reductions in brain activity. Such reductions are thought to reflect the decreased processing demands associated with processing of primed (compared to nonprimed) stimuli. A number of studies have demonstrated that perceptual priming is associated with reduced activity in extrastriate visual areas,[97–101] whereas conceptual priming is associated with reduced activation in left inferior prefrontal cortex.[102–104]

Taken together, the findings from behavioral studies of patients with neocortical lesions and neuroimaging studies in healthy individuals suggest that visuoperceptual priming is supported by occipital cortex and conceptual priming is supported by left infe-

rior prefrontal cortex. Intact perceptual and conceptual priming in amnesic patients is likely due to the preservation of these brain regions in amnesia.

Priming of Novel Information in Amnesia

Most of the priming tasks described thus far have used stimuli that are represented in long-term knowledge, i.e., words or drawings of objects that are familiar to participants. There has been a great deal of interest, however, in whether amnesic patients can show priming for novel stimuli, i.e., stimuli that lack preexisting representations in long-term knowledge. The motivation for this interest is a theory positing that spared priming in amnesia is due to activation mechanisms operating on premorbidly acquired knowledge representations.[69,105] According to this theory, when a stimulus is encountered in the study phase of a priming task, its representation in long-term knowledge is activated. During the test phase, such activation renders the stimulus more accessible and increases the likelihood (compared to nonprimed stimuli) that the stimulus will be identified or generated. By this view, amnesic patients should not show priming for novel stimuli because such stimuli do not have preexisting representations to be activated. Contrary to this prediction, amnesic patients have shown normal priming for novel stimuli such as pseudowords,[67,70,72,106] novel geometric patterns,[107,108] drawings of novel three-dimensional objects,[109] and photographs of unfamiliar faces.[110]

In a different approach to this question, Graf and Schacter[39] and Moscovitch and colleagues[111] developed paradigms to examine priming of novel word pairs (e.g., *anger-pattern*) in amnesia. Even though the constituent parts of such pairs are represented in long-term knowledge, the link between them is not. Thus, any priming that can be attributed to implicit memory for that link would constitute priming for novel information (or "new-associative priming"). In this sort of paradigm, subjects are exposed in the study phase to normatively unrelated word pairs (e.g., *anger-pattern, merchant-tribute*). In the subsequent test phase, subjects are exposed to pairs that had appeared in the study phase ("old" pairs, e.g., *anger-patterns*), to pairs formed by recombining words from the study phase ("recombined" pairs, e.g., *anger-tribute*), and to new, unstudied word pairs (e.g., *crying-topic*). The test phase might require word-stem completion (in which case the second item of each pair would consist of the three-letter beginning of a word), speeded reading, identification on very brief presentation, or speeded lexical decision. The measure of performance is the accuracy or speed of the response. For the present purposes, the critical comparison is between performance in the old condition and performance in the recombined condition. In both of these conditions, the constituents of each pair had appeared in the prior study phase; the conditions differ in that the novel pairing established in the study phase is preserved in the old condition but not in the recombined condition. Thus, any enhancement in performance in the old compared to the recombined condition would reflect new associative priming.

Studies that have used this paradigm with amnesic patients have yielded mixed results, with some studies reporting intact new-associative priming[111-113] and others reporting impaired new-associative priming in amnesia.[114-116] One way to reconcile these apparently contradictory findings is to consider the nature of the task on which amnesic patients have shown intact or impaired performance. Amnesic patients appear to show intact new-associative priming on tasks that require identification of briefly presented word pairs[112] (but see Ref. 117) or speeded identification (reading or lexical decision) of word pairs.[111,113] In at least one of these tasks (lexical decision), new-associative priming has been shown to be sensitive to study-test shifts in perceptual modality but insensitive to variations in level of semantic processing at study,[118,119] suggesting that the effect is perceptually based. Amnesic patients have shown impaired new-associative priming in word-stem completion,[114-116] an effect that appears to require semantic processing of word pairs in the study phase.[120] Thus, the status of new-associative priming in amnesia may depend upon the nature of the association to be primed, such that priming of new *perceptual* associations is intact in amnesia but priming of new *conceptual* associations is impaired.[121] Understanding the conditions under which amnesic patients can show implicit memory for novel associations may also be relevant to theories that assign a critical role to the hippocampus in binding together unrelated items in memory.[122]

In summary, the studies described above provide strong counterevidence to an activation account of spared priming in amnesia: amnesic patients show normal priming with pseudowords, orthographically illegal nonwords, novel patterns and objects, and at least some kinds of novel associations. Thus, it appears as though priming in amnesia is not limited to material that is premorbidly represented in long-term knowledge. Rather, amnesic patients can establish novel representations, and these representations can support normal priming effects.

CONCLUSION

Studies of spared and impaired memory function in amnesia have provided the empiric foundation for many of the theories that frame contemporary thinking about human memory. Evidence concerning the nature and extent of retrograde memory loss in amnesia elucidates the role of the hippocampus in the formation, maintenance, and retrieval of long-term memories. Examination of the relative integrity of episodic and semantic memory in amnesia sheds light on the potential neural separability of memory for personally experienced events and memory for facts about the world. Comparisons of recall and recognition performance in amnesia highlight the distinct contributions of recollection and familiarity to explicit memory performance and the distinct neural bases of those processes. Finally, the study of implicit memory effects in amnesia reveals the nature and localization of memory processes that operate outside of conscious awareness. In sum, behavioral studies in amnesia provide a powerful means to deepen our understanding of the nature and organization of normal human memory capacities.

REFERENCES

1. Zola-Morgan S, Squire LR: Neuroanatomy of memory. *Ann Rev Neurosci* 16:547–563, 1993.
2. Squire LR, Cohen NJ, Nadel L: The medial temporal region and memory consolidation: A new hypothesis, in Weingartner H, Parker ES (eds): *Memory Consolidation: Psychobiology of Cognition.* Hillsdale, NJ: Erlbaum, 1984, pp 185–210.
3. Squire LR, Alvarez P: Retrograde amnesia and memory consolidation: A neurobiological perspective. *Curr Opin Neurobiol* 5:169–177, 1995.
4. McClelland JL, McNaughton BL, O'Reilly RC: Why there are complementary learning systems in

the hippocampus and neocortex: Insights from the successes and failures of connectionist models of learning and memory. *Psychol Rev* 102:419–457, 1995.

5. Zola-Morgan S, Squire LR, Amaral DG: Human amnesia and the medial temporal region: Enduring memory impairment following a bilateral lesion limited to field CA1 of the hippocampus. *J Neurosci* 6:2950–2967, 1986.

6. Rempel-Clower NL, Zola SM, Squire LR, et al: Three cases of enduring memory impairment after bilateral damage limited to the hippocampal formation. *J Neurosci* 16:5233–5255, 1996.

7. Teng E, Squire LR: Memory for places learned long ago is intact after hippocampal damage. *Nature* 400:675–677, 1999.

8. Squire LR, Zola SM: Episodic memory, semantic memory, and amnesia. *Hippocampus* 8:205–211, 1998.

9. Alvarez P, Squire LR: Memory consolidation and the medial temporal lobe: A simple network model. *Proc Natl Acad Sci USA* 91:7041–7045, 1994.

10. Murre JMJ: TraceLink: A model of amnesia and consolidation of memory. *Hippocampus* 6:675–684, 1996.

11. Nadel L, Moscovitch M: Memory consolidation, retrograde amnesia and the hippocampal complex. *Curr Opin Neurobiol* 7:217–227, 1997.

12. Moscovitch M, Nadel L: Consolidation and the hippocampal complex revisited: In defense of the multiple-trace model. *Curr Opin Neurobiol* 8:297–300, 1998.

13. Nadel L, Samsonovich A, Ryan L, et al: Multiple trace theory of human memory: Computational, neuroimaging, and neuropsychological results. *Hippocampus* 10:352–368, 2000.

14. Nadel L, Moscovitch M: Hippocampal contributions to cortical plasticity. *Neuropharmacology* 37:431–439, 1998.

15. Nadel L, Moscovitch M: The hippocampal complex and long-term memory revisited. *Trends Cogn Sci* 5:228–230, 2001.

16. Nadel L, Bohbot V: Consolidation of memory. *Hippocampus* 11:56–60, 2001.

17. Squire LR, Clark RE, Knowlton BJ: Retrograde amnesia. *Hippocampus* 11:50–55, 2001.

18. Eichenbaum H, Cohen NJ: *From Conditioning to Conscious Recollection.* Oxford, UK: Oxford University Press, 2001.

19. Tulving E: Episodic and semantic memory, in Tulving E, Donaldson W (eds): *Organization of Memory.* New York: Academic Press, 1972, pp 381–403.

20. Tulving E: *Elements of Episodic Memory.* Oxford, UK: Oxford University Press, 1983.

21. Kinsbourne M, Wood F: Short-term memory processes and the amnesic syndrome, in Deutsch DD, Deutsch JA (eds): *Short-Term Memory.* New York: Academic Press, 1975, pp 258–291.

22. Warrington EK: The selective impairment of semantic memory. *Q J Exp Psychol* 27:635–657, 1975.

23. Shallice T: *From Neuropsychology to Mental Structure.* Cambridge, UK: Cambridge University Press, 1988.

24. Shimamura AP, Squire LR: A neuropsychological study of fact memory and source amnesia. *J Exp Psychol Learn Mem Cogn* 13:464–473, 1987.

25. Tulving E, Hayman CAG, MacDonald CA: Long-lasting perceptual priming and semantic learning in amnesia: A case experiment. *J Exp Psychol Learn Mem Cogn* 17:595–617, 1991.

26. Glisky EL, Schacter DL, Tulving E: Computer learning by memory-impaired patients: Acquisition and retention of complex knowledge. *Neuropsychologia* 24:313–328, 1986.

27. Glisky EL, Schacter DL: Long-term retention of computer learning by patients with memory disorders. *Neuropsychologia* 26:173–178, 1988.

28. Gabrieli JDE, Cohen NJ, Corkin S: The impaired learning of semantic knowledge following bilateral medial temporal-lobe resection. *Brain Cogn* 7:157–177, 1988.

29. Verfaellie M, Croce P, Milberg WP: The role of episodic memory in semantic learning: An examination of vocabulary acquisition in a patient with amnesia due to encephalitis. *Neurocase* 1:291–304, 1995.

30. Wood F, Ebert V, Kinsbourne M: The episodic-semantic memory distinction in memory and amnesia: Clinical and experimental observations, in Cermak LS (ed): *Human Memory and Amnesia.* Hillsdale, NJ: Erlbaum, 1982, pp 167–193.

31. Wood FB, Brown IS, Felton RH: Long-term follow-up of a childhood amnesic syndrome. *Brain Cogn* 10:76–86, 1989.

32. Ostergaard AL: Episodic, semantic and procedural memory in a case of amnesia at an early age. *Neuropsychologia* 25:341–357, 1987.

33. Vargha-Khadem F, Gadian DG, Watkins KE, et al: Differential effects of early hippocampal pathology on episodic and semantic memory. *Science* 277:376–380, 1997.

34. Gadian DG, Aicardi J, Watkins KE, et al: Developmental amnesia associated with early hypoxic-ischaemic injury. *Brain* 123:499–507, 2000.

35. Vargha-Khadem F, Gadian DG, Mishkin M: Dissociations in cognitive memory: The syndrome of developmental amnesia. *Philos Trans R Soc Lond* 356:1435–1440, 2001.

36. Ostergaard AL, Squire LR: Childhood amnesia and distinctions between forms of memory: A comment on Wood, Brown, and Felton. *Brain Cogn* 14:127–133, 1990.

37. Hamann SB, Squire LR: On the acquisition of new declarative knowledge in amnesia. *Behav Neurosci* 109:1027–1044, 1995.

38. Verfaellie M: Semantic learning in amnesia, in Boller F, Grafman J (eds): *Handbook of Neuropsychology,* 2d ed. Amsterdam: Elsevier, 2000, pp 335–354.

39. Graf P, Schacter DL: Implicit and explicit memory for new associations in normal and amnesic subjects. *J Exp Psychol Learn Mem Cogn* 11(3):501–518, 1985.

40. Mandler G: Recognizing: The judgment of previous occurrence. *Psychol Rev* 87:252–271, 1980.

41. Jacoby LL: Remembering the data: Analyzing interactive processes in reading. *J Verb Learn Verb Behav* 22:485–508, 1983.

42. Hirst W, Johnson MK, Kim JK, et al: Recognition and recall in amnesics. *J Exp Psychol Learn Mem Cogn* 12:445–451, 1986.

43. Hirst W, Johnson MK, Phelps AE, et al: More on recognition and recall in amnesics. *J Exp Psychol Learn Mem Cogn* 14:758–762, 1988.

44. Shimamura AP, Squire LR: Long-term memory in amnesia: Cued recall, recognition memory and confidence ratings. *J Exp Psychol Learn Mem Cogn* 14:763–770, 1988.

45. Haist F, Shimamura AP, Squire LR: On the relationship between recall and recognition memory. *J Exp Psychol Learn Mem Cogn* 18:691–702, 1992.

46. MacAndrew SBG, Jones GV, Mayes AR: No selective deficit in recall in amnesia. *Memory* 2:241–254, 1994.

47. Kopelman MD, Stanhope N: Recall and recognition memory in patients with focal frontal, temporal lobe and diencephalic lesions. *Neuropsychologia* 36:785–796, 1998.

48. Giovanello KS, Verfaellie M: The relationship between recall and recognition in amnesia: Effects of matching recognition between patients with amnesia and controls. *Neuropsychology* 15:444–451, 2001.

49. Hockley WA, Consoli A: Familiarity and recollection in item and associative recognition. *Mem Cogn* 27:657–664, 1999.

50. Gardiner JM, Java RJ: Forgetting in recognition memory with and without recollective experience. *Mem Cogn* 19:617–623, 1991.

51. Yonelinas AP, Kroll NEA, Dobbins I, et al: Recollection and familiarity deficits in amnesia: Convergence of remember-know, process dissociation, and receiver operating characteristic data. *Neuropsychology* 12:323–339, 1998.

52. Aggleton JP, Brown MW: Episodic memory, amnesia, and the hippocampal-anterior thalamic axis. *Behav Brain Sci* 425–489, 1999.

53. Brown MW, Aggleton JP: Recognition memory: What are the roles of the perirhinal cortex and hippocampus? *Nature Rev Neurosci* 2:51–61, 2001.

54. Mayes AR, Holdstock JS, Isaac CL, et al: Relative sparing of item recognition memory in a patient with adult-onset damage limited to the hippocampus. *Hippocampus.* 12:325–340, 2002.

55. Henke K, Kroll NEA, Hamraz B, et al: Memory lost and regained following bilateral hippocampal damage. *J Cogn Neurosci* 11:682–697, 1999.

56. Reed JM, Squire LR: Impaired recognition memory in patients with lesions limited to the hippocampal formation. *Behav Neurosci* 111:667–675, 1997.

57. Manns JR, Squire LR: Impaired recognition memory on the doors and people test after damage limited to the hippocampal region. *Hippocampus* 9:495–499, 1999.

58. Moscovitch M, Vriezen E, Goshen-Gottstein Y: Implicit tests of memory in patients with focal lesions and degenerative brain disorders, in Spinnler H, Boller F (eds): *Handbook of Neuropsychology.* Amsterdam: Elsevier, 1993, pp 133–173.

59. Schacter DL, Chiu C-YP, Ochsner KN: Implicit memory: A selective review. *Ann Rev Neurosci* 16:159–182, 1993.

60. Roediger HL, Weldon MS, Challis BH: Explaining dissociations between implicit and explicit measures of retention: A processing account, in Roediger HL, Craik FIM (eds): *Varieties of Memory and Consciousness: Essays in Honour of Endel Tulving.* Hillsdale, NJ: Erlbaum, 1989, pp 3–41.

61. Blaxton TA: Investigating dissociations among memory measures: Support for a transfer-appropriate processing framework. *J Exp Psychol Learn Mem Cogn* 15(4):657–668, 1989.

62. Clarke R, Morton J: Cross modality facilitation in tachistoscopic word recognition. *Q J Exp Psychol* 35A:79–96, 1983.

63. Jacoby LL, Dallas M: On the relationship between autobiographical memory and perceptual learning. *J Exp Psychol Genl* 110(3):306–340, 1981.

64. Rajaram S, Roediger HL: Direct comparison of four implicit memory tests. *J Exp Psychol Learn Mem Cogn* 19(19):765–776, 1993.

65. Blum D, Yonelinas AP: Transfer across modality in perceptual implicit memory. *Psychonom Bull Rev* 8:147–154, 2001.

66. Srinivas K, Roediger HL: Classifying implicit memory tests: Category association and anagram solution. *J Mem Lang* 29:389–412, 1990.

67. Keane MM, Gabrieli JDE, Mapstone HC, et al: Double dissociation of memory capacities after bilateral occipital-lobe or medial temporal-lobe lesions. *Brain* 118:1129–1148, 1995.

68. Hamann SB: Level-of-processing effects in conceptually driven implicit tasks. *J Exp Psychol Learn Mem Cogn* 16(6):970–977, 1990.

69. Cermak LS, Talbot N, Chandler K, et al: The perceptual priming phenomenon in amnesia. *Neuropsychologia* 23(5):615–622, 1985.

70. Haist F, Musen G, Squire LR: Intact priming of words and nonwords in amnesia. *Psychobiology* 19(4):275–285, 1991.

71. Hamann SB, Squire LR, Schacter DL: Perceptual thresholds and priming in amnesia. *Neuropsychology* 9:3–15, 1995.

72. Hamann SB, Squire LR: Intact priming for novel perceptual representations in amnesia. *J Cogn Neurosci* 9:699–713, 1997.

73. Graf P, Shimamura AP, Squire LR: Priming across modalities and priming across category levels: Extending the domain of preserved function in amnesia. *J Exp Psychol Learn Mem Cogn* 11:386–396, 1985.

74. Cermak LS, Verfaellie M, Chase KA: Implicit and explicit memory in amnesia: An analysis of data-driven and conceptually driven processes. *Neuropsychology* 9:281–290, 1995.

75. Vaidya CJ, Gabrieli JDE, Keane MM, et al: Perceptual and conceptual memory processes in global amnesia. *Neuropsychology* 9:580–591, 1995.

76. Keane MM, Gabrieli JDE, Monti LA, et al: Intact and impaired conceptual memory processes in amnesia. *Neuropsychology* 11:59–69, 1997.

77. Hyman BT, Van Hoesen GW, Damasio AR, et al: Alzheimer's disease: Cell-specific pathology isolates the hippocampal formation. *Science* 225:1168–1170, 1984.

78. Brun A, Englund E: Regional pattern of degeneration in Alzheimer's disease: Neuronal loss and histopathological grading. *Histopathology* 5:549–564, 1981.

79. Rogers J, Morrison JH: Quantitative morphology and regional and laminar distributions of senile plaques in Alzheimer's disease. *J Neurosci* 5(10):2801–2808, 1985.

80. Arnold SE, Hyman BT, Flory J, et al: The topographical and neuroanatomical distribution of neurofibrillary tangles and neuritic plaques in the cerebral cortex of patients with Alzheimer's disease. *Cereb Cortex* 1:1–6, 1991.

81. Esiri MM, Pearson RCA, Powell TPS: The cortex of the primary auditory area in Alzheimer's disease. *Brain Res* 366:385–387, 1986.

82. Lewis DA, Campbell MJ, Terry RD, et al: Laminar and regional distributions of neurofibrillary tangles and neuritic plaques in Alzheimer's disease: A quantitative study of visual and auditory cortices. *J Neurosci* 7(6):1799–1808, 1987.

83. Wilson RS, Sullivan M, deToledo-Morrell, et al: Association of memory and cognition in Alzheimer's disease with volumetric estimates of temporal lobe structures. *Neuropsychology* 10:459–463, 1996.

84. Keane MM, Gabrieli JDE, Fennema AC, et al: Evidence for a dissociation between perceptual and conceptual priming in Alzheimer's disease. *Behav Neurosci* 105(2):326–342, 1991.

85. Fleischman DA, Gabrieli JDE, Reminger S, et al: Conceptual priming in perceptual identification for patients with Alzheimer's disease and a patient with right occipital lobectomy. *Neuropsychology* 9:187–197, 1995.

86. Verfaellie M, Keane MM, Johnson G: Preserved priming in auditory perceptual identification in Alzheimer's disease. *Neuropsychologia* 38:1581–1592, 2000.

87. Moscovitch M: A neuropsychological approach to perception and memory in normal and pathological aging, in Craik FIM, Trehub S (eds): *Aging and Cognitive Processes.* New York: Plenum Press, 1982, pp 55–78.

88. Ober BA, Shenaut GK: Lexical decision and priming in Alzheimer's disease. *Neuropsychologia* 26(2):273–286, 1988.

89. Park SM, Gabrieli JDE, Reminger SL, et al: Preserved priming across study-test picture transformations in patients with Alzheimer's disease. *Neuropsychology* 12:340–352, 1998.

90. Gabrieli JDE, Vaidya CJ, Stone M, et al: Convergent behavioral and neuropsychological evidence for a distinction between identification and production forms of repetition priming. *J Exp Psychol Genl* 128:479–498, 1999.

91. Postle BR, Corkin S, Growdon JH: Intact implicit memory for novel patterns in Alzheimer's disease. *Learn Mem* 3:305–312, 1996.

92. Monti LA, Gabrieli JDE, Reminger SL, et al: Differential effects of aging and Alzheimer's disease upon conceptual implicit and explicit memory. *Neuropsychology* 10:101–112, 1996.

93. Brandt J, Spencer M, McSorley P, et al: Semantic activation and implicit memory in Alzheimer disease. *Alzheimer Dis Assoc Disord* 2:112–119, 1988.

94. Huff FJ, Mack L, Mahlmann J, et al: A comparison of lexical-semantic impairments in left hemisphere stroke and Alzheimer's disease. *Brain Lang* 34:262–278, 1988.

95. Salmon DP, Shimamura AP, Butters N, et al: Lexical and semantic priming deficits in patients with Alzheimer's disease. *J Clin Exp Neuropsychol* 10(4):477–494, 1988.

96. Gabrieli JDE, Fleischman DA, Keane MM, et al: Double dissociation between memory systems underlying explicit and implicit memory in the human brain. *Psychol Sci* 6:76–82, 1995.

97. Squire LR, Ojemann JG, Miezin FM, et al: Activation of the hippocampus in normal humans: A functional anatomical study of memory. *Proc Natl Acad Sci U S A* 89:1837–1841, 1992.

98. Buckner RL, Petersen SE, Ojemann JG, et al: Functional anatomical studies of explicit and implicit memory retrieval tasks. *J Neurosci* 15:12–29, 1995.

99. Schacter DL, Alpert NM, Savage CR, et al: Conscious recollection and the human hippocampal formation: Evidence from positron emission tomography. *Proc Natl Acad Sci USA* 93:321–325, 1996.

100. Badgaiyan RD, Posner MI: Time course of cortical activations in implicit and explicit recall. *J Neurosci* 17:4904–4913, 1997.

101. Lebreton K, Desgranges B, Landeau B, et al: Visual priming within and across symbolic format using a tachistoscopic picture identification task: A PET study. *J Cogn Neurosci* 13:670–686, 2001.

102. Demb JB, Desmond JE, Wagner AD, et al: Semantic encoding and retrieval in the left inferior prefrontal cortex: A functional MRI study of task difficulty and process specificity. *J Neurosci* 15:5870–5878, 1995.

103. Gabrieli JDE, Desmond JE, Demb JB, et al: Functional magnetic resonance imaging of semantic memory processes in the frontal lobes. *Psychol Sci* 7:278–283, 1996.

104. Wagner AD, Desmond JE, Demb JB, et al: Semantic repetition priming for verbal and pictorial knowledge: A functional MRI study of left inferior prefrontal cortex. *J Cogn Neurosci* 9:714–726, 1997.

105. Diamond R, Rozin P: Activation of existing memories in the amnesic syndromes. *J Abnorm Psychol* 93:98–105, 1984.

106. Keane MM, Gabrieli JDE, Noland JS, et al: Normal perceptual priming of orthographically illegal nonwords in amnesia. *J Int Neuropsychol Soc* 1:425–433, 1995.

107. Gabrieli JDE, Milberg W, Keane MM, et al: Intact priming of patterns despite impaired memory. *Neuropsychologia* 28(5):417–427, 1990.

108. Musen G, Squire LR: Nonverbal priming in amnesia. *Mem Cogn* 20:441–448, 1992.

109. Schacter DL, Cooper LA, Tharan M, et al: Preserved priming of novel objects in patients with memory disorders. *J Cogn Neurosci* 3:117–130, 1991.

110. Paller KA, Mayes AR, Thompson KM, et al: Priming of face matching in amnesia. *Brain Cogn* 18:46–59, 1992.

111. Moscovitch M, Winocur G, McLachlan D: Memory as assessed by recognition and reading time in normal and memory-impaired people with Alzheimer's disease and other neurological disorders. *J Exp Psychol Genl* 115:331–347, 1986.

112. Gabrieli JDE, Keane MM, Zarella MM, et al: Preservation of implicit memory for new associations in global amnesia. *Psychol Sci* 7:326–329, 1997.

113. Goshen-Gottstein Y, Moscovitch M, Melo B: Intact implicit memory for newly formed verbal associations in amnesic patients following single study trials. *Neuropsychology* 14:570–578, 2000.

114. Schacter DL, Graf P: Preserved learning in amnesic patients: Perspectives from research on direct priming. *J Clin Exp Neuropsychol* 8:727–743, 1986.

115. Mayes AR, Gooding P: Enhancement of word completion priming in amnesics by cueing with previously novel associates. *Neuropsychologia* 27(8):1057–1072, 1989.

116. Shimamura AP, Squire LR: Impaired priming of new associations in amnesia. *J Exp Psychol Learn Mem Cogn* 15:721–728, 1989.

117. Musen G, Squire LR: On the implicit learning of novel associations by amnesic patients and normal subjects. *Neuropsychology* 7(2):119–135, 1993.

118. Goshen-Gottstein Y, Moscovitch M: Repetition priming for newly formed and preexisting associations: Perceptual and conceptual influences. *J Exp Psychol Learn Mem Cogn* 21:1229–1248, 1995.

119. Goshen-Gottstein Y, Moscovitch M: Repetition priming effects for newly formed associations are perceptually based: Evidence from shallow encoding and format specificity. *J Exp Psychol Learn Mem Cogn* 21:1249–1262, 1995.

120. Schacter DL, Graf P: Effects of elaborative processing on implicit and explicit memory for new associations. *J Exp Psychol Learn Mem Cogn* 12(3):432–444, 1986.

121. Verfaellie M, Keane MM: Scope and limits of implicit memory in amnesia, in De Gelder B, De Haan EHF, Heywood CA (eds): *Out of Mind: Varieties of Unconscious Processes.* Oxford, UK: Oxford University Press, 2001.

122. Cohen NJ, Poldrack RA, Eichenbaum H: Memory for items and memory for relations in the procedural/declarative memory framework. *Memory* 5:131–178, 1997.

Chapter 26

CONFABULATION

Todd E. Feinberg
Joseph T. Giacino

Although no single definition of the term *confabulation* is universally agreed upon, confabulation can be broadly defined as an erroneous statement that is made without a conscious effort to deceive.[1] Korsakoff[2,3] first observed the tendency of patients with what is now known as Wernicke-Korsakoff syndrome to display both amnesia and confabulation ("pseudoreminiscences"). This syndrome was subsequently labeled *confabulation* by Kraepelin,[4] and many authors subsequently confirmed confabulation in Korsakoff's syndrome.[5–10] Although confabulation is usually associated with amnesia, the symptom occurs in a wide variety of neurologic and psychiatric conditions. This chapter addresses mainly confabulation associated with memory loss.

VARIETIES OF CONFABULATION

Kraeplin[11–13] distinguished two subtypes of confabulation. One variety, which he designated as *simple confabulation,* consisted in minor errors in content or temporal order. The other type, termed *fantastic confabulation,* comprised bizarre and patently impossible statements.[4] In a similar fashion, Bonhoeffer[5,6] distinguished between *momentary confabulation* due to the patient's efforts to cover a gap in memory and *fantastic confabulations,* which appeared to exceed the need to conceal or excuse such a gap. Berlyne[1] also found this distinction useful and suggested that momentary confabulation had to be provoked by questions from the examiner and that the content of such confabulations consisted of true memories that were temporally displaced. Van der Horst,[7] Williams and Rupp,[8] and Talland[9,10] previously suggested the notion that confabulations consisted of temporally displaced but veridical memories. Berlyne[1] suggested that fantastic confabu-

lations were not rooted in true memory and that their content was grandiose and wish-fulfilling.

Kopelman[14] reframed the two major catagories of confabulation while retaining the essential characteristics of the two types, and this terminology is in widest usage today. He distinguished *provoked confabulations* that were elicited specifically in response to questions that probed memory from *spontaneous confabulations* that were more grandiose, were more florid, and occurred without provocation. Kopelman found that provoked confabulatory errors of patients with Korsakoff's and Alzheimer's syndromes resembled those of healthy subjects whose memory was tested at prolonged retention intervals.

Feinberg[15] and Feinberg and Roane[16] suggested an alternative dichotomy within confabulatory subtypes. They suggest that there are two major varieties of confabulation. One form, which they called *neutral confabulation,* may occur in any domain (e.g., visual, somatosensory, memory) but is usually confined to that domain. This form of confabulation in part represents an exaggerated tendency of the sort of completion and filling in that occurs in normal perception or memory processes. Its occurrence is facilitated by impaired self-monitoring, but it is nondelusional and the material is not self-referential. Hence the designation *neutral.* Examples of neutral confabulation are visual completion in hemianopic, split-brain, and neglect patients. Some varieties of provoked confabulation in amnesic patients are also examples of neutral confabulation. The second variety is termed *personal confabulation.* The content of these confabulations is personal in the sense that the material is about the patient and the patient's defects or problems, not about particular stimuli or word associations that have no personal relevance for the patient. The confabulations are delusional beliefs that cut across sensory domains and are refractory to correction. In the final analysis, these designations for the varieties of confabulation are to a certain extent overlapping but emphasize different aspects of common underlying symptoms.

NEUROPSYCHOLOGICAL MECHANISMS OF CONFABULATION ASSOCIATED WITH AMNESIA

Over the last 30 years, various neuropsychological mechanisms have been proposed to account for confabulatory symptoms, although none have been universally accepted. Putative mechanisms underlying confabulation can generally be broken down into three categories: (1) amnestic-dysexecutive syndrome, (2) temporal/contextual displacement, and (3) deficient strategic retrieval.

While amnesia and confabulation frequently co-occur, amnesia and confabulation are partially dissociable symptoms. Both Talland[9] and Victor and coworkers[3] noted that in patients with Wernicke-Korsakoff syndrome, confabulation occurred most notably in the early stages of the disease, and Talland[9] described how, in the chronic phase of the illness, confabulation may recede from the clinical picture while notable memory impairment persists. Similarly, Alexander and Freedman[17] found that in patients who developed amnesia after rupture of an aneurysm of the anterior communicating artery (ACoA), confabulation cleared after recovery of weeks or months but amnesia might remain; Vilkki[18] also reported that only some of such patients with amnesia confabulate. The study of Mercer and associates[19] also found a lack of correlation between the degrees of amnesia and confabulation in a group of mixed etiologies.

While it is clear that amnesia in general and amnesia due to frontal lesions can occur without confabulation, whether confabulation occurs in the absence of memory impairment is more controversial. Some authors have suggested that confabulation does not require amnesia. Wyke and Warrington[20] made this argument with reference to a Korsakoff patient who showed visual completion to tachistoscopic stimuli in a fashion not attributable to memory impairment. They interpreted their findings as suggesting that confabulation per se was a primary symptom of Korsakoff's and not

a consequence of amnesia. Kapur and Coughlan[21] also reported, of their postaneurysm frontally damaged patient, that while memory was impaired, confabulation was prominent in spite of normal or near normal scores on tests of verbal and nonverbal recognition and paired-associate learning.

Deluca[4,22] argues that studies purporting to show that confabulation can occur without memory impairment,[23] particularly those studies that address this issue in patients with a ruptured ACoA aneurysm, did not sufficiently assess delayed recall. In support of this view, Deluca found that among six ACoA patients, only those with amnesia confabulated.[22]

Amnestic-Dysexecutive Syndrome

The majority of published studies concerning mechanisms of confabulation implicate some *combination* of memory impairment and executive dysfunction.[14,22,24–26] Stuss and coworkers,[24] in a series of five confabulatory patients, found evidence of frontal dysfunction superimposed upon a memory deficit, and Kopelman[14] also suggested that spontaneous confabulation was the result of the superimposition of frontal dysfunction on amnesia. Deluca[22] compared amnesic to nonamnesic patients after ACoA aneurysmal rupture. He found that confabulation occurred only in those patients with combined frontal and amnesic impairments.

Joseph[27] proposed that confabulated responses may arise from ideational disinhibition caused by injury to the frontal lobes. In this account, frontal disinhibition and behavioral overresponsiveness result in flooding and amplification of tangential and irrelevant associations. Consequently, pertinent information is overwhelmed and indiscriminate response selection produces confabulation. Among other shortcomings, this account does not explain why all patients with behavioral disinhibition do not confabulate or why some confabulatory patients do not evidence other signs of behavioral disinhibition.

Based on their analysis of 9 patients with confabulation following ACoA rupture, Fischer et al.[25] suggested that a common profile of executive deficits underlies confabulatory tendencies. These investigators reported that the 5 cases with severe spontaneous confabulation (i.e., unprovoked and persistent) had significantly greater perseveration and set-shifting deficits than the remaining 4 cases with provoked confabulation (i.e., reactive, transient). No significant between-group difference was found in the severity of memory encoding or retrieval deficits. The authors concluded that confabulation is dependent on the severity of executive dysfunction, particularly those functions involved in self-monitoring, and is not caused by memory impairment alone.

Deficient self-monitoring has also been causally linked to confabulation by Benson and colleagues.[28] Serial neuropsychological assessment and single photon emission computed tomography (SPECT) were performed across a 4-month period to monitor the resolution of confabulation in a 32-year-old woman who presented with acute Wernicke-Kosakoff's syndrome. On initial evaluation, basic attentional functions were intact, but performance was severely impaired on tests of simple and complex processing speed, free and cued recall, and verbal and design fluency. The initial SPECT scan showed focal hypoperfusion in the cingulate gyrus, orbitofrontal cortex, and mesial diencephalic region. On reevaluation 4 months later, the patient remained amnestic, but there were no further episodes of confabulation. Neuropsychometric findings were indicative of significant improvement on the executive measures but not on tests of memory. The change in executive functions occurred in association with recovery of perfusion of the cingulum to near normal levels on SPECT. The absence of improvement in memory was correlated with persistent mesial diencephalic hypoperfusion. In light of the simultaneous resolution of the confabulation and executive disturbance, the authors suggested that the confabulation was due to loss of self-monitoring, which, in turn, was secondary to hypoperfusion of the mesial and orbitofrontal regions.

Box and coworkers[29] also conducted longitudinal assessment of confabulation relative to cognitive functions but reported results that challenge the conclusions reached by Benson et al.[28] A 27-year-old woman presented with spontaneous confabulation and delusional misidentification following a traumatic brain injury. Cognitive assessment was completed on three occasions over a 4-month period. There was no consistent relationship between the presence of executive, memory, or visuoperceptual deficits and the emergence

or disappearance of confabulation. Specifically, confabulation emerged in the setting of severe impairments in executive (i.e., cognitive estimation, perseveration), memory (i.e., recall and recognition), and visuoperceptual (i.e., object recognition) functions but resolved on reevaluation 4 months later, despite significant, persistent cognitive deficits.

O'Connor and coworkers[30] completed neuropsychological assessment of a 74-year-old woman with a 10-year history of amnesia of unknown origin who developed Capgras' syndrome following a traumatic brain injury. Prior to the brain injury, neuropsychological evaluations showed global amnesia in the setting of superior intellectual and reasoning abilities. Subsequent to the injury, the patient presented with confabulatory delusions and there was dramatic decline on tests of mental flexibility and problem solving. Memory assessment was consistent with preinjury performance except that confabulated responses were noted for the first time. In view of the long-standing history of amnesia without confabulation and the simultaneous onset of reasoning deficits and confabulatory delusions, the authors argued that the confabulation was attributable to the convergence of impairments in reasoning (i.e., loss of critical attitude) and memory.

Although confabulation has frequently been shown to accompany combined deficits in memory and executive abilities, not all executive functions play a role. Cunningham and associates[31] reported that confabulation ratios (i.e., the number of confabulatory responses on formal tests of verbal and visuospatial recall divided by the total number of responses) were significantly greater in a group of high confabulators relative to low- and nonconfabulating groups. The high-confabulator group also performed significantly worse on tests of executive function involving sustained attention, set-shifting, and mental tracking. There was, however, no difference between groups on measures of concept formation, problem solving, and verbal fluency. These findings were construed as support for the combined-deficit model, which holds that memory and executive functions must be impaired for confabulation to develop, although specific components of the executive system must be implicated.

Lack of support for the combined-deficit model has been reported in a number of case studies. Kopelman and coworkers[32] investigated the nature of confabulatory erotic delusions in a 47-year-old woman who was diagnosed with schizophrenia. Neuropsychological test findings indicated superior intelligence and normal performance on tests assessing anterograde and retrograde memory and on all of the measures of executive function administered, including tests of verbal fluency, mental flexibility, and cognitive estimation. Based on these findings, the authors rejected the notion that executive dysfunction is a necessary component of confabulation.

Papagno and Baddeley[23] proposed that confabulation is contingent upon disruption of a particular component of the executive system. They described a 29-year-old patient who presented with florid confabulation and anosognosia following resection of a ruptured right subcortical frontoparietal arteriovenous malformation. Interestingly, the patient perfomed normally on four of six standardized memory tests. On interview, he was able to answer factual questions correctly but typically went on to embellish his responses with confabulated material. The authors characterized the underlying problem as a failure to discontinue the search process. The patient generally provided the correct information when it was requested but continued to supplement his initial answer with erroneous responses after exhausting his supply of valid information. This tendency was attributed to a specific aspect of self-monitoring responsible for evaluating the retrieval process and determining when it should be discontinued.

Temporal/Contextual Displacement

The temporal/contextual displacement model holds that confabulation results from inaccurate identification of the temporal order in which information is stored. Schnider and colleagues have completed a series of studies showing that confabulatory recall occurs when discrete elements of information become disconnected from their corresponding spatial and temporal contexts. Schnider et al.[33] described a 62-year-old woman who presented with global anterograde amnesia and confabulation on neuropsychometric assessment. Despite her amnesia, her test-induced confabulations almost exclusively represented actual or semantically related intrusions of material from prior evaluations conducted 4 months earlier. A series of experiments using recall and recognition paradigms were designed to determine whether the patient's memory failures stemmed from an inability to store new information or were due to lack of access to knowledge about where and when the information was acquired. Results indicated that despite very poor performance on free recognition tasks related to a high rate of false-positive errors, recognition discriminability improved significantly when an active information search strategy was imposed (i.e., use of a forced-choice response format). In addition, judgments concerning the personal (tester), temporal (order of presentation of stimuli), and spatial (place of testing) contexts in which the information was acquired were found to approximate chance level. The patient was also noted to perform normally on a recognition task that was not dependent upon contextual information (i.e., stimuli consisting of novel nonwords and nonsense designs). These findings support the premise that confabulation reflects an inability to label information contextually, thus producing pathologic fusion of unrelated memory elements.

In a second study using experimental paradigms similar to those described above, Schnider et al.[33] found a double dissociation in the memory profiles of spontaneous and provoked confabulators. When spontaneous confabulators were compared to amnesics with and without provoked confabulation, only the spontaneous confabulators failed to recognize the temporal order of stored information. Further, no correlation was found between the failure of temporal order recognition and provoked confabulation. Interestingly, there was no consistent relationship between performance on measures of executive function and confabulation. There were no significant differences in performance between spontaneous confabulators and other amnesics on six indices associated with executive dysfunction. The authors concluded that confabulation is based on a specific form of frontal dysfunction that causes impairment in temporal order discrimination and suggested that this disturbance is due to disconnection of the orbitofrontal cortex from the amygdala.

Further support for the premise that traditional symptoms of executive dysfunction do not account for confabulation was provided in a case report by Ptak and Schnider.[34] The authors described a 49-year-old male who became amnestic with spontaneous confabulation after sustaining rupture of the ACoA. Contrary to previous findings reported by these investigators, this patient did not demonstrate failure of temporal order recognition. In this study, the patient was given two runs of a recognition task for pictures. In the second run, administered 1 h after the first, the patient was required to distinguish between target stimuli from the first and second runs. Although target identification was low, there were no false-positive errors during either run, providing no evidence for temporal context confusion. The authors speculated that the absence of false-positive errors was related to the application of a very conservative recognition criterion, implicating strong reliance on self-monitoring strategies. This hypothesis was tested by repeating the same test with the admonition to avoid missing too many target items. In this condition, the number of false-positive errors exceeded the number of hits. It was concluded that the disturbance in temporal context order was masked by the patient's well-preserved capacity for self-monitoring. When monitoring processes were externally suppressed, temporal context confusion was released. These findings call into question the contribution of self-monitoring deficits to confabulation.

Additional evidence for a dissociation between confabulation and memory and executive functions comes from a longitudinal study of the evolution of spontaneous confabulation. Schnider et al.[35] performed neuropsychological reevaluations of 8 spontaneous confabulators 18 months after initial onset. Of these 8 patients, 3 stopped confabulating within 3 months, while 2 patients continued to confabulate for 2 or more years. Test results indicated that temporal context confusion, but not memory or executive performance, perfectly paralleled resolution of the confabulation. The duration of confabulation was also found to be related to the severity of orbitofrontal injury in this group.

Deficient Strategic Retrieval

In recent studies, confabulation has been directly tied to disruption of strategic retrieval processes.[26,36,37] These processes constitute problem-solving routines that are triggered when proximal cues are inadequate to retrieve the required information. Under normal conditions, memory demands initially engage automatic "associative" processes. During the associative process, proximal cues interact with previously stored

memories to produce memory traces. If the recovered trace is insufficient, a second retrieval process is activated to guide continuation of the search process. In opposition to the automatic associative retrieval process, strategic retrieval is conscious, effortful, and self-directed. This process is designed to locate the desired information or identify other appropriate cues that facilitate associative retrieval operations. Once the memory trace is retrieved, strategic processes evaluate the fit between the trace and the intended information. In this model, confabulation is presumed to be the result of a breakdown in strategic retrieval processes involved in memory search, temporal ordering, and output monitoring. The predisposition to confabulation increases when a particular cognitive subsystem (e.g., memory) is damaged and produces faulty output (e.g., failure to remember) in addition to impaired output monitoring (e.g., unawareness of response discrepancies).

While the strategic retrieval mechanism may appear similar to the temporal/contextual displacement model in explaining confabulation, there are important differences. Given its emphasis on temporal order and context-specific stimuli, the temporal/contextual displacement model predicts that confabulation should involve episodic but not semantic material. Dalla Barba has indeed shown that confabulation can be confined to the episodic memory system.[36] Using a questionnaire designed to elicit confabulation in a 75-year-old male diagnosed with Binswanger's encephalopathy, Dalla Barba found that confabulated responses occurred exclusively on questions related to episodic memory and not on items dependent upon the semantic system. He concluded that disruption of the episodic system causes faulty reporting of events, although the manner in which the event is reported depends upon the integrity of the semantic system. The greater the degree of semantic degradation, the more fantastic the confabulation. Conversely, Sandson and colleagues[38] described a 66-year-old male who sustained a left intracerebral hematoma. The patient presented with two distinct forms of confabulation. In addition to typical event-based confabulations, episodes of confabulation were also directly precipitated by semantic memory prompts. The latter occurred in response to questions concerning attributes of common objects and "definitions" of nonsense words. These confabulations occurred in the setting of literal and verbal paraphasic errors. The link between semantic confabulation and language disturbance in this case supports the premise that the probability of confabulation increases when specific cognitive subsystems are damaged along with strategic retrieval processes.

Laws and colleagues[39] argue that confabulation arises from imbalance or miscommunication between the autobiographical, semantic, and episodic components of the memory system rather than lack of access to these systems. This view also holds that the autobiographical system is organized around thematic frameworks that serve to index and reconstruct personally relevant information. Under normal circumstances, activation of a thematic framework (e.g., thinking about work) coactivates the semantic knowledge base to generate distinct memories (e.g., characteristics of individual coworkers), which concurrently activate the episodic system to retrieve past events associated with these individuals (e.g., "The day John and I got stuck in the airport in Boston"). When one of these components is damaged, an imbalance develops and the other components attempt to compensate for the deficiency. The remaining intact systems attempt to match the desired information requirements against preserved knowledge that is available within these systems. Personally relevant themes readily attract attention during the search process. Confabulation emerges from inappropriate binding of information from the three systems.

To illustrate the interrelationship among the three systems, Laws et al.[39] completed extensive neuropsychological assessment of a 39-year-old schizophrenic male who presented with multiple episodes of self-referential confabulation, including the belief that he was "Baron Caernarvon." This particular belief emerged following a dinner held at Caernarvon Castle that was attended by the patient. Assessment findings indicated that episodes of confabulation occurred (1) in response to names but not to faces, (2) primarily when the patient was acquainted with the topic but not when he was unfamiliar with it, and (3) more frequently for names of specific categories of people (e.g., politicians versus nonpoliticians). Of particular interest, the content of the confabulation was typically of personal and autobiographical relevance. These findings were interpreted as evidence that the confabulatory misidentification was not secondary to perceptual disturbance but rather that it was based largely on

preserved knowledge and was the result of compensatory albeit aberrant overreliance on specific personally relevant thematic frameworks. The authors suggest that repeated coactivation of information from these interdependent systems ultimately results in reinforcement of erroneously reconstructed events and acts to sustain the confabulation.

NEUROANATOMY OF AMNESIC CONFABULATION

The pathology of alcoholic patients with Wernicke-Korsakoff syndrome involves primarily the dorsomedial nucleus of the thalamus,[3] mamillary bodies,[40] both of these in combination,[41] or other thalamic nuclei.[42,43] Stuss and coworkers[24] found spontaneous confabulation of the "fantastical" variety in five patients with either head trauma, subarachnoid hemorrhage, or infarcts and found that this form of confabulation correlated with frontal dysfunction as judged by neurologic examination, computed tomography (CT)/electroencephalography (EEG), and neuropsychological test data.

As noted above, rupture of aneurysms of the ACoA have been noted to produce an amnestic syndrome that in some cases is accompanied by confabulation.[17,18,22,25,44–49] In the ACoA series of Alexander and Freedman,[17] 5 of 11 patients had the most marked and persistent confabulation. Of these 5 patients, 3 had right anterior cerebral artery (ACA) infarcts, a fourth had bilateral ACA territory infarcts (right greater than left), and the fifth had a right parietal infarct. Thus frontal and particularly right hemispheric regions were implicated. All patients had anterograde and retrograde amnesia. It was suggested that damage to basal forebrain, particularly the septal nuclei (which provide widespread cholinergic projections to cortical sites including hippocampus), might produce the amnesia. Vilkki's series[18] of ACoA patients also provided links between confabulation and frontal lobe damage; of 5 amnesic ACoA patients, 2 had profound confabulation; of these, 1 had bilateral frontobasal infarctions and the other had a right frontobasal subdural empyema treated surgically.

Damasio and coworkers[46] reported on several patients with spontaneous, "dreamlike" confabulations, all of whom had basal forebrain lesions including septal nuclei, nucleus accumbens, diagonal band, and medial substantia innominata. It was felt that the nucleus basalis was also probably involved. All patients had unilateral orbitofrontal lesions as well. The septal lesions were believed to be responsible for the amnesia due to interruption of connections with the hippocampus, amygdala, and parahippocampal gyrus. The anatomy of confabulation was not explored in this series. In another series of amnesic patients of mixed etiology, Baddeley and Wilson[47] found that among the 10 amnesics, there were 2 with confabulation. One had an ACoA and the other a head injury; both had bilateral frontal lesions. Interestingly, while neither of these patients differed from nonconfabulators on measures of delayed recall, both did significantly worse on measures of retrograde autobiographical memory. They attributed the confabulation to a dysexecutive syndrome due to frontal pathology.

Deluca and coworkers[4,22,48,49] provided additional support for the role of combined basal forebrain and frontal damage in producing confabulation in ACoA patients. Fischer and associates[25] reported on 9 ACoA patients divided into spontaneous (extended, grandiose) and provoked (limited, plausible) groups. While both groups had lesions of basal forebrain and anterograde amnesia, the spontaneous group had more extensive medial frontal and striatal pathology. They also showed more extensive retrograde amnesia and "executive deficits" on frontal-type tasks.

Finally, Schnider and Ptak[50] compared 6 patients with spontaneous confabulation to 12 nonconfabulatory amnesic patients. These authors found extensive overlap in the lesions of the confabulatory patients in the anterior limbic system, including medial orbitofrontal cortex, basal forebrain, amygdala, and perirhinal cortex or medial hypothalamus (Fig. 26-1).

a Spontaneous confabulators

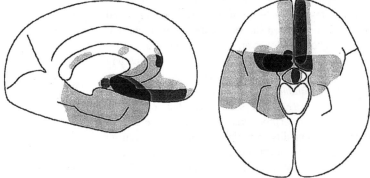

Figure 26-1
Lesion analysis of (a) spontaneous confabulators and (b) nonconfabulatory amnesics. Shaded areas represent paramedian lesions, dashed lines indicate lateral lesions. Straight parallel dashed lines in the lower part of the sagittal view in (b) indicate the composite axial slice used in the right column to indicate lesions of the (A) amygdala, (F) basal forebrain, (H) hippocampus, (HT) hypothalamus, and orbitofrontal cortex. (From Schnider and Ptak,[50] with permission.)

b Nonconfabulating amnesics

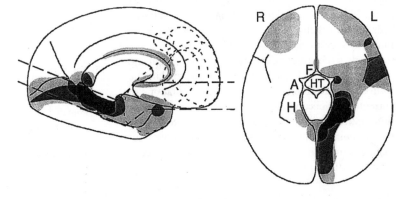

CONCLUSIONS

Most of the empiric evidence concerning neuropsychological mechanisms of confabulation is based on single case studies. Consequently, it is difficult to compare findings across studies because of significant differences in the operational definition of confabulation and variability in the design and procedures employed. Notwithstanding these differences, there appears to be some convergence among published findings:

1. *Memory impairment commonly but not necessarily accompanies confabulation.* This conclusion is tempered by the fact that most neuropsychometric measures tap episodic but not semantic memory processes. This leaves open the possibility that semantic memory impairment or disruption of the interface between the semantic and episodic systems is a prerequisite for confabulation.
2. *Executive dysfunction is a common but variable component of confabulatory syndromes.* Deficient self-monitoring, disinhibition, susceptibility to intrusive interference, inability to shift set, and impaired fluency have all been shown to correlate with confabulation. There is, however, no consistent relationship between the presence of any of these symptoms and the emergence or resolution of confabulation.
3. *Confabulation primarily involves disruption of retrieval processes.* It is not clear what specific aspect of the retrieval process is disturbed. Some evidence suggests an inability to retrieve temporal and contextual "tags" (versus difficulty retrieving the information itself), while other data support failure to regulate or disengage the search process.
4. *Direct damage or functional disconnection involving the ventromesial and orbitofrontal cortices is implicated in the majority of confabulation reports.* This region is believed to mediate cross-talk between limbic and prefrontal structures and appears to form the intersection of subjective experience with personal and social reasoning.[51] Lesions in this area may explain the fortuitous association of subjective representations of current experience with previously stored representations or imagined approximations and may account for the faulty selection and acceptance of episodic or semantic memory traces noted in empiric studies of confabulation. Unfortunately, traditional neuropsychological measures are relatively insensitive to the functional sequelae of ventromesial and orbitofrontal lesions.

REFERENCES

1. Berlyne N: Confabulation. *Br J Psychiatry* 120:31–39, 1972.
2. Victor M, Yakovlev PI: SS Korsakoff's psychic disorder in conjunction with peripheral neuritis: A translation of Korsakoff's original article with brief comments on the author and his contribution to clinical medicine. *Neurology* 5:394–406, 1955.
3. Victor M, Adams RD, Collins GH: *The Wernicke-Korsakoff Syndrome and Related Neurologic Disorders Due to Alcoholism and Malnutrition,* 2d ed. Philadelphia: Davis, 1989.
4. Deluca J: A cognitive neuroscience perspective on confabulation. *Neuropsychoanalysis* 3:3–16, 2001.
5. Bonhoeffer K: *Die akuten Geisteskrankheiten der Gewohnheitstrinker.* Jena: Gustav Fischer, 1901.
6. Bonhoeffer K: Der Korsakowsche Symptomenkomplex in seinen Beziehungen zu den verschiedenen Krankheitsformen. *Allg Z Psychiatry* 61:744–752, 1904.
7. Van der Horst L: Über die Psychologie des Korsakowsyndroms. *Monatschr Psychiatry Neurol* 83: 65–84, 1932.
8. Williams HW, Rupp C: Observations on confabulation. *Am J Psychiatry* 95:395–405, 1938.
9. Talland GA: Confabulation in the Wernicke-Korsakoff syndrome. *Nerv Ment Dis* 132:361–381, 1961.
10. Talland GA: *Deranged Memory.* New York: Academic Press, 1965.
11. Kraepelin E: *Lectures on Clinical Psychiatry.* Johnson T, transl. London: Baillière Tindall, 1904.
12. Kraepelin E: *Clinical Psychiatry: A Textbook for Students and Physicians.* Diefendorf AR, transl. New York: Macmillan, 1907.
13. Kraepelin E: *Dementia Praecox and Paraphrenia.* Barclay RM, transl. Edinburgh: E and S Livingstone, 1919.
14. Kopelman MD: Two types of confabulation. *Neurol Neurosurg Psychiatry* 43:461–463, 1980.
15. Feinberg TE: *Altered Egos: How the Brain Creates the Self.* New York: Oxford University Press, 2001.
16. Feinberg TE, Roane DM: Anosognosia, completion and confabulation: The neutral-personal dichotomy. *Neurocase* 3:73–85, 1997.
17. Alexander MR, Freedman M: Amnesia after anterior communicating artery aneurysm rupture. *Neurology* 34:752–757, 1984.

18. Vilkki J: Amnesic syndromes after surgery of anterior communicating artery aneurysms. *Cortex* 21:431–444, 1985.

19. Mercer B, Wapner W, Gardner H, Benson P: A study of confabulation. *Arch Neurol* 34:429–433, 1977.

20. Wyke M, Warrington E: An experimental analysis of confabulation in a case of Korsakoff's syndrome using a tachistoscopic method. *J Neurol Neurosurg Psychiatry* 23:327–333, 1960.

21. Kapur N, Coughlan AK: Confabulation and frontal lobe dysfunction. *Neurol Neurosurg Psychiatry* 43:461–463, 1980.

22. Deluca J: Predicting neurobehavioral patterns following anterior communicating artery aneurysm. *Cortex* 29:639–647, 1993.

23. Papagno C, Baddeley A: Confabulation in a dysexecutive patient: Implication for models of retrieval. *Cortex* 33:743–752, 1997.

24. Stuss DT, Alexander MP, Lieberman A, Levine H: An extraordinary form of confabulation. *Neurology* 28:1166–1172, 1978.

25. Fischer RS, Alexander MP, D'Esposito M, Otto R: Neuropsychological and neuroanatomical correlates of confabulation. *Clin Exp Neuropsychol* 17:20–28, 1995.

26. Moscovitch M, Melo B: Strategic retrieval and the frontal lobes: evidence from confabulation and amnesia. *Neuropsychologia* 35:1017–1034, 1997.

27. Joseph R: Confabulation and delusional denial: Frontal lobe and lateralized influences. *J Clin Psychol* 42:507–519, 1986.

28. Benson DF, Djenderedjian A, Miller BL, et al: Neural basis of confabulation. *Neurology* 46:1239–1243, 1996.

29. Box O, Laing H, Kopelman K: The evolution of spontaneous confabulation, delusional misidentification and a related delusion in a case of severe head injury. *Neurocase* 5:251–262, 1999.

30. O'Connor M, Walbridge M, Sandson T, et al: A neuropsychological analysis of Capgras syndrome. *Neuropsychiatry Neuropsychol Behav Neurol* 9(4):265–271, 1996.

31. Cunningham JM, Pliskin NH, Cassisi JE, et al: Relationship between confabulation and measures of memory and executive function. *J Clin Exp Neuropsychol* 19(6):867–877, 1997.

32. Kopelman MD, Guinan EM, Lewis PDR: Delusional memory, confabulation and frontal lobe dysfunction: A case study in De Clerambault's syndrome. *Neurocase* 1:71–77, 1995.

33. Schnider A, Gutbrod K, Hess CW, et al: Memory without context: Amnesia with confabulations after infarction of the right capsular genu. *J Neurol Neurosurg Psychiatry* 61:186–193, 1996.

34. Ptak R, Schnider A: Spontaneous confabulations after orbitofrontal damage: The role of temporal context confusion and self-monitoring. *Neurocase* 5:243–250, 1999.

35. Schnider A, Ptak R, von Daniken C, et al: Recovery from spontaneous confabulations parallels recovery of temporal confusion in memory. *Neurology* 55:74–83, 2000.

36. Dalla Barba G: Confabulation: knowledge and recollective experience. *Cogn Neuropsychol* 10(1):1–20, 1993.

37. Moscovitch M: Confabulation, in Schachter DL (ed): *Memory Distortion: How Minds, Brains and Societies Reconstruct the Past.* Cambridge, MA: Harvard University Press, 1995; p226–251.

38. Sandson J, Albert ML, Alexander MP: Confabulation in aphasia. *Cortex* 22:621–626, 1986.

39. Laws KR, McKenna PJ, McCarthy RA: Delusions about people. *Neurocase* 1:3439–362, 1995.

40. Barbizet J: Defect of memorizing of hippocampal-mammillary origin: A review. *Neurol Neurosurg Psychiatry* 26:127–135, 1963.

41. Weiskrantz L: Neuroanatomy of memory and amnesia: A case for multiple memory systems. *Human Neurobiol* 6:93–105, 1987.

42. Mair WGP, Warrington EK, Weiskrantz L: Memory disorder in Korsakoff's psychosis: A neuropathological and neuropsychological investigation of two cases. *Brain* 102:749–783, 1979.

43. Mayes AR, Meudell PR, Mann D, Pickering A: Location of lesions in Korsakoff's syndrome: Neuropsychological and neuropathological data on two patients. *Cortex* 24:367–388, 1988.

44. Talland GA, Sweet WH, Ballantine HT: Amnesic syndrome with anterior communicating artery aneurysm. *Nerv Ment Dis* 145:179–192, 1967.

45. Lindqvist G, Norlen G: Korsakoff's syndrome after operation on ruptured aneurysm of the anterior communicating artery. *Acta Psychiatr Scand* 42:24–34, 1966.

46. Damasio AR, Graff-Radford NR, Eslinger PJ, et al: Amnesia following basal forebrain lesions. *Arch Neurol* 42:263–271, 1985.

47. Baddeley AD, Wilson B: Amnesia, autobiographical memory, and confabulation, in Rubin DC (ed): *Autobiographical Memory.* Cambridge, England: Cambridge University Press, 1986.

48. Deluca J, Cicerone KD: Confabulation following aneurysm of the anterior communicating artery. *Cortex* 27:417–424, 1991.

49. Deluca J, Diamond BJ: Aneurysm of the anterior communicating artery: A review of neuroanatomical and

neuropsychologic sequelae. *Clin Exp Neuropsychol* 17:100–121, 1995.

50. Schnider A, Ptak R: Spontaneous confabulators fail to suppress currently irrelevant memory traces. *Nat Neurosci* 2:677–681, 1999.

51. Damasio A, Tranel D, Damasio H: Somatic markers and the guidance of behavior: Theory and preliminary testing, in Levin HS, Eisenberg HM, Benton AL (eds): *Frontal Lobe Function and Dysfunction*. New York: Oxford University Press, 1991, pp 217–229.

Chapter 27

SEMANTIC MEMORY IMPAIRMENTS

Martha J. Farah
Murray Grossman

Semantic memory refers to our general knowledge of the objects, people, and events of the world (Tulving, 1972). The knowledge that Paris is the capital of France, that birds have feathers, and that a desk is a piece of furniture exemplifies semantic memory. More particular knowledge, tied to an individual's personal experience, is considered *episodic memory* rather than semantic memory. Examples of the latter include the knowledge that you bought this book at a certain store or ate a certain food for breakfast this morning.

Neurologic disease and damage can affect semantic memory disproportionately. In this chapter the different forms of semantic memory impairment are reviewed, with attention to their etiologies, major behavioral features, and implications for the neural substrates and functional organization of semantic memory in the normal brain.

GENERALIZED IMPAIRMENT OF SEMANTIC MEMORY

Warrington (1975) first documented a pattern of preserved and impaired performance indicative of semantic memory impairment in a series of three patients suffering from progressive degenerative brain disease. Her subjects were relatively preserved on most measures of language and cognitive function but did poorly on tasks dependent on semantic memory, including confrontation naming, word-picture matching, and a verification task in which subjects were shown pictures or words and asked questions such as "Is it a bird?" or "Is it heavy?" In subsequent years a number of similar cases were reported, and the term *semantic dementia* was coined in the context of one such report (Snowden et al., 1989). Hodges and coworkers (1992) presented a wide-ranging study of five new cases of semantic dementia, reviewed the literature, and drew a number

of useful generalizations concerning the condition. A summary of their conclusions is presented here.

Semantic dementia may present initially as a language disorder whose most prominent feature is vocabulary loss, both expressive and receptive. Naming is minimally aided by phonemic cues, and naming errors tend to share a semantic relation with the correct name (e.g., "violin" for accordion, or "animal" for fox). In production, category fluency is severely impaired, and word definitions are improverished or wrong. Such patients have sometimes been described as having a fluent form of primary progressive aphasia (see Chaps. 16 and 17), but additional language testing and nonverbal semantic memory testing suggests that the underlying impairment is one of semantic memory knowledge rather than language. Syntax and phonology tend to be preserved, whereas entirely pictorial tasks that depend on knowledge of the depicted objects, such as sorting together semantically related objects or distinguishing real from imaginary objects, are failed. Although the formal assessment of episodic memory is difficult because of the loss of knowledge of word and picture meanings, Hodges and coworkers (Hodges et al., 1992) observe that at least some patients show significant preservation of autobiographical memories and practical day-to-day memory. The neuropathologic changes in semantic dementia are focused in the temporal lobes, often affecting the left more than the right, and semantic dementia has come to be regarded as a variant of frontotemporal lobar degeneration (see Chap. 32).

Another degenerative disease affecting semantic memory is Alzheimer's disease (AD) (Martin and Fedio, 1983; Bayles and coworkers, 1990; Chertkow and Bub, 1990; Hodges et al., 1992; Nebes, 1992; Grossman and Mickanin, 1994) although semantic memory is just one of many aspects of cognition impaired in AD, and initially some cases may present with only episodic memory impairment. To the extent that semantic memory is impaired in AD, pathologic changes in temporal cortex are responsible.

In recent years the study of semantic memory in neurologic patients has been complemented by a growing literature on semantic memory studied with functional neuroimaging in normal subjects (see Thompson-Schill, 2003, for a review). The temporal localization inferred from the cases of generalized semantic memory impairment, in degenerative conditions such as semantic dementia and AD, accords well with the conclusions emerging from the neuroimaging literature. For example, when Vandenberghe et al. (1996) mapped the regions active during different types of semantic tasks and presented via different modalities, regions in left temporal cortex were invariably activated. Using semantic priming as a marker for regions subserving semantics, Thompson-Schill et al. (1999) also found temporal activation.

In sum, semantic memory is at least partially dissociable from other forms of memory, language and cognition, and the dissociation is generally seen in the context of degenerative diseases. The neuropathology in these cases implicates temporal cortex, with some degree of lateralization to the left—a conclusion that finds growing support within the functional neuroimaging literature.

SELECTIVE IMPAIRMENTS OF SEMANTIC MEMORY

In addition to the generalized impairments of semantic memory described above, particular aspects of semanatic memory can be disproportionately impaired. These disorders suggest that semantic memory has an internal organization, with different components of semantics localized in different brain regions.

Category-Specific Semantic Memory Impairment

In some cases it appears that knowledge from certain semantic categories is disproportionately impaired, suggesting that the neural bases of semantic memory are subdivided by semantic category. The most common category-specific semantic memory impairment affects knowledge of living things.

The first report of impaired knowledge of living things was made by Warrington and Shallice (1984), who described three postencephalitic patients. Although the patients were generally impaired at tasks such as picture naming and defining words, they were dramatically worse when the pictures or words represented animals and plants than when they represented artifacts. In subsequent years numerous other reports appeared of similar patients, generally suffering damage to temporal cortex from herpes encephalitis, closed head injury, or, less frequently, cerebrovascular or degenerative disease. Category-specific disorders of semantic memory are distinct from the disorders described in the previous section, despite the implication of temporal brain regions in both, as neither semantic dementia (Hodges et al., 1992) nor AD (Tippett et al., 1996) routinely affects knowledge of living things more than nonliving.

The idea that certain brain regions are specialized for representing knowledge about living things has naturally aroused some skepticism and prompted a search for alternative explanations of apparently impaired knowledge of living things. The simplest alternative explanation is that the impairment is an artifact of the greater difficulty of retrieving knowledge about living things. It has been suggested that when difficulty is equated across living and nonliving test items, the selectivity of the semantic memory impairment disappears (Funnell and Sheridan, 1992; Stewart et al., 1992). However, the selectivity has been shown to persist in two cases when multiple measures of difficulty are accounted for (Farah et al., 1991), and the null results in other controlled studies are likely due to insufficient statistical power, as our reliable findings disappeared when we reduced our data set to the size of the other studies (Farah et al., 1996).

Cases of impaired knowledge of nonliving things with relatively spared knowledge of living things are rarer but have also been described (Warrington and McCarthy, 1983, 1987; Hillis and Caramazza, 1991; Sacchett and Humphreys, 1992). The lesions in these cases are confined to the left hemisphere. A precise intrahemispheric localization is not possible, as the lesions are typically large and relatively few cases have been reported, although the left temporal region again seems involved (Tippett et al., 1996). These patients provide the other half of a double dissociation with impaired knowledge of living things, thus adding further support to the hypothesis that category-specific semantic memory impairments are not simply due to the differential difficulty of particular categories.

Building on the hypothesis of Allport (1985), that semantic memory is subdivided into different sensorimotor modalities (e.g., visual knowledge, tactile knowledge, motor knowledge), Warrington and Shallice (1984) proposed a different kind of alternative explanation for category-specific knowledge deficits. They suggested that living and nonliving things may differ from one another in their reliance on knowledge from different sensorimotor modalities, with living things being known predominantly by their visual and other sensory attributes. Impaired knowledge of living things could result from an impairment of visual knowledge. Similarly, nonliving things might be known predominantly by their function, an abstract form of motoric representation, and impaired knowledge of nonliving things could result from an impairment of functional knowledge. This interpretation has the advantage of parsimony, in that it invokes a type of organization already known to exist in the brain—modality-specific organization—rather than invoking an organization based on semantic categories such as aliveness.

A computer simulation of semantic memory and its impairments has shown that a modality-specific organization can account for category-specific impairments, even the finding that functional knowledge of living things is impaired after visual semantic damage (Farah and McClelland, 1991). The latter finding is explained by the need for a certain "critical mass" of associated knowledge to help activate collaterally any one part of a distributed representation; if most of the representation of living things is visual and visual knowledge is damaged, then the remaining functional knowledge cannot be activated. The finding that visual knowledge of living things is the most impaired type of knowledge, with nonvisual knowledge of nonliving things the least impaired and visual nonliving and nonvisual living intermediate (Farah et al., 1989), is consistent with this fundamentally modality-specific view of semantic memory organization.

Nevertheless, the semantic impairment in some cases seems equally severe for visual and nonvisual knowledge of living things, while knowledge of even

the visual attributes of nonliving things is relatively preserved, implying that semantic memory is organized by category rather than, or in addition to, by modality of knowledge (Caramazza and Shelton, 1998; Farah and Rabinowitz, 2003). Findings from functional neuroimaging of normal subjects also offer evidence of both modality specificity in knowledge of living things (Thompson-Schill et al., 1999) and segregation of living things within the visual modality-specific semantic system (Chao and Martin, 1999). It now seems likely that the organization of semantic memory involves multiple levels of representation, some more closely related to the modality of the information represented and some more closely related to the semantic category.

A final point concerning category-specific impairments is that semantic memory is not the only functional system with a categorical internal structure, and this fact has led to some confusion. Within vision, the dissociability of face, object, and printed word recognition suggests the existence of subsystems whose specialization might be considered categorical. These subsystems differ crucially from those for living and nonliving things, however, in that they are required for visual recognition but not for more general knowledge retrieval. A visual object agnosic knows what a horse is and is simply unable to recognize it by sight. A patient with semantic memory impairment, in contrast, can neither recognize a horse by sight nor provide information of any kind about horses. Category-specific semantic memory impairments are also sometimes confused with category-specific impairments in name retrieval. The "fruit and vegetable" impairment observed in two cases (Hart et al., 1985; Farah and Wallace, 1992) affects naming only. As with more general anomias, the names are recognized when seen or heard, the objects themselves are recognized, and semantic information appears intact.

Modality-Specific Semantic Memory Impairment

There is a second way in which the phrase *modality-specific semantic memory* has been used in neuropsychology, and that is for components of semantic memory that are accessed *through* a particular input or output modality. According to this usage, visual semantics refers not to semantic knowledge of the visual appearance of objects but to the semantic knowledge of appearance, function, and so on that is accessed when an object is seen. The puzzling syndrome of "optic aphasia" has led some to conclude that semantic memory must have a modality-specific organization in this input-defined sense.

Optic aphasia consists of an impairment in naming visually presented stimuli in the face of relatively preserved naming of nonvisual stimuli and relatively preserved nonverbal demonstrations of visual recognition. It seems reasonable to assume that visual confrontation naming requires three major stages of processing: vision, semantics, and lexical retrieval. That is, it requires seeing the object clearly enough to access semantic knowledge of it and using that semantic knowledge of what the object is to retrieve its name. Paradoxically, the preserved nonvisual naming and nonverbal recognition performance of optic aphasics seem to exonerate all three stages.

A variety of attempts have been made to explain how an anomia could exist for visual stimuli only. An early and influential account takes the dissociations at face value and invokes separate modality-specific semantic memory systems for interpreting visual input and other modality inputs, so that optic aphasia can be explained as a disconnection between visual semantics (i.e., the semantic knowledge accessed by visual inputs) and verbal semantics (i.e., the semantic knowledge necessary to access a verbal output) (Beauvois, 1982). In recent years, more parsimonious alternative explanations of optic aphasia have been proposed (Plaut and Shallice, 1993; Sitton et al., 2000; see Chap. 7), thereby diminishing the need to hypothesize semantic systems specific for each input modality.

REFERENCES

Allport DA: Distributed memory, modular subsystems and dysphasia, in Newmans, Epstein R (eds): *Current Perspectives in Dysphasia*. Edinburgh: Churchill Livingstone, 1985.

Bayles KA, Tomoeda CK, Trosset MW: Naming and categorical knowledge in Alzheimer's disease: The process of semantic memory deterioration. *Brain Lang* 39:498–510, 1990.

Beauvois MF: Optic aphasia: A process of interaction between vision and language. *Philos Trans R Soc Lond* B 298:35–47, 1982.

Caramazza A, Shelton JR: Domain specific knowledge systems in the brain: The animate-inanimate distinction. *J Cogn Neurosci* 10:1–34, 1998.

Chao LL, Martin A: Cortical representation of perception, naming and knowledge of color. *J Cogn Neurosci* 11:25–35, 1999.

Chertkow H, Bub D: Semantic memory loss in dementia of Alzheimer's type: What do various measures measure? *Brain* 113:397–417, 1990.

Epstein R, DeYoe EA, Press DZ, et al: Neuropsychological evidence for a topographical learning mechanism in parahippocampal cortex. *Cogn Neuropsychol* 18:481–508, 2001.

Farah MJ: *Visual Agnosia: Disorders of Object Recognition and What They Tell Us About Normal Vision*. Cambridge, MA: MIT Press/Bradford Books, 1990.

Farah MJ, Hammon KH, Mehta Z, Ratcliff G: Category-specificity and modality-specificity in semantic memory. *Neuropsychologia* 27:193–200, 1989.

Farah MJ, McClelland JL: A computational model of semantic memory impairment: Modality-specificity and emergent category-specificity. *J Exp Psychol Genl* 120:339–357, 1991.

Farah MJ, McMullen PA, Meyer MM: Can recognition of living things be selectively impaired? *Neuropsychologia* 29:185–193, 1991.

Farah MJ, Meyer MM, McMullen PA: The living/nonliving dissociation is not an artifact: Giving an a priori implausible hypothesis a strong test. *Cogn Neuropsychol* 13:152–154, 1996.

Farah M, Rabinowitz C: Genetic and environmental influences on the organization of semantic memory in the brain: Is "living things" an innate category?" *Cogn Neuropsychol* 2003.

Farah MJ, Wallace MA: Semantically-bounded anomia: Implications for the neural implementation of naming. *Neuropsychologia* 30:609–621, 1992.

Funnell E, Sheridan J: Categories of knowledge? Unfamiliar aspects of living and non-living things. *Cogn Neuropsychol* 9:135–154, 1992.

Grossman M, Mickanin J: Picture comprehension and probable Alzheimer's disease. *Brain Cogn* 26:43–64, 1994.

Hart J, Berndt RS, Caramazza A: Category-specific naming deficit following cerebral infarction. *Nature* 316:439–440, 1985.

Hillis A, Caramazza C: Category-specific naming and comprehension impairment: A double dissociation. *Brain* 114:2081–2094, 1991.

Hodges JR, Patterson K, Oxbury S, Funnell E: Semantic dementia. *Brain* 115:1783–1806, 1992.

Hodges JR, Salmon DP, Butters N: Semantic memory impairment in Alzheimer's disease: Failure of access of degraded knowledge? *Neuropsychologia* 30:301–314, 1992.

Martin A, Fedio P: Word production and comprehension in Alzheimer's disease: The breakdown of semantic knowledge. *Brain Lang* 19:124–141, 1983.

Nebes RD: Cognitive dysfunction in Alzheimer's disease, in Craik FIM, Salthouse A (eds): *The Handbook of Aging and Cognition.* Hillsdale, NJ: Erlbaum, 1992.

Plaut DC, Shallice T: Perseverative and semantic influences on visual object naming errors in optic aphasia: A connectionist account. *J Cogn Neurosci* 5:89-117, 1993.

Sacchett C, Humphreys GW: Calling a squirrel a squirrel but a canoe a wigwam: A category-specific deficit for artifactual objects and body parts. *Cogn Neuropsychol* 9:73-86, 1992.

Shallice T: Impairments of semantic processing: Multiple dissociations, in Coltheart M, Sartori G, Job R (eds): *The Cognitive Neuropsychology of Language.* London: Erlbaum, 1987.

Sitton M, Mozer MC, Farah MJ: Superadditive effects of multiple lesions in a connectionist architecture: Implications for the neuropsychology of optic aphasia. *Psychol Rev* 709–734, 2000.

Snowden JS, Goulding PJ, Neary D: Semantic dementia: A form of circumscribed cerebral atrophy. *Behav Neurol* 2:167–182, 1989.

Stewart F, Parkin AJ, Hunkin NM: Naming impairments following recovery from herpes simplex encephalitis: Category specific? *Q J Exp Psychol* 44A:261–284, 1992.

Thompson-Schill SL: Neuroimaging studies of semantic memory: inferring "how" from "where." *Neuropsychologia*, 41:280–292, 2003.

Thompson-Schill SL, Aguirre GK, D'Esposito M, Farah MJ: A neural basis for category and modality specificity of semantic knowledge. *Neuropsychologia* 37:671–676, 1999.

Thompson-Schill SL, D'Esposito M, Kan IP: Effects of repetition and competition on prefrontal activity during word generation. *Neuron* 23:513–522, 1999.

Thompson-Schill SL, Gabrieli JD: Priming of visual and functional knowledge on a semantic classification task. *J Exp Psychol Learn Mem Cogn* 25:41–53, 1999.

Tippett LJ, Glosser G, Farah MJ: A category-specific naming deficit after temporal lobectomy. *Neuropsychologia.* 34:139–146, 1996.

Tippett LJ, Grossman M, Farah MJ: The semantic memory deficit of Alzheimer's disease: category-specific? *Cortex* 32:143–153, 1996.

Tulving E: Episodic and semantic memory, in Tulving E, Donaldson W (eds): *Organization of Memory.* New York: Academic Press, 1972.

Vandenberghe R, Price C, Wise R, et al: Functional anatomy of a common semantic system for words and pictures. *Nature* 383:254–256, 1996.

Warrington EK: The selective impairment of semantic memory. *Q J Exp Psychol* 27:635–657, 1975.

Warrington EK, McCarthy R: Category specific access dysphasia. *Brain* 106:859–878, 1983.

Warrington EK, McCarthy R: Categories of knowledge: Further fractionations and an attempted explanation. *Brain* 110:1273–1296, 1987.

Warrington EK, Shallice T: Category specific semantic impairments. *Brain* 107:829–854, 1984.

Chapter 28

ACALCULIA AND NUMBER PROCESSING DISORDERS

Stanislas Dehaene

The foundation for the amazing successes of our species in science and technology lies in our ability to do mathematics. Although little is known about the cerebral substrates of mathematics in general, one of its subareas, elementary arithmetic, has received considerable attention from cognitive neuroscientists. The present chapter reviews the organization of the number system from the point of view of cognitive neuropsychology. Brain lesions can selectively affect several components of the number processing system, revealing a highly organized brain architecture for arithmetic that is now being confirmed and refined by brain imaging methods. Current results indicate that (1) the number system is segregated from other symbolic processing systems at multiple levels; (2) parietal lobe lesions can interfere with the semantic component of number processing; (3) dissociations between operations are frequently observed, suggesting that multiple parietal circuits contribute to arithmetic; and (4) developmental disorders of calculation, possibly of genetic origin, can be traced to pre- or perinatal pathology often affecting the parietal lobe.

THE ISOLATION OF THE NUMBER PROCESSING SYSTEM

The specialization of the number processing system can be inferred from the observation that, at virtually all levels of processing, dissociations have been observed between numbers and the rest of language. For instance, high-level calculation abilities may be spared in patients with severe global aphasia (Rossor et al., 1995) or impaired short-term memory (Butterworth et al., 1996). At the visual identification level, pure alexic patients who fail to read words often show a largely preserved ability to read and process digits (Cohen and Dehaene, 1995; Déjerine, 1891; Déjerine, 1892). Con-

versely, a case of impaired number reading with preserved word reading is on record (Cipolotti et al., 1995). In the writing domain, severe agraphia and alexia may be accompanied by a fully preserved ability to write and read arabic numbers (Anderson et al., 1990). Even within the speech production system, patients who suffer from random phoneme substitutions, thus resulting in the production of an incomprehensible jargon, may produce jargon-free number words (Cohen et al., 1997).

Most importantly, numbers may doubly dissociate from other categories of words at the semantic level, suggesting the existence of a category-specific semantic system for numerical quantities. Spared calculation and number comprehension abilities have been described in patients with grossly deteriorated semantic processing (Thioux et al., 1998) or semantic dementia (Butterworth et al., 2001; Cappelletti et al., 2001). The converse dissociation is also on record. Cipolotti and coworkers (1991) first reported a striking case of a patient with a small left parietal lesion and an almost complete deficit in all spheres of number processing, sparing only the numbers 1 through 4, in the context of otherwise largely preserved language and semantic functions. Although such a severe degradation of the number system has never been replicated, other cases, discussed further below, confirm that the understanding of numbers and their relations can be specifically impaired in the context of preserved language and semantics (e.g., Dehaene and Cohen, 1997; Delazer and Benke, 1997).

THE CENTRAL ROLE OF THE PARIETAL LOBE AND ACALCULIA

The parietal lobe appears to play a central role in number processing. It has been known since the beginning of this century that parietal lesions, usually in the dominant hemisphere, can cause calculation deficits. Gerstmann (1940) reported the frequent co-occurence of agraphia, acalculia, finger agnosia, and left-right confusion in parietal cases, a tetrad of deficits referred to as Gerstmann's syndrome (although the elements of the syndrome are now known to be dissociable; see Benton, 1992). The lesions that cause acalculia of the Gerstmann's type are typically centered on the portion of the left intraparietal sulcus that sits immediately behind the angular gyrus (Brodman's area 39) (Mayer et al., 1999; Takayama et al., 1994). In many cases, the deficit can be extremely incapacitating. Patients may fail to compute operations as simple as 2 + 2, 3 − 1, or 3 × 9. Several characteristics indicate that the deficit arises at a rather abstract level of processing. First, patients may remain fully able to comprehend and to produce numbers in all formats. Second, they show the same calculation difficulties whether the problem is presented to them visually or auditorily and whether they have to respond verbally or in writing, or even merely have to decide whether a proposed operation is true or false. Thus, the calculation deficit is not due to an inability to identify the numbers or to produce the operation result. Rather, patients with inferior parietal lesions and acalculia of the Gerstmann type suffer from a category-specific impairment of the semantic representation and manipulation of numerical quantities (Dehaene and Cohen, 1995, 1997).

One patient, Mr. Mar (Dehaene and Cohen, 1997), experienced severe difficulties in calculation, especially with single-digit subtraction (75 percent errors). He failed on problems as simple as 3 − 1, with the comment that he no longer knew what the operation meant. His failure was not tied to a specific modality of input or output, because the problems were simultaneously presented visually and read out loud and because he failed in both overt production and covert multiple-choice tests. Moreover, he also erred on tasks outside of calculation per se, such as deciding which of two numbers is the larger (16 percent errors) or what number falls in the middle of two others (bisection task: 77 percent errors). He easily performed analogous comparison and bisection tasks in nonnumerical domains such as days of the week, months, or the alphabet (What is between Tuesday and Thursday? February and April? B and D?), indicating that he suffered from a category-specific deficit for numbers. This and similar

patients (Delazer and Benke, 1997; Takayama et al., 1994) suggest that parietal lesions can cause a selective disturbance to the central representation of numerical quantity.

BRAIN-IMAGING STUDIES OF NUMBER PROCESSING

The involvement of parietal cortex in number processing is confirmed by brain imaging studies in normal subjects. Roland and Friberg (1985) were the first to monitor blood-flow changes during calculation as opposed to rest. When subjects repeatedly subtracted 3 from a given number, activation increased bilaterally in inferior parietal and prefrontal cortex. These localizations were later confirmed using functional magnetic resonance imaging (fMRI) (Burbaud et al., 1995; Rueckert et al., 1996). A positron emission tomography (PET) study of multiplication and comparison of digit pairs revealed bilateral parietal activation confined to the intraparietal region (Dehaene et al., 1996), in agreement with lesion data. Several recent brain-imaging studies all confirm the involvement of bilateral parietal cortices in calculation (Burbaud et al., 1999; Chochon et al., 1999; Dehaene et al., 1999; Pesenti et al., 2000; Rueckert et al., 1996; Zago et al., 2001).

Several features of the inferior parietal contribution to number processing have been clarified by imaging methods. First, the parietal region is active whenever an arithmetic operation or the mere comprehension of the size of a number is called for (Chochon et al., 1999; Dehaene et al., 1999). Second, its activation is proportional to the number of calculations performed per unit of time (Menon et al., 2000). Third, its activation is independent of the particular input or output modalities used to convey the numbers, such as arabic or spelled-out numerals, suggesting that parietal cortex may be coding the abstract meaning of numbers rather than the numerical symbols themselves (Dehaene, 1996; Kiefer and Dehaene, 1997; Pinel et al., 2001). Fourth, the amount of activation correlates directly with the complexity of an arithmetic operation. Thus, event-related potentials (ERPs) and fMRI recordings in a number comparison task reveal that intraparietal activity is modulated by the numerical distance separating the numbers to be compared

(Dehaene et al., 1996; Pinel et al., 2001). Moreover, inferior parietal activity is larger and lasts longer during operations with large numbers than with small numbers (Kiefer and Dehaene, 1997; Stanescu-Cosson et al., 2000). Fifth, parietal activation during number processing can be found even when the subject is not aware of having been presented with a subliminal number (Dehaene et al., 1998; Naccache and Dehaene, 2001). I suggest that parietal cortices provide us with a "numerical intuition," a permanent and often implicit reference to the meaningful size of a numerical quantity in relation to others on the "mental number line" (Dehaene, 1992; Dehaene, 1997). Patients in whom this unconscious reference is impaired suffer a drastic loss of stable reference in the numerical domain.

DISSOCIATIONS BETWEEN OPERATIONS

Although the inferior parietal region seems to play a crucial role in number sense, it is important to note that it is not the only brain region involved in number processing in adults. The phrenologic notion that a single area can hold all the knowledge about an entire domain such as arithmetic has to give way to a more parallel view of number processing in the brain. Multiple brain areas are involved, whether for identifying arabic numerals, writing them down, understanding spoken number words, retrieving multiplication facts from memory, or organizing a sequence of multidigit calculations (Caramazza and McCloskey, 1987; Dehaene and Cohen, 1995; McCloskey and Caramazza, 1987; McCloskey et al., 1992). Correspondingly, a great variety of brain-lesioned patients with number processing deficits, too broad to be reviewed here, have been described.

One of the most striking dissociations occurs among different arithmetic operations. It is not rare for a patient to be much more severely impaired in multiplication than in subtraction (Cohen and Dehaene, 2000; Dagenbach and McCloskey, 1992; Dehaene and Cohen, 1997; Lampl et al., 1994; Pesenti et al., 1994), while other patients are much more impaired in subtraction than in multiplication (Dehaene and Cohen, 1997; Delazer and Benke, 1997). It may not be necessary, however, to postulate as many brain circuits as there are

arithmetical operations (although see van Harskamp and Cipolotti, 2001). Rather, such dissociations may reflect a basic distinction between overlearned arithmetic facts such as the multiplication table, which are stored in rote verbal memory, and the genuine understanding of number meaning that underlies non-table operations such as subtraction (Dehaene and Cohen, 1997; Delazer and Benke, 1997; Hittmair-Delazer et al., 1995). Indeed, patients with impaired multiplication often have associated aphasia and lesions within the left perisylvian areas (Cohen et al., 2000) or left basal ganglia (Dehaene and Cohen, 1997), while patients with impaired subtraction tend to have lesions in the left intraparietal region outside of language cortex per se.

Brain imaging has confirmed that different operations rely on partially dissociable parietal circuits, with bilateral intraparietal activation during subtraction and more posterior and left-lateralized subangular activation during multiplication (Chochon et al., 1999; Lee, 2000). Brain imaging also indicates that those parietal circuits are differentially called upon during exact calculation and approximation (Dehaene et al., 1999): exact calculation of addition problems is dependent on language and causes relatively greater activation of the left anterior inferior frontal region and the angular gyrus, while approximation of quantities is independent of language and causes greater activation of the bilateral intraparietal sulci. This finding may explain why some patients with severe deficits of exact calculation may remain able to compute approximations of the desired result (Dehaene and Cohen, 1991; Warrington, 1982).

HEMISPHERIC SPECIALIZATION

There is an as yet unresolved discrepancy between brain imaging and neuropsychological findings. On the one hand, the parietal activations during number processing tend to be bilateral, though often with increasingly greater left lateralization as the task requires exact calculation and arithmetic tables (e.g., Chochon et al., 1999). On the other hand, the lesion site for acalculia and Gerstmann's syndrome appears strictly lateralized to the dominant left parietal lobe. Although this is not fully understood yet, the issue may be partially clarified by studies of split-field presentations in callosal patients (Cohen and Dehaene, 1996; Gazzaniga and Hillyard, 1971; Gazzaniga and Smylie, 1984; Seymour et al., 1994). Those studies confirm that both hemispheres can process digits and quantities at the semantic level. When two digits are presented simultaneously *within* the same hemifield, split-brain patients experience no difficulty deciding whether they are the same or different (while their disconnection renders them completely unable to compare two digits *across* the two hemifields). Hence, both hemispheres can analyze digit shapes. Furthermore, both hemispheres can also point to the larger digit (or to the smaller), and both can classify digits or even two-digit numbers as larger or smaller than some reference. Hence, both hemispheres seem to possess a quantity representation of numbers.

There are, however, at least two striking differences between the numerical abilities of the left and the right hemispheres. First, digits presented to the left hemisphere can be named normally by the patients, but digits presented to the right hemisphere cannot. This is in keeping with the well-known lateralization of speech production abilities to the left hemisphere. Second, split-brain patients can calculate only with digits presented to their left hemisphere. When digits are presented to their right hemisphere, the patients fail with operations as simple as adding 2, multiplying by 3, subtracting from 10, or dividing by 2. This is the case even when they merely have to point to the correct result among several possible results or to indicate nonverbally whether a proposed result is correct or not. The only calculation ability that seems to be available to an isolated right hemisphere, at least occasionally, is approximation. A patient might not be able to decide whether $2 + 2$ makes 4 or 5, but might still easily notice that $2 + 2$ cannot make 9 (Cohen and Dehaene, 1996; Dehaene and Cohen, 1991). It has been suggested that the right hemisphere may have a special role in the "abstraction of numerical relations" (Langdon and Warrington, 1997).

DEVELOPMENTAL DYSCALCULIA

Deficits of number processing can be observed in adults with acquired brain lesions, but also in young children. Developmental dyscalculia, coarsely defined as a

failure on standardized tests of arithmetic independently of IQ or social factors, is not rare. Kosc (1974) reported an incidence of 6.4 percent in a sample of 375 children between the age of 10 and 12. Badian (1983) studied 1476 children between 7 and 14 years of age and observed that 2.7 percent had both reading and mathematical deficits, another 3.6 percent only had difficulties in mathematics, and yet another 2.5 percent only in reading. In another study in Great Britain, those figures were 2.3, 1.3, and 3.9 percent (Lewis et al., 1994). Other family members are frequently affected, suggesting that genetic factors may contribute to the disorder (Shalev et al., 2001).

A variety of systems of classification of developmental dyscalculia have been proposed. Badian (1983) used a terminology initially proposed for adult acalculia cases (Hécaen et al., 1961) to distinguish dyscalculia due to a reading or writing deficit, spatial dyscalculia due to an inability to organize the figures on a page, dyscalculia due to attentional disorders, and anarithmia proper. Kosc (1974) adopted a similar though more complex classification. Simpler categories were achieved by Temple (1991, 1994) on the basis of Caramazza and McCloskey's model of number processing (Caramazza and McCloskey, 1987; McCloskey and Caramazza, 1987; McCloskey et al., 1992). She distinguished dyscalculia due to a failure to process the number notations (e.g., difficulties in reading or in writing arabic numerals); arithmetic fact dyscalculia, or a failure to store and retrieve arithmetic tables; and procedural dyscalculia, or an inability to execute a multidigit calculation in the correct sequence. A particularly striking double dissociation between arithmetic fact and procedural dyscalculia was reported, strengthening the hypothesis that cases of developmental dyscalculia can be as selective as adult neuropsychological cases (Temple, 1991). A similar approach has been adopted to analyze a single case of number-notation dyscalculia (Sullivan et al., 1996) and two series of cases with various subtypes of developmental dyscalculia (Ashcraft et al., 1992; Sokol et al., 1994).

In a series of publications, Geary and colleagues have focused on developmental calculation deficits and have attempted to characterize their origins (Geary, 1990, 1993, 1994; Geary et al., 1992; Geary and Brown, 1991; Geary et al., 1991; Geary et al., 1986; Geary et al., 1987). In comparison to normal children, they report that dyscalculic children use immature calculation strategies, largely based on counting; make an improper choice of strategy; and show a slower evolution in their strategies with time. Dyscalculic children also have a poorer short-term memory span for digits (Geary et al., 1991; Hitch and McAuley, 1991). Most interestingly, some dyscalculic children may suffer from a lack of understanding of the counting principles proposed by Gelman and Gallistel (1978), suggesting that some of them at least may have a fundamental deficit in understanding the conceptual bases of arithmetic (Geary et al., 1992).

The notion that at least some children with developmental dyscalculia may suffer from a core conceptual deficit is supported by the existence of a "developmental Gerstmann syndrome" in children (Benson and Geschwind, 1970; Kinsbourne and Warrington, 1963; Spellacy and Peter, 1978; Temple, 1989; Temple, 1991). Like in adults, the calculation deficit is accompanied by most or all of the following symptoms: dysgraphia, left-right disorientation, and finger agnosia, which suggest a neurologic involvement of the parietal lobe. Interestingly, even in a sample of 200 normal children, a test of finger knowledge appears to be a better predictor of later arithmetic abilities than is a test of general intelligence (Fayol et al., 1998), again supporting a tight correlation between number knowledge and finger knowledge in the parietal lobe.

Very few imaging studies to date have been dedicated to developmental dyscalculia. Levy et al. (1999) report the case of an adult with lifelong isolated dyscalculia together with superior intelligence and reading ability, in whom the standard anatomic MRI appeared normal, yet MR spectroscopy techniques revealed a metabolic abnormality in the left inferior parietal area, exactly where a lesion would be expected in an adult Gerstmann syndrome case. Similarly, Isaacs and coworkers used voxel-based morphometry to compare gray matter density in adolescents born at equally severe grades of prematurity, half of whom suffered from dyscalculia (Isaacs et al., 2001). They found a single region of reduced gray matter in the left intraparietal sulcus, coinciding precisely with the site of fMRI activations during calculation in normal subjects. Those studies strengthen the hypothesis that early parietal dysfunction may underlie isolated developmental dyscalculia.

TURNER'S SYNDROME: DYSCALCULIA OF GENETIC ORIGIN?

If the parietal lobe involvement for arithmetic results at least in part from a genetic predisposition, then one would expect to find genetic diseases targeting the parietal region and causing dyscalculia. Although the search for such dyscalculias of genetic origin has only very recently begun, the possibility that Turner syndrome may conform to this typology has recently attracted attention. Turner syndrome is a genetic disorder characterized by partial or complete absence of one X chromosome in a female individual. The disorder occurs in approximately 1 girl in 2000 and is associated with well-documented physical disorders and abnormal estrogen production and pubertal development. The cognitive profile includes deficits in visual memory, visuospatial and attentional tasks, and social relations, in the context of a normal verbal IQ (Rovet, 1993). Most interestingly in the present context is the documentation of a mild to severe deficit in mathematics, particularly clear in arithmetic (Mazzocco, 1998; Rovet et al., 1994; Temple and Marriott, 1998). Anatomically, the data suggest possible bilateral parietooccipital dysfunction. A positron emission tomography study of five adult women demonstrated a glucose hypometabolism in bilateral parietal and occipital regions (Clark et al., 1990). Two anatomic MRI studies, one with 18 and the other with 30 affected women, demonstrated bilateral reductions in parietooccipital brain volume, together with other subcortical regions (Murphy et al., 1993; see also Reiss et al., 1993, 1995). Interestingly, the phenotype of Turner syndrome can differ depending on whether the remaining X chromosome is of paternal or maternal origin (Xm or Xp subtypes) (Bishop et al., 2000; Skuse, 2000; Skuse et al., 1997). Such a genomic imprinting effect was first demonstrated on tests of social competence (Skuse et al., 1997). It will be interesting to see if a similar effect exists in the arithmetic domain.

CONCLUSION

In this review, we have focused on the large empirical database of patients with number processing deficits. Detailed theoretical models of those deficits have been published (see, e.g., Caramazza and McCloskey, 1987; Dehaene and Cohen, 1995; McCloskey and Caramazza, 1987; McCloskey et al., 1992) and have been related to cognitive psychological, developmental, and animal research (Dehaene, 1997). As our knowledge of the normal and pathological organization of the number processing system increases, it may eventually become possible to design cognitive rehabilitation programs based on a more accurate anatomic and functional characterization of the impairment (for early attempts, see Girelli et al., 1996; Sullivan et al., 1996).

REFERENCES

Anderson SW, Damasio AR, Damasio H: Troubled letters but not numbers. Domain specific cognitive impairments following focal damage in frontal cortex. *Brain* 113, 749–766, 1990.

Ashcraft MH, Yamashita TS, Aram DM: Mathematics performance in left and right brain-lesioned children and adolescents. *Brain Cogn* 19:208–252, 1992.

Badian NA: Dyscalculia and nonverbal disorders of learning, in Myklebust HR (ed): *Progress in Learning Disabilities* New York: Stratton, 1983, vol 5, pp 235–264.

Benson DF, Geschwind N: Developmental Gerstmann syndrome. *Neurology* 20:293–298, 1970.

Benton AL: Gerstmann's syndrome. *Arch Neurol* 49:445–447, 1992.

Bishop DV, Canning E, Elgar K, et al: Distinctive patterns of memory function in subgroups of females with Turner syndrome: Evidence for imprinted loci on the X-chromosome affecting neurodevelopment. *Neuropsychologia* 38(5):712–721, 2000.

Burbaud P, Camus O, Guehl D, et al: A functional magnetic resonance imaging study of mental subtraction in human subjects. *Neurosci Lett* 273(3):195–199, 1999.

Burbaud P, Degreze P, Lafon P, et al: Lateralization of prefrontal activation during internal mental calculation: A functional magnetic resonance imaging study. *J Neurophysiol* 74:2194–2200, 1995.

Butterworth B, Cappelletti M, Kopelman M: Category specificity in reading and writing: The case of number words. *Nat Neurosci* 4(8):784–786, 2001.

Butterworth B, Cipolotti L, Warrington EK: Short-term memory impairment and arithmetical ability. *Q J Exp Psychol* 49A:251–262, 1996.

Cappelletti M, Butterworth B, Kopelman M: Spared numerical abilities in a case of semantic dementia. *Neuropsychologia* 39(11):1224–1239, 2001.

Caramazza A, McCloskey M: Dissociations of calculation processes, in Deloche G, Seron X (eds): *Mathematical Disabilities: A Cognitive Neuropsychological Perspective.* Hillsdale, NJ: Erlbaum, 1987, 221–234.

Chochon F, Cohen L, van de Moortele PF, Dehaene S: Differential contributions of the left and right inferior parietal lobules to number processing. *J Cogn Neurosci* 11:617–630, 1999.

Cipolotti L, Butterworth B, Denes G: A specific deficit for numbers in a case of dense acalculia. *Brain* 114:2619–2637, 1991.

Cipolotti L, Warrington EK, Butterworth B: Selective impairment in manipulating arabic numerals. *Cortex* 31:73–86, 1995.

Clark C, Klonoff H, Hadyen M: Regional cerebral glucose metabolism in Turner syndrome. *Can J Neurol Sci* 17:140–144, 1990.

Cohen L, Dehaene S: Number processing in pure alexia: The effect of hemispheric asymmetries and task demands. *Neurocase* 1:121–137, 1995.

Cohen L, Dehaene S: Cerebral networks for number processing: Evidence from a case of posterior callosal lesion. *Neurocase* 2:155–174, 1996.

Cohen L, Dehaene S: Calculating without reading: Unsuspected residual abilities in pure alexia. *Cogn Neuropsychol* 17(6):563–583, 2000.

Cohen L, Dehaene S, Chochon F, et al: Language and calculation within the parietal lobe: A combined cognitive, anatomical and fMRI study. *Neuropsychologia* 38:1426–1440, 2000.

Cohen L, Verstichel P, Dehaene S: Neologistic jargon sparing numbers: A category specific phonological impairment. *Cogn Neuropsychol* 14:1029–1061, 1997.

Dagenbach D, McCloskey M: The organization of arithmetic facts in memory: Evidence from a brain-damaged patient. *Brain Cogn* 20:345–366, 1992.

Dehaene S: Varieties of numerical abilities. *Cognition* 44:1–42, 1992.

Dehaene S: The organization of brain activations in number comparison: Event-related potentials and the additive-factors methods. *J Cogn Neurosci* 8:47–68, 1996.

Dehaene S: *The Number Sense.* New York: Oxford University Press, 1997.

Dehaene S, Cohen L: Two mental calculation systems: A case study of severe acalculia with preserved approximation. *Neuropsychologia* 29:1045–1074, 1991.

Dehaene S, Cohen L: Towards an anatomical and functional model of number processing. *Math Cogn* 1:83–120, 1995.

Dehaene S, Cohen L: Cerebral pathways for calculation: Double dissociation between rote verbal and quantitative knowledge of arithmetic. *Cortex* 33:219–250, 1997.

Dehaene S, Naccache L, Le Clec'H G, et al: Imaging unconscious semantic priming. *Nature* 395:597–600, 1998.

Dehaene S, Spelke E, Stanescu R, et al: Sources of mathematical thinking: Behavioral and brain-imaging evidence. *Science* 284:970–974, 1999.

Dehaene S, Tzourio N, Frak V, et al: Cerebral activations during number multiplication and comparison: A PET study. *Neuropsychologia* 34:1097–1106, 1996.

Déjerine J: Sur un cas de cécité verbale avec agraphie suivi d'autopsie. *Mem Soc Biol* 3:197–201, 1891.

Déjerine J: Contribution à l'étude anatomo-pathologique et clinique des différentes variétés de cécité verbale. *Mem Soc Biol* 4:61–90, 1892.

Delazer M, Benke T: Arithmetic facts without meaning. *Cortex* 33(4):697–710, 1997.

Fayol M, Barrouillet P, Marinthe X: Predicting arithmetical achievement from neuropsychological performance: A longitudinal study. *Cognition* 68:B63–B70, 1998.

Gazzaniga MS, Hillyard SA: Language and speech capacity of the right hemisphere. *Neuropsychologia* 9:273–280, 1971.

Gazzaniga MS, Smylie CE: Dissociation of language and cognition: A psychological profile of two disconnected right hemispheres. *Brain* 107:145–153, 1984.

Geary DC: A componential analysis of an early learning deficit in mathematics. *J Exp Child Psychol* 49:363–383, 1990.

Geary DC: Mathematical disabilities: Cognitive, neuropsychological and genetic components. *Psychol Bull* 114:345–362, 1993.

Geary DC: *Children's Mathematical Development.* Washington DC: American Psychological Association, 1994.

Geary DC, Bow-Thomas CC, Yao Y: Counting knowledge and skill in cognitive addition: A comparison of normal and mathematically disabled children. *J Exp Child Psychol* 54:372–391, 1992.

Geary DC, Brown SC: Cognitive addition: strategy choice and speed-of-processing differences in gifted, normal, and mathematically disabled children. *Dev Psychol* 27:398–406, 1991.

Geary DC, Brown SC, Samaranayake VA: Cognitive addition: A short longitudinal study of strategy choice and speed-of-processing differences in normal and mathematically disabled children. *Dev Psychol* 27:787–797, 1991.

Geary DC, Widaman KF, Little TD: Cognitive addition and multiplication: Evidence for a single memory network. *Mem Cogn* 14:478–487, 1986.

Geary DC, Widaman KF, Little TD, Cormier P: Cognitive addition: Comparison of learning disabled and academically normal elementary school children. *Cogn Dev* 2:249–269, 1987.

Gelman R, Gallistel CR: *The Child's Understanding of Number.* Cambridge, MA: Harvard University Press, 1978.

Gerstmann J: Syndrome of finger agnosia, disorientation for right and left, agraphia, and acalculia. *Arch Neurol Psychiatry* 44:398–408, 1940.

Girelli L Delazer M, Semenza C, Denes G: The representation of arithmetical facts: Evidence from two rehabilitation studies. *Cortex* 32(1):49–66, 1996.

Hécaen H, Angelergues R, Houillier S: Les variétés cliniques des acalculies au cours des lésions rétro-rolandiques: approche statistique du problème. *Rev Neurol* 105:85–103, 1961.

Hitch GJ, McAuley E: Working memory in children with specific arithmetical difficulties. *Br J Psychol* 82:375–386, 1991.

Hittmair-Delazer M, Sailer U, Benke T: Impaired arithmetic facts but intact conceptual knowledge—a single case study of dyscalculia. *Cortex* 31:139–147, 1995.

Isaacs EB, Edmonds CJ, Lucas A, Gadian DG: Calculation difficulties in children of very low birthweight: A neural correlate. *Brain* 124(Pt 9):1701–1707, 2001.

Kiefer M, Dehaene S: The time course of parietal activation in single-digit multiplication: Evidence from event-related potentials. *Math Cogn* 3:1–30, 1997.

Kinsbourne M, Warrington EK: The developmental Gerstmann syndrome. *Arch Neurol* 8: 490, 1963.

Kosc L: Developmental dyscalculia. *J Learn Disabil* 7:165–177, 1974.

Lampl Y, Eshel Y, Gilad R, Sarova-Pinhas I: Selective acalculia with sparing of the subtraction process in a patient with left parietotemporal hemorrhage. *Neurology* 44:1759–1761, 1994.

Langdon DW, Warrington EK: The abstraction of numerical relations: A role for the right hemisphere in arithmetic? *J Int Neuropsychol Soc* 3:260–268, 1997.

Lee KM: Cortical areas differentially involved in multiplication and subtraction: A functional magnetic resonance imaging study and correlation with a case of selective acalculia. *Ann Neurol* 48:657–661, 2000.

Levy LM, Reis IL, Grafman J: Metabolic abnormalities detected by H-MRS in dyscalculia and dysgraphia. *Neurology* 53:639–641, 1999.

Lewis C, Hitch GJ, Walker P: The prevalence of specific arithmetic difficulties and specific reading difficulties in 9- and 10-year-old boys and girls. *J Child Psychol Psychiatry* 35:283–292, 1994.

Mayer E, Martory MD, Pegna AJ, et al: A pure case of Gerstmann syndrome with a subangular lesion. *Brain* 122 (Pt 6):1107–1120, 1999.

Mazzocco MM: A process approach to describing mathematics difficulties in girls with Turner syndrome. *Pediatrics* 102(2 Pt 3):492–496, 1998.

McCloskey M, Caramazza A: Cognitive mechanisms in normal and impaired number processing, in Deloche G, Seron X (eds): *Mathematical Disabilities: A Cognitive Neuropsychological Perspective.* Hillsdale, NJ: Erlbaum, 1987, pp 201–219.

McCloskey M, Macaruso P, Whetstone T: The functional architecture of numerical processing mechanisms: Defending the modular model, in Campbell JID (ed): *The Nature and Origins of Mathematical Skills.* Amsterdam: Elsevier, 1992, pp 493–537.

Menon V, Rivera SM, White CD, et al: Dissociating prefrontal and parietal cortex activation during arithmetic processing. *Neuroimage* 12(4):357–365, 2000.

Murphy DG, DeCarli C, Daly E, et al: X-chromosome effects on female brain: A magnetic resonance imaging study of Turner's syndrome [see comments]. *Lancet* 342(8881):1197–1200, 1993.

Naccache L, Dehaene S: The priming method: imaging unconscious repetition priming reveals an abstract representation of number in the parietal lobes. *Cereb Cortex* 11(10):966–974, 2001.

Pesenti M, Seron X, van der Linden M: Selective impairment as evidence for mental organisation of arithmetical facts: BB, a case of preserved subtraction? *Cortex* 30(4):661–671, 1994.

Pesenti M, Thioux M, Seron X, De Volder A: Neuroanatomical substrates of arabic number processing, numerical comparison, and simple addition: a PET study. *J Cogn Neurosci* 12(3): 461–479, 2000.

Pinel P, Rivière D, Le Bihan D, Dehaene S: Modulation of parietal activation by semantic distance in a number comparison task. *Neuroimage* 14(5):1013–1026, 2001.

Reiss AL, Freund L, Plotnick L, et al: The effects of X monosomy on brain development: monozygotic twins discordant for Turner's syndrome. *Ann Neurol* 34(1):95–107, 1993.

Reiss AL, Mazzocco MM, Greenlaw R, et al: Neurodevelopmental effects of X monosomy: A volumetric imaging study. *Ann Neurol* 38(5):731–738, 1995.

Roland PE, Friberg L: Localization of cortical areas activated by thinking. *J Neurophysiol* 53:1219–1243, 1985.

Rossor MN, Warrington EK, Cipolotti L: The isolation of calculation skills. *J Neurol* 242(2):78–81, 1995.

Rovet J, Szekely C, Hockenberry MN: Specific arithmetic calculation deficits in children with Turner syndrome. *J Clin Exp Neuropsychol* 16(6):820–839, 1994.

Rovet JF: The psychoeducational characteristics of children with Turner syndrome. *J Learn Disabil* 26(5):333–341, 1993.

Rueckert L, Lange N, Partiot A, et al: Visualizing cortical activation during mental calculation with functional MRI. *Neuroimage* 3:97–103, 1996.

Seymour SE, Reuter-Lorenz PA, Gazzaniga MS: The disconnection syndrome: Basic findings reaffirmed. *Brain* 117:105–115, 1994.

Shalev RS, Manor O, Kerem B, et al: Developmental dyscalculia is a familial learning disability. *J Learn Disabil* 34:59–65, 2001.

Skuse DH: Imprinting, the X-chromosome, and the male brain: Explaining sex differences in the liability to autism. *Pediatr Res* 47(1):9–16, 2000.

Skuse DH, James RS, Bishop DV, et al: Evidence from Turner's syndrome of an imprinted X-linked locus affecting cognitive function [see comments]. *Nature* 387(6634):705–708, 1997.

Sokol SM, Macaruso P, Gollan TH: Developmental dyscalculia and cognitive neuropsychology. *Dev Neuropsychol* 10:413–441, 1994.

Spellacy F, Peter B: Dyscalculia and elements of the developmental Gerstmann syndrome in school children. *Cortex* 14:197–206, 1978.

Stanescu-Cosso, R, Pinel P, van de Moortele PF, et al: Cerebral bases of calculation processes: Impact of number size on the cerebral circuits for exact and approximate calculation. *Brain* 123:2240–2255, 2000.

Sullivan K S, Macaruso P, Sokol SM: Remediation of arabic number processing in a case of developmental dyscalculia. *Neuropsychol Rehabil* 6:27–53, 1996.

Takayama Y, Sugishita M, Akiguch I, Kimura J, et al: Isolated acalculia due to left parietal lesion. *Arch. Neurol* 51:286–291, 1994.

Temple CM: Digit dyslexia: A category-specific disorder in development dyscalculia. *Cogn Neuropsychol* 6:93–116, 1989.

Temple CM: Procedural dyscalculia and number fact dyscalculia: double dissociation in developmental dyscalculia. *Cogn Neuropsychol* 8:155–176, 1991.

Temple CM: The cognitive neuropsychology of the developmental dyscalculias. *Cah Psychol Cogn /Curr Psychol Cogn* 13:351–370, 1994.

Temple CM, Marriott AJ: Arithmetic ability and disability in Turner's syndrome: A cognitive neuropsychological analysis. *Dev Neuropsychol* 14:47–67, 1998.

Thioux M, Pillon A, Samson D, et al: The isolation of numerals at the semantic level. *Neurocase* 4:371–389, 1998.

van Harskamp NJ, Cipolotti L: Selective impairments for addition, subtraction and multiplication. Implications for the organisation of arithmetical facts. *Cortex* 37(3):363–388, 2001.

Warrington EK: The fractionation of arithmetical skills: A single case study. *Q J Exp Psychol* 34A:31–51, 1982.

Zago L, Pesenti M, Mellet E, et al: Neural correlates of simple and complex mental calculation. *Neuroimage* 13(2): 314–327, 2001.

Chapter 29

DISORDERS OF SKILLED MOVEMENTS: LIMB APRAXIA

Kenneth M. Heilman
Robert T. Watson
Leslie J. Gonzalez Rothi

Apraxia is an inability to correctly perform learned skilled movements. In part, it is defined by what it is not.[1] Patients with impaired motor performance induced by weakness, sensory loss, tremors, dystonia, chorea, ballismus, athetosis, myoclonus, ataxia, and seizures are not considered apraxic. Patients with severe cognitive, memory, motivational, and attentional disorders may have difficulty performing skilled motor acts because they cannot comprehend, cooperate, remember, or attend, but these deficits are also not considered apraxic.

Limb apraxia may be the most frequently unrecognized behavioral disorder associated with cerebral disease. It is most often associated with strokes and degenerative dementia of the Alzheimer type but also occurs with a variety of other diseases. For example, apraxia may be the presenting symptom and sign in corticobasal ganglionic degeneration.

Apraxia may go unrecognized for several reasons. The apraxia associated with strokes is often accompanied by weakness of the preferred arm. In attempting to perform skilled acts with the nonpreferred arm, apraxic patients may recognize that they are not performing well, but they may attribute their difficulty in performing skilled acts to the inexperience of this nondominant arm or to premorbid clumsiness of the nonpreferred arm. However, even when using their dominant limb, apraxic patients may be anosognosic for their apraxia[2] and therefore will not complain of a problem in performing skilled movements. Finally, many physicians and other health professionals do not test for limb apraxia and are not aware of the nature of the errors associated with it or that it may be a disabling disorder.

The types of limb apraxia are defined by the nature of errors made by the patient and the means by which these errors are elicited. Liepmann[3] subdivided limb apraxic disorders into three types: melokinetic (or limb kinetic), ideomotor, and ideational. In addition to discussing these forms of apraxia, three additional forms of apraxia are discussed below, which we have called *disassociation apraxia, conduction apraxia,* and *conceptual apraxia.*

APRAXIA TESTING

The physician must perform a thorough neurologic examination to be certain that abnormal performance is not induced by the nonapraxic motor, sensory, or cognitive disorders mentioned above. The presence of elemental motor defects does not prohibit apraxia testing; however, the examiner must interpret the results with the knowledge gained from the neurologic examination.

Both the right and left forelimbs should be tested independently. Patients should be requested to pantomime to verbal command (e.g., "Show me how you would use a pair of scissors"). All patients should also be asked to imitate the examiner's gestures. The examiner may want to perform both meaningful and meaningless gestures for the patient to imitate. Independent of the results of the pantomime and imitation tests, the patient should be given actual objects and tools and asked to demonstrate how to use the tool or object. One should test transitive movements (i.e., using a tool or instrument) and intransitive movements (i.e., communicative gestures not using tools, such as waving good-bye). When having a patient pantomime, in addition to giving verbal commands, the examiner may also want to show the patient a tool or a picture of the tool or object that the patient is required to pantomime. It may be valuable to see if the patient can recognize transitive and intransitive pantomimes performed by the examiner and discriminate between those that are well and poorly performed. To assess deftness (dexterity) the examiner measures speed, precision, and independent finger movement (e.g., rapid finger tapping; pegboard coin rotation between the thumb, index, and middle finger). The patient should be given a task that requires several motor acts in sequence. Finally, one may want to learn if the patient knows what tools operate on what objects (e.g., hammer and nail), what action is associated with each tool or object, and how to fabricate tools to solve mechanical problems.

LIMB KINETIC APRAXIA

In limb kinetic apraxia, there is a loss of the ability to make finely graded, precise, individual finger movements—a loss of deftness. Limb kinetic apraxia occurs primarily in the limb contralateral to a hemispheric lesion. Right-handed people who have left hemispheric dysfunction may also develop limb kinetic apraxia of their left ipsilesional forelimb.[4,5] Lawrence and Kuypers[6] demonstrated that monkeys with lesions confined to the corticospinal system show similar errors. We have noted that patients with convexity premotor lesions also have limb kinetic apraxia.

IDEOMOTOR APRAXIA

Clinical Findings

Patients with ideomotor apraxia (IMA) make the most errors when asked to pantomime transitive acts. They typically improve with imitation and may perform the best when using actual tools with actual objects.

We classify apraxic errors as errors of content or of production.[7] In order to be considered as having IMA, a patient should make primarily production errors. Content errors occur when a patient substitutes an incorrect but recognizable pantomime for the target pantomime. For example, when asked to pantomime using scissors, a patient may demonstrate hammering movements. Occasionally, a patient's performance is so profoundly impaired that the examiner cannot recognize the intent of the movements. When patients with

IMA pantomime, their pantomimes may be incorrectly produced, but the goal or intent of the act can usually be recognized as correct.

Patients with IMA make two major types of production errors: spatial and temporal. Spatial errors can be divided into several subtypes, including postural (or internal configuration), spatial movement, and spatial orientation. Regarding postural errors, Goodglass and Kaplan[8] noted that when patients with IMA are asked to pantomime, they often use a body part as the tool. For example, when these patients are asked to pantomime using a pair of scissors, they may use their fingers as if they were the blades. Many normal subjects make a similar error; therefore, it is imperative that the patient be instructed not to use a body part as a tool. Patients with IMA may continue to make errors using body parts as tools in spite of these instructions. Patients with IMA will often fail to position their hands as if they were holding the tool or object they were requested to pantomime.

When normal subjects are asked to use a tool, they will orient that tool to the target of that tool's action (whether real or imaginary). Patients with IMA often fail to orient their forelimbs to a real or imaginary target. For example, when asked to pantomime cutting a piece of paper in half with a scissors, rather than keeping the scissors oriented in the sagittal plane, the patient may orient the scissors laterally.[7]

When making spatial movement errors, patients with IMA will often make the correct core movement (e.g., twisting, pounding, cutting) but will not move their limb correctly through space.[7,9] These spatial movement errors are associated with incorrect joint movements such that the apraxic patients will stabilize a joint that should be moving and move joints that should be stabilized. For example, in pantomiming the use of a screwdriver, the patient with IMA may rotate his arm at the shoulder joint and fix his elbow. Shoulder rotation moves the hand in circles rather than rotating the hand on a fixed axis. When multiple joint movements must be coordinated, the patient may be unable to coordinate the movement to get the desired spatial trajectory. For example, when pantomiming sawing wood, the shoulder and elbow joints must be alternatively flexed and extended. When the joint movements are not well coordinated, the patient may make primarily chopping or stabbing movements.

Poizner and colleagues[9] have noted that patients with IMA may make timing errors, including a long delay before initiating a movement and brief multiple stops (stuttering movements). Patients with IMA often do not demonstrate a smooth sinusoidal hand speed when they perform cyclic movements, such as slicing bread with a knife.

Pathophysiology

Whereas in right-handed individuals, IMA is almost always associated with left hemisphere lesions, in left-handers IMA is usually associated with right hemisphere lesions. Ideomotor apraxia can be induced by lesions in a variety of structures, including the corpus callosum, inferior parietal lobe, and supplementary motor area (SMA). IMA has also been reported with subcortical lesions that involve basal ganglia and white matter. Below, each of these anatomic areas is discussed and an attempt is made to develop a model of how the brain mediates learned skilled motor activity of the limbs.

Corpus Callosum In 1907 Liepmann and Maas[10] described a patient with a right hemiparesis from a lesion of the pons and a lesion of the corpus callosum. This patient was unable to pantomime correctly to command with his left arm. Because this patient had a right hemiparesis, his right hand could not be tested. Since the work of Broca and Wernicke, neurologists have known that right-handers' left hemisphere is dominant for language. Liepmann and Maas could have attributed their patient's inability to pantomime to a disconnection between language and motor areas, such that the left hemisphere, which mediates comprehension of the verbal command, could not influence the right hemisphere, which is responsible for controlling the left hand. However, this patient could also not imitate gestures or use actual objects correctly, and language-motor disconnection could not account for these findings. Liepmann and Maas therefore posited that the left hemisphere of right-handers contains movement formulas (or spatiotemporal representations of movements) and that the callosal lesion disconnects these movement formulas from the motor areas of the right hemisphere.

Geschwind and Kaplan[11] as well as Gazzaniga and coworkers[12] found that their patients with callosal disconnection, unlike the callosal patient of Liepmann and Maas, could not correctly pantomime to command with the left hand but could imitate and correctly use actual objects with this hand, suggesting that the apraxia of callosal disconnection in these patients was induced by a language-motor disconnection. Watson and Heilman,[13] however, described a patient with an infarction of the body of the corpus callosum. This patient, however, had no weakness in her right hand and performed all tasks flawlessly with that hand; but with her left hand, she could not correctly pantomime to command, imitate, or use actual objects. Although early in her course she made content errors, she subsequently made the spatial and temporal errors associated with IMA. Her performance indicated that not only language but also movement representations were stored in the left hemisphere and her callosal lesion disconnected these movement representations from the right hemisphere.

Inferior Parietal Lobe Whereas Geschwind[9] proposed that the ideomotor apraxia associated with left-sided parietal lesions induced a language motor disconnection, Heilman and colleagues[14] and Rothi and coworkers[15] proposed that the movement representations or movement formulas were stored in the left parietal lobe of right-handers and that destruction of the left parietal lobe should induce not only a production deficit (apraxia) but also a gesture comprehension/discrimination disorder. Apraxia induced by premotor lesions, lesions of the pathways that connect premotor areas to motor areas, or the pathways that lead to the premotor areas from the parietal lobe may also cause a production deficit. In contrast to parietal lesions, however, these lesions should not induce gesture comprehension/discrimination disorders. Heilman and colleagues[14] and Rothi and associates[15] tested patients with anterior and posterior lesions and found that while both groups were apraxic, the patients with a damaged parietal lobe had comprehension-discrimination disturbances and those with more anterior lesions did not.

Liepmann proposed that handedness was related to the hemispheric laterality of the movement representations. It is not unusual, however, to see right-handed patients with left hemisphere lesions who are not apraxic. Although it is possible that these patients' lesions did not destroy a critical left hemisphere area, it is also possible that not all right-handers have movement representations stored entirely in their left hemisphere. Some people may have either bilateral movement representations or even right hemisphere representations. Apraxia from a right hemisphere lesion in a right-hander is rare but has been reported, suggesting that hand preference is not entirely determined by the laterality of the movement representations and may be multifactorial. Whereas the laterality of the movement formula may be the most important factor, there are other factors, including more elemental motor factors such as strength, speed, precision, attentional factors, and even environmental factors.

Supplementary Motor Area Muscles move joints, and motor nerves from the spinal cord activate these muscles. The motor nerves are activated by corticospinal neurons. The corticospinal tract neurons are, in turn, activated by neurons in the premotor areas.

For each specific skilled movement there is a set of spatial loci that must be traversed in a specific temporal pattern. We proposed that movement formulas that are represented in the inferior parietal lobe are stored in a three-dimensional supramodal code. Although Geschwind[11] thought that the convexity premotor cortex was important for praxis, its function in the control of praxis remains uncertain. The convexity premotor cortex may be important in motor learning or in adapting the program to environmental pertubations.

The medial premotor cortex or supplementary motor area (SMA), however, appears to play an important role in mediating skilled movements. Whereas electrical stimulation of the primary motor cortex induces simple movements, SMA stimulation induces complex movements of the fingers, arms, and hands. The SMA receives projections from parietal neurons and projects to motor neurons in the primary motor cortex. The SMA neurons appear to discharge before neurons in the primary motor cortex. Studies of cerebral blood flow, an indicator of synaptic activity, have revealed that a single repetitive movement increases activation of the contralateral motor cortex, but complex movements increase flow in the contralateral motor cortex and in SMA. When subjects remained still and thought about making complex movements, blood flow to the SMA increased but the blood flow to the motor

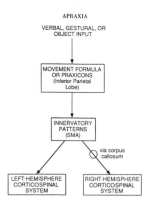

Figure 29-1
Diagrammatic model of ideomotor apraxia. SMA, supplementary motor area. (From Heilman and Rothi,[27] with permission.)

cortex remained unchanged. Watson and coworkers[16] reported several patients with left-sided mediofrontal lesions that included the SMA who demonstrated an ideomotor apraxia when tested with either arm. Unlike patients with parietal lesions, these patients could both comprehend and discriminate pantomimes.

The model we have discussed so far is illustrated in Fig. 29-1. The praxicon is a theoretical store of the temporospatial representations of learned skill movements. When a skilled act is being performed, these representations are transcoded into innervatory patterns by the SMA. When the right hand acts, the SMA programs the motor cortex (Brodmann's area 4) of the left hemisphere, and when the left hand acts, these innervatory patterns activate the motor regions of the right hemisphere via the corpus callosum.

Basal Ganglia and Thalamus Portions of the basal ganglia such as the putamen receive projections from premotor cortex including the SMA. Several investigators have reported that injury to the basal ganglia can induce IMA.[17,18] Pramstaller and Marsden,[19] however, thought that the evidence supporting the basal ganglia apraxia postulate was weak and that the apraxia reported to be associated with basal ganglia lesions was probably related to damage to other areas of the brain. More recently, Hanna-Pladdy not only reported additional patients with IMA from basal ganglia lesions but also demonstrated that these patients made primarily postural errors.

DeRenzi et al.[18] also reported that patients with thalamic lesions might demonstrate IMA. In regard to the intrathalamic localization, Shuren et al.[20] as well as Nadeau et al.[21] reported that these lesions might involve the pulvinar. The pulvinar thalamic nucleus projects primarily to the parietal lobe, where movement representation are stored, and these pulvinar lesions might interfere with the activation of these movement representations.

DISASSOCIATION APRAXIAS

Clinical Findings

Heilman[22] described several patients who, when asked to pantomime to command, looked at their open hands or would slowly pronate and supinate their arms but would not perform any recognizable action. Unlike the patients with ideomotor apraxia described above, these patients' imitations and use of objects were flawless. DeRenzi and colleagues[23] reported patients similar to those reported by Heilman[22] and also other patients who had a similar defect in other modalities. For example, when asked to pantomime in response to visual or tactile stimuli, they may have been unable to do so, but they could pantomime to verbal command.

Pathophysiology

While callosal lesions may be associated with an ideomotor apraxia, callosal disconnection may also cause disassociation apraxia. The subjects of Gazzaniga and associates[12] and the patients described by Geschwind and Kaplan[11] had disassociation apraxia. We posit that language in these patients was mediated by the left hemisphere and movement representations were bilaterally represented. A callosal lesion induced a dissociation between the portions of the left hemisphere, which are important in language comprehension, and the motor cortex of the right hemisphere, which controls the left hand. Thus, the patient with callosal disassociation apraxia will not be able to correctly carry out skilled learned movements of the left arm to command, but

he or she will be able to imitate and use actual objects with the left hand because these tasks do not require language and these patient's right hemisphere contains the movement formula as well as the other apparatus needed to transcode the time-space movement representations to motor acts.

Right-handed patients who have both language and movement formula represented in their left hemisphere may show a combination of disassociation and ideomotor apraxia with callosal lesions.[13] When asked to pantomime with their left hands, they may look at them and perform no recognizable movement (disassociation apraxia); but when imitating or using actual objects, they may demonstrate the spatial and temporal errors seen with ideomotor apraxia.

Left-handers may demonstrate an ideomotor apraxia without aphasia from a right hemisphere lesion. These left-handers are apraxic because their movement representations were stored in their right hemispheres and their lesions destroyed these representations.[24,25] These left-handers were not aphasic because language was mediated by their left hemispheres (as is the case in the majority of left-handers). If these left-handers had a callosal lesion, they may have demonstrated a disassociation apraxia of the left arm and an ideomotor apraxia of the right arm.

The disassociation apraxia described by Heilman[22] from left hemisphere lesions was unfortunately incorrectly termed "ideational apraxia." The patients reported by Heilman[22] and those of DeRenzi and associates[23] probably have an intrahemispheric language-movement formula, a visual-movement formula, or a somesthetic-movement formula disassociation. The locations of the lesions that cause these intrahemispheric disassociation apraxias are not known.

CONDUCTION APRAXIA

Clinical Findings

Ochipa and coworkers[26] reported a patient who was unlike patients with ideomotor apraxia because, rather than improving with imitation, this patient was more impaired when imitating than when pantomiming to command.

Pathophysiology

Because this patient with conduction apraxia could comprehend the examiner's pantomime and gestures, we believe that the patient's visual system could access the movement representations, or what we have termed *praxicons*,[27] and that the activated movement representations, or praxicons, could activate semantics. It is possible that decoding a gesture requires the accessing of different movement representations or praxicons than does programming an action. Therefore, Ochipa and colleagues[26] and Rothi and coworkers[28] suggested that there may be two different stores of movement representations, an input praxicon and output praxicon. In the verbal domain, a disconnection of the hypothetical input and output lexicons induces conduction aphasia; in the praxis domain, a disconnection between the input and output praxicons could induce conduction apraxia.

Whereas the lesions that induce conduction aphasia are usually in the supramarginal gyrus or Wernicke's area, the location of lesions that induce conduction apraxia are unknown.

IDEATIONAL APRAXIA

Unfortunately, there has been much confusion about the meaning of the term *ideational apraxia*. The inability to carry out a series of acts, an ideational plan, has been called ideational apraxia.[29,30] In performing a task that requires a series of acts, these patients have difficulty sequencing the acts in the proper order (for example, instead of cleaning the pipe, putting tobacco in the bowl, lighting the tobacco, and smoking, the patient might attempt to light the empty bowl, put the tobacco in the bowl, and then clean it). Pick[30] noted that most of the patients with this type of ideational apraxia have a dementing disease.

Whereas most patients with apraxia improve when they are using objects. DeRenzi and colleagues[31] reported patients who made errors with the use of actual objects. Although the inability to use actual objects may be associated with a conceptual disorder, a severe production disorder may also impair object use.[32] However, as discussed in the next section, production and conceptual disorders may be associated with different types of errors.

CONCEPTUAL APRAXIA

Clinical Findings

To perform a skilled act, two types of knowledge are needed: conceptual knowledge and production knowledge. Dysfunction of the praxis production system induces ideomotor apraxia. Defects in the knowledge needed to successfully select and use the tools or objects we term *conceptual apraxia*. Whereas patients with ideomotor apraxia make production errors (e.g., spatial and temporal errors), patients with conceptual apraxia make content and tool-selection errors. The patients with conceptual apraxia may not recall the types of actions associated with specific tools, utensils, or objects (tool–object action knowledge) and therefore make content errors.[33,34] For example, when asked to demonstrate the use of a screwdriver, either pantomining or using the tool, the patient may pantomime a hammering movement or use the screwdriver as if it were a hammer.

The patient with ideomotor apraxia may make production errors by moving the hand in circles rather than twisting the hand on its own axis. Although such patients make production errors by moving the hand in circles, they are demonstrating knowledge of the turning action of screwdrivers. Content errors (i.e., using a tool as if it were another tool) can also be induced by an object agnosia. However, Ochipa and associates[35] reported a patient who could name tools (and therefore was not agnosic) but often used them inappropriately.

Patients with conceptual apraxia may be unable to recall which specific tool is associated with a specific object (tool–object association knowledge). For example, when shown a partially driven nail, they may select a screwdriver rather than a hammer from an array of tools. This conceptual defect may also be in the verbal domain, such that when an actual tool is shown to a patient with conceptual apraxia, the patient may be able to name it (e.g., hammer); but when the patient is asked to name or point to a tool when its function is discussed, he or she cannot. The patient may also be unable to describe the functions of tools.

Patients with conceptual apraxia may also have impaired mechanical knowledge. For example, if they are attempting to drive a nail into a piece of wood and there is no hammer available, they may select a screwdriver rather than a wrench or pliers (which are hard, heavy, and good for pounding).[35] Mechanical knowledge is also important for tool development, and patients with conceptual apraxia may be unable to develop tools correctly.[35]

Pathophysiology

Liepmann[3] thought that conceptual knowledge was located in the caudal parietal lobe, and DeRenzi and Luccelli[33] placed it in the temporoparietal junction. The patient reported by Ochipa and coworkers[34] was left-handed and rendered conceptually apraxic by a lesion in the right hemisphere, suggesting that both production and conceptual knowledge have lateralized representations and that such representations are contralateral to the preferred hand. Further evidence that these conceptual representations are stored in the hemisphere contralateral to the preferred hand comes from a study of right-handed patients who had unilateral strokes of either their right or left hemisphere. This study revealed that left hemisphere but not right hemisphere injury is associated with conceptual apraxia.[36] We also studied a patient who had a callosal disconnection and demonstrated conceptual apraxia and ideomotor apraxia of her nonpreferred (left) hand.[13] Conceptual apraxia, however, is most commonly seen in degenerative dementia of the Alzheimer type.[35] Ochipa and colleagues noted that the severity of conceptual and ideomotor apraxia did not always correlate. The observation that patients with ideomotor apraxia may not demonstrate conceptual apraxia and patients with conceptual apraxia may not demonstrate ideomotor apraxia provides support for the postulate that the praxis production and praxis conceptual systems are independent. For normal function, however, these two systems must interact.

CONCLUSIONS

Lesions of the motor cortex and perhaps convexity premotor cortex induces a loss of hand deftness called limb-kinetic apraxia. In right handed people left hemisphere injury can cause ipsilateral deficits.

Movement representations (praxicons) are stored in the left inferior parietal lobe of right-handers. These representations code the spatial and temporal patterns of learned skilled movements. Injury to the left parietal lobe induces a production deficit in both hands termed ideomotor apraxia. Patients with ideomotor apraxia make spatial and temporal errors. Patients with injury to these representations are not only impaired at pantomiming, imitating, and using actual objects but also cannot discriminate between well- and poorly performed gestures. These patients may also not be able to comprehend gestures. Patients with injury to premotor cortex and the basal ganglia also have IMA but these patients can discriminate and comprehend gestures.

There are patients who are more impaired at imitation of gestures than they are when gesturing to command (conduction apraxia), suggesting that movement representations (praxicons) may be divided into input and output subdivisions. In conduction apraxia, there is a dissociation between these input and output praxicons.

In order to perform learned skilled acts, abstract movement representations have to be transcoded into motor programs. This transcoding appears to be performed by a premotor (supplementary motor area)—basal ganglia (putamen-globus pallidus-thalamus) system. Injuries to the brain that interrupt the connections between the movement representations stored in the parietal lobe and the portions of the brain that develop the innervatory patterns or the parts of the brain that allow the innervatory patterns to gain access to the motor system may also produce a praxis production deficit (ideomotor apraxia).

A patient may have intact representations of learned skilled movements but have modality-specific deficits in accessing these representations. For example, a patient with dissociation apraxia may be unable to pantomime to command but be able to pantomime correctly when seeing the tool.

Finally, some patients, when pantomiming or using actual tools, may make content errors. Whereas spatial and temporal errors are related to deficits in the praxic production system, content errors are related to deficits in a hypothetical praxis conceptual system or action semantics. Dysfunction of this system, termed *conceptual apraxia,* may produce deficits of associative knowledge, such as tool-action or tool-object knowledge (i.e., knowing that a hammer is used to pound and that a hammer is associated with a nail). Defects in action semantics may also be associated with deficits in mechanical knowledge (i.e., knowing how to use alternative tools and how to fabricate tools).

REFERENCES

1. Geschwind N: Disconnection syndromes in animals and man. *Brain* 88:237–294, 585–644, 1965.
2. Rothi LJG, Mack L, Heilman KM: Unawareness of apraxic errors. *Neurology* 40(suppl 1):202, 1990.
3. Liepmann H: Apraxia. *Erbgn Ges Med* 1:516–543, 1920.
4. Heilman KM, Meador KJ, Loring DW: Hemispheric asymmetries of limb-kinetic apraxia: A loss of deftness. *Neurology* 55:523–526, 2000.
5. Hanna-Pladdy B, Daniels SK, Fieselman MA, et al: Praxis lateralization: Errors in right and left hemisphere stroke. *Cortex* 37:219–230, 2001.
6. Lawrence DG, Kuypers HGJM: The functional organization of the motor system in the monkey. *Brain* 91:1–36, 1968.
7. Rothi LJG, Mack L, Verfaellie M, et al: Ideomotor apraxia: Error pattern analysis. *Aphasiology* 2:381–387, 1988.
8. Goodglass H, Kaplan E: Disturbance of gesture and pantomime in aphasia. *Brain* 86:703–720, 1963.
9. Poizner H, Mack L, Verfaellie M, et al: Three dimensional computer graphic analysis of apraxia. *Brain* 113:85–101, 1990.
10. Liepmann H, Mass O: Fall von Linksseitiger Agraphie und Apraxie bei Rechsseitiger Lahmung. *Z Psychol Neurol* 10:214–227, 1907.
11. Geschwind N, Kaplan E: A human cerebral disconnection syndrome. *Neurology* 12:675–685, 1962.
12. Gazzaniga M, Bogen J, Sperry R: Dyspraxia following diversion of the cerebral commisures. *Arch Neurol* 16:606–612, 1967.
13. Watson RT, Heilman KM: Callosal apraxia. *Brain* 106:391–403, 1983.
14. Heilman KM, Rothi LJ, Valenstein E: Two forms of ideomotor apraxia. *Neurology* 32:342–346, 1982.
15. Rothi LJG, Heilman KM, Watson RT: Pantomime comprehension and ideomotor apraxia. *J Neurol Neurosurg Psychiatry* 48:207–210, 1985.
16. Watson RT, Fleet WS, Rothi LJG, Heilman KM: Apraxia and the supplementary motor area. *Arch Neurol* 43:787–792, 1986.
17. Agostoni E, Coletti A, Orlando G, Tredici G: Apraxia in deep cerebral lesions. *J Neurol Neurosurg* Psychiatry 46(9):804–808, 1983.
18. DeRenzi E, Faglioni P, Scarpa M, Crisi G: Limb apraxia in patients with damage confined to the left basal ganglia and thalamus. *J Neurol Neurosurg Psychiatry* 49(9):1030–1038, 1986.
19. Pramstaller PP, Marsden CD: The basal ganglia and apraxia. *Brain* 119(pt 1):319–340, 1996.
20. Shuren JE, Maher LM, Heilman KM: Role of the pulvinar in ideomotor praxis. *J Neurol Neurosurg Psychiatry* 57(10):1282–1283, 1994.
21. Nadeau SE, Roeltgen DP, Sevush S, et al: Apraxia due to a pathologically documented thalamic infarction. *Neurology* 44(11):2133–2137, 1994.
22. Heilman KM: Ideational apraxia–A re-definition. *Brain* 96:861–864, 1973.
23. DeRenzi E, Faglioni P, Sorgato P: Modality-specific and supramodal mechanisms of apraxia. *Brain* 105:301–312, 1982.
24. Heilman KM, Coyle JM, Gonyea EF, Geschwind N: Apraxia and agraphia in a left-hander. *Brain* 96:21–28, 1973.
25. Valenstein E, Heilman KM: Apraxic agraphia with neglect induced paragraphia. *Arch Neurol* 36:506–508, 1979.
26. Ochipa C, Rothi LJG, Heilman KM: Conduction apraxia. *J Clin Exp Neuropsychol* 12:89, 1990.
27. Heilman KM, Rothi LJG: Apraxia, in Heilman KM, Valenstein E (eds): *Clinical Neuropsychology*, 3d ed. New York: Oxford University Press, 1993.
28. Rothi LJG, Ochipa C, Heilman KM: A cognitive neuropsychological model of limb praxis. *Cogn Neuropsychol* 8:443–458, 1991.
29. Marcuse H: Apraktiscke Symotome bein linem Fall von seniler Demenz. *Zentralbl Mervheik Psychiatr* 27:737–751, 1904.
30. Pick A: *Studien über Motorische Apraxia und ihre Mahestenhende Erscheinungen*. Leipzig: Deuticke, 1905.
31. DeRenzi E, Pieczuro A, Vignolo L: Ideational apraxia: A quantitative study. *Neuropsychologia* 6:41–52, 1968.
32. Zangwell OL: L'apraxie ideatorie. *Nerve Neurol* 106:595–603, 1960.
33. DeRenzi E, Lucchelli F: Ideational apraxia. *Brain* 113:1173–1188, 1988.
34. Ochipa C, Rothi LJG, Heilman KM: Ideational apraxia: A deficit in tool selection and use. *Ann Neurol* 25:190–193, 1989.
35. Ochipa C, Rothi LJG. Heilman KM: Conceptual apraxia in Alzheimer's disease. *Brain* 115:1061–1071, 1992.
36. Heilman KM, Maher LM, Greenwald ML, Rothi LJG: Conceptual apraxia from lateralized lesions. *Neurology* 49:457–464, 1997.

Chapter 30

CALLOSAL DISCONNECTION*

Kathleen Baynes
Michael S. Gazzaniga

BRIEF HISTORICAL BACKGROUND

Appropriate Techniques Required to Demonstrate Disconnection Phenomena

Although the anatomic prominence of the corpus callosum suggested to early neuroanatomists that it played a key role in human cognition, actual demonstration of its function was difficult to accomplish. The first attempts to surgically separate the two hemispheres were undertaken by Van Wagenen in the 1940s.[1] The hope was that patients with debilitating epileptic seizures would have some relief if electric activity could not spread from one hemisphere to the other via the callosum. In this series of patients, unfortunately, there was inconsistent evidence of improved seizure control. Moreover, despite administration of a battery of standard neuropsychological tests before and after surgery, no consistent cognitive effects were observed.[2,3] The enormous band of fibers connecting the two hemispheres seemed to have an insignificant functional role, and section of the corpus callosum as a treatment for epilepsy was abandoned.

During the 1950s, Sperry and Meyers discovered in animals that it was necessary to use special techniques that isolated the acquisition of new information to a single hemisphere to see the radical behavioral effects of callosal section.[4,5] Although their work was accomplished with cats, the lessons learned there were applied to the evaluation of a new series of surgeries initiated by Bogen and Vogel in the 1960s.[6,7] In addition, Geschwind's work on disconnection syndromes indicated that more profound changes should result from the interruption of fiber tracts than had been observed

in the earlier series.[8] Bogen and Vogel surmised that perhaps the early callosotomies had been ineffective because they failed to include the other cerebral commissures; therefore a new series of commissurotomies was planned that included the anterior commissure. In light of the work of Sperry and Geschwind, a more sophisticated investigation of cognitive changes was included.

When the new series was initiated, careful evaluation of cognitive function of each hemisphere was undertaken using brief (tachistoscopic) presentations to assure that stimuli were displayed to only one hemisphere.[8] Once the callosum is completely sectioned, information cannot be easily shared between the two hemispheres. Eye movements, however, can cause a loss of lateralization. The work in the 1970s eliminated this possibility by displaying words and pictures for 150 ms or less, faster than the eye can move from the central fixation point to the display.[9] Later, special contact lenses, eye-tracking techniques, and lateral fixation techniques would be used as well.[10,11]

These initial studies confirmed assertions that the left hemisphere (LH) was dominant for language whereas the right could neither name nor describe objects presented to it visually or tactually, although it could perform certain visuospatial tasks. Current eye-tracking techniques permit visual displays with extended durations, thus allowing more precise observations.[11] Theoretical and methodologic advances continue to develop our understanding of perceptual, cognitive, mnemonic, and linguistic processes and their integration into coherent thought and behavior. Such techniques provide unique means of testing hemispheric hypotheses and enriching our understanding of neurologic and neuropsychological symptoms, from alexia to alien-hand sign, as well as yielding insights to the evolution of lateralized processing and the understanding of consciousness.

* **ACKNOWLEDGMENTS:** Supported in part by NIH/NIDCD grant R01 DC04442 to KB and NIH/NINDS grant P01 NS17778 to MSG and the John S. McDonnell Foundation.

LANGUAGE

One of the most striking of the split-brain observations was the ability of the mute right hemisphere (RH) to understand spoken language and read single words. It was apparent that the right hemisphere could respond to some simple verbal commands and read single words as long as a verbal response was not required. This ability facilitated the demonstration of two hemispheres responding independently to stimuli and generated excitement in fields from neurology to philosophy. The demonstration of this basic phenomenon required as little as a blindfold or screen to keep the dominant LH in the dark and a response method to permit the nondominant right hemisphere a nonverbal means of expression.

Basic language skills appeared to be present in the RH of all of the Bogen and Vogel series of splits, suggesting that the RH might play a larger role in language than had been expected.[7,12,13] Theories implicating the RH in errors made by dyslexic and aphasic patients abounded,[14,15] but the RH was given little credit for being more than an error generator when the LH was weakened or damaged or when developmental lateralization processes had gone awry. However, in the larger Wilson-Roberts series initiated in the 1970s, the presence of even rudimentary RH language was much less frequent. By 1983, of the 28 completed callosotomies, only 3 patients had documented RH language. Today the series stands at about 40 callosotomies (Roberts DW: Personal communication, 2001), but those three remain the only ones with sufficient RH language to participate in tachistoscopic experiments. Over time, the population from which the callosotomy candidates are drawn has changed, which may influence the frequency with which RH language occurs. Increased ability to identify and remove focal areas that initiate seizure activity has led to a greater number of focal surgeries, with only a few patients with very severe and often diffuse seizure activity being considered for split-brain surgery. Such severe illness often leaves the patients with decreased mental capacity and limited reading ability prior to surgery. Only one new patient with robust RH reading has been added to the active testing group since the mid-1980s.[16–18] Hence, most of these observations regarding RH language are based on

a small but well-studied group of patients. The degree to which they generalize to the neurologically normal population remains a matter of speculation. However many functional magnetic resonance imaging (fMRI) studies have demonstrated RH activation during some language tasks in normal subjects, and RH activation appears to be important during some stage of recovery from LH stroke.[19,20]

In those patients with RH language capacity, semantic and conceptual information appears to be more adequately represented in the RH than is phonological and syntactic information. The lexicon or vocabulary of the RH appears to be similar to, albeit somewhat smaller than, the corresponding LH lexicon.[21] Both hemispheres can make a variety of semantic judgments, recognizing categorical, functional, and associative relations among words. The ability to discriminate word from nonword letter strings is limited but possible,[22,23] which suggests that the visual word form is represented in the RH of these patients. One way to conceptualize the right/left difference is in terms of a static lexicon and a productive grammar.[24] The lexicon stores information about the meaning and associations of words and is present in both hemispheres. In contrast, the grammar that contains rules for generating new sentences which communicate meaning is present only in the LH.

Limited Control of Speech and Grammar in the Isolated Right Hemisphere

In the same way as grammar allows the combination of words into sentences, phonology allows the combination of the sounds of a language in a meaningful way to create words or lexical items. Both processes present difficulties for the RH. Although the RH possesses some limited phonological competence and can both generate and understand limited speech, it shows very little ability to perform any of the letter-to-sound tasks used to test phonological competence. It has difficulty with the identification of written rhymes or even selecting pictures with rhyming names.[25,26] There is better evidence for some ability to discriminate auditory phonemes,[27] but this would be the minimal competence expected to support auditory comprehension in the RH. Moreover, some higher-level influences on perception of auditory sounds can be demonstrated using manipulations like the McGurk effect, in which the perception of an auditory sound is altered by viewing a speaker pronouncing a different sound.[27] These basic perceptual integrations can be accomplished by the RH, whereas those required to decode sound from written language do not appear to be possible.

Nor does the linguistic prowess of the RH extend to the use of grammatical rules for the comprehension and production of sentences. Although the RH can distinguish between grammatical and ungrammatical sentences, the ability to use grammatical information is limited in other tasks such as sentence/ picture matching.[21,28] Hence, it appears that a rapid, almost reflexive judgment about grammar is possible, but a decision that requires decoding of the meaning carried by grammar is not. Likewise, although the RH can sometimes make single-word verbal responses to words and pictures, there is no evidence of the ability to use grammar to combine words to generate more complex, sentence length responses. Passive use of both phonological and grammatical knowledge in the RH in the absence of generative use may indicate that both phonology and grammar depend upon LH output mechanisms to be used productively.

Right Hemisphere Reading

Right hemisphere reading proceeds more slowly than LH reading and may use a different mode of processing.[29] A right hemisphere lexicon has been suggested as the source of certain reading errors in deep dyslexic[14,30] and pure dyslexic patients[31,32] (see Chaps. 17 and 20). Although insensitivity to grammar and poor print-to-sound skills in the RH of these patients is consistent with some aspects of these claims, both left and right hemispheres appear to be capable of generating the range of errors found in deep dyslexia.[33] The language profile seen in callosotomy patients is more consistent with the profile reported by Coslett and Saffran[31,32] for the preserved reading of their pure alexic patients than with that reported for deep dyslexic patients.

Perhaps more interesting are the claims that the RH lexicon is needed to support a variety of metalinguistic tasks, from interpretation of humor to metaphor

to indirect requests.[34-37] One source for these problems might be RH differences in semantic representation and/or processing.[38,39] Lateralized presentations to normal readers show that whereas the right visual field/left hemisphere (RVF/LH) shows priming for a variety of relations between words after reading short paragraphs, the left visual field/right hemisphere (LVF/RH) shows priming only for primarily lexical relations, not those that are dependent on grammatical information.[40] Moreover, the LH of split-brain patients shows priming for all of these relations as well. It is possible that the spreading of lexical activation without grammar is sufficient to facilitate some discourse-level processes and may support some other metalinguistic functions as well.

MEMORY

Recall and Recognition Memory Following Callosotomy

Changes in mnemonic capacity after callosotomy may reflect discrete processing capacities in the isolated hemispheres. Loss of general memory capacity as measured by standardized tests has been reported for some patients,[41,42] whereas Clark and Geffen[43] suggested that discrepancies in memory function reported after callosotomy might be due to involvement of the hippocampal commissure. Phelps and coworkers[44] have observed a decrement in both visual and verbal recall following posterior callosal section, which may damage the hippocampal commissure, but preserved or even improved memory after anterior callosal section, which does not. Recognition memory was relatively intact in both groups. Kroll and colleagues[45,46] reported that complete callosotomy interferes with the binding of visual and verbal material, yielding error patterns similar to those of hippocampally lesioned patients.

There appear to be hemisphere-specific changes in the accuracy of memory processes that may be useful in understanding the behavior of some neurologically impaired patients. The LH appears to make greater use of general knowledge schemas to explain perceptions and experiences and to use them to "interpret" events[47] than does the RH, and this predilection has an impact on the accuracy of memory.[44] When subjects were presented with a series of pictures that represented common events (i.e., getting up in the morning or making cookies) and were then asked, several hours later, to identify whether pictures in another series had appeared in the original series, both hemispheres were equally accurate in recognizing previously viewed pictures and rejecting novel, unrelated ones. Only the RH, however, correctly rejected pictures in the second set that were not previously viewed but were semantically congruent with pictures from the first set. The LH incorrectly "recalled" significantly more of these semantically congruent lures as having occurred in the first set, presumably because they fit into the schema it had constructed regarding the event. This finding is consistent with the hypothesis that there is an LH "interpreter" that constructs theories to assimilate perceived information into a comprehensible whole.[48,49] As a result, however, the elaborative processing involved has a deleterious effect on the accuracy of perceptual recognition. This has been confirmed by Metcalfe and colleagues and extended to include verbal material.[50]

HEMISPHERIC DOMINANCE

The Left Hemisphere as Interpreter

The LH is considered to be the "dominant" hemisphere in most right-handed people. The term *dominant* is usually taken to mean language-dominant, but Gazzaniga has suggested that the LH is not only superior in terms of language function but also in the ability to make simple inferences and to interpret its own behavior and emotions.[51] It is, in fact, the "intelligent" hemisphere. It is unclear whether these functions are dependent upon the development of generative language skills or if they arise independently. Nonetheless, such observations strongly indicate that the LH is not only more able than the RH to express itself verbally but that it plays a dominant role in interpreting behavior and providing a rationale for events in the world. Taking the evolutionary view, Gazzaniga and colleagues suggest that the corpus callosum allowed the evolution of these lateralized skills to occur and enabled the development of consciousness.[49,52]

Evolution of Dominance

One of the most perplexing and recalcitrant questions about the neural representation of cognition is the basis for hemispheric lateralization. Although the split-brain model confirmed that the LH is language dominant and the RH is better at many visuospatial tasks, it is clear that both hemispheres share many capacities and possess at least rudimentary skills in both verbal and nonverbal domains. One insightful approach to this problem is under investigation by Paul Corballis and colleagues.[52–56]

Corballis suggests that the corpus callosum has played a role in the evolution of lateralized skills in what was previously a symmetrical system.[52] The inhibitory power of the corpus callosum allowed new skills associated with language to develop in the LH, while prior visuospatial abilities were maintained in the RH. Hence, certain low-level visual effects are common to both hemispheres (i.e., luminance[56,57] and binocular rivalry[58]), whereas other visual processes that require spatial localization are present only in the RH (i.e., size and orientation discrimination[56] and perceptual matching[59]). Corballis further suggests that this division may reflect the what/where system's association with the dorsal and ventral pathways.[56] Although still under investigation, such a view provides an interesting perspective from which to examine visuospatial function.

Visuospatial Functions

The expected right hemispheric superiority in visuospatial function has been demonstrated in callosotomy patients,[6,60] but the LH has some visuospatial skills as well. In fact, superior use of visual imagery using a letter-based task has been demonstrated in the LH.[61] Although the use of tactile information to build spatial representations of abstract shapes also appears to be better developed in the RH,[60] tasks such as block design from the Wechsler Adult Intelligence Scale (WAIS), which are typically associated with the right parietal lobe, appear to require integration between hemispheres in some patients.[62] This observation is compatible with neuropsychological observations that document different types of visuospatial errors associated with lesions to the right and left hemispheres.

As noted above, Corballis and colleagues have tried to explain the distribution of skills in the two hemispheres by comparing visual tasks that vary in their dependence on high-level spatial processing for completion. The RH shows competence for all of the tested visual tasks, regardless of whether there is a strong need for spatial processing. In contrast, the LH shows competence only for those tasks and effects that depend upon luminance, timing, or some other lower-level perceptual information. Hence, this line of investigation is finding increasing support for the view that the hemispheres share the capacity for basic perceptual processing, whereas the RH dominance becomes more apparent as higher-level spatial information is required.

INTERHEMISPHERIC INTEGRATION OF PERCEPTION AND ATTENTION

Hemispheric Isolation of Visual and Tactile Information

When appropriate lateralization procedures are followed (see Fig. 30-1), visual and tactile perception can be isolated to each hemisphere. Although split subjects can make accurate same/different judgments about visual material that has been isolated to one hemisphere or the other, they cannot make comparisons between the two hemifields. Performance is at or near chance levels when words or pictures are presented in different visual fields for same/different judgments.[63-65] Despite reports of integration of higher-order information following callosotomy,[66,67] such reports have not always proved replicable or explicable through the patient's strategic maneuvers.[65,68,69] At present, it appears that if visual or tactile information is presented so that it is initially perceived by only one hemisphere, the perception remains isolated within that hemisphere.

The animal literature, however, has documented that information from areas close to the visual midline is shared by both hemispheres.[70,71] It appears that this observation is also true for the human species in an area no more than 2 degrees from the vertical meridian.[72] Although represented, the visual information in this area has little utility, as neither detailed shape comparisons nor brief displays could be reliably compared across the meridian.[73]

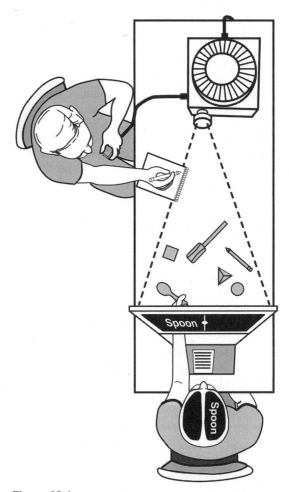

Figure 30-1
Tachistoscopic method of data collection from split-brain patients used in original studies. Current studies use computers and eye-tracking technology to control display and timing of lateralized stimuli.

Sharing of Attentional Control

Although both higher cognitive function and basic perceptual information appear to be isolated within each hemisphere, there is some evidence for sharing control of visual attention. The hemispheres appear to share control of the "attentional spotlight" via their subcortical connections. That is, if attention is directed to a particular position in the visual field by a cue in one field, that information can be used by both hemispheres.[64,74]

Nonetheless, explicit interfield comparisons of spatial location cannot be made accurately,[64] nor can attention be simultaneously directed to different points in each visual field.[75]

It also appears that attentional resources are limited despite the "splitting" of consciousness. Holtzman demonstrated that increasing processing demands in one hemisphere had a deleterious effect on the other hemisphere.[76] Nonetheless, in comparison with normal subjects, there was less decrement in a dual-task condition for callosotomized subjects.[77] Thus, though the two hemispheres may compete for cognitive resources, there is evidence for independence of function. This latter finding is consistent with the observation of Luck and coworkers[78] that visual search is independently mediated by both hemispheres. Using a standard spatial cuing paradigm that incorporated a bilateral cue to assess the influence of information presented to one hemisphere on the performance of the other, Mangun and colleagues[79] demonstrated differential processing of spatial cues, with only the LVF (right-hand) trials yielding an advantage for validly cued trials. Although the failure to find an RVF advantage for valid trials is at odds with other results,[74,80] it is consistent with a view of the RH as dominant in terms of spatial attention (see Chaps. 14 and 15).

Apparent inconsistencies uncovered in untangling the ways in which the hemispheres compete for attentional resources has suggested to some researchers that there are different types of attention that engage the hemispheres differently at different levels of processing. Kingstone and colleagues[81,82] have suggested that reflexive or exogenous orienting engages each hemisphere independently but that voluntary (or endogenous) orienting involves competition between the hemispheres for a single resource pool. Luck and Hillyard[83] emphasize that differences in mechanisms utilized at different processing stages determine the ways in which attentional resources are used.

SPECIFICITY OF CALLOSAL FIBERS

In human studies, observations regarding functional specificity of callosal fibers arise from three different sources. First, callosal sections are completed in two different stages, usually anterior first, allow-

ing for observation of functional differences in partially resected patients. Second, development of high-resolution imaging techniques like MRI has permitted verification of the fibers resected during callosotomy and identification of inadvertently spared fibers. Finally, some strokes leave patients with clearly defined lesions of parts of the callosum. Examination of differences in transfer ability in these three groups allows better understanding of specificity of transfer.

It has long been observed that separating up to two-thirds of the anterior callosum leads to little if any change in abilities.[84] If the anterior split continues far enough, disruption of the ability to transfer sensory and position information from hand to hand will be observed. In contrast, the section of the splenium disrupts the transfer of visual information between the hemispheres, which isolates lateralized visual input in a single hemisphere. After posterior section, although explicit identification and naming of LVF stimuli is not possible, some transfer of higher order information may occur.[85]

CONCLUSIONS

Although the behaving being is remarkably intact following callosotomy, investigation reveals hemispheric capacities that refine and confirm hypotheses based on normal subjects and patients with focal lesions. The isolated RH usually cannot read, write, or speak, despite displaying a variety of cognitive behaviors. Dissociations like left-handed tactile anomia or agraphia may be an indication of less competence in language output in the RH. However, the ability to comprehend auditory and visual language may be present in the RH and may contribute to the presentation of aphasic and alexic patients. Recent observations indicate that the RH may participate in long-term recovery from aphasia.[19] Perhaps of greater interest, however, is the study of callosotomy patients to investigate the hemispheric bases of cognition and the integration of diverse perceptual, sensory, and emotional information into a single behavioral plan. The important role played by the LH in allowing the organism to observe and interpret its own actions and emotional states was first recognized in this population. Insights regarding the components of perception, attention, and language continue to arise from this population and to inform our models of normal perceptual and cognitive processing.

REFERENCES

1. Van Wagenen WP, Herren RY: Surgical division of commissural pathways in the corpus callosum: Relation to spread of an epileptic attack. *Arch Neurol Psychiatry* 44:740–759, 1940.

2. Akelaitis AJ: Studies on the corpus callosum: Higher visual functions in each homonymous field following complete section of corpus callosum. *Arch Neurol Psychiatry* 45:788–796, 1941.

3. Akelaitis AJ: A study of gnosis, praxis, and language following section of the corpus callosum and anterior commissure. *J Neurosurg* 7:94–102, 1944.

4. Meyers RE: Function of the corpus callosum in intraocular transfer. *Brain* 79:358, 1956.

5. Meyers RE, Sperry RW: Interhemisperic communication through the corpus callosum: Mnemonic carry-over between the hemispheres. *Arch Neurol Psychiatry* 80:298–303, 1958.

6. Bogen, JE, Gazzaniga MS: Cerebral commissurotomy in man: Minor hemisphere dominance for certain visuospatial functions. *J Neurosurg* 23:394–399, 1965.

7. Sperry RW et al: Interhemispheric relationships: The neocortical commissures; syndromes of hemisphere disconnection, in Vinken PJ, Bruyn GW (eds): *Handbook of Clinical Neurology*. New York: Wiley, 1969, vol 4, pp 273–290.

8. Geschwind N: Disconnection syndromes in animals and man. Part I. *Brain* 88:237–294, 1965.

9. Gazzaniga MS: *The Bisected Brain*. New York: Appleton-Century-Crofts, 1970.

10. Zaidel E: A technique for presenting lateralized visual input with prolonged exposure. *Vision Res* 15:283–289, 1974.

11. Gazzaniga MS: Principles of human brain organization derived from split-brain studies. *Neuron* 14:217–288, 1995.

12. Gazzaniga MS et al: Some functional effects of sectioning the cerebral commissures in man. *Proc Natl Acad Sci U S A* 48:1765–1769, 1962.

13. Levy J et al: Expressive language in the surgically separated minor hemisphere. *Cortex* 7:49–58, 1971.

14. Coltheart M: Deep dyslexia: A right-hemisphere hypothesis, in Coltheart M et al (eds): *Deep Dyslexia*. London: Routledge, 1980.

15. Coltheart M: Disorders of reading and their implications for models of normal reading. *Vis Lang* 15:246–286, 1981.

16. Baynes K et al: Modular organization of cognitive systems masked by interhemispheric integration. *Science* 280:902–905, 1998.

17. Eliassen JC et al: Direction information coordinated via the posterior third of the corpus callosum during bimanual movements. *Exp Brain Res* 128:573–577, 1999.

18. Eliassen JC et al: Anterior and posterior callosal contributions to simultaneous bimanual movements of the hands and fingers. *Brain* 123:2501–2511, 2000.

19. Weiller C: Imaging recovery from stroke. *Exp Brain Res* 123:13–17, 1998.

20. Weiller C et al: Recovery from Wernicke's aphasia: A positron emission tomographic study. *Ann Neurol* 37:723–732, 1995.

21. Gazzaniga MS et al: Profiles of right hemisphere language and speech following brain bisection. *Brain Lang* 22:206–220, 1984.

22. Baynes K, Eliassen JC: The visual lexicon: Its access and organization in commissurotomy patients, in Beeman M, Chiarello C (eds): *Right Hemisphere Language Comprehension*. Hillsdale NJ: Erlbaum, 1998, pp 79–104.

23. Eviatar Z, Zaidel E: The effects of word length and emotionality on hemispheric contributions to lexical decision. *Neuropsychologia* 29:415–428, 1991.

24. Pinker S: *The Language Instinct*. New York: Morrow, 1994.

25. Sidtis JJ et al: Variability in right hemisphere language function after callosal section: Evidence for a continuum of generative capacity. *J Neurosci* 1:323–331, 1981.

26. Zaidel E, Peters AM: Phonological encoding and ideographic reading by the disconnected right hemisphere: Two case studies. *Brain Lang* 14:205–234, 1981.

27. Baynes K et al: Hemispheric contributions to the integration of visual and auditory information in speech perception. *Percept Psychophys* 55:633–641, 1994.

28. Baynes K, Gazzaniga MS: Right hemisphere language: Insights into normal language mechanisms? in Plum F (ed): *Language, Communication, and the Brain*. New York: Raven Press, 1988.

29. Reuter-Lorenz PA, Baynes K: Modes of lexical access in the callosotomized brain. *J Cogn Neurosci* 4(2):155–164, 1992.

30. Schweiger A et al: Right hemisphere contribution to lexical access in an aphasic with deep dyslexia. *Brain Lang* 37:73–89, 1989.

31. Coslett HB, Saffran E: Evidence for preserved reading in "pure alexia." *Brain* 112:327–359, 1989.

32. Coslett HB, Saffran EM: Reading and the right hemisphere: Evidence from acquired dyslexia, in Beeman M, Chiarello C. (eds): *Right Hemisphere Language Comprehension: Perspectives from Cognitive Neuroscience.* Hillsdale, NJ: Erlbaum, 1998, pp 105–132.

33. Baynes K et al: Emergence of access to speech in a disconnected right hemisphere. *Soc Neurosci Abstr* 19: 1809, 1993.

34. Brownell HH: Appreciation of metaphoric and connotative word meaning by brain-damaged patients, in Chiarello C (ed): *Right Hemisphere Contributions to Lexical-Semantics.* New York: Springer-Verlag, 1988, pp 18–31.

35. Brownell HH et al: Inference deficits in right brain-damage. *Brain Lang* 22:310–321, 1986.

36. Gardner H, Denes G: Connotative judgments by aphasic patients on a pictorial adaptation of the semantic differential. *Cortex* 9:183–196, 1973.

37. Hirst W et al: Constraints on the processing of indirect speech acts: Evidence from aphasiology. *Brain Lang* 23:26–33, 1984.

38. Beeman M: Course semantic coding and discourse comprehension, in Beeman M, Chiarello C (eds): *Right Hemisphere Language Comprehension.* Hillsdale, NJ: Erlbaum, 1998, pp 255–284.

39. Chiarello C: On codes of meaning and the meaning of codes: Semantic access and retrieval within and between hemispheres, in Beeman M, Chiarello C (eds): *Right Hemisphere Language Comprehension.* Hillsdale, NJ: Erlbaum, 1998, pp 141–160.

40. Long DL, Baynes K: Discourse representation in the two cerebral hemispheres. *J Cogn Neurosci* 14(2):228–242, 2002.

41. Zaidel D, Sperry RW: Memory impairment after commissurotomy in man. *Brain* 97:263–272, 1974.

42. Zaidel E: Language functions in the two hemispheres following complete cerebral commissurotomy and hemispherectomy, in Boller F, Grafman G (eds): *Handbook of Neuropsychology.* Amsterdam: Elsevier, 1990, vol 4, pp 115–150.

43. Clark CR, Geffen GM: Corpus callosum surgery and recent memory. *Brain* 112:165–175, 1989.

44. Phelps EA, Gazzaniga MS: Hemispheric differences in mnemonic processing: The effects of left hemisphere interpretation. *Neuropsychologia* 30:293–297, 1992.

45. Kroll NEA et al: Cohesion failure as a source of memory illusions. *Mem Lang* 35:176–196, 1996.

46. Jha AP et al: Memory encoding following commissurotomy. *J Cogn Neurosci* 9:143–159, 1997.

47. Gazzaniga MS: *The Social Brain.* New York: Basic Books, 1985.

48. Funnell MG et al (eds): *Hemispheric Interactions and Specializations: Insights From the Split Brain.* Amsterdam: Elsevier, 2000.

49. Gazzaniga MS: Cerebral specialization and interhemispheric communication: Does the corpus callosum enable the human condition? *Brain* 123:1293–1326, 2000.

50. Metcalfe J et al: Right hemisphere memory superiority: studies of a split-brain patient. *Psychol Sci* 6(3):157–164, 1995.

51. Gazzaniga MS: Consciousness and the cerebral hemispheres, in Gazzaniga MS (ed): *The Cognitive Neurosciences.* Cambridge, MA: MIT Press, 1995, pp 1391–1400.

52. Corballis PM et al: An evolutionary perspective on hemispheric asymmetries. *Brain Cogn* 43:112–117, 2000.

53. Corballis PM et al: Illusory contour perception and amodal boundary completion: Evidence of a dissociation following callosotomy. *J Cogn Neurosci* 11:459–466, 1999.

54. Corballis PM et al: A dissociation between spatial and identity matching in callosotomy patients. *Neuroreport* 10(10):2183–2187, 1999.

55. Corballis PM et al: An investigation of the line motion effect in a callosotomy patient. *Brain Cogn* 48(2–3):327–332, 2002.

56. Corballis PM et al: Hemispheric asymmetries for simple visual judgments in the split brain. *Neuropsychologia* 40(4):401–410, 2002.

57. Forster B et al: Effect of luminance on successive discrimination in the absence of the corpus callosum. *Neuropsychologia* 38:441–450, 2000.

58. O'Shea RP, Corballis PM: Binocular rivalry between complex stimuli in split-brain observers. *Brain Mind.* In press.

59. Funnell MG et al: A deficit in perceptual matching in the left hemisphere of a callosotomy patient. *Neuropsychologia* 37:1143–1154, 1999.

60. Milner B, Taylor L: Right hemisphere superiority in tactile pattern recognition after cerebral commissurotomy: Evidence for non-verbal memory. *Neuropsychologia* 10:1–15, 1972.

61. Farah MJ et al: A left hemisphere basis for visual mental imagery? *Neuropsychologia* 23:115–118, 1985.

62. Gazzaniga MS: Organization of the human brain. *Science* 245:947–952, 1989.

63. Baynes K et al: The emergence of the capacity to name left visual field stimuli in a callosotomy patient:

Implications for functional plasticity. *Neuropsychologia* 33(10):1225–1242, 1995.

64. Holtzman JD et al: Dissociation of spatial information for stimulus localization and the control of attention. *Brain* 104:861–872, 1981.

65. Seymour S et al: The disconnection syndrome: Basic findings reaffirmed. *Brain* 117:105–115, 1994.

66. Sergent J: Unified response to bilateral hemispheric stimulation by a split-brain patient. *Nature* 305(27):800–802, 1983.

67. Sergent J: Furtive incursions into bicameral minds. *Brain* 113:537–568, 1990.

68. Corballis MC: Can commissurotomized subjects compare digits between the visual fields? *Neuropsychologia* 32:1475–1486, 1994.

69. Kingstone A, Gazzaniga MS: Subcortical transfer of higher order information in the split-brain patient: More illusory than real? *Neuropsychology* 9:321–328, 1995.

70. Fukuda Y et al: Nasotemporal overlap of crossed and uncrossed retinal ganglion cell projections in the Japanese monkey (*Macaca fuscata*). *J Neurosci* 9:2353–2373, 1989.

71. Stone J: The naso-temporal division of the monkey retina. *J Comp Neurol* 135:585–600, 1966.

72. Fendrich R et al: Naso-temporal overlap at the retinal vertical meridian: Investigations with a callosotomy patient. *Neuropsychologia* 34:637–646, 1996.

73. Fendrich R, Gazzaniga MS: Evidence of foveal splitting in a commissurotomy patient. *Neuropsychologia* 27(3):273–281, 1989.

74. Holtzman JD et al: Spatial orientation following commissural section, in Parasuraman R, Davies DR (eds): *Varieties of Attention.* New York: Academic Press, 1984, pp 375–394.

75. Holtzman JD: Interactions between cortical and subcortical visual areas: Evidence from human commissurotomy patients. *Vis Res* 24:801–813, 1984.

76. Holtzman JD, Gazzaniga MS: Dual task interactions due exclusively to limits in processing resources. *Science* 218:1325–1327, 1982.

77. Holtzman JD, Gazzaniga MS: Enhanced dual task performance following callosal commissurotomy in humans. *Neuropsychologia* 23:315–321, 1985.

78. Luck SJ et al: Independent hemispheric attentional systems mediate visual search in split-brain patients. *Nature* 342:543–545, 1989.

79. Mangun GR et al: Monitoring the visual world: Hemispheric asymmetries and subcortical processes in attention. *J Cogn Neurosci* 6:265–273, 1994.

80. Reuter-Lorenz PA, Fendrich R: Orienting attention across the vertical meridian: Evidence from callosotomy patients. *J Cogn Neurosci* 2:232–238, 1990.

81. Enns J, Kingstone A: Hemispheric cooperation in visual search: Evidence from normal and split-brain observers, in Christman S (ed): *Cerebral Asymmetries in Sensory and Perceptual Processes.* Amsterdam: North-Holland, 1997, pp 197–231.

82. Kingstone A et al: Paying attention to the brain: The study of selective visual attention in cognitive neuroscience, in Burak J, Enns J (eds): *Attention, Development, and Psychopathology.* New York: Guilford, 1997, pp 263–287.

83. Luck SJ, Hillyard SA: The operation of selective attention at multiple stages of processing: Evidence from human and monkey electrophysiology, in Gazzaniga MS (ed): *The Cognitive Neurosciences.* Cambridge, MA: MIT Press, 1999, pp 687–700.

84. Risse GL et al: Interhemispheric transfer in patients with incomplete section of the corpus callosum: Anatomic verification with magnetic resonance imaging. *Arch Neurol* 46:437–443, 1989.

85. Sidtis JJ et al: Cognitive interaction after staged callosal section: Evidence for transfer of semantic activation. *Science* 212:344–346, 1981.

Part V

NONFOCAL ETIOLOGIES:
DEMENTIAS AND
DEVELOPMENTAL DISORDERS

Chapter 31

ALZHEIMER'S DISEASE*

William Milberg
Regina McGlinchey-Berroth

Alzheimer's disease (AD) is the most common dementing illness affecting older adults. It was the first to be identified and clearly defined clinically, and more is known about the pathology, genetics, and molecular biology of AD than about any other degenerative dementia. It has also received a great deal of attention from investigators interested in defining its clinical neuropsychological character and trying to relate these observations to normal models of cognition. Yet progress in this latter enterprise has been slow and marked in some cases by a surprising amount of disagreement about even fundamental theoretical issues. There are several good reasons for the lack of consensus. First, the experimental paradigms and theoretical constructs of experimental and cognitive psychology rest on the assumption that neural functions are represented focally and are for the most part independent or modular. The field of cognitive neuropsychology was founded on this assumption and has indeed provided powerful tools for the description and analysis of syndromes that are based on single focal lesions or lesions of a single neural syndrome. For example, deficits in language, memory, and vision following stroke or other focal lesions have been very effectively studied using the paradigms of cognitive neuropsychology. Patients with AD may suffer from deficits in all of these domains simultaneously, making it more difficult to conclude that deficits on an experimental task are solely attributable to a single domain.

Second, cognitive neuropsychology rests on the assumption that the underlying lesion itself is ablative. That is, the entire function residing in a circumscribed area of brain tissue has been removed via an ablative lesion. The "lesion" of AD is likely not to be ablative, at least in the stages that allow patients to be sufficiently intact to perform psychological tasks.

While it is true that AD patients do suffer from neural atrophy, this does not appear to be a factor that distinguishes AD from many other disorders. Neural atrophy appears in such diseases as Huntington's chorea, Parkinson's disease, schizophrenia, and alcoholism as well as others.[1] Neural atrophy can also be present to the same extent in older normal adults without AD. None of these other populations have been associated with the extensive semantic memory disorder described in patients with AD.

Furthermore, for most patients, neural atrophy appears to be more important later in the course of the disorder, appearing as a consequence of pathophysiologic factors specific to AD that occur early in the disease. In a longitudinal study, Fox et al.[2] measured cerebral atrophy in clinically normal individuals who were at high risk for developing AD. Blinded assessment of the scans revealed "the appearance of diffuse cerebral and medial temporal lobe atrophy in subjects *only once they were clinically affected*" (our italics) by the clinical signs of dementia. These patients, however, did show preclinical cognitive decline on neuropsychological measures well before the appearance of detectable atrophy or clinically significant dementia. This finding suggests that incipient pathologic changes were occurring in these patients before atrophy itself could be observed.

In fact, the critical early marker for the disorder is the effect on synaptic connectivity caused by neuritic plaques and neurofibrillary tangles.[3-6] There is now considerable evidence that affected neurons sprout new dystrophic neural connections.[7] Last, there is increasing evidence that the reduction of such

* **ACKNOWLEDGMENT**: This research was supported by Department of VA Medical Research Service VA Merit Review Awards to Regina McGlinchey-Berroth and William Milberg.

neurotransmitters as acetylcholine has the effect of demodulating existing neural connections by increasing the likelihood of activation (for a review see Ref. 8).

A more realistic model of the pathology of AD should at least make some reference to the changes and disregulation of connectivity that characterize the disease during its early stages. In fact, very recently there have been some attempts to develop models of the pathology of AD that are more closely derived from the notion that connectivity is disrupted.[8,9] In these models, the pathologic mechanism is an interruption of the modulation of activation rather than a loss of activation per se. For example, Hasselmo[8] has suggested that the mechanism underlying the advancement of AD within the nervous system is what he terms "runaway synaptic modification," a cascade of synaptic overactivation that gradually induces pathology in ever increasing areas of a neural network. Models such as Hasselmo's have not been applied to the problem of providing an account for the neuropsychological deficits of AD, but they at least represent a biologically plausible pathologic mechanism that does not rely on the notion of degraded knowledge to account for functional deficits.

A third reason for the lack of theoretical consensus, and perhaps the one causing the most difficulty, is that the clinical syndrome of AD is in itself an evolving phenomenon, potentially changing its fundamental nature as the disease progresses. While the early stages of the disease may be accompanied by extensive neural disconnection affecting strategic focal regions, the later stages of the disease may indeed be more ablative in nature, though more neural regions and systems may be affected.

With these issues in mind we review below two areas of cognitive function that have been most intensively investigated: semantic memory and attention.

SEMANTIC MEMORY IN ALZHEIMER'S DISEASE

Semantic memory encompasses our general knowledge of word meanings and categories (see Chap. 27). Martin and Fedio made what was probably the first strong theoretical statement regarding semantic memory in AD.[10] Based on logic first outlined by Warrington and others,[11,12] they argued that AD patients' consistent pattern of deficits on a number of language tasks could be attributed to a "disruption in the organization of semantic knowledge" or a "loss of semantic knowledge." Subsequently, the view favored by Martin and Fedio was widely echoed by other laboratories,[13–15] who continued to document AD patients' poor performance on a variety of tasks designed to directly assess the integrity of their semantic knowledge base (i.e., facts, word meanings, etc.).

Nebes and colleagues[16] were the first to challenge the semantic loss or degradation view by using a semantic priming paradigm that had previously uncovered evidence of preserved semantic processing in aphasic patients.[17] This paradigm differed in an important way from those used in most of the previous studies examining the semantic memory of patients with AD. Specifically, the priming paradigm assessed semantic knowledge indirectly or implicitly by observing changes in the time and accuracy with which individuals performed simple word-nonword decisions (lexical decisions) or in overlearned language tasks such as word reading. This was in contrast to prior studies that asked patients to directly access and retrieve semantic information or make explicit judgments upon that information. Having set out to support further the already overwhelming case for degraded representations (R.D. Nebes, personal communication, July 14, 1998), the investigators were surprised to find that AD patients showed normal sensitivity to semantic relationships (i.e., semantic priming).[16,18] Since the initial reports by Nebes and colleagues, these findings have also been extended and replicated in a number of laboratories.[19–24] It was the assumption of these investigators that the presence of preserved semantic priming constituted a prima facie case that AD patients suffered not from a degradation or loss of semantic knowledge but from a loss of retrieval or other attentionally mediated access processes.[21]

There is no question that these two theoretical positions have had considerable heuristic value, galvanizing a great deal of research focused on an important clinical issue. There is also little question that this work provided a foundation for the emergence of semantic memory as a topic central to the field of experimental clinical neuropsychology. It is therefore disconcerting that the theoretical dividing lines drawn by these views have changed little since Nebes reviewed what was already a fully formed debate a decade ago.[25] The lack of evolution toward a theoretical common ground suggests that there must be something singularly unconvincing about the constituent positions of an explanatory dichotomy that has allowed for more steadfast and unrelenting partisanship than a congressional debate on taxes. With only a little reflection, it becomes evident that each position has both empiric and logical disadvantages that have prevented the development of a consensus on how to describe the pathology of semantic memory of AD.

The primary empiric disadvantage of each of these theoretical positions is that neither knowledge degradation nor retrieval-based models can account for the wide range of experimental phenomenon characterizing the semantic memory deficit of AD. This probably derives from the fact that each position has primarily drawn support from a specific and limited set of experimental paradigms. For example, most studies that provide evidence for degraded knowledge or degraded representations have used tasks that require explicit access or direct judgments to be made upon semantic information (e.g., word reading, picture identification, providing definitions, category attribute ranking or judgment, matching category members or features to objects, etc.). On the other hand, most of the studies that have concluded that semantic knowledge is preserved in AD have relied almost entirely on implicit measures like the semantic priming paradigm. The alliance of paradigm with theory has been so nearly complete in this literature as if to establish a virtual operational identity between the two.

One important exception was a study by Chertkow and coworkers,[26] who assessed implicit priming performance relative to explicit performance on a variety of semantic knowledge tasks. Using this multimeasure approach, they documented a critical observation regarding a possible priming abnormality in patients with AD. They found larger-than-normal priming or "hyperpriming" in patients with AD. This effect was most pronounced for exemplars from categories found to be "degraded" in the tasks requiring more explicit access to semantic knowledge. They thereby operationalized degraded knowledge as a failure to perform normally on explicit semantic tasks. Because of this

association, they concluded that "hyperpriming" was a reflection of degraded knowledge.

The study by Chertkow et al.[26] represents one of the only attempts to reconcile direct/explicit and indirect/implicit semantic memory measures and to document potential abnormalities in both kinds of tasks. Though hyperpriming has been offered as a possible example of an implicit phenomenon that could be associated with knowledge degradation, the arguments of Chertkow and colleagues depends on the acceptance of the assumption that failure of a semantic judgment task can be caused only by degradation of knowledge. As we discuss below, failure to perform on tasks requiring the use of semantic knowledge does *not* necessarily implicate the unavailability of that information, since the performance of these tasks requires the participation of retrieval operations and other attentionally mediated functions.

Furthermore, "knowledge degradation" theories predict a reduction of priming for all semantic relationships. For example, computational models of semantic memory in AD simulate the differential loss of weak compared to strong semantic relationships by the addition of "noise" or to a random loss of nodes or internodal connectivity (see Chap. 7).[27,28] In these models, all relationships are degraded, but weaker associates may drop below threshold before stronger associates. There is indeed evidence that weak semantic associates may produce less reliable priming effects in patients with AD than normal adults.[29,30]

Hyperpriming is but one of several patterns of results obtained with implicit measures of semantic knowledge that presents an empiric challenge to both degradation and retrieval accounts. Recall that the data of Chertkow et al.[26] contrast to the initial findings of Nebes et al.,[16] who found normal semantic priming effects. Indeed, some studies showed priming effects of a normal magnitude,[16,18] still others showed diminished priming,[21,30] and some have even shown negative priming.[19,31]

Ober and Shenaut[24] have suggested that variations in the magnitude of semantic priming effects may be due to the degree to which automatic and controlled processing contribute to performance in a particular semantic priming experiment. In a metanalysis of approximately 21 priming studies conducted between 1984 and 1991, Ober and Shenaut concluded that hyperpriming was observed only in those experiments that employed "a pairwise, long stimulus onset asynchrony (SOA) priming paradigm, with relatedness proportions from 0.33 to 0.67." They speculated that such conditions allowed for controlled processing to contribute to performance. In contrast, normal priming was observed in experimental paradigms using "short-SOA, pairwise paradigms, or continuous paradigms" that only allowed automatic processing to contribute to performance. They interpreted these results as an indication that automatic processes are intact in AD, leading to normal magnitude priming effects during these conditions. They hypothesized that controlled processing is the central impairment of semantic memory in AD, leading to abnormal hyperpriming. Though in principle Ober and Shenaut's claim may be true, the automatic-controlled dichotomy does not account for the fact that some studies show reduced priming for prime-target relationships that do not have a strong associative relationship.[29,30] It also does not account for that fact that AD patients may also show "negative priming."[19,31]

In addition to their ties to limited sets of empiric phenomena, the degradation and retrieval-based theoretical positions require the acceptance of either vague or questionable assumptions and logic. First consider the retrieval-based account of the semantic memory deficits in AD. Though retrieval processes or other attentionally mediated processes may be involved in both explicit and implicit semantic tasks, these constructs are at best vague and do not provide a blueprint to account for the wide variety of deficits that have been consistently documented in AD patients. The phenomenon of hyperpriming is an important example. To posit a retrieval-based account of hyperpriming as due to impaired controlled processes is at best descriptive because, in the context of a semantic priming paradigm, there are at least two candidate processes that could be responsible for variations in priming effects at long SOAs: prime-target expectancies[32] and postlexical checking.[33] Both involve the retrieval or recognition of the semantic relationship between prime and target to help reduce response time in making target-based responses to related word targets. We know from the explicit studies that AD patients have an impaired ability to retrieve semantic information. The inability to retrieve or recognize prime-target relations

should *reduce, not increase,* attentionally mediated or controlled-based priming. A controlled-based account of hyperpriming must posit a deficit based on a greater-than-normal tendency or ability to retrieve and/or predict semantically based relationships between prime and target. Such an explanation is at best counterintuitive, though it is possible, as we argue, that under some circumstances highly overlearned semantic associations may attain abnormally salient status for patients with AD. As such, it may be possible to describe a controlled processing mechanism to account for hyperpriming, but such a description has not been forthcoming.

Another empiric difficulty with controlled processing–based accounts is that, at least in the context of semantic priming tasks, these processes are never directly measured or observed. The operation of controlled processes is only indirectly observed by varying experimental conditions (such as SOA or relatedness proportion) that would merely allow such processes to occur. There has yet to be a direct demonstration of controlled processing abnormalities in a semantic priming task in AD patients. The difficulty in operationalizing such constructs (as retrieval and controlled processing) probably accounts for the fact that they have failed to find their way into formal models of the pathology of semantic memory.

Although the construct of knowledge degradation may be more easily operationalized than that of retrieval or controlled processes, acceptance of this position is based on the assumption that performance on semantic memory tasks is solely dependent on the availability of knowledge structures. This leads to the related premise that performance deficits on semantic tasks are functionally equivalent to "degraded representations." This logic was first advanced by Warrington and Shallice,[12] who suggested that certain criteria could be used to infer the presence of deficits in stored information by comparing performance to criterial patients (e.g., agnosics or aphasics), for whom such deficits could be assumed to be true.

More recently, several laboratories have explored specific processes intrinsic to the retrieval of semantic information without implicating retrieval per se. The most intriguing example of this type of approach is in the work of Balota and his colleagues,[20,34,35] who have suggested that dysfunction in inhibitory control systems contributes to the impairments seen in attention, semantic memory, and language comprehension in AD. This position is appealing because it is quite specific as an account of deficits on tasks requiring explicit retrieval of semantic information without the inherent difficulties of knowledge degradation–based accounts. However, this model also asserts that facilitatory processes are preserved (e.g., Ref. 34). As described, the phenomena of hyperpriming and negative priming suggest that semantic facilitation is not always normal in AD. Although inhibitory control may still work as an account for a variety of judgment-based deficits, it remains to be seen whether the data from implicit tasks may ultimately be incorporated into this type of model.

Milberg et al.[36] recently proposed that small disruptions in the rate and peak levels of activation (caused by alterations in the time constant of the function relating activation to time) can be used to account for a wide variety of implicit and explicit data as well as some of the critical phenomena that are considered clinical benchmarks of the semantic memory disorder of AD (see Ref. 31). The gain/decay hypothesis suggests that variations in the strength of association will lead to empirically different consequences than variations in the time constant. This simple change has many specific empiric implications, accounting for both implicit and explicit semantic memory findings.

ATTENTION IN AD

Most studies investigating attentional processing in AD (and in normal individuals) have adopted the paradigm and basic premises of Posner's attentional orienting task.[37,38] Posner and colleagues proposed a model of attentional orienting consisting of three component processes: (1) disengagement of attention from the current focus, (2) moving or shifting of attention to a new focus, and (3) engagement of attention at the new focus. These shifts of attention can occur overtly, meaning that eye movements accompany them, or they can occur covertly, without eye movements. Posner and his colleagues proposed that facilitation of response times (RTs) at the validly cued location reflects the RT savings in having already oriented to the target location based on the cue, whereas the lengthened RTs to invalidly cued targets are due to the time required to disengage and reorient attention from an incorrect to a correct spatial location.[39,40]

Using this logic, investigators have examined the phenomenon of inhibition of return (IOR) in patients with AD. *IOR* refers to a tendency to inhibit the orienting of attention to a previously attended location; a very early visual attentional biasing mechanism thought to automatically orient the visual system to novel stimuli in the environment. A number of studies investigating IOR using cuing paradigms have indicated that this function is intact in patients with AD (e.g., Ref. 34), but that it can break down in the context of more complex processing requirements.[41]

In a classic demonstration, Parasuraman and colleagues[42] investigated AD patients' ability to orient their attention spatially. It was found that AD patients were not impaired in their ability to focus attention to a validly cued target location (indicated by RT benefits that did not differ between AD patients and controls) but were markedly impaired in their ability to shift attention from an invalidly cued location to a new location (greater costs), particularly with centrally located cues (that initiate more effortful shifts) and at longer SOAs. This "disengage deficit" has been replicated in numerous, more complex visual search tasks and may be most pronounced for AD patients in conjunction searches in which the precue does not precisely indicate the correct location of the target, suggesting a restriction in the dynamic range of spatial attention in AD.[43–45]

Taken together, these studies suggest that AD patients can use the advanced information provided by a cue to select stimuli, but also that their ability to shift the focus of attention from a cued location to an unexpected location is greatly compromised. This story is complicated, however, by the findings of Duncan et al.[46] This target detection experiment was similar to the study of Parasuraman et al.[42] in that targets were lateralized and preceded by valid, invalid, and neutral cues with varying SOAs. Consistent with the earlier study, the data indicated that control participants showed significant benefits for valid cues and significant costs for invalid cues. The AD patients, however, showed significant benefits for valid cues but no significant costs from invalid cues. In fact, AD patients were actually *faster* to respond to invalid cues than normal (see also Freed et al.,[47] who found a subgroup of AD patients who responded "anomalously" to targets following an invalid cue in that they were faster to respond in the invalid compared to valid condition). A possible reconciling factor between the study of Duncan and colleagues and that of Parasuraman et al. is that in the latter study patients had a mean score on the Folstein Mini-Mental State Exam (MMSE) of 21.3. The sample of patients in the study of Duncan et al. had a mean MMSE score of 18.6, and there was a significant positive correlation between MMSE and costs. Thus it is possible that our patients were functionally more impaired and manifesting a greater inhibitory deficit (see below).

The "Posner paradigm" has also been used extensively to investigate selective attention. Selective attention refers to a set of mechanisms that function to limit or focus the stream of incoming information from the environment that subsequently receives more elaborative processing. In this way, stimuli in the environment are either "selected" for more elaborative processing,[37,48–50] or they can passively decay over time,[51,52] or they are actively suppressed.[53–55]

The concepts of selection and inhibition in attentional functioning have been examined across a broad range of tasks, from simple target detection to semantic activation. Overall, this research has indicated that the selection component of attention remains relatively intact in patients with AD, but there is a selective impairment in the inhibitory component that, while present to some degree in "normal aging," is more severe in patients with AD.

For example, in an early study, Nebes and Brady[56] asked subjects to detect a target letter in an array of six letters. The target letter was always black, but on half of the trials, four of the distractors were red (reducing the relevant distractors to only two). The difference between search times for targets in mixed distractor arrays compared to all-black arrays was similar in their patients and their control subjects, indicating intact selection.

Sullivan and coworkers[35] investigated selective attention in a group of AD patients, age-matched normal controls, and young controls using a priming paradigm similar to that developed by Tipper and colleagues.[53,54] Sullivan et al. found that AD patients could successfully discriminate a target from a distractor (indicating intact selection) but were disproportion-

ately impaired relative to the young and age-matched normal controls in their ability to inhibit distracting information.

In a similar study, Grande et al.[57] used a semantic priming task in which two vertically aligned drawings of objects (one orange, one blue) served as the priming stimuli and object names served as target stimuli. Subjects attended to the drawing of only one color and read aloud a centrally presented word target that was the name of either the attended object, the unattended object, or an object unrelated to either in the prime display. Normal control participants showed semantic facilitation only for target items that were the name of the attended prime object, while AD patients demonstrated facilitation for both the attended and unattended prime objects. Grande et al. suggested that these findings were due to an impairment in AD patients that resulted in semantic activation of information that is normally inhibited.

Duncan et al.[46] also examined semantic facilitation and inhibition in a priming task. In this experiment, precues indicated the probable location of a critical priming stimulus (left or right visual field) that always appeared with a nonsense priming stimulus in the opposing visual field. The target stimuli were centrally presented words that could be either semantically related, unrelated, or neutral with regard to the priming stimulus. Findings indicated that for normal control participants, the cue was sufficient to orient attention only to the validly cued primes; semantic facilitation was observed only following validly cued primes. AD patients, however, showed significant semantic facilitation regardless of the validity of the cue. This finding was interpreted to indicate a deficit in the ability of AD patients to inhibit semantic information appearing at an invalidly cued location.

Further support for an inhibitory breakdown in AD comes from studies utilizing the Stroop task. In general, a number of studies have reported that older control subjects are slowed in the incongruent condition (greater interference effect) to a greater extent than are younger subjects,[58–60] but that AD patients are disproportionately slowed compared to age-matched normal control participants.[61,62] These studies support the notion of an inhibitory dysfunction in normal aging and an accelerated breakdown in inhibition in patients with AD.

REFERENCES

1. Hopkins A: *Clinical Neurology: A Modern Approach.* London: Oxford University Press, 1993.
2. Fox NC, Warrington EK, Seiffer AL, et al: Presymptomatic cognitive deficits in individuals at risk of familial Alzheimer's disease—a longitudinal prospective study. *Brain* 121:1631-1639, 1998.
3. Callahan LM, Coleman PD: Neurons bearing neurofibrillary tangles are responsible for selected synaptic deficits in Alzheimer's disease. *Neurobiol Aging* 16(3):311–314, 1995.
4. Cook IA, Leuchter AF: Synaptic dysfunction in Alzheimer's disease: clinical assessment using quantitative EEG. *Behav Brain Res* 78:15–23, 1996.
5. Dickson DW, Crystal HA, Bevona C, et al: Correlations of synaptic and pathological markers with cognition of the elderly. *Neurobiol Aging* 16(3):285–304, 1995.
6. Nielson KA, Cummings BJ, Cotman CW: Constructional apraxia in Alzheimer's disease correlates with neuritic neuropathology in occipital cortex. *Brain Res* 741(1–2):284–293, 1996.
7. Clinton J, Blackman SE-A, Royston MC, et al: Differential synaptic loss in the cortex in Alzheimer's disease: A study using archival material. *Neuroreport* 5: 497–500, 1994.
8. Hasselmo ME: Runaway synaptic modification in models of cortex: Implications for Alzheimer's disease. *Neur Netw* 7(1):13–40, 1994.
9. Ruppin E, Horn D, Levy N, et al: Computational studies of synaptic alterations in Alzheimer's disease, in Reggia JA, Ruppin E, Berndt RS (eds): *Neural Modeling of Brain and Cognitive Disorders*. Singapore: World Scientific, 1996, pp 63–87.
10. Martin A, Fedio P: Word production and comprehension in Alzheimer's disease: The breakdown of semantic knowledge. *Brain Lang* 19:124–141, 1983.
11. Warrington EK: The selective impairment of semantic memory. *Q J Exp Psychol* 27:635–657, 1975.
12. Warrington EK, Shallice T: Semantic access dyslexia. *Brain* 102:43–63, 1979.
13. Bayles KA, Tomoeda CK, Trosset MW: Naming and categorical knowledge in Alzheimer's disease: The process of semantic memory deterioration. *Brain Lang* 39:498–510, 1990.
14. Grober E, Buschke H, Kawas C, et al: Impaired ranking of semantic attributes in dementia. *Brain Lang* 26(2):276–286, 1985.
15. Hodges JR, Salmon DP, Butters N: Semantic memory impairment in Alzheimer's disease: Failure of access or degraded knowledge. *Neuropsychologia* 30(4):301–314, 1992.
16. Nebes RD, Martin DC, Horn LC: Sparing of semantic memory in Alzheimer's disease. *J Abnorm Psychol* 93(3):321–330, 1984.
17. Milberg W, Blumstein S: Lexical decision and aphasia: Evidence for semantic processing. *Brain Lang* 14:371–385, 1981.
18. Nebes RD, Boller F, Holland A: Use of semantic context by patients with Alzheimer's disease. *Psychol Aging* 1(3):261–269, 1986.
19. Albert M, Milberg W: Semantic processing in patients with Alzheimer's disease. *Brain Lang* 37:163–171, 1989.
20. Balota DA, Duchek JM: Semantic priming effects, lexical repetition effects, and contextual disambiguation effects in healthy aged individuals and individuals with senile dementia of the Alzheimer's type. *Brain Lang* 40:181–201, 1991.
21. Ober BA, Shenaut GK: Lexical decision and priming in Alzheimer's disease. *Neuropsychologia* 26(2):273–286, 1988.
22. Ober BA, Shenaut GK, Jagust WJ, et al: Automatic semantic priming with various category relations in Alzheimer's disease and normal aging. *Psychol Aging* 6(4):647–660, 1991.
23. Ober BA, Shenaut GK, Reed BR: Assessment of associative relations in Alzheimer's disease: evidence for preservation of semantic memory. *Aging Cogn* 2(4):254–267, 1995.
24. Ober BA, Shenaut GK: Semantic priming in Alzheimer's disease: Meta-analysis and theoretical evaluation, in Allen PA, Bashore TR (eds): *Age Differences in Word and Language Processing*. Amsterdam: North Holland, 1995.
25. Nebes RD: Semantic memory in Alzheimer's disease. *Psychol Bull* 106(3):377–394, 1989.
26. Chertkow J, Bub D, Seidenberg M: Priming and semantic memory loss in Alzheimer's Disease. *Brain Lang* 36:420–446, 1989.
27. Devlin JT, Andersen ES, Seidenberg MS: Category coordinate errors in a dynamic system: Simulating the naming errors in Alzheimer's disease. *Brain Lang* 65(1):81–83, 1998.
28. Tippett LJ, McAuliffe S, Farah MJ: Preservation of categorical knowledge in Alzheimer disease: A computational account. *Memory* 3:519–533, 1995.
29. Glosser G, Friedman RB: Lexical but not semantic priming in Alzheimer's disease. *Psychol Aging* 6:522–527, 1991.

30. Glosser G, Friedman RB, Grugan PK, et al: Lexical semantic and associative priming in Alzheimer's disease. *Neuropsychology* 12(2):218–224, 1998.

31. McGlinchey-Berroth R, Milberg WP: Preserved semantic memory structure in Alzheimer's disease, in Cerella J et al (eds): *Adult Information Processing: Limits on Loss.* San Diego: Academic Press, 1993, pp 407–422.

32. Neely JH: Semantic priming effects in visual word recognition: a selection review of current findings and theories, in Besner D, Humphreys GW (eds): *Basic Processes in Reading: Visual Word Recognition.* Hillsdale, NJ: Erlbaum, 1991.

33. de Groot AMB: Primed lexical decision: Combined effects of proportion of related prime-target pairs and the stimulus-onset asynchrony of prime and target. *Q J Exp Psychol* 96:29–44, 1984.

34. Faust ME, Balota DA, Duchek JM, et al: Inhibitory control during sentence comprehension in individuals with dementia of the Alzheimer's type. *Brain Lang* 57:225–253, 1997.

35. Sullivan MP, Faust ME, Balota DA: Identity negative priming in older adults and individuals with dementia of the Alzheimer's type. *Neuropsychology* 9(4):1–19, 1995.

36. Milberg WP, McGlinchey-Berroth R, Duncan K, et al: Evidence for alterations in the dynamics of semantic activation in Alzheimer's disease: The gain/decay hypothesis of a disorder of semantic memory. *J Int Neuropsychol Soc* 5:641–658, 1999.

37. Posner MI, Cohen Y: Components of visual orienting, in Bouma H, Bouwhuis D (eds): *Attention and Performance X.* Hillsdale, NJ: Erlbaum, 1984, pp 531–556.

38. Posner MI, Inhoff AW, Friedrich FJ, et al: Isolating attentional systems: A cognitive-anatomical analysis. *Psychobiology* 15(2):107–121, 1987.

39. Posner MI: Structures and functions of selective attention, in Boll T, Bryant B (eds): *Master Lectures in Clinical Neuropsychology.* Washington DC: American Psychological Association, 1988.

40. Posner MI, Peterson S: The attentional system of the human brain. *Annu Rev Neurosci* 13:25–42, 1990.

41. Langley LK, Fuentes LJ, Hochhalter AK, et al: Inhibition of return in aging and Alzheimer's disease: Performance as a function of task demands and stimulus timing. *J Clin Exp Neuropsychol* 23(4):431–446, 2001.

42. Parasuraman R, Greenwood PM, Haxby JV, et al: Visuospatial attention in dementia of the Alzheimer type. *Brain* 115:711–733, 1992.

43. Greenwood PM, Parasuraman R, Alexander GE: Controlling the focus of spatial attention during visual search: Effects of advanced aging and Alzheimer's disease. *Neuropsychologia* 11(3):3–12, 1997.

44. Parasuraman R, Greenwood PM, Alexander GE: Selective impairment of spatial attention during visual search in Alzheimer's disease. *Neuroreport* 6(14):1861–1864, 1995.

45. Parasuraman R, Greenwood PM, Alexander GE: Alzheimer's disease constricts the dynamic range of spatial attention in visual search. *Neuropsychologia* 38(8):1126–1135, 2000.

46. Duncan K, Tunick R, McGlinchey-Berroth R, et al: Covert attention and semantic priming in Alzheimer's disease. Presented at the 27th Annual Meeting of the International Neuropsychological Society, Boston, 1999.

47. Freed DM, Corkin S, Growden JH, et al: Selective attention in Alzheimer's disease: Characterizing cognitive subgroups of patients. *Neuropsychologia* 27(3):325–339, 1989.

48. Houghton G, Tipper P: A model of inhibitory mechanisms in selective attention, in Dagenbach D, Carr TH (eds): *Inhibitory Processes in Attention, Memory, and Language.* San Diego, CA: Academic Press, 1994, pp 53–112.

49. Kahneman D: *Attention and Effort.* Englewood Cliffs, NJ: Prentice-Hall, 1973.

50. Shiffrin RM, Schneider W: Controlled and automatic human information processing: II. Perceptual learning, automatic attending, and a general theory. *Psychol Rev* 84(2):127–190, 1977.

51. Broadbent DE: *Decision and Stress.* London: Academic Press, 1971.

52. Kahneman D, Treisman A: Changing views. of attention and automaticity, in Parasuraman R, Davies R, Beatty J (eds): *Varieties of Attention.* New York: Academic Press, 1984.

53. Tipper SP, Cranston M: Selective attention and priming: Inhibitory and facilitory effects of ignored primes. *Q J Exp Psychol* 37A:591–611, 1985.

54. Tipper SP: The negative priming effect: Inhibitory priming by ignored objects. *Q J Exp Psychol* 37A:571–590, 1985.

55. Tipper SP, Driver J: Negative priming between pictures and words in a selective attention task: Evidence for semantic processing of ignored stimuli. *Mem Cogn* 16(1):64–70, 1988.

56. Nebes RD, Brady CB: Focused and divided attention in Alzheimer's disease. *Cortex* 25(2):305–315, 1989.

57. Grande LJ, McGlinchey-Berroth R, Milberg W, et al: Facilitation of unattended semantic information in Alzheimer's disease: Evidence from a selective attention task. *Neuropsychology* 10(4):475–484, 1996.

58. Cohn NB, Dustman RE, Bradford DC: Age-related decrements in Stroop color test performance. *J Clin Psychol* 40:1244–1250, 1984.

59. Comalli PE, Wapner S, Werner H: Interference effects of Stroop Color-Word Test in childhood, adulthood, and aging. *J Genet Psychol* 100:47–53, 1962.

60. Panek P, Rush M, Slade L: Locus of age-Stroop interference relationships. *J Genet Psychol* 25:201–216, 1984.

61. Fisher LM, Freed DM, Corkin S: Stroop color-word test performance in patients with Alzheimer's disease. *J Clin Exp Neuropsychol* 12(5):745–758, 1990.

62. Speiler DH, Balota DA, Faust ME: Stroop performance in younger adults, healthy older adults and individuals with senile dementia of the Alzheimer's type. *J Exp Psychol Hum Percept Perform* 22(2):461–479, 1996.

Chapter 32

FRONTOTEMPORAL DEMENTIA

Mario F. Mendez

Frontotemporal lobar degeneration (FTLD) is a broad category of degenerative disease that emcompasses frontotemporal dementia (FTD) and variants including primary progressive aphasia and semantic dementia. Beginning in 1892, Arnold Pick described a series of patients with dementia and circumscribed lobar atrophy, particularly of the left temporal lobe.[1] Alzheimer and Altman went on to describe prominent lobar atrophy of gray and white matter and argentophilic intraneuronal inclusions known as Pick's bodies. On neuropathologic examination, however, most patients with FTD lack these pathognomonic Pick bodies necessary for the clinicopathologic diagnosis of "Pick's disease." In fact, FTD is not a single entity but part of a spectrum of disorders that have in common circumscribed and progressive atrophy of the frontotemporal lobes (Table 32-1).[2–4] Converging evidence now suggests that these FTLDs are "taupathies," stemming from tau protein abnormalities in the brain.[2]

EPIDEMIOLOGY

The FTLDs are the second most common degenerative dementia[5] after Alzheimer's disease (AD). FTD is especially common when the age of onset is less than 65 years.[4] The age of onset of FTD averages about 56 to 58 years, with a range beginning as young as 22; the average duration of the disease is 8 to 11 years, with motor variants having a shorter, more malignant course.[4,5] Males and females are equally affected, and the main risk factor is familial; 42 to 50 percent of patients with FTD have a first-degree relative with a FTD.[6,7]

FTD CLINICAL FEATURES

In most patients with FTD, personality changes are dramatic symptoms, and these usually precede or overshadow the cognitive disabilities.[5] Clinical Consensus Criteria for diagnosing FTD include a progressive course, qualitative impairments in social interactions, quantitative changes in personal regulation, impaired emotional ability or blunting, and loss of insight (Table 32-2).[4] Patients lose social tact and become socially intrusive and inappropriate. They are often disinhibited, with impulsive behavior; apathetic, with decreased initiative; or both. FTD patients lack empathy and appear emotionally shallow and indifferent. Other emotional changes include depression, mania, lability, anger, and irritability.[5] As the disease progresses, FTD patients neglect their hygiene and may wander unclothed or urinate or defecate in public. In addition, FTD patients tend toward decreased verbal output, later progressing to complete mutism.

Prominent compulsive-like behaviors are other manifestations of this disease.[8] Perseverative and stereotyped behaviors encompass simple repetitive acts, and verbal or motor stereotypies such as lip smacking, hand rubbing or clapping, counting aloud, and humming. They also encompass complex repetitive motor routines such as wandering a fixed route, collecting and hoarding objects, counting money, and rituals involving unusual toileting behavior, oral behaviors, singing the same songs, touching, grabbing, or superstitious acts.

In midstages of FTD, bilateral temporal lobe involvement with damage to the amygdalar nuclei predisposes to the Klüver-Bucy syndrome.[4,5] This syndrome

Table 32-1
Frontotemporal dementia (FTD) and its variants

FTD, bilateral frontotemporal involvement
  FTD, lacking distinctive histology on neuropathology
  FTD, with Pick bodies and Pick cells on
    neuropathology

Primary progressive aphasia from asymmetrical left
  hemisphere frontotemporal lobar degeneration (FTLD)

Semantic dementia from asymmetrical temporal lobe FTLD

FTD with motor neuron disease or amyotrophic
  lateral sclerosis

FTD with parkinsonism linked to chromosome 17
  (FTDP-17)

Corticobasal ganglionic degeneration (CBGD)

Table 32-2
Consensus clinical diagnostic features of FTD[4]

I. Core diagnostic features (all must be present)
  A. Insidious onset and gradual progression
  B. Early decline in social interpersonal conduct
  C. Early impairment in regulation of personal conduct
  D. Early emotional blunting
  E. Early loss of insight

II. Supportive diagnostic features
  A. Behavioral disorder
    1. Decline in personal hygiene and grooming
    2. Mental rigidity and inflexibility
    3. Distractibility and impersistence
    4. Hyperorality and dietary changes
    5. Perseverative and stereotyped behavior
    6. Utilization behavior
  B. Speech and language: Altered speech output
    (aspontaneity and economy of speech, press of
    speech), stereotypy of speech, echolalia,
    perseveration, mutism
  C. Physical signs: Primitive reflexes, incontinence,
    akinesia, rigidity, tremor, low and labile blood
    pressure
  D. Investigations
    1. Neuropsychology: impaired frontal tests without
    amnesia or perceptual deficits
    2. EEG: normal on conventional EEG despite
    clinically evident dementia
    3. Brain imaging: predominant frontal and/or
    anterior temporal abnormality

Source: From Neary et al.,[4] with permission.

includes hypermetamorphosis or the compulsion to attend and touch every visual stimulus, hyperorality and altered dietary changes, altered sexual behavior, visual agnosia, and placidity. Hypermetamorphosis is the compulsion to attend to any visual stimulus. Patients are driven to explore and manipulate objects, particularly with their mouths. Hyperorality results in overeating and the eating of inedible items; it may require restraints to prevent suffocation.[9]

On neuropsychologic testing, frontal-executive functions are compromised early, memory is less impaired, and occipitoparietal functions are relatively preserved.[10] Frontal-executive functions such as planning and follow-through, set shifting and sequencing, and judgment are abnormal. Memory is eventually compromised, but there is relative preservation of recognition memory compared to free recall. Visuospatial functions, however, remain intact in most patients. As the disease advances, patients develop global cognitive impairments and compromised activities of daily living.

On neurologic examination, abnormalities are usually confined to the presence of primitive reflexes such as grasp, snout, and sucking reflexes. In subsets of FTD patients, however, the neurologic examination discloses dysarthria, dysphagia, fasciculations, muscle wasting, parkinsonism, ideomotor apraxia, or dystonia.

FTLD Variants: Primary Progressive Aphasia, Semantic Dementia, and Motor Variants

Investigators have identified several variants of FTLD.[11,12] The left hemisphere–predominant patients have early speech and language difficulty or a primary progressive aphasia syndrome (see below) but otherwise normal behavioral status. In contrast, the right hemisphere–predominant patients have preserved speech and language but prominent personality changes. In addition to the usual frontotemporal combination, there are patients with predominant frontal or predominant temporal involvement.[12] The predominant frontal patients have more dysexecutive cognitive changes and the predominant temporal patients may have elements of the Klüver-Bucy syndrome or of semantic dementia (see below).

Table 32-3

Consensus clinical criteria for progressive nonfluent aphasia

I. Core diagnostic features
  A. Insidious onset and gradual progression
  B. Nonfluent spontaneous speech with at least one of the following: agrammatism, phonemic paraphasias, anomia

II. Supportive diagnostic features
  A. Speech and language
    1. Stuttering or oral apraxia
    2. Impaired repetition
    3. Alexia, agraphia
    4. Early preservation of word meaning
    5. Late mutism
  B. Behavior
    1. Early preservation of social skills
    2. Late behavioral changes similar to FTD
  C. Physical signs: late contralateral primitive reflexes, akinesia, rigidity, and tremor
  D. Investigations
    1. Neuropsychology: nonfluent aphasia without amnesia or perceptual disorder
    2. EEG: normal or minor asymmetrical slowing
    3. Brain imaging (structural and/or functional): asymmetric abnormality predominantly affecting dominant (usually left) hemisphere

Source: From Neary et al.,[4] with permission.

Table 32-4

Consensus clinical criteria for semantic dementia

I. Core diagnostic features
  A. Insidious onset and gradual progression
  B. Language disorder characterized by
    1. Progressive, fluent, empty spontaneous speech
    2. Loss of word meaning, manifest by impaired naming and comprehension
    3. Semantic paraphasias *and/or*
  C. Perceptual disorder characterized by
    1. Prosopagnosia: impaired recognition of identity of familiar faces *and/or*
    2. Object agnosia: impaired recognition of object identity
  D. Preserved perceptual matching and drawing reproduction
  E. Preserved single-word repetition
  F. Preserved ability to read aloud and write to dictation orthographically regular words

II. Supportive diagnostic features
  A. Speech and language: Press of speech, idiosyncratic word usage, absence of phonemic paraphasias, surface dyslexia and dysgraphia, preserved calculation
  B. Behavior: Loss of sympathy and empathy, narrowed preoccupations, parsimony
  C. Physical signs: Absent or late primitive reflexes, akinesia, rigidity, and tremor
  D. Investigations: Neuropsychology: Profound semantic loss, manifest in failure of word comprehension and naming and/or face and object recognition; preserved phonology, syntax, perceptual/spatial skills, memorizing. EEG: normal; Brain imaging: predominant anterior temporal abnormality-symmetrical or asymmetrical

Source: From Neary et al.,[4] with permission.

Some patients with FTLD lateralized to the left hemisphere present with an isolated primary progressive aphasia (PPA) for at least 2 years before other clinical manifestations appear.[13] PPA is characterized by difficulty in verbal expression, anomia, and shortened phrase length in the presence of relative preservation of comprehension (Table 32-3).[4] Speech is hesitant, broken, telegraphic (agrammatism), dysarthric, and effortful. There may be phonologic (phonemic paraphasic) errors, particularly in repetition, a decreased repetition span, and comparably impaired reading and writing. PPA that progresses anteriorly to affect frontal functions is usually associated with FTD, but the syndrome is etiologically heterogeneous, with some patients found at postmortem to have had AD.[13]

Another asymmetrical FTLD variant is semantic dementia (Table 32-4).[4] In this syndrome, which some consider to be a semantic form of PPA, speech production is fluent, but there are deficiencies in single-word comprehension. There may be semantic paraphasias characterized by the replacement of correct words with semantically related ones. Reading is consistent with surface dyslexia; there is preserved ability to read phonologically, with regular spelling-to-sound correspondence, but difficulty reading orthographically irregular words. The rest of the cognitive profile in semantic dementia reflects early profound semantic loss in other domains with preservation of other cognitive abilities. There may be impairments of object meaning or identity (object agnosia) or of the recognition of familiar faces (prosopagnosia). These are not perceptual disturbances, because patients can match objects and demonstrate normal performance on perceptual matching for identity. These patients usually have a temporal variant of FTLD affecting the inferior and middle temporal gyri,[14] and they can have other FTLD-spectrum findings such as motor neuron disease.[15]

Motor variants of FTLD include FTD with motor neuron disease or amyotrophic lateral sclerosis (ALS-FTD), FTD with parkinsonism linked to chromosome 17 (FTDP-17), and corticobasal ganglion degeneration (CBGD). Approximately 10 percent of FTD patients have accompanying ALS with prominent bulbar involvement and a rapid disease course.[16] In some cases, FTD with parkinsonism occurs as a hereditary autosomal dominant disorder linked to chromosome 17q21-22.[17] These FTDP-17 patients make up about 13 to 14 percent of those with a positive family history of FTD, and, in addition to early parkinsonism, manifest a more rapidly progressive course and an earlier age of onset than most FTD patients.[18] Finally, the combination of FTD with asymmetrical involvement of the parietal lobe and basal ganglia plus brainstem basophilic (corticobasal) inclusions may be identical with the syndrome of CBGD. These patients have asymmetrical parkinsonism, myoclonus, ideomotor apraxia, and an "alien limb" that feels foreign with involuntary, semipurposeful movements.[19]

DIFFERENTIAL DIAGNOSIS

Clinicians diagnose FTD after excluding other conditions that can present with similar behavioral changes, such as primary psychiatric disease and other frontally predominant dementias. Other diseases involving the frontal or frontal and temporal lobes include AD with frontal features, vascular dementia, normal-pressure hydrocephalus, neurosyphilis, AIDS dementia, Huntington's disease, Creutzfeldt-Jakob disease, adult-onset neuronal intranuclear hyaline inclusion disease, adult polyglucason body disease, and frontotemporal mass lesions.

During life, FTD is most commonly confused with AD.[5] In early AD, there is amnesia with preserved social skills and personal propriety; in early FTD,

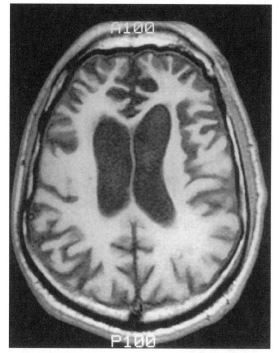

A

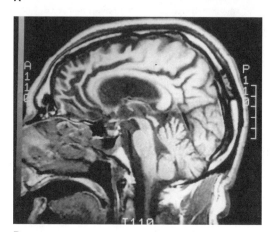

B

Figure 32-1
Magnetic resonance imaging scans of patient with frontotemporal dementia proven to be Pick's disease on autopsy. T1-weighted horizontal (A) and sagittal (B) images demonstrating frontotemporal atrophy.

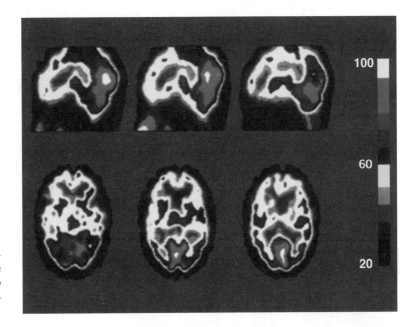

Figure 32-2
Single photon emission computed tomography (SPECT) scans of patient with Pick's disease demonstrating frontal hypometabolism.

there are interpersonal and other personality changes with the relative preservation of memory.[5] In these early stages, FTD patients also perform significantly better than the AD patients on elementary drawings and calculations.[20] Loss of personal awareness, eating changes or hyperorality, stereotyped and perseverative behavior, progressive reduction of speech rather than fluent logorrhea, and preserved spatial orientation differentiated 100 percent of patients with FTD from those with AD.[21]

NEUROIMAGING

There are no definitive laboratory tests for FTD, but neuroimaging can help confirm the presence of this syndrome. Although absent early, most FTD patients eventually show frontotemporal atrophy, which is often asymmetrical, on computed tomography (CT) or magnetic resonance imaging (MRI) (Fig. 32-1). In contrast, AD patients have more generalized atrophy with smaller hippocampal formations.[22,23] Functional imaging is more sensitive than structural imaging for the diagnosis of FTD. Single photon emission computed tomography (SPECT) and positron emission tomography (PET) show decreased regional cerebral blood

flow and hypometabolism in the frontal cortex and anterior temporal lobes (Fig. 32-2).[24] In contrast, SPECT and PET scans show predominant posterior temporoparietal changes in AD.[24] Patients with the PPA and semantic dementia show asymmetrical changes in the left hemisphere or temporal lobes, respectively (Fig. 32-3).

NEUROPATHOLOGIC FEATURES

At autopsy, the brains of patients with FTD show a lobar distribution of atrophy involving the frontal lobes, temporal lobes, or both. Coronal sections reveal deep sulci and knife-edged gyri in the atrophic areas (Fig. 32-4). An abrupt transition may be evident between involved and uninvolved cortical regions, and there is a tendency for sparing of the precentral gyrus and the posterior one-third of the superior temporal gyrus. The cortical degeneration mainly involves the gray matter. Further studies of FTD patients disclose Pick bodies in about 20 to 25 percent, motor neuron changes in 10 percent, early parkinsonian changes in 3 to 4 percent, and CBGD in a small percentage.[2,16,17,19,25]

There are several major histopathologic variants of FTLD.[25] First, the most common is a nonspecific

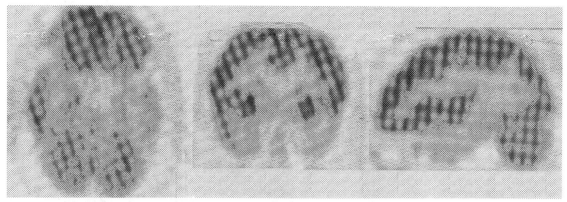

Figure 32-3

Fluorodeoxyglucose positron emission tomography (PET) of patient with semantic dementia demonstrating bilateral anterior temporal hypoperfusion, greater on the left. This image was greatly magnified.

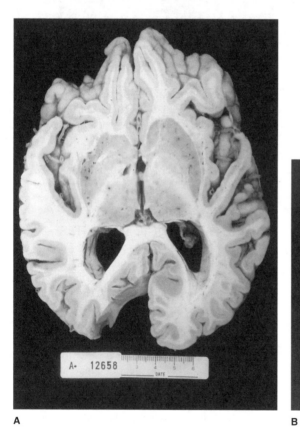

A

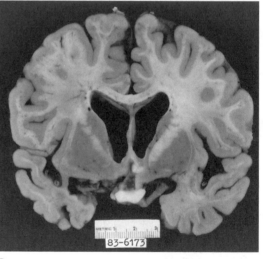

B

Figure 32-4

Gross neuropathologic features of Pick's disease demonstrating disproportionate atrophy of the frontal (A) and temporal (B) lobes (Courtesy of Drs. Linda Chang and Bruce L. Miller.)

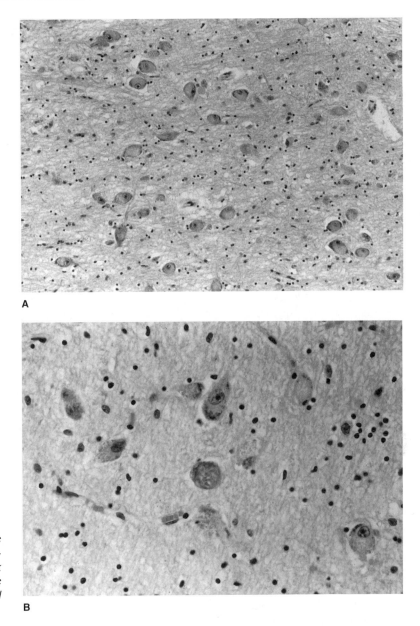

Figure 32-5
Microscopic neuropathologic features of Pick's disease demonstrating neocortical Pick bodies. These intracytoplasmic inclusions have a dark rim and displace the nuclei laterally.

frontotemporal atrophy "lacking distinctive histology." There is neuronal loss and astrogliosis with spongiosis (minute cavities or microvacuolation) of the outer, supragranular layers (II to III) of the frontotemporal cortex, with variable involvement of subcortical and limbic structures. Second, in addition to these changes, there may be pathognomonic changes of Pick's disease. These include severe frontotemporal atrophy often with "knife-like" gyri, ballooned neurons or Pick cells, and tau-positive, ubiquitin-positive Pick bodies (Fig. 32-5). Pick bodies are spherical, argentophilic intraneuronal inclusions consisting of straight 10- to 20-nm neurofilaments and constricted 160-nm fibrils, particularly concentrated in neocortical layers II to III and V to VI and in the granular layer of the dentate gyrus and CA1 sector of the hippocampus.[26] Third, there may be evidence of additional involvement of anterior horn cells with or without ubiquitin-positive inclusions. Finally, smaller numbers of FTLD patients have involvement of the substantia nigra, striatopallidum, parietal cortex, thalamus, and other structures.

The neurotransmitter's changes primarily involve serotonin. There are decreases in serotonin receptors and in postsynaptic serotonin.[27] On the other hand, choline acetyltransferase activity is comparable with that of normal controls, and scopolamine infusion may not improve memory in FTD. Cerebrospinal fluid and brain tissue studies suggest that dopamine is relatively spared but somatostatin is decreased.

PATHOPHYSIOLOGY

The underlying cause of FTLD is unknown, but genetic factors are strongly implicated. A positive family history of a similar dementia in a first-degree relative is present in as many as 38 to 50 percent of patients with FTD.[6,7] Analysis of the frequency of apolipoprotein alleles in patients with FTD indicates an increased frequency of the $\varepsilon 4$ allele, but this is not as strong as for AD.[7,28] Most molecular studies have shown autosomal dominant mutations on chromosome 17[17]; however, there is an FTD pedigree with trinucleotide repeat expansions linked to chromosome 3.[29]

The chromosome 17 mutations involve primarily the gene for tau protein. The most common known tau mutations are located in the microtubular binding domain of tau and are either missplicing mutations in the intronic "stem-loop" site following exon 10 or missense mutations in or outside the exon 10 coding region.[30] These mutations may result in neuronal damage from hyperphosphorylation of tau and disruption of its microtubular binding and stabilization properties.[31] Hyperphosphorylated tau impairs microtubule function and axonal transport, leading to inability to bind to microtubules and allowing the abnormal tau to aggregate into wide, twisted, ribbon-like filaments. In patients with FTDP-17, one common mechanism leading to this abnormal tau function and aggregation is an increase in the ratio of the tau protein isoform with four microtubular binding repeats over the three repeat isoforms.

Another mechanism for abnormal tau expression in some FTDP-17 patients results from mutations located outside the exon 10 region, which lead to neuronal inclusions with both 4R and 3R tau isoforms, similar to the paired helical and straight filaments seen in AD.

TREATMENT

Currently, there is no specific treatment for FTD. In addition to managing the general aspects of dementia, the management of these patients focuses on behavioral interventions. Given the decreased serotonin receptor binding in FTD, many of the behavioral symptoms of FTD may respond to selective serotonin reuptake inhibitors (SSRIs).[32] Marked disinhibition, aggressive behavior, or verbal outbursts may respond to small doses of risperidone or quetiapine, trazodone, or to anticonvulsants such as carbamazepine and valproate. There is no evidence of benefit, however, from the acetylcholinesterase inhibitors used for AD. Patients with PPA and semantic dementia may respond to speech therapy techniques. Methods for the effective treatment of FTLD patients require much more research and investigation. In the future, drugs directed at altering the pathophysiology, such as the abnormally phosphorylated tau residues, may be the key to treating the FTLD disorders.

REFERENCES

1. Kertesz A, Kalvach P: Arnold Pick and German neuropsychiatry in Prague. *Arch Neurol* 53:935, 1996.
2. Kertesz A, Davidson W, Munoz DG: Clinical and pathological overlap between frontotemporal dementia, primary progressive aphasia and corticobasal degeneration: The Pick complex. *Dement Geriatr Cogn Disord* 10:46, 1999.
3. Pasquier F, Lebert F, Lavenu I, et al: The clinical picture of frontotemporal dementia: Diagnosis and follow-up. *Dement Geriatr Cogn Disord* 10:10, 1999.
4. Neary D, Snowden JS, Gustafson L, et al: Frontotemporal lobar degeneration: A consensus on clinical diagnostic criteria. *Neurology* 51:1546, 1998.
5. Mendez MF, Selwood A, Mastri AR, et al: Pick's disease versus Alzheimer's disease: A comparison of clinical characteristics. *Neurology* 43:289, 1993.

6. Chow TW, Miller BL, Hayashi VN, et al: Inheritance of frontotemporal dementia. *Arch Neurol* 56:817, 1999.

7. Stevens M, van Duijn CM, Kamphorst W, et al: Familial aggregation in frontotemporal dementia. *Neurology* 50:1541, 1998.

8. Mendez MF, Perryman KM, Miller BL, et al: Compulsive behaviors as presenting symptoms of frontotemporal dementia. *J Geriatr Psychiatry Neurol* 10:154, 1997.

9. Mendez MF, Foti DJ: Lethal hyperoral behavior from the Klüver-Bucy syndrome. *J Neurol Neurosurg Psychiatry* 62:293, 1997.

10. Hodges JR, Gurd JM: Remote memory and lexical retrieval in a case of frontal Pick's disease. *Arch Neurol* 51:821, 1994.

11. Miller BL, Chang L, Mena I, et al: Progressive right frontotemporal degeneration: Clinical, neuropsychological, and SPECT characteristics. *Dementia* 4:204, 1993.

12. Edwards-Lee T, Miller BL, Benson DF, et al: The temporal variant of frontotemporal dementia. *Brain* 120:1027, 1997.

13. Mesulam MM: Primary progressive aphasia. *Ann Neurol* 49:425, 2001.

14. Mummery CJ, Patterson K, Price CJ, et al: A voxel-based morphometry study of semantic dementia: Relationship between temporal lobe atrophy and semantic memory. *Ann Neurol* 47:36, 2000.

15. Rossor MN, Revesz T, Lantos PL, et al: Semantic dementia with ubiquitin-positive tau-negative inclusion bodies. *Brain* 123:267, 2000.

16. Neary D, Snowden JS, Mann DM: Cognitive change in motor neurone disease/amyotrophic lateral sclerosis (MND/ALS). *J Neurol Sci* 180:15, 2000.

17. Wilhelmsen KC: Chromosome 17-linked dementias. *Cell Mol Life Sci* 54:920, 1998.

18. Basun H, Almkvist O, Axelman K, et al: Clinical characteristics of a chromosome 17-linked rapidly progressive familial frontotemporal dementia. *Arch Neurol* 54:539, 1997.

19. Jendroska K, Rossor MN, Mathias CJ, et al: Morphological overlap between corticobasal degeneration and Pick's disease: A clinicopathological report. *Mov Disord* 10:111, 1995.

20. Mendez MF, Cherrier M, Perryman KM, et al: Frontotemporal dementia versus Alzheimer's disease: Differential cognitive features. *Neurology* 47:1189, 1996.

21. Miller BL, Ikonte C, Ponton M, et al: A study of the Lund-Manchester research criteria for frontotemporal dementia: Clinical and single-photon emission CT correlations. *Neurology* 48:937, 1997.

22. Frisoni GB, Beltramello A, Geroldi C, et al: Brain atrophy in frontotemporal dementia. *J Neurol Neurosurg Psychiatry* 61:157, 1996.

23. Kitagaki H, Mori E, Yamaji S, et al: Frontotemporal dementia and Alzheimer disease: Evaluation of cortical atrophy with automated hemispheric surface display generated with MR images. *Radiology* 208:431, 1998.

24. Duara R, Barker W, Luis CA: Frontotemporal dementia and Alzheimer's disease: Differential diagnosis. *Dement Geriatr Cogn Disord* 10:37, 1999.

25. Jackson M, Lowe J: The new neuropathology of degenerative frontotemporal dementias. *Acta Neuropathol* 91:127, 1996.

26. Hof PR, Bouras C, Perl DP, et al: Quantitative neuropathologic analysis of Pick's disease cases: Cortical distribution of Pick bodies and coexistence with Alzheimer's disease. *Acta Neuropathol* 87:115, 1994.

27. Francis PT, Holmes C, Webster MT, et al: Preliminary neurochemical findings in non-Alzheimer dementia due to lobar atrophy. *Dementia* 4:172, 1993.

28. Geschwind D, Karrim J, Nelson SF, et al: The apolipoprotein E epsilon 4 allele is not a significant risk factor for frontotemporal dementia. *Ann Neurol* 44:134, 1998.

29. Brown J: Chromosome 3-linked frontotemporal dementia. *Cell Mol Life Sci* 54:925, 1998.

30. Goedert M, Crowther RA, Spillantini MG: Tau mutations cause frontotemporal dementias. *Neuron* 21:955, 1998.

31. Arawaka S, Usami M, Sahara N, et al: The tau mutation (val337met) disrupts cytoskeletal networks of microtubules. *Neuroreport* 10:993, 1999.

32. Swartz JR, Miller BL, Lesser IM, et al: Frontotemporal dementia: Treatment response to serotonin selective reuptake inhibitors. *J Clin Psychiatry* 58:212, 1997.

Chapter 33

DEMENTIA IN PARKINSON'S DISEASE, HUNTINGTON'S DISEASE, AND RELATED DISORDERS*

Diane M. Jacobs
Gilberto Levy
Karen Marder

OVERVIEW

This chapter describes the epidemiology, clinical characteristics, and pathology of dementia in Parkinson's disease, Huntington's disease, progressive supranuclear palsy, corticobasal ganglionic degeneration, multiple system atrophy, and spinocerebellar ataxia. Each of these conditions is associated with degeneration of subcortical nuclei and is characterized by prominent motor symptomatology; the presence of cognitive change or dementia varies somewhat depending upon the specific condition. Although some cognitive characteristics are associated more with one of these disorders than another, in general they share a common neuropsychological profile often referred to as subcortical dementia or subcorticofrontal dysfunction.

Examples of cognitive symptoms associated with these disorders include slowed information processing, impaired attention and executive functioning, and poor memory retrieval in the context of relatively preserved encoding and consolidation. Primary language abilities are also typically preserved. A summary of cognitive characteristics is provided in Table 33-1. This pattern of performance is distinct from that associated with "cortical dementias" (e.g., Alzheimer disease), which are characterized by amnesia, aphasia, and agnosia. The subcorticofrontal dysfunction associated with these disorders can be explained by damage to connections between subcortical structures (in the basal ganglia, basal forebrain, brainstem, and cerebellum) and neocortical association areas.

* **ACKNOWLEDGMENTS:** This work was supported by federal grant NS36630 and the Parkinson's Disease Foundation.

PARKINSON'S DISEASE

Epidemiology

Idiopathic Parkinson's disease (PD) is characterized clinically by tremor at rest, rigidity, bradykinesia, and postural instability. Accuracy of clinical diagnosis is improved by additional characteristics, such as asymmetrical onset and the absence of atypical features suggestive of a parkinsonian disorder other than PD.[1] PD affects approximately 1 per 1000 persons.[2] The prevalence of PD increases with advancing age, affecting 1.6 percent of those over 65 years of age.[3] The average incidence rate of PD is about 10 per 100,000 person-years of observation.[2,4]

Estimates of the prevalence of dementia among PD patients vary widely, from under 10 percent to over 80 percent.[5-8] The type of assessment of cognitive impairment (nonstandardized clinical examination versus screening cognitive tests or neuropsychological battery) and the diagnostic criteria for dementia partly account for this variation. In community-based studies, which provide less biased estimates than hospital-based studies, dementia as defined by the *Diagnostic and Statistical Manual of Mental Disorders,* revised third edition (DSM-III-R)[9] criteria is present in about 20 to 40 percent of PD patients assessed with either the Mini-Mental State Examination or a neuropsychological battery.[10-15]

The risk of incident dementia among patients with PD is increased compared to that of individuals of the same age without PD, ranging from 1.7- to 5.9-fold.[13,16-18] Estimates of the incidence rate of dementia in PD range from 42.6 to 112.5 per 1000 person-years of observation.[13,18-22] The identification of dementia

Table 33-1
*Neuropsychological characteristics of dementia in degenerative disease**

	Alzheimer's disease	Parkinson's disease	Huntington's disease	Progressive supranuclear palsy	Corticobasal ganglionic degeneration
Orientation	Impaired	Normal	Normal	Normal	Normal
Memory					
Immediate recall	Impaired	Impaired	Impaired	Normal–mildly impaired	Normal–mildly impaired
Delayed recall	Severely impaired	Impaired	Impaired	Normal–mildly impaired	Normal–mildly impaired
Delayed recognition	Severely impaired	Normal	Normal	Normal	Normal
Percent retained[†]	0–50	50–80‡	50–80‡	50–80‡	50–80‡
Executive functions/problem solving	Severely impaired	Severely impaired‡	Severely impaired	Severely impaired‡	Severely impaired
Language					
Naming	Severely impaired; anomia, paraphasia	Normal–mildly impaired; anomia	Normal; visual misperceptions	Normal; visual misperceptions	Normal–mildly impaired
Verbal fluency	Impaired	Severely impaired	Severely impaired	Severely impaired	Severely impaired
Visuospatial skills	Impaired	Impaired	Severely impaired	Impaired	Impaired
Praxis	Normal	Normal	Normal	Normal	Severely impaired; asymmetrical

*Distinct neuropsychological characteristics are most commonly observed when overall severity of dementia is mild.
[†] Percent retained = (delayed recall/immediate recall) × 100.
‡Executive functions often are disproportionately impaired relative to other cognitive abilities.

in patients with PD is of clinical significance for several reasons. First, dementia is the single most important factor limiting standard pharmacotherapy of PD.[23] Second, cognitive impairment in PD affects quality of life,[24] contributes to caregiver distress,[25] and has been associated with nursing home placement.[26] Last, the development of dementia has been associated with reduced survival in patients with PD.[27−30]

Among PD patients, risk factors for developing dementia include advancing age, severity of extrapyramidal motor signs, depressive symptoms, and levodopa-induced psychosis or confusional states.[11,13,18,20,22,31−37] Low education was significantly associated with dementia in PD in one study.[38] This may suggest a nonspecific effect of education in the expression of cognitive impairment, given the association of lower education with Alzheimer's disease.[39] Some studies have shown a higher frequency of dementia in males with PD[17,22,38,40,41]; in females, an inverse association between estrogen replacement therapy and dementia in PD has been reported.[42] An association of a family history of dementia[41] and Alzheimer's disease[43] with dementia in PD has been found. However, with the exception of one study,[44] no increased frequency of the ApoE-ε4 allele was found in demented PD patients.[45−48] While an inverse association between smoking and PD has been consistently demonstrated, a positive association was observed between smoking and dementia in the setting of PD.[31,49]

Cognitive Characteristics

Cognitive impairment occurs frequently in patients with PD, even in the absence of overt dementia. Estimates of the prevalence of neuropsychological abnormalities among nondemented patients with PD indicate that as many as 93 percent[50] experience some difficulty on tests requiring speeded mental processing, attention, and executive functioning, abstract reasoning, visuospatial skills, recall memory, and verbal fluency. Often these impairments are subtle and do not interfere with daily functioning. This mild or relatively circumscribed cognitive dysfunction, which is evident in many patients with PD, does not progress to frank dementia in all affected individuals. As described above, cognitive impairment sufficient to warrant a diagnosis of dementia occurs in 20 to 40 percent of PD patients.[10−15]

Whether dementia in PD represents a worsening of the cognitive symptoms present in nondemented PD patients or the introduction of additional cognitive deficits is a matter of some controversy and has implications regarding the pathophysiology of dementia in PD. Girotti et al.,[51] for example, observed that demented PD patients had more severe and widespread cognitive deficits than nondemented patients, but mostly on those measures that already discriminated nondemented PD patients from control subjects. In contrast, Stern et al.[52] concluded that although cognitive problems preceding dementia in PD patients continue to worsen with the onset of dementia, there is also a qualitative shift in the pattern of cognitive deficits, with substantial broadening and worsening of memory dysfunction as dementia emerges.

The dementia associated with PD is generally characterized by predominant impairment on tests of executive functioning (e.g., planning, initiating, sequencing, monitoring, and shifting between responses; adapting to novel situations; abstract reasoning), visuospatial and visuomotor skills, free recall memory, and verbal fluency. Language functions other than verbal fluency typically are relatively preserved, as are orientation, cued recall, and recognition memory. Impairment of executive functions—particularly on measures requiring response initiation, planning, set-shifting, and ability to benefit from feedback—may be disproportionately severe relative to deficits in other cognitive domains.

Performance on neuropsychological tests of memory yields important clues as to the nature of the memory deficit in PD. Specifically, memory in Parkinson dementia is associated with impaired ability to retrieve information from memory stores.[53,54] The ability to register, store, and consolidate new memories, however, is relatively preserved. As a result, performance on tests requiring free recall is impaired, while cued recall or recognition memory may be relatively intact. Another way of examining this phenomenon is by examining retention of recently learned material over time, often referred to as "savings" scores. Although initial level of recall may be low for PD patients, retention of material after a delay interval typically is commensurate with the level of initial recall; that is, there is little forgetting over time (i.e., good "savings"). In contrast, patients with Alzheimer's disease rapidly forget recently learned material, often retaining less than half of initially recalled material after an interval of only a few minutes. While the memory impairment associated with PD is considered primarily a retrieval deficit, Alzheimer's disease is characterized by deficient encoding or consolidation of new information. The encoding deficit of Alzheimer's disease reflects the prominent pathology of the hippocampus and entorhinal cortex associated with this disorder,[55-57] while the poor retrieval of new information by PD patients may be secondary to executive dysfunction (i.e., inability to plan and initiate systematic searches of memory stores) and reflects dysfunction of subcorticofrontal circuits.[58]

There is mounting evidence that many of the cognitive impairments observed in Parkinson patients, including poor memory and visuospatial functioning, are associated with limited or slowed processing resources that characterize cognition in PD.[59-61] For example, Stebbins et al.[61] found significant group differences between PD patients and normal control subjects on tests of explicit memory (i.e., free recall, cued recall, and delayed recognition) and working memory (i.e., listening span and digit ordering); however, once the effects of psychomotor processing speed were removed from the analysis, group differences were no longer significant. Similarly, Pillon et al.[60] concluded that impaired memory for spatial locations observed in PD results mainly from a disturbance of strategic processes and from decreased attentional resources.

Pathology

The pathologic hallmark of PD is loss of pigmented cells in the substantia nigra and other pigmented brainstem nuclei. Lewy bodies are found within remaining neurons in the affected areas.[62,63] Small numbers of cortical Lewy bodies have also been described as a constant finding in PD cases in neuropathologic series.[64,65] The pattern of neuropsychological deficit typical of dementia in PD, including prominent impairment on "frontal-lobe" or executive tasks, has been attributed to subcortical degeneration of dopaminergic (medial substantia nigra and ventral tegmental area),[66-68] noradrenergic (locus ceruleus),[68-70] and cholinergic (nucleus basalis of Meynert)[71-75] structures. Other pathologic entities that have been proposed as the neuropathologic basis for dementia in PD include

concomitant Alzheimer's disease[76-78] and dementia with Lewy bodies.[79,80] Recently, α-synuclein was found to be a major component of Lewy bodies, leading to the description of PD as a "synucleinopathy."[81] Two studies using α-synuclein immunostaining found a stronger association of cortical Lewy bodies than Alzheimer cortical changes with dementia in PD.[82,83]

HUNTINGTON'S DISEASE

Epidemiology

Huntington's disease (HD) is characterized by an extrapyramidal movement disorder, cognitive, and psychiatric impairment. The movement disorder includes impairment in both involuntary movements (chorea, dystonia, tremor, and rigidity) and voluntary movements (saccadic and smooth pursuit, gait, and speech). Impairment in memory, executive function, and visuomotor skills may be seen. Psychiatric impairment may include irritability, depression, mania, psychosis, and obsessive-compulsive disorder.[84-86]

There are currently 30,000 individuals in the United States who have HD and an additional 150,000 who are at risk by virtue of having a parent with HD. In North America and western Europe, the prevalence of HD is 4 to 7 per 100,000,[87] while among African blacks, Japanese, Chinese, and Finnish, the prevalence is tenfold lower due to a lower CAG repeat length.[88] The mean age of onset is from 36 to 45 years, but it has been reported as early as age 2 and as late as age 90.[84] Death occurs on average 15 to 20 years after onset (usually dated from the onset of the extrapyramidal movement disorder). Approximately 6 percent of HD presents before the age of 20. This form of the disease is known as juvenile HD or the Westphal variant.[84]

HD is an autosomal dominant disorder and the disease gene was localized to chromosome 4p16.3 in 1983.[89] In 1993, when the mutation was identified,[90] direct testing became a possibility for any at-risk individual. HD alleles range from 36 to 121 repeats, with the vast majority exhibiting repeat lengths $\geq$40 (mean 42 to 46).[91] A highly significant negative correlation between age of onset of HD and length of the repeat has been demonstrated, such that higher polyglutamine repeat length is associated with earlier age of onset.[92,93]

This negative correlation is strongest for those with a high number of repeats, who generally have juvenile HD (>60 repeats). The correlation is weaker for alleles within the range of 40 to 50 repeats, which constitutes the majority of HD alleles. Because repeat length accounts for approximately 50 percent of the variance in age of onset,[92,94] there may be other genes[92,95,96] or environmental modifiers[97] that affect the age of onset.

Cognitive dysfunction is a common feature of HD; however, the severity of impairment does vary from patient to patient. The juvenile onset form is associated with severe and rapidly progressive dementia, while cognitive dysfunction is relatively mild and slowly progressive in patients with onset of motor symptoms after age 50.[98] The dementia associated with midlife onset of HD, the most frequent presentation, is intermediate between the juvenile and late onset in terms of severity and rapidity of course. Degree of dementia is closely associated with severity of motor involvement.[99]

Cognitive Characteristics

A metanalysis of 36 studies published between 1980 and 1997 confirmed the characterization of HD as a prototypical subcortical dementia.[100] Specifically, dementia in HD is characterized by impaired performance on tests of learning and memory, attention and executive functions, and visuospatial skills. Patients typically are very slow to initiate responses. As in PD, language functions are relatively preserved in patients with HD with the exception of verbal fluency, which can be markedly impaired.

The memory impairment of HD, like that of PD, is characterized by poor performance on tests of recall memory. Nevertheless, rates of retention from immediate to delayed testing are relatively preserved[101]; that is, once something is learned, it is retained in long-term memory. This is further demonstrated by the fact that performance of HD patients on memory tests using a recognition format improves dramatically. These findings suggest that the memory impairment of HD, as in PD, is characterized by impaired retrieval of stored information. Specifically, patients have difficulty initiating and organizing spontaneous retrieval strategies.

Since the discovery of the genetic mutation for HD in 1993, there have been several studies comparing cognitive functioning of presymptomatic gene carriers who have no motor or psychiatric symptoms to non–gene carriers. These studies have yielded mixed results, with some finding significant differences on measures of memory[102] as well as attention and problem solving[103] while others found no differences on neuropsychological testing between these two groups.[104] Differences in test selection, small sample sizes, and the cross-sectional methodology of many of these studies undoubtedly contribute to these disparate findings. Variation in gene repeat length may be associated with cognitive symptomatology, although there have been conflicting findings in this regard.[102,105] Longitudinal analyses of gene carriers suggest that abnormalities on neuropsychological testing are more evident as conversion to clinical disease nears.[105,106] Nevertheless, impairments on tests of executive function (i.e., Symbol-Digit and Stroop Tests) may be observed as long as 2 years before the onset of clinically significant motor signs.[106] These findings suggest that, at least in some individuals, cognitive change may be the earliest manifestation of disease onset.

Pathology

The core pathologic feature of HD is atrophy of the caudate, putamen, and deep layers of the cortex. Striatal degeneration begins dorsomedially and extends ventrolaterally, such that neuronal loss in the caudate precedes neuronal loss in the putamen and ventral striatum.[107] Striatal medium spiny neurons are selectively impaired. These GABAergic projection neurons, which also express D1 and D2 receptors, make up 90 percent of all striatal neurons.[108] In contrast, large aspiny cholinergic interneurons that are adjacent to the medium spiny neurons are preserved until late in the illness.[109]

HD is one of nine triplet repeat disorders caused by expansion of a trinucleotide repeat (CAG) that codes for glutamine.[110,111] All share certain features: (1) they are neurodegenerative—in all, there is neuronal cell death in an overlapping set of brain regions including basal ganglia, cortex, brainstem, and cerebellum; (2) with the exception of spinobulbar muscular atrophy, which is x-linked recessive, they are autosomal dominant; (3) despite widespread tissue distribution of the protein both centrally and peripherally, the affected region is primarily in the brain; (4) they show genetic anticipation (the earlier onset of disease in succeeding generations, which has long been observed in HD, particularly when disease is inherited from the father); and (5) neuronal intranuclear inclusions have been found in most (HD, dentatorubropallidoluysian atrophy, spinobulbar muscular atrophy, and spinocerebellar ataxias 1, 3, and 7).

PROGRESSIVE SUPRANUCLEAR PALSY

Epidemiology

Clinical characteristics of progressive supranuclear palsy (PSP) include early gait impairment and postural instability with falls, supranuclear ophthalmoplegia primarily affecting vertical gaze, dysarthria, dysphagia, and axial and nuchal rigidity.[112–115] Litvan et al.[114] found that supranuclear downward gaze abnormalities and postural instability with unexplained falls were the best predictors of the diagnosis of PSP pathologically proven. Conversely, the absence of supranuclear gaze palsy is a common reason for the misdiagnosis of PSP as PD.[116] In two studies, the prevalence of PSP has been estimated as 1.4 and 6.4 per 100,000.[117,118] Incidence rates of PSP have ranged from 0.3 to 1.1 per 100,000 person-years.[119–122] Age and male gender may be risk factors for PSP.[117,119,121–124] Mean age at onset in most series is between 60 and 70 years,[113,115,117,124,125] and median duration of disease from onset to death ranges from 5 to 10 years.[113,117,121,124]

Dementia commonly occurs in individuals with PSP. Cognitive or behavioral symptoms were reported in 7 of the 9 cases described by Steele and colleagues.[112] Subsequent estimates of the prevalence of dementia in PSP range from 50 to 80 percent.[113,116,121,126,127] Diagnostic criteria for dementia are likely to influence prevalence estimates of dementia in PSP. Daniel et al.[116] found that only 10 out of 17 autopsy cases of PSP were demented using DSM-III-R criteria, which requires memory impairment. In a study by Pillon et al.,[126] dementia was defined as performance on a global cognitive score at least two standard deviations lower than that of a control group. If the global cognitive score included tests of attention, orientation, memory, and reasoning,

the prevalence of dementia in PSP was 58 percent; if the global cognitive score additionally included frontal lobe tests, the prevalence of dementia increased to 71 percent.

Cognitive Characteristics

Comparisons of cognitive functioning in PSP, PD, and multiple system atrophy (MSA) generally have found that cognitive decline is more frequent and severe in PSP than either PD or MSA.[126,128–130] For example, Pillon et al.[126] reported that dementia, defined by a global intellectual performance two standard deviations lower than mean control values, was diagnosed in 58 percent of patients with PSP but only 18 percent of those with PD. Despite differences in the frequency and severity of cognitive dysfunction, however, the neuropsychological pattern of cognitive compromise in PSP, PD, and MSA is similar.

PSP is considered a prototypical subcortical dementia. In fact, the seminal paper on cognition in PSP by Albert et al.[131] was among the first to introduce the term *subcortical dementia*. Albert et al.[131] described forgetfulness, slowed thought processes, emotional or personality changes, and impaired ability to manipulate acquired knowledge as typical cognitive changes in PSP. Executive dysfunction is a prominent feature at all stages of the disease course.[126,132] Although performance on relatively simple attentional tasks may be normal, performance on more complex tasks—such as those requiring sequencing, mental flexibility, abstraction, and reasoning—is severely impaired. PSP patients score lower on tests of executive and frontal lobe functions than PD patients matched for overall level of intellectual deterioration.[126] Slowness of information processing in PSP is pervasive and marked. Dubois et al.[133] found processing time in patients with PSP to be increased, even relative to patients with PD. Albert et al.[131] reported that when patients were allowed additional time to respond (sometimes as long as 4 to 5 min for a single question), their performance improved by as much as 50 percent. Verbal fluency is generally very severely impaired; however, other language functions remain preserved, and paraphasic errors are uncommon. Although language is relatively preserved, severe dysarthria often impairs communicative ability.[134] The memory disorder of PSP is generally mild.[135] Although PSP patients may be impaired on memory tasks requiring free recall, they are able to benefit from retrieval cues and perform normally on tests of cued recall.[136]

Pathology

Cell loss and neurofibrillary changes occur in various regions of the basal ganglia, brainstem, and cerebellum in PSP, including the pallidum, striatum, subthalamic nucleus, substantia nigra, red nucleus, superior colliculi, nuclei cuneiformis and subcuneiformis, periaqueductal gray matter, pontine tegmentum, and the dentate nucleus.[112,137–139] Involvement of the cholinergic pedunculopontine nucleus[140,141] and nucleus basalis of Meynert[142] as well as neurofibrillary degeneration in the cerebral cortex[143,144] have also been reported in PSP. Together with corticobasal ganglionic degeneration and Pick's disease, PSP is now classified as a "tauopathy."[145] The neurofibrillary tangle in PSP differs from that in Alzheimer's disease and consists of straight filaments composed almost entirely of four-repeat tau protein.[145] Both the A0 allele, a dinucleotide repeat polymorphism of the gene coding for tau, and the A0/A0 genotype are significantly overrepresented in PSP patients versus controls.[146,147] Higgins et al.[148] have also identified an extended 5′-tau haplotype consisting of four single nucleotide polymorphisms (SNP) that are associated with the disease phenotype in sporadic PSP.

CORTICOBASAL GANGLIONIC DEGENERATION

Epidemiology

Corticobasal ganglionic degeneration (CBGD) is an uncommon disorder characterized by asymmetrical akinetic-rigid syndrome, limb ideomotor apraxia, focal dystonia or myoclonus, alien limb sign, cortical sensory loss, tremor, supranuclear gaze palsy, postural instability, and gait impairment.[149–152] Signs and symptoms are often strikingly asymmetrical. Asymmetrical signs and symptoms and late postural instability and

falls help distinguish CBGD from PSP, while marked apraxia, alien limb sign, and poor response to levodopa distinguish CBGD from PD.[153] The alien limb sign is defined as a feeling that one limb is foreign or "has a will of its own," together with involuntary motor activity; spontaneous levitation and posturing may be more common in CBGD than in alien limb sign due to cerebrovascular disease.[154]

The low sensitivity (<50 percent) of the clinical diagnosis of CBGD suggests that this disorder is underdiagnosed.[153] Mean age at onset in clinical and pathologic series is between 60 and 65 years, and median duration of disease from onset to death is 6 to 8 years.[152,153,155] Cases of CBGD reported in the literature have been sporadic, but two families presenting with dementia and with a neuropathologic diagnosis of CBGD have been described.[156] Although dementia or behavioral manifestations were not a prominent feature in the initial report of this disorder,[149,150] subsequent studies have reported pathologically proven CBGD manifesting as dementia, frontal lobe symptomatology, or progressive aphasia.[157–159] In a pathologic series of 13 patients with CBGD followed in movement disorders or memory clinics, 9 presented with dementia, suggesting that dementia may be a common initial manifestation of CBGD.[160]

Cognitive Characteristics

The neuropsychological profile of dementia associated with CBGD is characterized by a prominent dysexecutive syndrome; deficient dynamic motor control (e.g., bimanual coordination, temporal organization); asymmetrical praxis disorders; and poor free recall but intact cued recall and recognition memory.[136] Massman et al.[161] found a dissociation in neuropsychological functioning between CBGD and Alzheimer's disease patients matched for dementia severity, such that CBGD patients performed significantly better than Alzheimer's disease patients on tests of immediate and delayed verbal recall memory, whereas Alzheimer's disease patients (with or without extrapyramidal symptoms) performed better on tests of praxis, finger-tapping speed, and motor programming. Both groups were severely impaired on tests of sustained attention/mental control and verbal fluency, and mildly impaired on tests of confrontation naming. Similarly, Pillon et al.[136] found that CBGD patients, like patients with PSP, had more severe executive dysfunction than Alzheimer's disease patients, while Alzheimer disease patients were more impaired on tests of learning and memory than either CBGD or PSP.

The presence of apraxia is among the most frequent and distinguishing behavioral features of CBGD. Leiguarda et al.[162] assessed praxis in the least affected limb of 10 patients with CBGD and found that 70 percent of patients were impaired on tests of ideomotor apraxia (e.g., waving goodbye, using a hammer), 30 percent had both ideomotor apraxia and ideational apraxia (i.e., inability to complete multistep purposeful tasks), and none showed buccofacial apraxia. Ideomotor praxis correlated significantly with scores on the Mini-Mental State Examination and Picture Arrangement subtest of the Wechsler Adult Intelligence Scale, which requires planning and abstract reasoning. It is not uncommon that patients can accurately describe an action (e.g., using a key to open a door) that they are completely unable to perform.

Pathology

CBGD is characterized pathologically by atrophy of frontal and parietal cortex, often greater contralateral to the side of the body, with pronounced motor involvement, cortical cell loss, gliosis, swollen and achromatic neurons, neuropil threads, and sometimes neurofibrillary tangles. Basophilic inclusions, cell loss, and gliosis are observed in the substantia nigra and other subcortical structures, including the thalamus, striatum, pallidum, subthalamic nucleus, red nucleus, and dentate nucleus.[138,149,150,157] As in the case of PSP, CBGD brains contain tau-immunoreactive neuronal and glial inclusions composed predominantly of four-repeat tau protein.[145,163] Despite a significant neuropathologic overlap, there are morphological and regional differences between CBGD and PSP.[163] Glial inclusions have been reported to be relatively specific; astrocytic plaques and tufted astrocytes are seen in CBGD and PSP, respectively.[144,164] A tau haplotype overrepresented in PSP has also been associated with CBGD, suggesting a similar genetic background for these disorders.[165,166]

MULTIPLE SYSTEM ATROPHY

Epidemiology

The term *multiple system atrophy* (MSA) encompasses striatonigral degeneration, Shy-Drager syndrome, and sporadic olivopontocerebellar atrophy but excludes familial autosomal dominant olivopontocerebellar atrophy. The clinical features of MSA include parkinsonism and cerebellar, pyramidal, and autonomic dysfunction in different combinations.[167] Some clinical features are useful in distinguishing MSA from PD, including poor response to levodopa, absence of levodopa-induced confusion, speech or bulbar dysfunction, falls, and absence of dementia up to death.[168] The prevalence of MSA has been estimated as 4.4 per 100,000 in one study.[118] Mean age of onset ranges from 50 to 55 years old, and median survival estimates range from 5 to 10 years.[167,169,170] Dementia seems to be a most unusual manifestation of MSA. In a review of 203 pathologically proven cases of MSA, severe intellectual impairment was described in only 1 case and moderate intellectual impairment in 4 cases during the course of the disease.[169]

Cognitive Characteristics

Although clinically significant dementia is not a common symptom associated with MSA, a number of studies have reported neuropsychological abnormalities in patients with these disorders.[128,129,171–173] Most of these investigations have examined patients with probable striatonigral degeneration–type illness. While there have been reports of global impairment on neuropsychological testing in MSA patients compared to control subjects,[129] the majority of studies have found a relatively circumscribed dysexecutive syndrome, as evidenced by poor performance on tests of attentional set shifting, spatial working memory, speeded mental processing, visuospatial organization, abstract reasoning, constructional skill, and verbal fluency.[128,171–173] These deficits have been observed in the context of relatively preserved memory, language, visual perception, and general intellectual functioning.[171,173] The pattern of cognitive dysfunction in MSA is similar to that observed in patients with PD and not as severe as that seen in patient with PSP.[129,173] Studies comparing PD and

MSA patients suggest that patients with MSA are more impaired on tests of verbal fluency[129] and motor movement time,[172] while PD patients are more impaired on the Wisconsin Card Sorting Test.[173]

Pathology

Pathologically, MSA is characterized by cell loss and gliosis in the striatum, pallidum, substantia nigra, locus ceruleus, inferior olives, pontine nuclei, cerebellar Purkinje cells, and intermediolateral cell columns of the spinal cord.[169] The description of oligodendroglial cytoplasmic and other inclusions, which contain α-synuclein, has linked MSA to PD as a synucleinopathy.[81,174]

SPINOCEREBELLAR ATAXIA

Spinocerebellar ataxia (SCA) is an autosomal dominant disorder characterized clinically by progressive gait and limb ataxia and dysarthria. Additional clinical features are characteristic of specific genotypes, as several different mutations, mostly CAG repeat expansions (see "Huntington's Disease," above), have been identified in SCA.[111] Cognition in SCA is characterized by poor performance on tests of attention and executive functioning, despite normal learning, memory, and general intellectual functioning.[175–177] These findings suggest that cognitive deficits in patients with SCA reflect disruption of subcorticofrontal pathways.

REFERENCES

1. Hughes AJ, Ben Shlomo Y, Daniel SE, Lees AJ: What features improve the accuracy of clinical diagnosis in Parkinson's disease: A clinicopathologic study. *Neurology* 42:1142–1146, 1992.
2. Mayeux R, Marder K, Cote LJ, et al: The frequency of idiopathic Parkinson's disease by age, ethnic group, and sex in northern Manhattan, 1988–1993 [published erratum appears in *Am J Epidemiol* 143:528, 1996]. *Am J Epidemiol* 142:820–827, 1995.
3. de Rijk MC, Tzourio C, Breteler MM, et al: Prevalence of parkinsonism and Parkinson's disease in Europe: The EUROPARKINSON Collaborative Study. European Community Concerted Action on the Epidemiology of Parkinson's disease. *J Neurol Neurosurg Psychiatry* 62:10–15, 1997.
4. Bower JH, Maraganore DM, McDonnell SK, Rocca WA: Incidence and distribution of parkinsonism in Olmsted County, Minnesota, 1976–1990. *Neurology* 52:1214–1220, 1999.
5. Brown RG, Marsden CD: How common is dementia in Parkinson's disease? *Lancet* 2:1262–1265, 1984.
6. Cummings JL: Intellectual impairment in Parkinson's disease: Clinical, pathologic, and biochemical correlates. *J Geriatr Psychiatry Neurol* 1:24–36, 1988.
7. Dubois B, Boller F, Pillon B, Agid Y: Cognitive deficits in Parkinson's disease, in Boller F, Grafman J (eds): *Handbook of Neuropsychology*. Amsterdam: Elsevier, 1991, pp 195–240.
8. Marder K, Mayeux R: The epidemiology of dementia in patients with Parkinson's disease. *Adv Exp Med Biol* 295:439–445, 1991.
9. American Psychiatric Association: *Diagnostic and Statistical Manual of Mental Disorders,* 3d rev ed (DSM-III-R). Washington, DC: American Psychiatric Press, 1987.
10. Ebmeier KP, Calder SA, Crawford JR, et al: Dementia in idiopathic Parkinson's disease: Prevalence and relationship with symptoms and signs of parkinsonism. *Psychol Med* 21:69–76, 1991.
11. Mayeux R, Denaro J, Hemenegildo N, et al: A population-based investigation of Parkinson's disease with and without dementia. Relationship to age and gender. *Arch Neurol* 49:492–497, 1992.
12. Tison F, Dartigues JF, Auriacombe S, et al: Dementia in Parkinson's disease: A population-based study in ambulatory and institutionalized individuals. *Neurology* 45:705–708, 1995.
13. Marder K, Tang MX, Cote L, et al: The frequency and associated risk factors for dementia in patients with Parkinson's disease. *Arch Neurol* 52:695–701, 1995.
14. Aarsland D, Tandberg E, Larsen JP, Cummings JL: Frequency of dementia in Parkinson disease. *Arch Neurol* 53:538–542, 1996.
15. Giladi N, Treves TA, Paleacu D, et al: Risk factors for dementia, depression and psychosis in long-standing Parkinson's disease. *J Neural Transm (Budapest)* 107:59–71, 2000.
16. Rajput AH, Offord KP, Beard CM, Kurland LT: A case-control study of smoking habits, dementia, and other illnesses in idiopathic Parkinson's disease. *Neurology* 37:226–232, 1987.

17. Breteler MM, de Groot RR, van Romunde LK, Hofman A: Risk of dementia in patients with Parkinson's disease, epilepsy, and severe head trauma: A register-based follow-up study. *Am J Epidemiol* 142:1300–1305, 1995.

18. Aarsland D, Andersen K, Larsen JP, et al: Risk of dementia in Parkinson's disease: A community-based, prospective study. *Neurology* 56:730–736, 2001.

19. Mayeux R, Chen J, Mirabello E, et al: An estimate of the incidence of dementia in idiopathic Parkinson's disease. *Neurology* 40:1513–1517, 1990.

20. Biggins CA, Boyd JL, Harrop FM, et al: A controlled, longitudinal study of dementia in Parkinson's disease. *J Neurol Neurosurg Psychiatry* 55:566–571, 1992.

21. Mahieux F, Fenelon G, Flahault A, et al: Neuropsychological prediction of dementia in Parkinson's disease. *J Neurol Neurosurg Psychiatry* 64:178–183, 1998.

22. Hughes TA, Ross HF, Musa S, et al: A 10–year study of the incidence of and factors predicting dementia in Parkinson's disease. *Neurology* 54:1596–1602, 2000.

23. Mayeux R: A current analysis of behavioral problems in patients with idiopathic Parkinson's disease. *Mov Disord* 4 (Suppl 1):S48–S56, 1989.

24. Schrag A, Jahanshahi M, Quinn N: What contributes to quality of life in patients with Parkinson's disease? *J Neurol Neurosurg Psychiatry* 69:308–312, 2000.

25. Aarsland D, Larsen JP, Karlsen K, et al: Mental symptoms in Parkinson's disease are important contributors to caregiver distress. *Int J Geriatr Psychiatry* 14:866–874, 1999.

26. Aarsland D, Larsen JP, Tandberg E, Laake K: Predictors of nursing home placement in Parkinson's disease: A population-based, prospective study. *J Am Geriatr Soc* 48:938–942, 2000.

27. Mindham RH, Ahmed SW, Clough CG: A controlled study of dementia in Parkinson's disease. *J Neurol Neurosurg Psychiatry* 45:969–974, 1982.

28. Marder K, Leung D, Tang M, et al: Are demented patients with Parkinson's disease accurately reflected in prevalence surveys? A survival analysis. *Neurology* 41:1240–1243, 1991.

29. Piccirilli M, D'Alessandro P, Finali G, Piccinin GL: Neuropsychological follow-up of parkinsonian patients with and without cognitive impairment. *Dementia* 5:17–22, 1994.

30. Roos RA, Jongen JC, van der Velde EA: Clinical course of patients with idiopathic Parkinson's disease. *Mov Disord* 11:236–242, 1996.

31. Ebmeier KP, Calder SA, Crawford JR, et al: Clinical features predicting dementia in idiopathic Parkinson's disease: A follow-up study. *Neurology* 40:1222–1224, 1990.

32. Stern Y, Marder K, Tang MX, Mayeux R: Antecedent clinical features associated with dementia in Parkinson's disease. *Neurology* 43:1690–1692, 1993.

33. Piccirilli M, Piccinin GL, Agostini L: Characteristic clinical aspects of Parkinson patients with intellectual impairment. *Eur Neurol* 23:44–50, 1984.

34. Elizan TS, Sroka H, Maker H, et al: Dementia in idiopathic Parkinson's disease. Variables associated with its occurrence in 203 patients. *J Neural Transm* 65:285–302, 1986.

35. Starkstein SE, Mayberg HS, Leiguarda R, et al: A prospective longitudinal study of depression, cognitive decline, and physical impairments in patients with Parkinson's disease. *J Neurol Neurosurg Psychiatry* 55:377–382, 1992.

36. Starkstein SE, Bolduc PL, Mayberg HS, et al: Cognitive impairments and depression in Parkinson's disease: A follow-up study. *J Neurol Neurosurg Psychiatry* 53:597–602, 1990.

37. Guillard A, Chastang C, Fenelon G: Etude a long terme de 416 cas de maladie de Parkinson. Facteurs de pronostic et implications therapeutiques. *Rev Neurol* 142:207–214, 1986.

38. Glatt SL, Hubble JP, Lyons K, et al: Risk factors for dementia in Parkinson's disease: effect of education. *Neuroepidemiology* 15:20–25, 1996.

39. Katzman R: Education and the prevalence of dementia and Alzheimer's disease. *Neurology* 43:13–20, 1993.

40. Guillard A, Chastang C: Maladie de Parkinson. Les facteurs de pronostic a long terme. *Rev Neurol* 134:341–354, 1978.

41. Marder K, Flood P, Cote L, Mayeux R: A pilot study of risk factors for dementia in Parkinson's disease. *Mov Disord* 5:156–161, 1990.

42. Marder K, Tang MX, Alfaro B, et al: Postmenopausal estrogen use and Parkinson's disease with and without dementia. *Neurology* 50:1141–1143, 1998.

43. Marder K, Tang MX, Alfaro B, et al: Risk of Alzheimer's disease in relatives of Parkinson's disease patients with and without dementia. *Neurology* 52:719–724, 1999.

44. Arai H, Muramatsu T, Higuchi S, et al: Apolipoprotein E gene in Parkinson's disease with or without dementia. *Lancet* 344:889, 1994.

45. Marder K, Maestre G, Cote L, et al: The apolipoprotein epsilon 4 allele in Parkinson's disease with and without dementia. *Neurology* 44:1330–1331, 1994.

46. Koller WC, Glatt SL, Hubble JP, et al: Apolipoprotein E genotypes in Parkinson's disease with and without dementia. *Ann Neurol* 37:242–245, 1995.

47. Inzelberg R, Chapman J, Treves TA, et al: Apolipoprotein E4 in Parkinson disease and dementia: new data and meta-analysis of published studies. *Alzheimer Dis Assoc Disord* 12:45–48, 1998.

48. Whitehead AS, Bertrandy S, Finnan F, et al: Frequency of the apolipoprotein E epsilon 4 allele in a case-control study of early onset Parkinson's disease. *J Neurol Neurosurg Psychiatry* 61:347–351, 1996.

49. Levy G, Tang MX, Cote LJ, et al: Do risk factors for Alzheimer's disease predict dementia in Parkinson's disease? An exploratory study. *Mov Disord.* 17:250–257, 2002.

50. Pirozzolo FJ, Hansch EC, Mortimer JA, et al: Dementia in Parkinson disease: A neuropsychological analysis. *Brain Cogn* 1:71–83, 1982.

51. Girotti F, Soliveri P, Carella F, et al: Dementia and cognitive impairment in Parkinson's disease. *J Neurol Neurosurg Psychiatry* 51:1498–1502, 1988.

52. Stern Y, Richards M, Sano M, Mayeux R: Comparison of cognitive changes in patients with Alzheimer's and Parkinson's disease. *Arch Neurol* 50:1040–1045, 1993.

53. Helkala EL, Laulumaa V, Soininen H, Riekkinen PJ: Recall and recognition memory in patients with Alzheimer's and Parkinson's diseases. *Ann Neurol* 24:214–217, 1988.

54. Taylor AE, Saint-Cyr JA, Lang AE: Memory and learning in early Parkinson's disease: Evidence for a "frontal lobe syndrome." *Brain Cogn* 13:211–232, 1990.

55. Hyman BT, Van Horsen GW, Damasio AR, Barnes CL: Alzheimer's disease: Cell-specific pathology isolates the hippocampal formation. *Science* 225:1168–1170, 1984.

56. Van Hoesen GW, Hyman BT, Damasio AR: Entorhinal cortex pathology in Alzheimer's disease. *Hippocampus* 1:1–8, 1991.

57. Braak H, Braak E: Evolution of the neuropathology of Alzheimer's disease. *Acta Neurol Scand Suppl* 165:3–12, 1996.

58. Taylor AE, Saint-Cyr JA, Lang AE: Frontal lobe dysfunction in Parkinson's disease. The cortical focus of neostriatal outflow. *Brain* 109:845–883, 1986.

59. Bondi MW, Kaszniak AW, Bayles KA, Vance KT: Contributions of frontal system dysfunction to memory and perceptual abilities in Parkinson's disease. *Neuropsychology* 7:89–102, 1993.

60. Pillon B, Deweer B, Vidailhet M, et al: Is impaired memory for spatial location in Parkinson's disease domain specific or dependent on "strategic" processes? *Neuropsychologia* 36:1–9, 1998.

61. Stebbins GT, Gabrieli JD, Masciari F, et al: Delayed recognition memory in Parkinson's disease: A role for working memory? *Neuropsychologia* 37:503–510, 1999.

62. Gibb WR, Scott T, Lees AJ: Neuronal inclusions of Parkinson's disease. *Mov Disord* 6:2–11, 1991.

63. Jellinger K: New developments in the pathology of Parkinson's disease. *Adv Neurol* 53:1–16, 1990.

64. Hughes AJ, Daniel SE, Blankson S, Lees AJ: A clinicopathologic study of 100 cases of Parkinson's disease. *Arch Neurol* 50:140–148, 1993.

65. Duyckaerts C, Gaspar P, Costa C, et al: Dementia in Parkinson's disease. Morphometric data. *Adv Neurol* 60:447–455, 1993.

66. Rinne JO, Rummukainen J, Paljarvi L, Rinne UK: Dementia in Parkinson's disease is related to neuronal loss in the medial substantia nigra. *Ann Neurol* 26:47–50, 1989.

67. Paulus W, Jellinger K: The neuropathologic basis of different clinical subgroups of Parkinson's disease. *J Neuropathol Exp Neurol* 50:743–755, 1991.

68. Zweig RM, Cardillo JE, Cohen M, et al: The locus ceruleus and dementia in Parkinson's disease. *Neurology* 43:986–991, 1993.

69. Mann DM, Yates PO: Pathological basis for neurotransmitter changes in Parkinson's disease. *Neuropathol Appl Neurobiol* 9:3–19, 1983.

70. Cash R, Dennis T, L'Heureux R, et al: Parkinson's disease and dementia: Norepinephrine and dopamine in locus ceruleus. *Neurology* 37:42–46, 1987.

71. Gaspar P, Gray F: Dementia in idiopathic Parkinson's disease. A neuropathological study of 32 cases. *Acta Neuropathol* 64:43–52, 1984.

72. Nakano I, Hirano A: Parkinson's disease: Neuron loss in the nucleus basalis without concomitant Alzheimer's disease. *Ann Neurol* 15:415–418, 1984.

73. Tagliavini F, Pilleri G, Bouras C, Constantinidis J: The basal nucleus of Meynert in idiopathic Parkinson's disease. *Acta Neurol Scand* 70:20–28, 1984.

74. Whitehouse PJ, Hedreen JC, White CL III, Price DL: Basal forebrain neurons in the dementia of Parkinson disease. *Ann Neurol* 13:243–248, 1983.

75. Dubois B, Pillon B, Lhermitte F, Agid Y: Cholinergic deficiency and frontal dysfunction in Parkinson's disease. *Ann Neurol* 28:117–121, 1990.

76. Hakim AM, Mathieson G: Dementia in Parkinson disease: A neuropathologic study. *Neurology* 29:1209–1214, 1979.

77. Boller F, Mizutani T, Roessmann U, Gambetti P: Parkinson disease, dementia, and Alzheimer disease: Clinicopathological correlations. *Ann Neurol* 7:329–335, 1980.

78. Bancher C, Braak H, Fischer P, Jellinger KA: Neuropathological staging of Alzheimer lesions and intellectual status in Alzheimer's and Parkinson's disease patients. *Neurosci Lett* 162:179–182, 1993.

79. Kosaka K, Tsuchiya K, Yoshimura M: Lewy body disease with and without dementia: A clinicopathological study of 35 cases. *Clin Neuropathol* 7:299–305, 1988.

80. McKeith IG, Galasko D, Kosaka K, et al: Consensus guidelines for the clinical and pathologic diagnosis of dementia with Lewy bodies (DLB): Report of the consortium on DLB international workshop. *Neurology* 47:1113–1124, 1996.

81. Galvin JE, Lee VM, Trojanowski JQ: Synucleinopathies: Clinical and pathological implications. *Arch Neurol* 58:186–190, 2001.

82. Hurtig HI, Trojanowski JQ, Galvin J, et al: Alpha-synuclein cortical Lewy bodies correlate with dementia in Parkinson's disease. *Neurology* 54:1916–1921, 2000.

83. Mattila PM, Rinne JO, Helenius H, et al: Alpha-synuclein-immunoreactive cortical Lewy bodies are associated with cognitive impairment in Parkinson's disease. *Acta Neuropathol* 100:285–290, 2000.

84. Folstein SE: *Huntington's Disease. A Disorder of Families*. Baltimore: The Johns Hopkins University Press, 1989.

85. Rosenblatt A, Leroi I: Neuropsychiatry of Huntington's disease and other basal ganglia disorders. *Psychosomatics* 41:24–30, 2000.

86. De Marchi N, Mennella R: Huntington's disease and its association with psychopathology. *Harvard Rev Psychiatry* 7:278–289, 2000.

87. Harper PS: The epidemiology of Huntington's disease. *Hum Genet* 89:365–376, 1992.

88. Squitieri F, Andrew SE, Goldberg YP, et al: DNA haplotype analysis of Huntington disease reveals clues to the origins and mechanisms of CAG expansion and reasons for geographic variations of prevalence. *Hum Mol Genet* 3:2103–2114, 1994.

89. Gusella JF, Wexler NS, Conneally PM, et al: A polymorphic DNA marker genetically linked to Huntington's disease. *Nature* 306:234–238, 1983.

90. The Huntington's Disease Collaborative Research Group: A novel gene containing a trinucleotide repeat that is expanded and unstable on Huntington's disease chromosomes. *Cell* 72:971–983, 1993.

91. Albin RL, Tagle DA: Genetics and molecular biology of Huntington's disease. *Trends Neurosci* 18:11–14, 1995.

92. Brinkman RR, Mezei MM, Theilmann J, et al: The likelihood of being affected with Huntington disease by a particular age, for a specific CAG size. *Am J Hum Genet* 60:1202–1210, 1997.

93. The American College of Medical Genetics/American Society of Human Genetics Huntington Disease Genetic Testing Working Group: ACMG/ASHG statement. Laboratory guidelines for Huntington disease genetic testing. *Am J Hum Genet* 62:1243–1247, 1998.

94. Andrew SE, Goldberg YP, Kremer B, et al: The relationship between trinucleotide (CAG) repeat length and clinical features of Huntington's disease. *Nat Genet* 4:398–403, 1993.

95. Kremer B, Almqvist E, Theilmann J, et al: Sex-dependent mechanisms for expansions and contractions of the CAG repeat on affected Huntington disease chromosomes. *Am J Hum Genet* 57:343–350, 1995.

96. Rubinsztein DC, Leggo J, Chiano M, et al: Genotypes at the GluR6 kainate receptor locus are associated with variation in the age of onset of Huntington disease. *Proc Natl Acad Sci U S A* 94:3872–3876, 1997.

97. Sudarsky L, Myers RH, Walshe TM: Huntington's disease in monozygotic twins reared apart. *J Med Genet* 20:408–411, 1983.

98. Bird ED: The brain in Huntington's chorea. *Psychol Med* 8:357–360, 1978.

99. Brandt J, Strauss ME, Larus J, et al: Clinical correlates of dementia and disability in Huntington's disease. *J Clin Neuropsychol* 6:401–412, 1984.

100. Zakzanis KK: The subcortical dementia of Huntington's disease. *J Clin Exp Neuropsychol* 20:565–578, 1998.

101. Troster AI, Butters N, Salmon DP, et al: The diagnostic utility of savings scores: Differentiating Alzheimer's and Huntington's diseases with the logical memory and visual reproduction tests. *J Clin Exp Neuropsychol* 15:773–788, 1993.

102. Hahn-Barma V, Deweer B, Durr A, et al: Are cognitive changes the first symptoms of Huntington's disease? A study of gene carriers. *J Neurol Neurosurg Psychiatry* 64:172–177, 1998.

103. Kirkwood SC, Siemers E, Hodes ME, et al: Subtle changes among presymptomatic carriers of the Huntington's disease gene. *J Neurol Neurosurg Psychiatry* 69:773–779, 2000.

104. de Boo GM, Tibben AA, Hermans JA, et al: Memory and learning are not impaired in presymptomatic individuals with an increased risk of Huntington's disease. *J Clin Exp Neuropsychol* 21:831–836, 1999.

105. Campodonico JR, Codori AM, Brandt J: Neuropsychological stability over two years in asymptomatic carriers of the Huntington's disease mutation. *J Neurol Neurosurg Psychiatry* 61:621–624, 1996.

106. Paulsen JS, Zhao H, Stout JC, et al: Clinical markers of early disease in persons near onset of Huntington's disease. *Neurology* 57:658–662, 2001.

107. Vonsattel JP, Myers RH, Stevens TJ, et al: Neuropathological classification of Huntington's disease. *J Neuropathol Exp Neurol* 44:559–577, 1985.

108. Graveland GA, Williams RS, DiFiglia M: Evidence for degenerative and regenerative changes in neostriatal spiny neurons in Huntington's disease. *Science* 227:770–773, 1985.

109. Ferrante RJ, Kowall NW, Richardson EP Jr: Proliferative and degenerative changes in striatal spiny neurons in Huntington's disease: A combined study using the section-Golgi method and calbindin D28k immunocytochemistry. *J Neurosci* 11:3877–3887, 1991.

110. Ross CA: Intranuclear neuronal inclusions: A common pathogenic mechanism for glutamine-repeat neurodegenerative diseases? *Neuron* 19:1147–1150, 1997.

111. Subramony SH, Filla A: Autosomal dominant spinocerebellar ataxias ad infinitum? (letter; comment). *Neurology* 56:287–289, 2001.

112. Steele JC, Richardson JC, Olszweski J: Progressive supranuclear palsy. *Arch Neurol* 10:333–358, 1964.

113. Maher ER, Lees AJ: The clinical features and natural history of the Steele-Richardson-Olszewski syndrome (progressive supranuclear palsy). *Neurology* 36:1005–1008, 1986.

114. Litvan I, Agid Y, Jankovic J, et al: Accuracy of clinical criteria for the diagnosis of progressive supranuclear palsy (Steele-Richardson-Olszewski syndrome). *Neurology* 46:922–930, 1996.

115. Litvan I, Agid Y, Calne D, et al: Clinical research criteria for the diagnosis of progressive supranuclear palsy (Steele-Richardson-Olszewski syndrome): Report of the NINDS-SPSP international workshop. *Neurology* 47:1–9, 1996.

116. Daniel SE, de Bruin VM, Lees AJ: The clinical and pathological spectrum of Steele-Richardson-Olszewski syndrome (progressive supranuclear palsy): A reappraisal. *Brain* 118:759–770, 1995.

117. Golbe LI, Davis PH, Schoenberg BS, Duvoisin RC: Prevalence and natural history of progressive supranuclear palsy. *Neurology* 38:1031–1034, 1988.

118. Schrag A, Ben Shlomo Y, Quinn NP: Prevalence of progressive supranuclear palsy and multiple system atrophy: A cross-sectional study. *Lancet* 354:1771–1775, 1999.

119. Radhakrishnan K, Thacker AK, Maloo JC, et al: Descriptive epidemiology of some rare neurological diseases in Benghazi, Libya. *Neuroepidemiology* 7:159–164, 1988.

120. Rajput AH, Offord KP, Beard CM, Kurland LT: Epidemiology of parkinsonism: Incidence, classification, and mortality. *Ann Neurol* 16:278–282, 1984.

121. Bower JH, Maraganore DM, McDonnell SK, Rocca WA: Incidence of progressive supranuclear palsy and multiple system atrophy in Olmsted County, Minnesota, 1976 to 1990. *Neurology* 49:1284–1288, 1997.

122. Golbe LI: The epidemiology of progressive supranuclear palsy. *Adv Neurol* 69:25–31, 1996.

123. Kristensen MO: Progressive supranuclear palsy—20 years later. *Acta Neurol Scand* 71:177–189, 1985.

124. Litvan I, Mangone CA, Mckee A, et al: Natural history of progressive supranuclear palsy (Steele-Richardson-Olszewski syndrome) and clinical predictors of survival: A clinicopathological study. *J Neurol Neurosurg Psychiatry* 60:615–620, 1996.

125. Santacruz P, Uttl B, Litvan I, Grafman J: Progressive supranuclear palsy: A survey of the disease course. *Neurology* 50:1637–1647, 1998.

126. Pillon B, Dubois B, Ploska A, Agid Y: Severity and specificity of cognitive impairment in Alzheimer's, Huntington's, and Parkinson's diseases and progressive supranuclear palsy. *Neurology* 41:634–643, 1991.

127. Collins SJ, Ahlskog JE, Parisi JE, Maraganore DM: Progressive supranuclear palsy: Neuropathologically based diagnostic clinical criteria. *J Neurol Neurosurg Psychiatry* 58:167–173, 1995.

128. Robbins TW, James M, Owen AM, et al: Cognitive deficits in progressive supranuclear palsy, Parkinson's disease, and multiple system atrophy in tests sensitive to frontal lobe dysfunction. *J Neurol Neurosurg Psychiatry* 57:79–88, 1994.

129. Monza D, Soliveri P, Radice D, et al: Cognitive dysfunction and impaired organization of complex motility in degenerative parkinsonian syndromes. *Arch Neurol* 55:372–378, 1998.

130. Soliveri P, Monza D, Paridi D, et al: Neuropsychological follow-up in patients with Parkinson's disease, striatonigral degeneration-type multisystem atrophy, and progressive supranuclear palsy. *J Neurol Neurosurg Psychiatry* 69:313–318, 2000.

131. Albert ML, Feldman RG, Willis AL: The "subcortical dementia" of progressive supranuclear palsy. *J Neurol Neurosurg Psychiatry* 37:121–130, 1974.

132. Litvan I: Cognitive disturbances in progressive supranuclear palsy. *J Neural Transm Suppl* 42:69–78, 1994.

133. Dubois B, Pillon B, Legault F, et al: Slowing of cognitive processing in progressive supranuclear palsy. A comparison with Parkinson's disease. *Arch Neurol* 45:1194–1199, 1988.

134. Podoll K, Schwarz M, Noth J: Language functions in progressive supranuclear palsy. *Brain* 114:1457–1472, 1991.

135. Milberg W, Albert M: Cognitive differences between patients with progressive supranuclear palsy and Alzheimer's disease. *J Clin Exp Neuropsychol* 11:605–614, 1989.

136. Pillon B, Blin J, Vidailhet M, et al: The neuropsychological pattern of corticobasal degeneration: Comparison with progressive supranuclear palsy and Alzheimer's disease. *Neurology* 45:1477–1483, 1995.

137. Jellinger K, Riederer P, Tomonaga M: Progressive supranuclear palsy: Clinicopathological and biochemical studies. *J Neural Transm Suppl* 111–128, 1980.

138. Hauw JJ, Daniel SE, Dickson D, et al: Preliminary NINDS neuropathologic criteria for Steele-Richardson-Olszewski syndrome (progressive supranuclear palsy). *Neurology* 44:2015–2019, 1994.

139. Litvan I, Hauw JJ, Bartko JJ, et al: Validity and reliability of the preliminary NINDS neuropathologic criteria for progressive supranuclear palsy and related disorders. *J Neuropathol Exp Neurol* 55:97–105, 1996.

140. Hirsch EC, Graybiel AM, Duyckaerts C, Javoy-Agid F: Neuronal loss in the pedunculopontine tegmental nucleus in Parkinson disease and in progressive supranuclear palsy. *Proc Natl Acad Sci U S A* 84:5976–5980, 1987.

141. Zweig RM, Whitehouse PJ, Casanova MF, et al: Loss of pedunculopontine neurons in progressive supranuclear palsy. *Ann Neurol* 22:18–25, 1987.

142. Tagliavini F, Pilleri G, Gemignani F, Lechi A: Neuronal loss in the basal nucleus of Meynert in progressive supranuclear palsy. *Acta Neuropathol* 61:157–160, 1983.

143. Vermersch P, Robitaille Y, Bernier L, et al: Biochemical mapping of neurofibrillary degeneration in a case of progressive supranuclear palsy: Evidence for general cortical involvement. *Acta Neuropathol* 87:572–577, 1994.

144. Bergeron C, Pollanen MS, Weyer L, Lang AE: Cortical degeneration in progressive supranuclear palsy. A comparison with cortical-basal ganglionic degeneration. *J Neuropathol Exp Neurol* 56:726–734, 1997.

145. Morris HR, Lees AJ, Wood NW: Neurofibrillary tangle parkinsonian disorders—tau pathology and tau genetics. *Mov Disord* 14:731–736, 1999.

146. Conrad C, Andreadis A, Trojanowski JQ, et al: Genetic evidence for the involvement of tau in progressive supranuclear palsy. *Ann Neurol* 41:277–281, 1997.

147. Higgins JJ, Litvan I, Pho LT, et al: Progressive supranuclear gaze palsy is in linkage disequilibrium with the tau and not the alpha-synuclein gene. *Neurology* 50:270–273, 1998.

148. Higgins JJ, Golbe LI, De Biase A, et al: An extended 5'-tau susceptibility haplotype in progressive supranuclear palsy. *Neurology* 55:1364–1367, 2000.

149. Rebeiz JJ, Kolodny EH, Richardson EP Jr: Corticodentatonigral degeneration with neuronal achromasia: A progressive disorder of late adult life. *Trans Am Neurol Assoc* 92:23–26, 1967.

150. Rebeiz JJ, Kolodny EH, Richardson EP Jr: Corticodentatonigral degeneration with neuronal achromasia. *Arch Neurol* 18:20–33, 1968.

151. Kompoliti K, Goetz CG, Boeve BF, et al: Clinical presentation and pharmacological therapy in corticobasal degeneration. *Arch Neurol* 55:957–961, 1998.

152. Rinne JO, Lee MS, Thompson PD, Marsden CD: Corticobasal degeneration. A clinical study of 36 cases. *Brain* 117:1183–1196, 1994.

153. Litvan I, Agid Y, Goetz C, et al: Accuracy of the clinical diagnosis of corticobasal degeneration: a clinicopathologic study. *Neurology* 48:119–125, 1997.

154. Doody RS, Jankovic J: The alien hand and related signs. *J Neurol Neurosurg Psychiatry* 55:806–810, 1992.

155. Wenning GK, Litvan I, Jankovic J, et al: Natural history and survival of 14 patients with corticobasal degeneration confirmed at postmortem examination. *J Neurol Neurosurg Psychiatry* 64:184–189, 1998.

156. Brown J, Lantos PL, Roques P, et al: Familial dementia with swollen achromatic neurons and corticobasal inclusion bodies: a clinical and pathological study. *J Neurol Sci* 135:21–30, 1996.

157. Bergeron C, Pollanen MS, Weyer L, et al: Unusual clinical presentations of cortical-basal ganglionic degeneration. *Ann Neurol* 40:893–900, 1996.

158. Lang AE: Cortical basal ganglionic degeneration presenting with "progressive loss of speech output and orofacial dyspraxia." (letter; comment). *J Neurol Neurosurg Psychiatry* 55:1101, 1992.

159. Lippa CF, Cohen R, Smith TW, Drachman DA: Primary progressive aphasia with focal neuronal achromasia. *Neurology* 41:882–886, 1991.

160. Grimes DA, Lang AE, Bergeron CB: Dementia as the most common presentation of cortical-basal ganglionic degeneration. *Neurology* 53:1969–1974, 1999.

161. Massman PJ, Kreiter KT, Jankovic J, Doody RS: Neuropsychological functioning in cortical-basal ganglionic degeneration: Differentiation from Alzheimer's disease. *Neurology* 46:720–726, 1996.

162. Leiguarda R, Lees AJ, Merello M, et al: The nature of apraxia in corticobasal degeneration. *J Neurol Neurosurg Psychiatry* 57:455–459, 1994.

163. Feany MB, Mattiace LA, Dickson DW: Neuropathologic overlap of progressive supranuclear palsy, Pick's disease and corticobasal degeneration. *J Neuropathol Exp Neurol* 55:53–67, 1996.

164. Komori T, Arai N, Oda M, et al: Astrocytic plaques and tufts of abnormal fibers do not coexist in corticobasal degeneration and progressive supranuclear palsy. *Acta Neuropathol* 96:401–408, 1998.

165. Di Maria E, Tabaton M, Vigo T, et al: Corticobasal degeneration shares a common genetic background with progressive supranuclear palsy. *Ann Neurol* 47:374–377, 2000.

166. Houlden H, Baker M, Morris HR, et al: Corticobasal degeneration and progressive supranuclear palsy share a common tau haplotype. *Neurology* 56:1702–1706, 2001.

167. Wenning GK, Ben Shlomo Y, Magalhaes M, et al: Clinical features and natural history of multiple system atrophy. An analysis of 100 cases. *Brain* 117:835–845, 1994.

168. Wenning GK, Ben Shlomo Y, Hughes A, et al: What clinical features are most useful to distinguish definite multiple system atrophy from Parkinson's disease? *J Neurol Neurosurg Psychiatry* 68:434–440, 2000.

169. Wenning GK, Tison F, Ben Shlomo Y, et al: Multiple system atrophy: A review of 203 pathologically proven cases. *Mov Disord* 12:133–147, 1997.

170. Ben Shlomo Y, Wenning GK, Tison F, Quinn NP: Survival of patients with pathologically proven multiple system atrophy: a meta-analysis. *Neurology* 48:384–393, 1997.

171. Robbins TW, James M, Lange KW, et al: Cognitive performance in multiple system atrophy. *Brain* 115 Pt 1:271–291, 1992.

172. Testa D, Fetoni V, Soliveri P, et al: Cognitive and motor performance in multiple system atrophy and Parkinson's disease compared. *Neuropsychologia* 31:207–210, 1993.

173. Pillon B, Gouider-Khouja N, Deweer B, et al: Neuropsychological pattern of striatonigral degeneration: comparison with Parkinson's disease and progressive supranuclear palsy. *J Neurol Neurosurg Psychiatry* 58:174–179, 1995.

174. Jaros E, Burn DJ: The pathogenesis of multiple system atrophy: past, present, and future. *Mov Disord* 15:784–788, 2000.

175. Storey E, Forrest SM, Shaw JH, et al: Spinocerebellar ataxia type 2: Clinical features of a pedigree displaying prominent frontal-executive dysfunction. *Arch Neurol* 56:43–50, 1999.

176. Maruff P, Tyler P, Burt T, et al: Cognitive deficits in Machado-Joseph disease. *Ann Neurol* 40:421–427, 1996.

177. Gambardella A, Annesi G, Bono F, et al: CAG repeat length and clinical features in three Italian families with spinocerebellar ataxia type 2 (SCA2): Early impairment of Wisconsin Card Sorting Test and saccade velocity. *J Neurol* 245:647–652, 1998.

Chapter 34

MENTAL RETARDATION

Kytja K. S. Voeller

Mental retardation (MR) as defined by the American Association of Mental Retardation (AAMR) comprises an array of clinical syndromes with onset before age 18 years, "...characterized by significantly subaverage intellectual functioning, existing concurrently with related limitations in two or more of the following applicable adaptive skill areas: communication, self-care, home living, social skills, community use, self-direction, health and safety, functional academics, leisure and work."[1]

Examining each component of this definition, "significantly subaverage" implies that general cognitive ability, measured by an individually administered, standardized test, falls below a specific point. Although previously set at −2 standard deviations (SDs) below the mean, the cutoff point was raised in the 1992 AAMR definition from 70 to 75. Sattler[2] points out that it is also important to take into consideration the statistical properties of the specific test that is used. That is, "below −2 standard deviations" (SD) in tests with an SD of 15 (e.g., the Wechsler series) results in an IQ of 69 or less, whereas those with an SD of 16 (e.g., the Stanford-Binet) will result in an IQ of 67 or less.

The severity of MR is not specified in the AAMR definition, but the American Psychiatric Association (APA) identifies four levels of severity (Mild, IQ 50 or 55 to 70; Moderate 35 or 40 to 50 to 55, Severe 20 or 25 to 35 to 40, Profound < 20 to 25) and a "severity unspecified" category, indicating a strong presumption of MR, but the patient cannot be tested in a formal manner.[3]

Although intelligence is determined by a combination of genetic and environmental factors, recent studies that control statistically for effects of intrafamilial environments strongly support the notion that genetic factors have a profound influence on cognition and behavior.[4,5] Genetic effects on regional brain volumes have been demonstrated in a study of monozygotic (MZ) and dizygotic (DZ) twin

pairs. Thompson et al. demonstrated that gray matter volumes and cortical volumes in frontal association areas and those subserving language (including Broca's and Wernicke's areas) appear to be under a greater degree of genetic control than sensorimotor and parietal association cortices.[6] Correlations in MZ twins for frontal and language association cortices were in the range of 95 to 100 percent ($p < 0.0001$), in contrast to more a modest 60 to 70 percent ($p < 0.05$) correlations in DZ twins. These authors were able to demonstrate a highly significant correlation between frontal gray matter and Spearman's g ($p < 0.0044$) after controlling for other factors.

NEUROBIOLOGICAL FACTORS IN MENTAL RETARDATION

The majority of cases of MR result from a perturbation of early brain development that is influenced to a variable and usually modest extent by environmental factors. With the exception of brain injury occurring either pre- or postnatally, most cases of MR result from genetic anomalies.

How do various genetic syndromes result in MR? There are many different specific causes of MR, but they can be grouped into two general classes: (1) a disruption of neuronal migration and/or (2) "dysgenetic dendrites" or "sick synapses."* Disorders of neuronal

---

* A special subclass of structural brain malformations are associated with inborn errors of metabolism. For example, hypoplastic temporal lobes are found in association with glutaric aciduria (both type 1 and type 2). Dysplasia of the corpus callosum is a very common anomaly, being found in maternal phenylketonuria, Menkes' syndrome, and numerous other metabolic disorders. (This subject was reviewed in detail by Nissenkorn A, Michelson M, Ben-Zeev B, et al.: Inborn errors of metabolism: A cause of abnormal brain development. *Neurology* 56:1265, 2001.)

differentiation and migration often result in structural malformations that are visible to the naked eye, whereas disruption of the proliferation of dendrites and synapses may result in anomalies that are more subtle and obvious only with morphometric measurements or histologic techniques.

Dendritic spines receive the bulk of the excitatory glutamatergic inputs that regulate synaptic plasticity, a process that underlies not only early in brain development but also learning and memory throughout life. Although dendrites were originally viewed as relatively immutable structures, the notion that they moved ("twitched") was proposed by Crick in 1982[7] and confirmed by direct observation somewhat later.[8] Dendrites turn out to be remarkably plastic structures, and dendritic spines and associated synapses can be remodeled in a matter of seconds.[9] These changes are dependent on the polymerization and depolymerization of actin in the spines, which is regulated by small GTPases from the Rho family that are highly expressed in neurons. For example, one of these GTPases, RacV12, increases spine density, reduces spine size, and may facilitate development of new spines; another–RhoAV14–reduces spine density and length and may block spine formation and maintenance, suggesting that density and spine size are independent.[10] Neurotransmitters also play an important role in regulating brain growth during early development and then, postnatally, are involved in neural transmission.[11] Thus, any disruption of the genes governing these multiple processes that are involved in building a brain is likely to result in some form of cognitive dysfunction if not frank MR. Thus, it is not surprising that Golgi studies have revealed a number of abnormalities in both the morphology and branching patterns of dendrites in a number of MR syndromes.[12] Moreover, in some cases, the brain is subjected to a double whammy in the sense that not only is the initial connectivity disrupted but the ability to learn new information is severely compromised by the same process. A challenge in this area is to be able to link the genetic perturbation to the specific pattern of cognitive dysfunction.

In the pages that follow, I will briefly describe a limited number of common MR syndromes and discuss relevant neurobehavioral and neurobiologic features.

LISSENCEPHALY

Lissencephaly reflects a disturbance of migration early in brain development, so that neurons do not reach their normal ultimate positions in the brain. There are four cortical layers, and the brain is smooth and lacks normal sulcal and gyral markings. Affected children are microcephalic; they have severe spasticity, profound MR, intractable seizures, and usually die at an early age. There are two forms, one involving the *LIS1* gene located on chromosome 17p13.3.[13] Although the precise role of LIS1 is unclear, this is a highly conserved protein that likely is involved in neuroblast proliferation, migration, and dendritic development.[14] Mild forms of lissencephaly—at least one with an IQ in the average range—present with pachygyria restricted to posterior cortical regions. These are associated with missense mutations of the *LIS1* gene.[15] The other—*double cortin*—(*DCX or XLIS*) gene—is located at Xq22.3-q23.[16] Few male fetuses survive. Carrier females have a highly variable phenotype, presumably due to X-inactivation, with some 20 percent having average-range intelligence, with mild to severe MR in the remaining 80 percent.[17] Seizures are very common. The brain has a relatively normal external appearance, with six cortical layers, but there is a band of heterotopic gray matter lying between the ventricles and the cortex (the "double cortex") or subcortical band heterotopia. The DCX protein is expressed from 9 to 20 gestational weeks, most intensely during the period of neuronal migration, and plays a critical role in stabilizing microtubule formation and nucleokinesis.[18]

RETT'S SYNDROME

Rett's syndrome (RS) is an X-linked disorder with a prevalence of 1 in 10,000 to 15,000 females. Only about 1 percent of RS cases are familial. Most cases (70 to 80 percent) arise from de novo mutations of the methyl-CpG-binding protein 2 (MECP2) gene, which has been mapped to Xq28.[19] Mutations, which mainly occur in the paternal germ line,[20] involve nonsense, missense, and frameshift mutations.

It was originally believed that RS occurred almost exclusively in females. In the classic situation, the affected girl is normal at birth and develops normally until 3 to 4 months, when a deceleration of head growth becomes apparent. Delayed somatic growth, followed by loss of milestones and language, emerges around 6 and 18 months. A characteristic hand-washing stereotypy appears, with ataxia as well as gait and limb apraxia. Affected girls are typically severely retarded and without language; they have severe seizures and periods of hyperpnea as well as impaired somatic growth and often present an autistic façade. However, it is now known that the phenotypic spectrum is much broader than previously imagined and encompasses males as well as females, with preserved language or only mild learning problems. In these females, X-inactivation may play an important role in the clinical phenotype. Males who have the MECP2 mutation and Klinefelter's syndrome (XXY) or whose mothers are mosaic for the mutation often present with a clinical picture similar to that of the more classic RS phenotype.[21]

What is the pathophysiology of RS? The early deceleration of head growth coupled with neuroimaging studies suggest a failure of the normal exuberant growth of the neuropil in early childhood. The MECP2 gene is a highly conserved gene that is expressed in both fetal and brain and is involved in transcriptional silencing of genes restricting synaptic proliferation.[22] Johnston et al.[23] have suggested that since these restrictive genes are not inhibited, normal synaptic expansion does not occur.

RUBINSTEIN-TAYBI SYNDROME

RTS is a syndrome characterized by severe MR, growth retardation, a characteristic facial appearance, broad thumbs and toes, and cardiac abnormalities. Behaviors reminiscent of bipolar disorder have been reported in RTS.[24] The RTS gene has been localized to 16p13.3. The gene encoding cAMP response element-binding binding protein (CREBBP) (a ubiquitously expressed transcriptional coactivator and histone acetyl transferase which regulates the expression of numerous other genes) is localized to this region. Impaired synaptic proliferation in RTS appears to result from a mutation in CREBBP. CREB also plays an important role in long term memory (LTM) formation, a process that has many similarities to synaptic plasticity.[25] Although yet to be demonstrated in human subjects with RTS, a

mouse model has been shown to be deficient in LTM but not STM storage.[26]

CRETINISM

Cretinism results from a lack of thyroid hormone (TH) during early brain development. Although rare in the United States, there are endemic pockets of cretinism around the world where iodine deficiency leads to the full-blown syndrome. Cretins have IQs in the 20 to 40 range, impaired somatic growth, sensorineural hearing loss, deaf-mutism, spasticity and hyperreflexia (particularly in the lower extremities), and retained primitive reflexes. Even in cases of equivalent iodine deficiency, the clinical severity can vary. It has been suggested that the presence of the APOE ε4 allele, which has TH-binding properties, is a risk factor for iodine-deficient cretinism.[27] When cretinism is treated early and vigorously, brain development and ultimate intellectual function can be normal but usually somewhat below that of siblings. The IQ often declines with age. Visuospatial and attentional deficits are noted, with relative preservation of verbal ability. Those receiving early treatment often perform within the average range in reading and spelling but often experience greater difficulty with arithmetic.[28]

TH regulates the transcription and the rate of gene expression during brain development both by direct effects on specific genes and indirect effects on "downstream" genes. TH impacts neuronogenesis, neuronal migration, dendritic and synaptic proliferation (in part through effects on the small GTPase system[29]), and myelinization. Although all these processes ultimately do occur, even in the brain deprived of TH, and the gross morphology of the brain is not anomalous, the normal timing of brain development is disrupted.[30]

NONSYNDROMIC X-LINKED MENTAL RETARDATION

Boys with nonsyndromic X-linked MR (XMR) have no characteristic somatic features except for MR. They represented something of an enigma in the past, but at this point at least seven genes have been cloned, all of which play an important role in dendritic pro-liferation and synapse formation through either direct or indirect effects on the Rho GTPases and the actin cytoskeleton.[31] MECP2 has been identified as one of the genes.[32]

DOWN'S SYNDROME

Down's syndrome (DS) (trisomy 21) is the most common genetic cause of MR, occurring in 1 out of every 700 live births. In women aged 45 to 49 years, the prevalence increases to 5 per 100. The DS phenotype is characterized by a small, brachycephalic head, epicanthic folds, upward-slanting palpebral fissures, Brushfield spots, protruding tongue, and transverse palmar creases. Persons with DS are at increased risk for congenital heart disease, duodenal atresia, seizures, and immunologic and hematologic problems (particularly leukemia).

The IQ of children with DS ranges from <40 to the average range. The mean IQ of children with trisomy is generally lower (52 ± 14.6) compared to those with mosaic DS (67 ± 13.8).[33] Language (particularly syntax)[34] and verbal memory[35] are typically impaired, with relative strengths in the visuospatial and social areas. Children with DS are typically friendly and sociable. They perform relatively well on Theory of Mind tasks.[36] Compared to an age- and IQ-matched group of boys with fragile-X syndrome, boys with DS performed somewhat better on tasks requiring visual attentional control and inhibition, although relative to a normal IQ group their performance was impaired.[37]

Alzheimer's dementia (AD) is a significant risk in adults with DS: the average age of onset of dementia is in the range of 50 to 55 years. By age 40, the DS brain has neurofibrillary tangles and senile plaques similar to those seen in AD. Atrophy of the medial temporal lobe can be observed before the onset of clinically apparent memory loss.[38] However, amyloid deposition starts earlier and is much more widespread in DS than AD[39] and can be observed even in the 21-week-old fetus.[40] The APOE $\varepsilon 4$ genotype represents an additional and independent risk factor.[41]

The brain in DS is small, with disproportionately small cerebellar, brainstem, frontal lobe, and hippocampal volumes and atrophy of the superior temporal gyrus.[42,43] In children with DS, amygdalar volume, when corrected for total brain volume, did not differ from that of controls, but hippocampal volumes were significantly smaller.[44]

Although DS is one of the oldest and best-studied of the MR syndromes, the pathophysiology has yet to be worked out. The mouse trisomy 16 model, which shares many of the genes with human trisomy 21, has been helpful in elucidating the underlying pathophysiology. Current information points to a restriction of dendritic proliferation starting in midgestation. By 22 weeks of gestation in the human fetus, anomalies of cortical lamination are noted.[45] One possible explanation is that cytokines resulting from amyloid deposition during fetal brain development disrupt the process of dendritic expansion. Another is that nerve growth factor transfer is deficient, resulting in degeneration of cholinergic input to the basal forebrain.[46]

FRAGILE-X SYNDROME

Fragile-X syndrome (FRAX) occurs in 1 out of every 2000 to 5000 live births and is the most common form of inherited MR. Adult males with FRAX have a characteristic long, narrow face, large dysmorphic ears, a prominent jaw, and macroorchidism. The neuropsychiatric phenotype is characterized by hyperactivity, impaired social relatedness, social anxiety, gaze avoidance, and stereotypies that appear "autistic." These behavioral and physical attributes are not as prominent in young boys. IQ ranges from normal to profound MR and declines in early puberty.[47]

Carrier females have few somatic features and a milder cognitive phenotype but manifest deficits in working memory as well as impaired visuospatial and prefrontal executive function. Social anxiety, hyperarousal, attention problems, and stereotypic movements are often seen. IQ is variable.[48]

Neuroimaging studies reveal an enlarged fourth ventricle, with decrease in size of the cerebellar vermis (especially lobules VI and VII), and enlarged caudate nuclei.[49] In each case, these measurements are most striking in FRAX males, with carrier females falling in an intermediate status between affected males and controls. There is an association between decreased vermis size and IQ.[50]

FRAX results from an expansion of an unstable CGG trinucleotide repeat,[51] which causes transcriptional silencing of the FMR1 gene (located at Xq27.3) by methylation. Silencing occurs when the number of CGG trinucleotide repeats within the initial (5′) untranslated portion of the gene reaches 200 or more. The average person has no more than 50 CGG repeats, whereas in persons with FRAX, CGG repeats range from 200 to over 1000. The FMR1 gene regulates the production of FMR protein (FMRP), a protein found in many cells, FMRP, which is prominently expressed in neurons and plays a critical role in the transport and regulation of mRNA. FMRP increases rapidly in the normal synapse in response to neuronal stimulation.[52] Histologic studies of the brains of humans with FRAX and of *fmr-1* knockout mice reveal abnormal dendritic spine morphology.[53] In the developing brain, decreased or absent FMRP results in impaired synaptic plasticity; in the adult, learning and memory are disrupted.

In carrier females, there is a relationship between IQ and CGG repeats. The mean group IQ of those with CGG repeats greater than 200 was 89.4 in comparison to a mean IQ of 107 in those with CGG repeats below 200. Dyer-Friedman et al. studied the relationship of home environment to genetic factors and found that mean parental IQ contributed strongly to the variance of the cognitive outcome, particularly verbal and attentional abilities in girls with FRAX, whereas in males the mean parental IQ contributed only to the performance IQ and processing scale scores. Surprisingly, they could not demonstrate a strong correlation between FMRP and cognitive outcomes in either males or females.[54] Kwon et al. studied female FRAX carriers and demonstrated that there was a correlation between neural activation in the middle frontal gyrus on a visuospatial working memory task and the level of FMRP expression and activation of various areas of the frontal lobe, suggesting that FMRP may play a dynamic role in modulating brain activation in response to working memory load.[55]

PRADER-WILLI SYNDROME

Prader-Willi syndrome (PWS) has a prevalence of 1 in 10,000 to 1 in 25,000. Persons with PWS are of short stature and severely obese; they have small hands and feet, almond-shaped eyes, and hypogonadism. IQ can range from the retarded to low-average range, but language is often particularly impaired. At birth, children with PWS are hypotonic and undergrown. Around age 2, they develop a voracious appetite and gain weight rapidly. As they mature, it becomes increasingly hard for their care providers to limit food intake. Older children and adults are prone to display tantrums, OCD-spectrum behaviors, and skin-picking.[56] PWS results from an absence of expression of paternally active genes in 15q11-q13 ("PWS critical region"). In 70 percent of the cases this is the result of a deletion on paternal chromosome 15. In 30 percent of the cases both chromosomes come from the mother, a case of *uniparental disomy* (UPD).

ANGELMAN'S SYNDROME

Children with Angelman's syndrome (AS) appear normal at birth, but their subsequent development is severely delayed and many children with AS never speak. They are often microcephalic and hypopigmented relative to other members of their families. There is prominent motor dysfunction, hyperactivity, hyperarousability, and a seizure disorder that is hard to control. Because patients with AS smile almost continuously, AS has been dubbed the "happy puppet" syndrome. AS involves the same deletion at 15q11-q13 as PWS, but it is due to an absence of expression of maternally active genes. Four distinct genetic mechanisms have been identified: paternal UPD, an imprinting defect, a large insterstitial deletion of 15q11-q13, and a mutation in the E3ubiquitin protein ligase gene. A fifth type does not have any identifiable genetic mechanisms. Deletion patients are the most severely affected, while those with a mutation of the ubiquitin gene or an imprinting defect have a milder phenotype and do not differ substantially from one another.[57]

TURNER'S SYNDROME

Turner's syndrome occurs in about 1 out of every 5000 live female births. Babies with TS have a short, webbed neck, low hairline, low-set ears, ptosis, micrognathia, a high-arched palate, and an atypical facies. Older girls and women are short, and a percentage have ovarian failure. There is an increased incidence of coarctation of the aorta. IQ ranges from normal to mild MR. Verbal skills are typically a strength, and there is often a verbal > performance gap.[58] These children typically manifest both visuospatial and executive function deficits, characterized by inattention and impulsivity. This pattern is reminiscent of dysfunction of the frontal-parietal system (the "where" system). Arithmetic skills are often poor. Neither estrogen nor normal hormonal function improves cognitive performance, and cognitive deficits remain stable into adulthood.

There are a variety of different genotypic patterns in TS. About 50 percent of TS have an absent X chromosome (45XO) and 10 to 15 percent are XO/XX mosaics. TS is rarely inherited, but this does occur.[59]

Reiss and colleagues reported a particularly instructive study of twins discordant for TS.[60] Both twins had superior full-scale IQs and the verbal IQs were within 3 points of each other, but there was a 25 point V>P discrepancy in the XO twin. The Perceptual Organization index of the XO twin was 21 points lower than that of the unaffected twin, with impaired performance on visuospatial, attentional, and executive function tasks relative to the normal twin. Mild atrophy with decreased gray matter was noted on the XO twin's MRI.

CHROMOSOME 22q11.2–DELETION SYNDROME

The chromosome 22q11.2–deletion syndrome (Chr 22q11.2) includes velocardiofacial syndrome, DiGeorge syndrome, and conotruncal face syndrome; it involves a spectrum of serious cardiovascular malformations as well as immunologic and endocrinologic disorders. Most patients have a characteristic facial appearance, with abnormalities of the palate and ears, but some do not. It is quite common, occurring in 1 in 2000 to 4000 live births. IQ ranges from mild MR to normal but there is a high incidence of learning disabilities and borderline IQ, with a pattern of declining IQ scores with maturation. In a group of 4-year-olds, the mean IQ obtained on the Stanford-Binet IQ was 87; it was 84 on the Leiter International Performance Test. On the WISC-R, 8-year-olds obtained a mean verbal IQ of 76 and a mean Performance IQ of 79; this IQ was about the

same in a group of 13-year-olds. Young children often present with speech and language problems,[61,62] but deficits in the visuospatial domain, including memory, are prominent. Impaired reading comprehension and arithmetic are often noted.[63]

Chr 22q11.2 is overrepresented in psychiatric samples—there is a higher incidence of ADHD, OCD, and bipolar disorder[64] as well as schizophrenia (in fact, Chr 22q11.2 appears to be the highest known risk factor for schizophrenia).[65] Interestingly, the 22q11 deletion includes the catechol O-methyltransferase (COMT) gene. COMT inactivates catecholamine neurotransmitters. A common polymorphism (the COMT108[met] variant) leads to a reduction of COMT activity. Patients who are homozygous for the COMT108[met] variant or have Chr 22q11.2 and the COMT108[met] variant on the allele that is not deleted have reduced levels of COMT, with a resulting increase in circulating catecholamines. This group is at very high risk for neuropsychiatric disorders. A knockout mouse model shows defective sensorimotor gating as well as learning and memory defects.[66] Graf et al.[67] reported that treatment with metyrosine, a competitive inhibitor of tyrosine hydroxylase that reduces brain dopamine and subsequent stages of the catecholamine pathway, resulted in modest improvements in the neuropsychiatric status of these patients.

MRI morphometric studies have revealed reduced total brain volume and reduced volumes of left parietal lobe and right cerebellum.[68] A high incidence of midline anomalies (cavum vergae) and atrophy were reported in schizophrenics.[69] Polymicrogyria have also been noted.[70] These markers for disturbed neuronal migration may reflect the impact of the disordered catecholamine levels during early brain development.

This syndrome has been mapped to a deletion on chromosome 22q11.2, involving some 30 genes. Eliez et al. have reported that patients who inherit the deletion on the maternal chromosome have reduced gray matter volumes compared to normal controls and those inheriting the deletion from their fathers.[71]

WILLIAMS' SYNDROME

Williams' syndrome (WS) is a rare type of MR, with an incidence of 1 in 25,000. Hypercalcemia and supravalvular stenosis are often detected in the neonatal period. Early motor and language development is delayed. As they mature, persons with WS acquire sophisticated vocabularies and elaborate syntactic structures and often demonstrate average range performance on language tasks. Social skills are relatively intact—they are gregarious (if not overly friendly), and object recognition and face-processing are cognitive strengths.[72] WS is associated with significantly impaired visuospatial function and prefrontal deficits—characterized by impulsivity and impaired attention. IQs range from 40 to 100 with a mean of about 60.[73]

On gross examination and MRI morphometric studies, the brain in WS is only slightly reduced in size (13 percent) compared to that of controls. The shape of the brain is unusual, with a marked reduction in the volume of the parieto-occipital area, and a decrease in the size of the splenium. The cerebellum is normal in size except for some enlargement of the vermis.[74,75] The gyral pattern is generally normal, but the central sulcus and some gyri in the dorsal area are anomalous.[76] Microscopic examination reveals a normal cytoarchitectonic structure with subtle changes—diminished neuronal cell packing density and increased glia. Columnar organization is reduced, particularly in the posterior region.[77] The difference between the relatively normal structure of the ventral, perisylvian, and anterior regions of the brain and the subtle anomalies observed in dorsal and posterior areas is consistent with the symmetry in cognitive function in WS. That is, functions of the ventral pathway are relatively intact whereas those subserved by the dorsal pathway are defective.

The genetic anomaly has been identified as a submicroscopic deletion on chromosome 7q11.23[78] Several genes in this region are expressed in the brain and play prominent roles in brain development. These are LIM kinase-1 (a protein tyrosine kinase), STX1-A (involved in synaptic development), and FZD9 (previously known as FZD3—the human homologue of the drosophila "frizzled" gene). It has been suggested that these genes may be related to the cognitive and morphologic features of WS, but subsequent reports have shown that the typical WS cognitive phenotype occurs in persons with small deletions that do not include these genes.[79,80]

SUMMARY

This brief review of some of the MR syndromes has attempted to portray the remarkable variety of the neurocognitive profiles which are seen in these syndromes and discuss the pathophysiology with particular attention to some of the neurogenetic aspects. In the next decade we can look forward to dramatic advances in our understanding of how these genetic anomalies result in differences in cognitive profile, brain structure, and behavior. However, it is apparent that there is considerable variability in the genetic aspect of these syndromes and one cannot predict the outcome in most cases from the genotype. Thus, clinicians need to conduct detailed neurocognitive examinations in order to define the cognitive strengths and weaknesses of these patients. For the clinician, the challenge is to be aware of the genetic features of these syndromes but at the same time understand the functional abilities of the specific patient. This will enable the clinician to provide the patient with appropriate and carefully tailored adaptive and cognitive strategies and to control adverse environmental factors so that persons with MR can function at an optimal level.

REFERENCES

1. American Association on Mental Retardation: *Mental Retardation: Definition, Classification, and Systems of Supports,* 9th ed. Washington DC: AAMR, 1992.
2. Sattler JM: *Assessment of Children. Behavioral and Clinical Applications,* 4th ed. San Diego, CA: Jerome M. Sattler, 2002.
3. American Psychiatric Association: *Diagnostic and Statistical Manual of Mental Disorders: Text Revision,* 4th ed. (DSM-IV-TR). Washington, DC: American Psychiatric Association, 2000.
4. McClearn GE, Johansson B, Berg S, et al: Substantial genetic influence on cognitive abilities in twins 80 or more years old. *Science* 276:1560:1997.
5. Tramo MJ, Loftus WC, Stukel TA, et al: Brain size, head size, and intelligence quotient in monozygotic twins. *Neurology* 50:1246, 1998.
6. Thompson PM, Cannon, TD, Narr KL, et al: Genetic influences on brain structure. *Nat Neurosci* 4:1253, 2001.
7. Crick F: Do spines twitch? *Trends Neurosci* 5:44, 1982.

8. Dunaevsky A, Tashiro A, Majewska A, et al: Developmental regulation of spine motility in mammalian CNS. *Proc Natl Acad Sci U S A* 96:13438, 1999.

9. Fischer M, Kaech S, Knutti D, et al: Rapid actin-based plasticity in dendritic spines. *Neuron* 20:847, 1998.

10. Tashiro A, Minden A, Yuste R: Regulation of dendritic spine morphology by the rho family of small GTPases: Antagonistic roles of rac and rho. *Cereb Cortex* 10:927, 2000.

11. Levitt P, Harvey JA, Friedman E, et al: New evidence for neurotransmitter influences on brain development. *Trends Neurosci* 20:269, 1997.

12. Marín-Padilla M: Structural abnormalities of the cerebral cortex in human chromosomal aberrations. A Golgi study. *Brain Res* 44:625, 1972.

13. Lo Nigro C, Chong SS, Smith ACM, et al: Point mutations and an intragenic deletion in *LIS1*, the lissencephaly causative gene in isolated lissencephaly sequence and Miller-Dieker syndrome. *Hum Mol Genet* 6:157:1997.

14. Liu Z, Steward R, Luo L: Drosophila *Lis1* is required for neuroblast proliferation, dendritic elaboration and axonal transport. *Nat Cell Biol* 2:776, 2000.

15. Leventer RJ, Cardoso C, Ledbetter DH, et al: *LIS1* missense mutations cause milder lissencephaly phenotypes including a child with normal IQ. *Neurology* 57:416, 2001.

16. Ross ME, Allen KM, Srivastava AK, et al: Linkage and physical mapping of X-linked lissencephaly/SBH *XLIS*: A gene causing neuronal migration defects in human brain. *Hum Mol Genet* 6:555, 1997.

17. Dobyns WB, Andermann E, Andermann F, et al: X-linked malformations of neuronal migration. *Neurology* 47:331, 1996.

18. Qin J, Mizuguchi M, Itoh M, et al: Immunohistochemical expression of doublecortin in the human cerebrum: Comparison of normal development and neuronal migration disorders. *Brain Res* 863:225, 2000.

19. Amir RE, Van den Veyver IB, Wan M, et al: Rett syndrome is caused by mutations in X-linked MeCP2, encoding methyl-CpG-binding protein 2. *Nat Genet* 23:185, 2001.

20. Girard M, Couvert P, Carrié A, et al: Parental origin of de novo MECP2 mutations in Rett syndrome. *Eur J Hum Genet* 9:231, 2001.

21. Schanen C: Rethinking the fate of males with mutations in the gene that causes Rett syndrome. *Brain Dev* 23:S144, 2001.

22. Nan X, Ng HH, Johnson CA, et al: Transcriptional repression by the methyl-CpG-binding protein MeCP2 involves a histone deacetylase complex. *Nature* 393:386, 1998.

23. Johnston MV, Jeon O-H, Pevsner J, et al: Neurobiology of Rett syndrome: A genetic disorder of synapse development. *Brain Dev* 23:S206, 2001.

24. Hellings JA, Hossain S, Martin JK, et al: Psychopathology, GABA, and the Rubinstein-Taybi syndrome: A review and case study. *Am J Med Genet* 8:114, 2001.

25. Wang HY, Zhang FC, Cao JJ, et al: Apolipoprotein E is a genetic risk factor for fetal iodine deficiency disorder in China. *Mol Psychiatry* 5:363, 2000.

26. Oike Y, Hata A, Mamiya T, et al: Truncated CBP protein leads to classical Rubinstein-Taybi syndrome phenotypes in mice: Implications for a dominant-negative mechanism. *Hum Mol Genet* 8:387, 1999.

27. Wang HY, Zhang FC, Cao JJ, et al: Apolipoprotein E is a genetic risk factor for fetal iodine deficiency disorder in China. *Mol Psychiatry* 5:363:2000.

28. Rovet J: Congenital hypothyroidism, in Rourke BP (ed): *Syndrome of Nonverbal Learning Disabilities: Neurodevelopmental Manifestations*. New York: Guilford Press, 1995; pp 255–281.

29. Vargiu P, Morte B, Manzano J, et al: Thyroid hormone regulation of rhes, a novel Ras homolog gene expressed in the striatum. *Brain Res Mol Brain Res* 94:1, 2000.

30. Madeira MD, Paula-Barbosa MM: Reorganization of mossy fiber synapses in male and female hypothyroid rats: A stereological study. *J Comp Neurol* 337:334, 1993.

31. Ramakers GJA: Rho proteins, mental retardation and the cellular basis of cognition. *Trends Neurosci* 25:191, 2002.

32. Couvert P, Bienvenu T, Aquaviva C, et al: ME CP2 is highly mutated in X-linked mental retardation. *Hum Mol Genet* 10:941, 2001.

33. Fishler K, Koch R, Donnell GN: Comparison of mental development in individuals with mosaic and trisomy 21 Down's syndrome. *Pediatrics* 58:744, 1976.

34. Bellugi U, Bihrle A, Jernigan T, et al: Neuropsychological, neurological, and neuroanatomical profile of Williams syndrome. *Am J Hum Genet Suppl* 6:115, 1990.

35. Brugge KL, Nichols SL, Salmon DP, et al: Cognitive impairment in adults with Down's syndrome: Similarities to early cognitive changes in Alzheimer's disease. *Neurology* 44:232, 1994.

36. Baron-Cohen S, Leslie AM, Frith U: Does the autistic child have a "theory of mind"? *Cognition* 21:37, 1985.

37. Wilding J, Cornish K, Munir F: Further delineation of the executive deficit in males with fragile-X syndrome. *Neuropsychologia* 40, 1343, 2002.

38. Krasuski JS, Alexander GE, Horwitz B, et al: Relation of medial temporal lobe volumes to age and memory function in nondemented adults with Down's syndrome:

Implications for the prodromal phase of Alzheimer's disease. *Am J Psychiatry* 159:74–81, 2002.

39. Hof PR, Couras C, Perl DP, et al: Age-related distribution of neuropathologic changes in the cerebral cortex of patients with Down's syndrome: Quantitative regional analysis and comparison with Alzheimer's disease. *Arch Neurol* 52:379, 1995.

40. Teller JK, Russo C, DeBusk LM, et al: Presence of soluble amyloid beta-peptide precedes amyloid plaque formation in Down's syndrome. *Nat Med* 2:93, 1996.

41. Hyman BT, West HL, Rebeck GW, et al: Neuropathological changes in Down's syndrome hippocampal formation. *Arch Neurol* 52:373, 1995.

42. Kemper TL: Down syndrome, in Peters A, Jones EG (eds): *Cerebral Cortex. IX: Normal and Altered States of Function.* New York: Plenum Press, 1991, vol 9, p 511.

43. Pinter JD, Eliez S, Schmitt JE, et al: Neuroanatomy of Down's syndrome: A high-resolution MRI study. *Am J Psychiatry* 158:1659, 2001.

44. Pinter JD, Brown WE, Eliez S, et al: Amygdala and hippocampal volumes in children with Down syndrome: A high resolution MRI study. *Neurology* 56:972, 2001.

45. Schmidt-Sidor B, Wisniewski KE, Shepard T, et al: Brain growth in Down syndrome subjects 15 to 22 weeks of gestational age and birth to 60 months. *Clin Neuropathol* 9:181, 1990.

46. Cooper JD, Salehi A, Delcroix JD, et al: Failed retrograde transport of NGF in a mouse model of Down's syndrome: Reversal of cholinergic neurodegenerative phenotypes following NGF infusion. *Proc Natl Acad Sci U S A* 98:10439, 2001.

47. Hodapp RM, Dykens EM, Hagerman R, et al: Developmental implications of changing trajectories of IQ in males with fragile X syndrome. *J Am Acad Child Adolesc Psychiatry* 29:214, 1990.

48. Rousseau F, Heitz D, Tarleton J, et al: A multicenter study on genotype-phenotype correlations in the fragile X syndrome, using direct diagnosis with probe StB123.3: The first 2,253 cases. *Am J Hum Genet* 55:225, 1994.

49. Eliez S, Blasey CM, Freund LS, et al: Brain anatomy, gender and IQ in children and adolescents with fragile X syndrome. *Brain* 124:1610, 2001.

50. Mostofsky SH, Mazzocco MMM, Aakalu G, et al: Decreased cerebellar posterior vermis size in fragile X syndrome. Correlation with neurocognitive performance. *Neurology* 50:121, 1998.

51. Oberlé I, Rousseau F, Heitz D, et al: Instability of a 550-base pair DNA segment and abnormal methylation in fragile X syndrome. *Science* 252:1097, 1991.

52. Weiler IJ, Irwin SA, Klintsova AY, et al: Fragile X mental retardation protein is translated near synapses in response to neurotransmitter activation. *Proc Natl Acad Sci U S A* 94:5395, 1997.

53. Nimchinsky EA, Oberlander AM, Svoboda K: Abnormal development of dendritic spines in FMR1 knock-out mice. *J Neurosci* 21:5139, 2001.

54. Dyer-Friedman J, Glaser B, Hessi D, et al: Genetic and environmental influences on the cognitive outcomes of children with fragile X syndrome. *J Am Acad Child Adolesc Psychiatry* 41:237, 2002.

55. Kwon H, Menon V, Eliez S, et al: Functional neuroanatomy of visuospatial working memory in fragile X syndrome: Relation to behavioral and molecular measures. *Am J Psychiatry* 158:1040, 2001.

56. Dimitropoulos A, Feurer ID, Butler MG, et al: Emergence of compulsive behavior and tantrums in children with Prader-Willi syndrome. *Ment Retard* 106:39, 2001.

57. Lossie AC, Whitney MM, Amidon D, et al: Distinct phenotypes distinguish the molecular classes of Angelman syndrome. *J Med Genet* 38:834, 2001.

58. Temple CM, Carney RA: Intellectual functioning of children with Turner syndrome: A comparison of behavioural phenotypes. *Dev Med Child Neurol* 35:691, 1993.

59. Leichtman D, Schmickel R, Gelehrntner T, et al: *Ann Intern Med* 89:473, 1978.

60. Reiss AL, Freund L, Plotnick L, et al: The effects of X monosomy on brain development: Monozygotic twins discordant for Turner's syndrome. *Ann Neurol* 34:95, 1993.

61. Solot CB, Knightly C, Handler SD, et al: Communication disorders in the 22q11.2 microdeletion syndrome. *J Commun Disord* 33:187, 2000.

62. Bearden CE, Woodin MR, Wang PP, et al: The neurocognitive phenotype of the 22q11.2 deletion syndrome: Selective deficit in visual-spatial memory. *J Clin Exp Neuropsychol* 23:447, 2001.

63. Golding-Kushner KJ, Weller G, Shprintzen RJ: Velo-cardio-facial syndrome: Language and psychological profiles. *J Craniofac Genet Dev Biol* 5:259, 1985.

64. Papolos DR, Faedda GL, Veit S, et al: Bipolar spectrum disorders in patients diagnosed with velo-cardio-facial syndrome: Does a hemizygous deletion of chromosome 22q11 result in bipolar affective disorder? *Am J Psychiatry* 153:1541, 1996.

65. Murphy KC, Jones LA, Owen NH: High rates of schizophrenia in adults with velo-cardio-facial syndrome. *Arch Gen Psychiatry* 56:940–945, 1999.

66. Paylor R, McIlwain KL, McAninch R, et al: Mice deleted for the DiGeorge/velocardiofacial syndrome region show abnormal sensorimotor gating and learning and memory impairments. *Hum Mol Genet* 20:2645, 2001.

67. Graf WD, Unis AS, Yates CM, et al: Catecholamines in patients with 22q11.2 deletion syndrome and the low-activity COMT polymorphism. *Neurology* 57:410, 2001.
68. Eliez S, Schmitt JE, White CD, et al: Children and adolescents with velocardiofacial syndrome, a volumetric MRI study. *Am J Psychiatry* 157:409, 2000.
69. Chow EW, Mikulis DJ, Zipursky RB, et al: Qualitative MRI findings in adults with 22q11 deletion syndrome and schizophrenia. *Biol Psychiatry* 157:409, 1999.
70. Cramer SC, Schaefer PW, Krishnamoorthy KS: Microgyria in the distribution of the middle cerebral artery in a patient with DiGeorge syndrome. *J Child Neurol* 11:494, 1996.
71. Eliez S, Antonarakis SE, Morris MA, et al: Parental origin of the deletion 22qll.2 and brain development in velocardiofacial syndrome. *Arch Gen Psychiatry* 58:64, 2001.
72. Tager-Flusberg H, Boshart J, Baron-Cohen S: Reading the windows to the soul: Evidence for domain-specific sparing in William's syndrome. *J Cogn Neurosci* 10:631, 1998.
73. Bellugi U, Lictenberger L, Mills D, et al.: Bridging cognition, the brain and molecular genetics: Evidence from Williams syndrome. *Trends Neurosci* 22:197, 1999.
74. Wang PP, Hesselink JR, Jernigan TL, et al: Specific neurobehavioral profile of Williams' syndrome is associated with neocerebellar hemispheric preservation. *Neurology* 42:1999, 1992.
75. Schmitt JE, Eliez S, Warsofsky IS, et al: Enlarged cerebellar vermis in Williams syndrome. *J Psychiatr Res* 35:225, 2001.
76. Galaburda AM, Schmitt JE, Atlas SW, et al: Dorsal forebrain anomaly in Williams syndrome. *Arch Neurol* 58:1865, 2001.
77. Galaburda AM, Wang PP, Bellugi U, et al: Cytoarchitectonic anomalies in a genetically based disorder. Williams syndrome. *Neuroreport* 5:753, 1994.
78. Ewart AK, Morris CA, Atkinson D, et al: Hemizygosity at the elastin locus in a developmental disorder. Williams syndrome. *Nat Genet* 5:11, 1993.
79. Botta A, Novelli G, Mari A, et al: Detection of an atypical 7q11.23 deletion in Williams syndrome patients which does not include the STX1A and FZd3 genes. *J Med Genet* 36:478, 1999.
80. Tassabehji M, Metcalfe K, Karmiloff-Smith A, et al: Williams syndrome: use of chromosomal microdeletions as a tool to dissect cognitive and physical phenotypes. *Am J Hum Gen* 64:118, 1999.

Chapter 35

ATTENTION DEFICIT HYPERACTIVITY DISORDER*

Bruce F. Pennington
Nomita Chhabildas

A syndrome involving hyperactivity in children was first described over 150 years ago by Heinrich Hoffman,[1] a German physician, who wrote a humorous poem describing the antics of "fidgety Phil who couldn't sit still." Somewhat later, Still[2] described the main problem in this syndrome as a deficiency in "volitional inhibition" or "a defect in moral control." As we will see, problems with inhibition continue to be central to current conceptions of ADHD. However, much work remains to be done to determine whether inhibition deficits can truly account for symptom presentation in ADHD or whether other deficits are at the core of the disorder.

Whether there is brain dysfunction in ADHD and how to characterize it have been confusing and controversial issues in the history of ADHD research. The notion that childhood hyperactivity was a brain disorder was promoted by Strauss and Lehtinen,[3] based on similarities with the behavior of children who had suffered brain damage because of encephalitis. Unfortunately, this analogy led to some muddled terminology, whereby children with hyperactivity were described as having "minimal brain damage" or "minimal brain dysfunction." These terms are misleading for several reasons: (1) the large majority of children with ADHD have a developmental disorder, not acquired brain damage; (2) the damage or dysfunction to the brain implied in these labels was not documented directly but only inferred from behavioral symptoms that could have many different causes; (3) many children with acquired brain damage do not have hyperactivity[4]; and (4) these terms were vague and overinclusive and thus

impeded progress in delineating distinct neuropsychological syndromes affecting learning and behavior in childhood. As detailed below, there is now much more direct evidence that ADHD is related to brain dysfunction that is substantially heritable, although we are still learning about the neurobiology of ADHD.

ADHD is now more clearly defined and better understood than it once was, yet it remains a somewhat broad and controversial diagnosis. Over half of children who meet diagnostic criteria for ADHD qualify for a comorbid diagnosis,[5] and the list of comorbid disorders includes conduct disorder, depression, anxiety, Tourette's disorder, dyslexia, and bipolar disorder. Moreover, children with autism, schizophrenia, and mental retardation frequently exhibit the symptoms of ADHD, although the DSM-IV stipulates that their more serious primary diagnosis excludes an ADHD diagnosis. So more research is needed to understand the basis of these comorbidities and to define purer subtypes of ADHD.

DEFINITION

DSM-IV[6] defines ADHD with two distinct but correlated dimensions of symptoms, those involving *inattention* (e.g., making careless mistakes and not paying close attention to details, forgetfulness, difficulty organizing tasks and activities, and failure to begin or complete tasks that require sustained mental effort) and those comprising *hyperactivity-impulsivity* (e.g., excessive fidgeting, locomotion, or talking; interrupting or intruding in conversations, games, and other situations). With two dimensions, there are thus three possible subtypes of ADHD: a predominantly inattentive subtype, a predominantly hyperactive-impulsive subtype, and a combined subtype. Someone who meets the

* **ACKNOWLEDGMENTS:** This work was supported by NICHD grants HD27802 and HD04024, an NIMH grant, MH38820, as well as by the second author's NRSA fellowship, MH12017.

diagnostic cutoff (six of nine symptoms) for a single dimension qualifies for that subtype; someone who meets this cutoff on both dimensions qualifies for the combined subtype. Additional requirements for the diagnosis include that the symptoms (1) must cause a clinically significant impairment in adaptive functioning, (2) are inconsistent with developmental level (e.g., not just secondary to mental retardation), (3) have been present for at least 6 months with an onset of some symptoms before age 7, (4) are present in two or more settings, and (5) are not better accounted for by another mental disorder (pervasive developmental disorder, psychosis, or a mood, anxiety, dissociative, or personality disorder). As pointed out below, there is more empirical support for the construct validity of the inattentive and combined subtypes than for the hyperactive-impulsive subtype.

EPIDEMIOLOGY

Attention deficit hyperactivity disorder (ADHD) is one of the most common chronic disorders of childhood, with a 6-month prevalence of 3 to 5 percent among school-aged children according to recent epidemiologic studies.[7] Of course, prevalence depends on definition and definitions vary in how pervasive they require the ADHD symptoms to be. In a careful epidemiologic study that required pervasiveness across three different reporters—parents, teachers, and a physician—the prevalence was only 1.2 percent.[8] Sex ratios in referred samples have been reported to be as high as 9:1 (males:females), but an epidemiologic study found a sex ratio of 3:1.[9] Thus, as in other disorders such as reading disability (RD), males are more likely to be referred than females. Because much of the research on ADHD has relied on referred samples, we currently know much more about ADHD in males than in females.

ADHD has been found across social classes and cultures. There are higher rates of ADHD in lower social classes, but these differences are no longer found once comorbid conditions, such as conduct disorder, are controlled for (see review, Ref. 10). Roughly comparable rates of ADHD have been found in studies in the United States, Japan, and India, with a somewhat higher rate in Germany.[10] At times, there can be

dramatic differences in prevalence even between very similar cultures (i.e., the United States and the United Kingdom) simply due to differences in diagnostic criteria and practice.[7]

In terms of natural history, the age of onset is usually in toddlerhood, with a peak age of onset between ages 3 and 4.[11] Symptoms of ADHD may appear earlier, even in utero. It is becoming clearer that ADHD is a chronic disorder across the life span[12] and that many of the tasks of adult development are disrupted by ADHD because sustained effort, planning, and organization are central to many adult responsibilities.

ETIOLOGY

The exact etiology of ADHD is still unknown. However, recent progress in understanding the genetics of developmental disorders (see Chap. 38), as well as developmental cognitive neuroscience more generally, has taught us a fair amount about genes and brain pathways that may be involved in the disorder. Thus, ADHD represents a success story for a neuroscience approach to understanding psychopathology. This section comprises a review of evidence that ADHD is familial, moderately heritable, and may be influenced by two genes that affect dopamine neurotransmission. Environmental influences on ADHD are also discussed.

Familiality

The rate of ADHD in families of ADHD male probands has been found to be over seven times the rate of the disorder in nonpsychiatric control families[13]; a later study reported a similar increase in risk among relatives of female probands.[14,15]

Heritability

Stevenson[16] found a heritability of 0.76 for ADHD in his twin study, and numerous other twin studies have found similar results, both for the diagnosis of ADHD as well as for individual differences in ADHD symptomatology.[17–24] Although extreme scores on both the defining dimensions of ADHD, inattention (IA) and hyperactivity-impulsivity (HI), are moderately heritable, this appears to *not* be the case for the

HI dimension once the correlation between the two dimensions is accounted for.[23] That is, extreme scores on the IA dimension are moderately heritable regardless of the level of HI symptoms in the proband (i.e., both the inattentive and combined subtypes of ADHD are moderately heritable). However, extreme scores on the HI dimension were *not* significantly heritable ($h^2g = 0.08$) when probands were not also extreme on IA. These results suggest the etiology of the HI subtype is largely nongenetic and differs from the etiology of the other two subtypes.

Mode of Transmission There has been one segregation analysis of ADHD,[15] which found autosomal dominant transmission with considerably reduced penetrance of the hypothesized major gene. Although this suggests that there may be loci of sizable effect, the genetic etiology of ADHD is very unlikely to be due to just one gene.

Gene Locations Efforts to identify specific genes influencing ADHD illustrate the potential power of the candidate gene association approach. This approach usually depends on a hypothesis derived from an understanding of the neurobiology of the disorder. We know that the primary drug used to treat ADHD, methylphenidate (Ritalin), is a dopamine agonist, and that it achieves this effect by blocking the dopamine transporter, a receptor on the presynaptic neuron involved in the reuptake of dopamine in the synapse. Hence, blocking reuptake increases the dopamine available in the synapse. Since receptors are coded for by genes, a gene for a dopamine transporter or genes for other dopamine receptors are reasonable candidate genes in ADHD.

Molecular genetic research on ADHD has focused on dopamine genes, particularly a dopamine transporter gene (DAT1) and DRD4, one of the dopamine receptors. Since both of these dopamine genes are polymorphic (they have frequently occurring allelic variations), they could be tested as candidates in association studies.

The 10-copy allele of DAT1 was significantly associated with ADHD in a study of 53 families.[25] This finding has now been replicated in two separate samples,[26,27] although it is not significant in all samples.[28-30]

An allele of the DRD4 gene that contains a seven-repeat base-pair sequence was shown to be significantly associated with novelty-seeking behavior, which prompted the hypothesis that it might also be linked to impulsive behavior seen in ADHD.[31,32] Indeed, numerous studies have now found an association between the DRD4 allele and ADHD,[33-37] although again this result is not significant in all studies.[28,38]

A recent metanalysis of all available studies of the association between ADHD and DRD4[39] concluded that the association between the two is indeed real, although small in magnitude.

Although these are exciting findings, there are complications that still need to be resolved. Counterintuitively, the risk allele of the DAT1 gene is *more* frequent than the nonrisk allele in the general population, a result that may well hold for many alleles associated with psychopathology. Second, the effect size of each of these risk alleles is small. Finally, as discussed further on, one study[40] found that presence of the DRD4 risk allele was *not* associated with the neuropsychological deficits that characterize ADHD.

In sum, there will likely be other risk alleles that influence ADHD, and this influence may vary by ADHD subtype, whether these be DSM-IV subtypes or those defined by comorbidities.

Other evidence for genetic influence on ADHD or its symptoms comes from their association with known genetic syndromes, including Turner's syndrome (45, X) in females; 47, XYY in males; fragile X syndrome; neurofibromatosis; and early treated PKU (reviewed in Ref. 41).

Environmental Influences

There are several known bioenvironmental correlates of ADHD, including fetal alcohol exposure, environmental lead, and pediatric head injury (reviewed in Ref. 41). Since that review, it has become clear that maternal smoking in pregnancy is associated with an increased risk of ADHD in offspring (see review in Ref. 10). However, exposure to these bioenvironmental risk factors is not randomly assigned and, for some of them, we have evidence that exposure is correlated with ADHD in the parent or child, which may be genetically mediated. At the same time, it seems implausible that the dramatic ADHD symptoms observed clinically in fetal alcohol syndrome or pediatric head injury can be entirely explained by such a confound. Instead, it might be better to conceptualize at least some of these bioenvironmental risk factors as examples of gene-environment correlations: the presence of the ADHD genotype increases exposure to environmental risk factors that exacerbate the ADHD phenotype.

We do not have evidence that the social environment, in particular parenting practices, can directly cause ADHD. At the same time, there is no doubt that the social environment influences the course of ADHD, in particular whether ADHD develops into another disruptive behavior disorder.

BRAIN MECHANISMS

The hypothesis of frontal lobe dysfunction in ADHD has been advanced by several researchers[42-47] based on the observation that frontal lesions in both experimental animals and human patients sometimes produce hyperactivity, distractibility, and/or impulsivity, alone or in combination.[48-50] Of course, lesions in other parts of the brain can also produce these symptoms. The evidence that supports frontal-striatal dysfunction in ADHD is reviewed below.

Structural Studies

With regard to brain structure, earlier work[51,52] found no evidence of structural differences in computed tomography (CT) studies of ADHD children and colleagues. Hynd and colleagues,[53] however, using magnetic resonance imaging (MRI), did find absence of the usual R>L frontal asymmetry in ADHD children. They contrasted ADHD subjects with both dyslexics and controls; the frontal finding was present in both clinical groups but did not differentiate between them, even though the dyslexic group was selected to be non-ADHD. There is an association between the right frontal lobe and measures of sustained attention, so this neuroanatomic difference has theoretical relevance to ADHD. This lack of frontal asymmetry in ADHD has been replicated in two other studies.[54,55] Abnormalities of caudate volume have also been found across numerous studies of ADHD.[54-57] In addition, the globus pallidus has been found to be significantly smaller in

those with ADHD.[54,58,59] These structural studies support developmental differences in frontal-striatal structures known to be important in action selection.

The hypothesis that these structural differences were related to deficits in action selection was tested in a study by Casey et al.[60] They correlated performance on three separate inhibition tasks with measures of prefrontal cortex and basal ganglia volume. The three inhibition tasks, which were designed to tap response inhibition at different stages of attentional processing, were all impaired in the children with ADHD when compared to controls. Furthermore, prefrontal cortex, caudate, and globus pallidus volumes correlated significantly with task performance. Of course, this correlation does not prove cause. Such a finding could be a *result* of ADHD or just a correlate of ADHD.

However, brain structure differences in ADHD are not exclusively in the prefrontal cortex and basal ganglia. Decreased areas in different regions of the corpus callosum have been observed in several studies,[53,54,61-63] as well as smaller total cerebral volume and a smaller cerebellum.[54]

Functional Studies

In terms of brain function, electrophysiologic measures have supported the hypothesis of CNS underarousal in at least a subgroup of hyperactive children.[64] Likewise, Lou and coworkers,[65] using regional cerebral blood flow, found decreased blood flow to the frontal lobes in ADHD children, which increased after the children received methylphenidate. This treatment also decreased blood flow to the motor cortex and primary sensory cortex, "suggesting an inhibition of function of these structures, seen clinically as less distractibility and decreased motor activity during treatment" (Ref. 65, p. 829). These investigators replicated this result in an expanded sample[66]; in this second report they emphasize the basal ganglia as the locus of reduced blood flow in ADHD. Zametkin et al.[67] used positron emission tomography (PET) to study the parents of ADHD children, who themselves had residual-type ADHD. They found an overall reduction in cerebral glucose utilization, particularly in right frontal areas, but increased utilization in posterior medio-orbital areas. A second study by this group[68] investigating teenagers with

ADHD replicated some but not all of those findings. This second study found significant reductions in the ADHD group in normalized glucose metabolism in 6 of 60 brain regions, including the left anterior frontal lobe. Metabolism in that region correlated inversely with ADHD symptom severity across the combined sample of patients and controls. Since hyperfrontality of blood flow is characteristic of the normal brain, hypofrontality in ADHD could explain the low central arousal found in the electrophysiologic studies.

Other studies have demonstrated decreased blood flow in ADHD subjects both in prefrontal regions and the striatum.[69] More recently, functional magnetic resonance imaging (fMRI) has demonstrated similar results, showing hypoperfusion in the right caudate nucleus, which was ameliorated after treatment with methylphenidate.[70]

Neurochemical Studies

In terms of brain biochemistry, Shaywitz and colleagues[71] found lower levels of homovanillic acid (HVA—the main dopamine metabolite) in the cerebrospinal fluid of ADHD children compared to controls. This could also lend support to a frontal theory of ADHD, as dopamine has a preponderant distribution in the frontal regions of the cortex. Moreover, a well-validated animal model of ADHD involves dopamine depletion.[52]

In summary, one plausible theory of brain mechanisms in ADHD is as follows. The symptoms of ADHD are caused by functional hypofrontality, which in turn is caused by either structural and/or biochemical changes in the prefrontal lobes and striatum and is detectable as reduced frontal blood flow. Biochemically, the cause would be low dopamine levels, which methylphenidate treatment reverses at least in part.

Unfortunately, the story is not that simple. One study found that some dopamine agonists were not effective in treating hyperactive children,[72] whereas certain dopamine *antagonists* did have unexpected beneficial effects in children with ADHD.[47] Both of these results are opposite to what would be predicted by the dopamine depletion hypothesis. So the neurochemical mechanisms may be more complex, although the ubiquitous problem of heterogeneity in ADHD samples is another explanation.

Zametkin and Rapoport[47] argue that no single neurotransmitter is exclusively involved in the pathogenesis of ADHD, both because stimulant medications always affect more than one neurotransmitter and because of the multiple interrelations among specific catecholamines and their precursors and metabolites. They and Oades[73] both argue that the combined action of dopaminergic and noradrenergic systems should be considered in the biology of ADHD.

Obviously, much more research is needed, preferably using familial samples that are as phenotypically homogeneous as possible. The associations between ADHD and the DAT1 and DRD4 alleles will begin to allow neurobiologic research to focus on genetic subtypes of ADHD.

NEUROPSYCHOLOGY

There is a fairly extensive literature on cognitive processes in ADHD, which has become more explicitly neuropsychological in the hypotheses tested. Virginia Douglas has been a pioneer in this area, establishing that there is a distinctive cognitive phenotype in ADHD that needs to be explained. She and others have found that children with ADHD are impaired on tasks requiring vigilance, systematic search, and motor control and inhibition but are unimpaired on tasks tapping basic verbal and nonverbal memory functions.[74]

Neuropsychological studies of ADHD have mainly focused on the frontal lobe or executive function (EF) hypothesis, for reasons discussed earlier. A number of researchers have proposed an EF deficit theory of ADHD.[41,75–79]

We recently reviewed published studies of EFs in ADHD.[80] We found that 15 of 18 studies found a significant difference between ADHD subjects and controls on one or more EF measures. A total of 60 EF measures were used across studies; for 40 of these (67 percent), there was significantly worse performance in the ADHD group. In contrast, *none* of the 60 measures was significantly better in the ADHD group. The most consistently impaired domain of EF was inhibition; in contrast, children with ADHD were less likely to be impaired at set-shifting or working memory. In addition, children with ADHD in these studies were generally unimpaired on measures of verbal memory, other verbal processes, or visuospatial processing. They were fairly consistently impaired on measures of vigilance (GDS) and perceptual speed (Coding and Digit Symbol), but these measures would be expected to be influenced by an inhibitory deficit.

Although there are many different meanings of the term *inhibition* in psychology, inhibition in this case is "intentional motor inhibition,"[81] which requires consciously restraining a dominant or prepotent motor response. The inhibitory process is thought to be primarily mediated by higher cognitive processes and thus is thought to require prefrontally mediated executive function.

The most widely researched measure of this type of inhibition in the domain of ADHD is the stop signal paradigm.[82] In this paradigm, a subject is taught a particular response and then later told to inhibit the very same response on the subset of trials signaled by a beep. The paradigm allows for the computation of the stop signal reaction time (SSRT), or the time it takes to inhibit a response. In a recent meta-analysis of studies using the stop task,[83] consistent deficits were demonstrated in groups with ADHD, providing evidence that children with ADHD are impaired in their ability for response inhibition. Nigg[84] also recently demonstrated inhibitory deficits in children with ADHD combined type using the stop signal paradigm. Deficits on the task were specific to ADHD and not associated with comorbid reading or behavior problems. Furthermore, a study by Aman and coworkers[85] demonstrated that deficits of children with ADHD on the stop task were normalized when the children had taken methylphenidate.

These findings that children with ADHD consistently have slower SSRTs than control children, that this deficit is specific to ADHD, and that it is reversed by stimulant medication are all consistent with the hypothesis that ADHD is caused by a slow inhibitory process. However, this interpretation is clouded by the fact that children with ADHD often have slower "go" reaction times as well. Some researchers (e.g., Ref. 86 and Swanson, personal communication) suggest that rather than a specific inhibitory deficit, ADHD is characterized by slower and more variable reaction times, which would produce the pattern of performance observed in groups with ADHD on the stop task and on a variety of other tasks.

More generally, although the executive or inhibitory deficit theory of ADHD has considerable support,

there are nonetheless several important threats to its validity. Perhaps the most important threat is the amount of variance in ADHD symptoms that EF measures can account for. The most sensitive measures of EF with regard to ADHD, as discussed previously, tend to be those that tap inhibition, such as the stop task and continuous performance tasks.[87–89] However, when comparing performance of those with ADHD and controls, even these measures produce effect sizes that are relatively small, ranging from about .5 to 1.5.[80,84,90] This effect is much smaller than the effect size of the typical difference in symptoms of ADHD between the two groups, which is usually in the range of 2.5 to 3.5. In addition, correlations between behavior ratings of attention and impulsivity do not correlate highly with EF measures, typically being in the range of 0.15 to 0.30.[91] These limited correlations mean that an EF deficit, as currently measured, cannot totally account for the symptoms that define the disorder.

There are several competing explanations to account for these relatively small effect sizes. One possibility is that children with ADHD are a substantially heterogeneous group, and some but not all have primary deficits in inhibition. In addition, differences within or among samples in ADHD subtype, age, gender, and prevalence of comorbid disorders could also affect the findings.

A second possibility is that EF deficits are not the primary deficit in ADHD but instead are just a correlate of the actual, underlying deficit. There are a number of competing motivational and arousal theories of ADHD, and they all argue that the primary deficit in ADHD is not a cognitive one. For instance, Sonuga-Barke et al.[92] argue that the underlying difference in ADHD is not a deficit of inhibition but rather a preference to shorten delay. Other competing theories of ADHD argue that state regulation, regulation of arousal, or motivation may truly be the critical deficit in children with ADHD.[93–96] These authors view the inhibition deficit as being secondary to a more primary difficulty in another area. Therefore, in the appropriate circumstances, children with ADHD should be able to inhibit responses. A recent study by Kuntsi and associates[97] compared performance of children with ADHD and control children on tasks of inhibition, working memory, and delay aversion. Children with ADHD performed more poorly than control children on some of the working memory measures and on the delay aversion task. In contrast, this study found no group differences on the inhibition measures from the stop signal paradigm. However, on the stop signal task, children with ADHD had slower "go" reaction times. The authors suggest these results could be consistent with a state-regulation theory of ADHD,[86] as this response style could reflect a lack of consistent effort.

Yet a third possibility is that there are two (or more) primary deficits in ADHD, which may interact. In this case, each deficit by itself would account for a relatively small proportion of the variance in ADHD symptoms.

Another threat to the validity of an EF theory of ADHD comes from a recent study relating molecular measures to executive measures in ADHD.[40] Since the seven-repeat allele of the DRD4 receptor is significantly associated with ADHD, the next link in an EF theory of ADHD would be to test whether this gene is linked to the hypothesized underlying psychological deficit in ADHD, the EF deficit. Such a finding would provide a comprehensive explanation of symptom presentation in ADHD using an EF framework: Variations in dopamine genes lead to reduced dopaminergic function in the prefrontal cortex and basal ganglia, thereby impairing executive functions, particularly inhibition, and thus producing the behavioral symptoms of ADHD. So, from an EF framework, the presence of the seven-repeat allele should be significantly associated not only with ADHD but also with deficits in EF.

To test this theory, Swanson and colleagues compared subgroups of ADHD children with and without the seven-repeat allele on a series of EF tasks. Directly *opposite* to prediction, only children in the seven-absent group were impaired on EF tasks, whereas those with the DRD4 risk allele performed very similarly to controls on all EF measures in the study. This finding is inconsistent with an EF theory of ADHD or is at least inconsistent with the hypothesis that the DRD4 receptor mediates the EF deficits.

However, this study had a relatively small sample size (with 13 children in the seven-present group and 19 children in the seven-absent group) and needs to be replicated. In addition, the presence of the DRD4 seven-repeat allele is not necessary for a diagnosis of ADHD and is clearly not the only genetic locus contributing to the phenotype of ADHD. It is possible that EF deficits in ADHD are instead related to another

genetic locus, such as the DAT1 allele or to an interaction among several alleles. It is also possible that the DRD4 receptor is significantly related only to a particular subtype of ADHD, the inattentive subtype. A recent study[35] found that the seven-repeat allele of DRD4 was associated more strongly with the predominantly inattentive subtype rather than the combined subtype of ADHD. In the study of Swanson et al., however, only children with the combined subtype of ADHD were studied.

Another study used a behavioral genetic approach to examine the relationship between ADHD and EF deficits and obtained some support for a state-regulation conceptualization of ADHD.[98] This study tested whether hyperactivity shared common genetic factors with underlying psychological processes found to be related to ADHD in previous work.[98] Since ADHD is highly heritable, a primary psychological deficit accounting for symptom presentation would be expected to be coheritable with the ADHD diagnosis. The study only found significant evidence of shared genetic factors between hyperactivity and variability of response time, whereas there was not evidence of shared genetic influence on measures of working memory, inhibition, or delay aversion. These results do not support an EF theory but could support a state-regulation account of ADHD.

In sum, despite converging evidence in support of an EF theory of ADHD, there are several important threats to the validity of this theory, including the low effect sizes obtained in studies using inhibition paradigms, competing explanations for the underlying deficit (such as motivational, delay aversion, and state-regulation perspectives), and the inconsistent genetic findings just discussed.[40,98]

TREATMENT

The treatment of ADHD has recently been reviewed.[7] Here, the main points of that review are summarized. The use of psychostimulant drugs such as methylphenidate (Ritalin), dextroamphetamine (Dexedrine), and pemoline (Cylert) to treat ADHD is the most thoroughly researched application of psychopharmacology in child psychiatry. The efficacy and safety of these drugs in treating ADHD has now been well established. About 75 to 90 percent of children with ADHD show a favorable treatment response with psychostimulant medication. The side effects of psychostimulants are generally mild, especially compared to other psychopharmacologic treatments, and usually abate with time and changes in dose. These side effects include decreased sleep and appetite, jitteriness, stomachaches, and headaches.

There are ongoing public controversies about the diagnosis and treatment of ADHD, not all of which are supported by research. Earlier concerns about growth retardation, precipitation of a tic disorder, psychostimulants becoming drugs of abuse, overdiagnosis of ADHD, or overprescription of psychostimulant drugs have not been supported by research, but some of these concerns could become real problems in the future. There is nonetheless valid concern about the misdiagnosis of ADHD. Not all practitioners prescribing stimulant medication for ADHD have the time or the training to make this demanding differential diagnosis accurately.

Psychosocial treatments for ADHD mainly consist of behavioral intervention techniques for parents and teachers to help them better manage these children, who can be very disruptive in a classroom or family. Such treatments are particularly important for children who do not respond to medication or whose parents prefer not to use medication. In general, the efficacy of psychosocial treatments for improving ADHD symptoms is (1) less than that of psychostimulants[99] and (2) greater for teachers than parents.

The question naturally arises as to whether the combination of psychostimulant and behavioral interventions would be more efficacious than either alone. A recent large study funded by the National Institute of Mental Health addressed this question. This 3-year multimodal treatment of ADHD study[100] compared four treatment conditions: medication alone, behavioral intervention alone, a combination of the two, and no treatment beyond what is already typically provided in the community. The behavioral intervention was intensive, involving parent training, school intervention, and summer treatment in a camp setting. The medication management was more intensive than what would typically be provided in a community setting. Subjects were randomly assigned to one of the four conditions, treated for 14 months, and followed for 22 months after that. There was a large main effect of medication treatment on ADHD symptoms, for which the addition of the behavioral intervention produced no added benefit. However, the behavioral intervention did improve outcome in some nonsymptom areas.

There are also several nonconventional therapies for ADHD, including the Feingold diet and EEG biofeedback, which have not been supported by careful treatment studies.

REFERENCES

1. Hoffman H: *Der Struwelpeter: Oder lustige Geschichten und drollige Bilder.* Leipzig: Insel-Verlag, 1845.
2. Still GF: Some abnormal psychical conditions in children. *Lancet* 1:1008–1012, 1163–1168, 1077–1082, 1902.
3. Strauss A, Lehtinen L: *Psychopathology and Education of the Brain-Injured Child.* New York: Grune & Stratton, 1947.
4. Rutter M, Quinton, D: Psychiatric disorders: Ecological factors and concepts of causation, in McGurk H (ed): *Ecological Factors in Human Development.* Amsterdam: North-Holland, 1977, pp 173–187.
5. Biederman J, Faraone, SV, Keenan K, et al: Further evidence for family-genetic risk factors in attention deficit hyperactivity disorder. Patterns of comorbidity in probands and relatives in psychiatrically and pediatrically referred samples. *Arch Gen Psychiatry* 49:728–738, 1992.
6. *Diagnostic and Statistical Manual of Mental Disorders,* 4th ed (DSM-IV). Washington, DC: American Psychiatric Association, 1994.
7. Satcher D: *Mental Health: A Report of the Surgeon General.* http://www.mentalhealth.org/specials/surgeongeneralreport, 1999.
8. Spreen O, Tupper D, Risser A, et al: *Human Developmental Neuropsychology.* New York: Oxford University Press, 1984.
9. Szatmari P, Offord DR, Boyle M: Correlates, associated impairments, and patterns of service utilization of children with attention deficit disorders: Findings from the Ontario Child Health Study. *J Child Psychol Psychiatry* 30:205–217, 1989.
10. Barkley RA: Attention-deficit/hyperactivity disorder, in Mash EJ, Barkley RA (eds): *Child Psychopathology.* New York: Guilford Press, 1996; pp 63–112.
11. Palfrey JS, Levine MD, Walker DK, et al: The emergence of attention deficits in early childhood: A

prospective study. *J Dev Behav Pediatr* 6:339–348, 1985.

12. Gittleman R, Mannuzza S, Shenker R, et al: Hyperactive boys almost grown up. *Arch Gen Psychiatry* 42:937–947, 1985.

13. Biederman J, Faraone SV, Keenan K, et al: Family-genetic and psychosocial risk factors in DSM III attention deficit disorder. *J Am Acad Child Adolesc Psychiatry* 29:526–533, 1990.

14. Faraone S, Biederman J, Keenan K, et al: A family genetic study of girls with DSM-III attention deficit disorder. *Am J Psychiatry* 148:112–117, 1991.

15. Faraone S, Biederman J, Chen WJ, et al: Segregation analysis of attention deficit hyperactivity disorder: Evidence for single major gene transmission. *Psychiatr Genet* 2:257–275, 1992.

16. Stevenson J: Evidence for a genetic etiology in hyperactivity in children. *Behav Genet* 2:337–344, 1992.

17. Eaves L, Silberg J, Meyer J, et al: Genetics and developmental psychopathology: 2. The main effects of genes and environment on behavioral problems in the Virginia Twin Study of Adolescent Behavioral Development. *J Child Psychol Psychiatry* 38:965–980, 1997.

18. Gillis JJ, Gilger JW, Pennington BF, et al: Attention deficit disorder in reading-disabled twins: Evidence for a genetic etiology. *J Abnorm Child Psychol* 20(3):303–331, 1992.

19. Gjane H, Stevenson J, Sundet J: Genetic influence on parent-reported attention-related problems in a Norwegian general population twin sample. *J Am Acad Child Adolesc Psychiatry* 35:588–596, 1996.

20. Levy F, Hay D, McStephen M, et al: Attention-deficit hyperactivity disorder: A category or a continuum? A genetic analysis of a large-scale twin study. *J Am Acad Child Adolesc Psychiatry* 36:737–744, 1997.

21. Sherman D, Iacono W, McGue M: Attention-deficit/hyperactivity disorder dimensions: A twin study of inattention and impulsivity/hyperactivity. *J Am Acad Child Adolesc Psychiatry* 36:745–753, 1997.

22. Thapar A, McGuffin P: Are anxiety symptoms in childhood heritable? *J Child Psychol Psychiatry*, 36:439–447, 1995.

23. Willcutt EG, Pennington BF, DeFries JC: A twin study of the etiology of comorbidity between reading disability and attention-deficit/hyperactivity disorder. *Am J Med Genet (Neuropsychiatr Gene)* 96:293–301, 2000.

24. Willerman L: Activity level and hyperactivity in twins. *Child Dev* 44:288–293, 1973.

25. Cook EH, Stein MA, Krasowski MD, et al: Association of attention deficit disorder and the dopamine transporter gene. *Am J Hum Genet* 56:993–998, 1995.

26. Gill M, Daly G, Heron S, et al: Confirmation of association between attention deficit hyperactivity disorder and a dopamine transporter polymorphism. *Mol Psychiatry* 2:311–313, 1997.

27. Waldman ID, Rowe DC, Abramowitz A, et al: Association of the dopamine transporter gene (DAT1) and attention deficit hyperactivity disorder in children (abstr). *Am J Hum Genet* 59:A25, 1996.

28. Asherson P, Virdee V, Curran S, et al: Association of DSM-IV attention deficit hyperactivity disorder and monoamine pathway genes. *Am J Med Genet* 81:549, 1998.

29. LaHoste G, Wigal S, Glabe C, et al: Dopamine related genes and attention deficit hyperactivity disorder. Paper presented at the annual meeting of the Society for the Neurosciences, San Diego, CA, November 1995.

30. Poulton K, Holmes J, Hever T, et al: A molecular genetic study of hyperkinetic disorder/attention deficit hyperactivity disorder. *Am J Med Gen* 81:458, 1998.

31. Benjamin J, Li L, Patterson C, et al: Population and family association between the D4 dopamine receptor gene and measures of novelty seeking. *Nat Genet* 12:81–84, 1996.

32. Ebstein R, Novick O, Umansky R, et al: Dopamine D4 receptor (DRD4) exon III polymorphism associated with the human personality trait of novelty seeking. *Nat Gene* 12:78–80, 1996.

33. Faraone SV, Biederman J, Weiffenbach B, et al: Dopamine D4 gene 7-repeat allele and attention-deficit hyperactivity disorder. *Am J Psychiatry* 156:768–770, 1999.

34. LaHoste GJ, Swanson JM, Wigel SB, et al: Dopamine D4 receptor gene polymorphism is associated with attention deficit hyperactivity disorder. *Mol Psychiatry* 1(2):121–124, 1996.

35. Rowe DC, Stever G, Giedinghagen LN, et al: Dopamine DRD4 receptor polymorphism and attention deficit hyperactivity disorder. *Mol Psychiatry* 3:419–426, 1998.

36. Smalley SL, Bailey JN, Palmer GG, et al: Evidence that the dopamine D4 receptor is a susceptibility gene in attention deficit hyperactivity disorder. *Mol Psychiatry* 3:427–430, 1998.

37. Swanson J, Sunhora GA, Kennedy JL, et al: Association of the dopamine receptor D4 (DRD4) gene with a refined phenotype of attention deficit hyperactivity disorder (ADHD): A family based approach. *Mol Psychiatry* 3:38–41, 1998.

38. Castellanos FX, Lau E, Tayebi N, et al: Lack of an association between a dopamine-4 receptor polymorphism and attention-deficit/hyperactivity disorder:

Genetic and brain morphometric analyses. *Mol Psychiatry* 3:431–434, 1998.

39. Faraone SV, Doyle AE, Mick E, et al: Meta-analysis of the association between the 7-repeat allele of the dopamine D4 receptor gene and attention deficit hyperactivity disorder. *Am J Psychiatry* 158:1052–1057, 2001.

40. Swanson J, Oosterlaan J, Murias M, et al: Attention deficit/hyperactivity disorder children with a 7-repeat allele of the dopamine receptor D4 gene have extreme behavior but normal performance on critical neuropsychological tests of attention. *Proc Natl Acad Sci U S A* 97:4754–4759, 2000.

41. Pennington BF: *Diagnosing Learning Disorders: A Neuropsychological Framework*. New York: Guilford Press, 1991.

42. Gualtieri CT, Hicks RE: Neuropharmacology of methylphenidate and a neural substrate for childhood hyperactivity. *Psychiatr Clin North Am* 6:875–892, 1985.

43. Mattes JA: The role of frontal lobe dysfunction in childhood hyperkinesis. *Comp Psychiatry* 21:358–369, 1989.

44. Pontius AA: Dysfunctional patterns analogous to frontal lobe system and caudate nucleus syndromes in some groups of minimal brain dysfunction. *J Am Med Women Assoc* 28:285–292, 1973.

45. Rosenthal RH, Allen TW: An examination of attention, arousal and learning dysfunctions of hyperkinetic children. *Psychol Bull* 85:689–715, 1978.

46. Stamm JS, Kreder SV: Minimal brain dysfunction: Psychological and neuropsychological disorders in hyperkinetic children, in Gazzaniga MS (ed), *Handbook of Behavioral Neurology: Neuropsychology*. New York: Plenum Press, 1979, vol 2, pp 119–150.

47. Zametkin AJ, Rapoport JL: The pathophysiology of attention deficit disorders, in Lahey BB, Kadzin AE (eds): *Advances in Clinical Child Psychology*. New York: Plenum Press, 1986. pp 177–216.

48. Fuster JM: *The Prefrontal Cortex: Anatomy, Physiology and Neuropsychology of the Frontal Lobe*, 2d ed. New York: Raven Press, 1989.

49. Levin HS, Eisenberg HM, Benton AL: *Frontal Lobe Function and Dysfunction*. New York: Oxford University Press, 1991.

50. Stuss DT, Benson DF: *The Frontal Lobes*. New York: Raven Press, 1986.

51. Harcherick DF, Cohen DJ, Ort S, et al: Computed tomographic brain scanning in four neuropsychiatric disorders of childhood. *Am J Psychiatry* 142:731–737, 1985.

52. Shaywitz SE, Shaywitz BA, Cohen DJ, et al: Monoaminergic mechanisms in hyperactivity, in Rutter M (ed): *Developmental Neuropsychiatry*. New York: Guilford Press, 1983.

53. Hynd GW, Semrud-Clikeman M, Lorys AR, et al: Brain morphology in developmental dyslexia and attention deficit disorder/hyperactivity. *Arch Neurol* 47:919–926, 1990.

54. Castellanos FX, Giedd JN, Marsh WL, et al: Quantitative brain magnetic resonance imaging in attention-deficit/hyperactivity disorder. *Arch Gen Psychiatry* 53:607–616, 1996.

55. Filipek PA, Semrud-Clikeman M, Steingard RJ, et al: Volumetric MRI analysis comparing attention deficit hyperactivity disorder with normal controls. *Neurology* 48:589–601, 1997.

56. Hynd GW, Hern KL, Novey ES, et al: Attention deficit hyperactivity disorder and asymmetry of the caudate nucleus. *J Child Neurol* 8:339–347, 1993.

57. Mataro M, Garcia-Sanchez C, Junque C, et al: Magnetic resonance imaging measurement of the caudate nucleus in adolescents with attention-deficit hyperactivity disorder and its relationship with neuropsychological and behavioral measures. *Arch Neurol* 54:963–968, 1997.

58. Aylward EH, Reiss AL, Reader MJ, et al: Basal ganglia volumes in children with attention-deficit hyperactivity disorder. *J Child Neurol* 11:112–115, 1996.

59. Singer HS, Reiss AL, Brown JE, et al: Volumetric MRI changes in basal ganglia of children with Tourette's syndrome. *Neurology* 43:950–956, 1993.

60. Casey BJ, Castellanos FX, Giedd JN, et al: Implication of right frontostriatal circuitry in response inhibition and attention deficit hyperactivity disorder. *J Am Acad Child Adolesc Psychiatry* 36:374–383, 1997.

61. Baumgardner TL, Singer HS, Denckla MB, et al: Corpus callosum morphology in children with Tourette syndrome and attention deficit hyperactivity disorder. *Neurology* 4:477–482, 1996.

62. Giedd JN, Castellanos FX, Casey BJ, et al: Quantitative morphology of the corpus callosum in attention deficit hyperactivity disorder. *Am J Psychiatry* 151:665–669, 1994.

63. Semrud-Clikeman M, Filipek PA, Biederman J, et al: Attention-deficit hyperactivity disorder: Magnetic resonance imaging morphometric analysis of the corpus callosum. *J Am Acad Child Adolesc Psychiatry* 33:875–881, 1994.

64. Ferguson HB, Rappaport JL: Nosological issues and biological validation, in Rutter M (ed): *Developmental*

64. *Neuropsychiatry.* New York: Guilford Press, 1993, pp 369–384.

65. Lou HC, Henriksen L, Bruhn P: Focal cerebral hypoperfusion in children with dysphasia and/or attention deficit disorder. *Arch Neurol* 41:825–829, 1984.

66. Lou HC, Henriksen L, Bruhn P: Striatal dysfunction in attention deficit and hyperkinetic disorder. *Arch Neurol* 46:48–52, 1989.

67. Zametkin AJ, Nordahl TE, Gross M, et al: Cerebral glucose metabolism in adults with hyperactivity of childhood onset. *N Engl J Med* 323:1361–1366, 1990.

68. Zametkin AJ, Liebenauer LL, Fitzgerald GA, et al: Brain metabolism in teenagers with attention-deficit hyperactivity disorder. *Arch Gen Psychiatry* 50:333–340 1993.

69. Amen DG, Paldi JH, Thisted RA: Brain SPECT imaging. *J Am Acad Child Adolesc Psychiatry* 32:1080–1081, 1993.

70. Teicher MH, Polcari A, English CD, et al: Dose-dependent effects of methylphenidate on activity, attention, and magnetic resonance imaging measures in children with ADHD (abstr). *Society Neurosci Abstr* 22:1191, 1996.

71. Shaywitz BA, Cohen DJ, Bowers MB: CSF monoamine metabolites in children with minimal brain dysfunction: Evidence for alteration of brain dopamine. *J Pediatr* 90:67–71, 1977.

72. Mattes JA, Gittelman R: A pilot trial of amantadine in hyperactive children. Paper presented at the NCDEU meeting, Key Biscayne, FL, 1979.

73. Oades RD: Attention deficit disorder with hyperactivity: The contribution of catecholaminergic activity. *Prog Neurobiol* 29:365–391, 1987.

74. Douglas VI: Cognitive deficits in children with attention deficit disorder with hyperactivity, in Bloomingdale LM, Sergeant J (eds): *Attention Deficit Disorder: Criteria, Cognition, Intervention.* Elmsford, NY: Pergamon Press, 1988.

75. Barkley RA: *Attention-Deficit Hyperactivity Disorder: A Handbook for Diagnosis and Treatment.* New York: Guilford Press, 1990.

76. Barkley RA: Behavioral inhibition, sustained attention, and executive functions: Constructing a unifying theory of ADHD. *Psychol Bull* 121:65–94, 1997.

77. Conners CK, Wells KC: *Hyperkinetic Children: A Neuropsychological Approach.* Beverly Hills, CA: Sage, 1986.

78. Douglas VI: Attention and cognitive problems, in Rutter M (ed): *Developmental Neuropsychiatry.* New York: Guilford Press, 1983, pp 280–329.

79. Schachar RJ, Tannock R, Logan G: Inhibitory control, impulsiveness, and attention deficit hyperactivity disorder. *Clin Psychol Rev* 13:721–739, 1993.

80. Pennington BF, Ozonoff S: Executive functions and developmental psychopathology. *J Child Psychol Psychiatry* 37:51–87, 1996.

81. Nigg JT: On inhibition/disinhibition in developmental psychopathology: Views from cognitive and personality psychology and a working inhibition taxonomy. *Psychol Bull* 126:1–27, 2000.

82. Logan GD, Cowan WB, Davis KA: On the ability to inhibit simple and choice reaction time responses: A model and a method. *J Exp Psychol Hum Percept Perform* 10:276–291, 1984.

83. Oosterlaan J, Sergeant JA: Response inhibition in ADHD, CD, comorbid ADHD + CD, anxious and normal children: A meta-analysis of studies with the stop task. *J Child Psych Psychiatry* 39:411–426, 1998.

84. Nigg JT: The ADHD response inhibition deficit as measured by the stop task: Replication with DSM-IV combined type, extension, and qualification. *J Abnor Child Psychol* 27:391–400, 1999.

85. Aman CJ, Roberts RJ, Pennington BF: A neuropsychological examination of the underlying deficit in attention deficit hyperactivity disorder: Frontal lobe versus right parietal lobe theories. *Dev Psychol* 34:956–969, 1998.

86. Van der Meere J: The role of attention, in Sandberg S (ed): *Hyperactivity Disorders of Childhood.* Cambridge, England: Cambridge University Press, 1996, pp 111–148.

87. Barkley RA, Grodzinsky G, DuPaul G: Frontal lobe functions in attention deficit disorder with and without hyperactivity: A review and research report. *J Abnorm Child Psychol* 20:163–188, 1992.

88. Halperin J, Wolfe L, Pascualvaca D, et al: Differential assessment of attention and impulsivity in children. *J Am Acad Child Adolesc Psychiatry* 27:326–329, 1988.

89. Losier B, McGrath P, Klein R: Error patterns on the continuous performance test in non-medicated and medicated samples of children with and without ADHD: A meta-analytic review. *J Child Psychol Psychiatry* 37:971–987, 1996.

90. Chhabildas N, Pennington BF, Willcutt EG: A comparison of the cognitive deficits in the DSM-IV subtypes of ADHD. *J Abnorm Child Psychol* 29:529–540, 2001.

91. Nigg JT, Hinshaw SP, Carte E, et al: Neuropsychological correlates of childhood attention deficit hyperactivity disorder: Explainable by comorbid disruptive behavior or reading problems? *J Abnorm Psychol* 107:468–480, 1998.

92. Sonuga-Barke EJS, Taylor E, Sembi S, et al: Hyperactivity and delay aversion: I. The effect of delay on choice. *J Child Psychol Psychiatry* 33:387–398, 1992.

93. Borger N, van der Meere JJ, Ronner, A, et al: Heart rate variability and sustained attention in ADHD. *J Abnorm Child Psychol* 27:25–33, 1999.

94. Douglas VI: Can Skinnerian theory explain attention deficit disorder? A reply to Barkley, in Bloomingdale LM, Sergeant JA (eds): *Attention Deficit Disorder: Current Concepts and Emerging Trends in Attentional and Behavioral* Disorders of Childhood. Elmsford, NY: Pergamon Press, 1989, pp 235–254.

95. Sanders AF: Towards a model of stress and performance. *Acta Psychol* 53:61–97, 1983.

96. Sergeant JA, van der Meere JJ: Convergence of approaches in localizing the hyperactivity deficit, in Lahey BB, Kazdin AE (eds): *Advancements in Clinical Child Psychology*. New York: Plenum Press, 1990; vol 13, pp 207–245.

97. Kuntsi J, Oosterlaan J, Stevenson J: Psychological mechanisms in hyperactivity: I. Response inhibition deficit, working memory impairment, delay aversion, or something else? *J Child Psychol Psychiatry* 42:199–210, 2001.

98. Kuntsi J, Stevenson J: Psychological mechanisms in hyperactivity: II. The role of genetic factors. *J Child Psychol Psychiatry* 42:211–219, 2001.

99. Pelham WE Jr, Wheeler T, Chronis A: Empirically supported psychosocial treatments for attention deficit hyperactivity disorder. *J Clin Child Psychol* 27:190–205, 1998.

100. MTA Cooperative Group: A 14- month randomized clinical trial of treatment strategies for attention-deficit/hyperactivity disorder. *Arch Gen Psychiatry* 56:1073–86, 1999.

Chapter 36

AUTISM AND RELATED CONDITIONS

Nancy J. Minshew
Jessica A. Meyer

INTRODUCTION

Classification

The diagnostic category of Pervasive Developmental Disorders (PDD) refers to autism and related disorders whose features share qualities referred to as autistic-like. These disorders are now commonly referred to as Autism Spectrum Disorders (ASD) because this term is more meaningful, but the term PDD is entrenched in legislation and educational policy and so is likely to remain in official use. These terms are used interchangeably and both were chosen to encompass the full range of intellectual functioning associated with these disorders, from severe and profound mental retardation to IQ scores in the superior range. Even "mild" forms have by definition a severe impact on adaptive function.

The PDDs are diagnosed clinically by abnormalities in social reciprocity, verbal and nonverbal language and its use for communication, imaginative play, and restricted and repetitive behavioral patterns and interests. The current diagnostic classification for PDD in the *Diagnostic and Statistical Manual for Mental Disorders*, 4th ed, Text Revision (DSM-IV-TR),[1] includes Autistic Disorder, Asperger's Disorder, Pervasive Developmental Disorder Not Otherwise Specified (PDDNOS), Childhood Disintegrative Disorder (CDD), and Rett's Disorder.

Rett's disorder presents with regression or global neurologic deterioration in the first or second year of life, which is the sole basis for its potential confusion with autism. It is otherwise a very different disorder, being characterized by decelerating head growth, microcephaly, loss of voluntary hand movements and walking if acquired, periodic breathing, and difficulty swallowing. It is also a disorder of females. Childhood disintegrative disorder is defined by regression or neurologic deterioration between 2 and 12 years of age, typically after sentence language has been established. Given the wide age span of these cases, CDD is likely to be related to diverse neurologic degenerative disorders, the most commonly now recognized of which is adrenoleukodystrophy. Because of these key differences from the other PDDs, clinical discussions of PDD usually refer to autistic disorder, Asperger's disorder, and PDDNOS only.

There are two diseases that produce the syndrome of autism above chance association—tuberous sclerosis and fragile-X syndrome; autistic symptoms are common among those with these diseases. A third condition, the Nonverbal Learning Disabilities Syndrome (NLD) or the Syndrome of the Developmental Learning Disabilities of the Right Hemisphere, is probably a subset of the PDDs rather than a separate syndrome, but it was originally described on the basis of a neuropsychological profile of right hemisphere deficits. Social dysfunction was described as part of this syndrome but was not well characterized.

A diverse and large group of diseases has been associated with cases of autism. Within each disease, autism is a rare occurrence. These cases account for less than 10 percent of autism, and the percentage is directly related to the stringency of the diagnostic criteria used.

Prevalence

The prevalence of autism is substantially higher than in the past. In 1980, the prevalence of the PDDs—e.g., autism and PDDNOS—was estimated at 20 per 10,000. Three studies in the last 2 years have estimated the prevalence of Autistic Disorder, Asperger's Disorder, and PDDNOS at 58, 63, and 67/10,000.[2–4] This corresponds to 1 per 150 to 1 per 170 births. Although it has been suggested that this increase is due to overdiagnosis, these studies were conducted by internationally acknowledged autism experts using state-of-the-art research diagnostic instruments. A second explanation proposed for this increase is that autism was previously underdiagnosed. The correction of the underdiagnosis of the past is not, however, sufficient to account for the tremendous increase in cases that is being seen internationally. The exact timing of the rise in prevalence is unknown but appears to be about a decade old. There is an overall ratio of 3 or 4 to 1 in terms of male:female predominance for the PDDs, but the male predominance is much higher at the higher-IQ end of the spectrum, approaching 15 to 1.

Genetics

Autism is now generally acknowledged to be a polygenetic disorder resulting from three or four interacting liability genes, with the particular genes differing between cases and thus complicating their identification.[5] It is estimated that as many as 20 autism liability genes exist. Heritability is estimated at 90 percent. The recurrence risk is about 6 percent, though both lower and higher numbers are proposed. Approximately 1 to 4 percent of cases have identifiable chromosome 15 abnormalities.[6,7] Genome-wide linkage studies of sibling pair families have provided support for involvement of chromosomes 7q, 2q, and 16p.[8]

CLINICAL SYNDROME

Clinical distinctions between the PDDs are largely defined in terms of deviations from autism. Most of the distinctions, other than the absence of developmental language delay in Asperger's disorder, are based on less severe symptoms than those expected for an individual of the same age and IQ with autism. Such clinical distinctions are not reliably attainable outside of a research setting and are not clinically important. The clinical emphasis should be on whether the person

has a PDD, because it is the quality of the symptoms that necessitates an entirely different approach to intervention from that used in any other disability. The diagnostic evaluation should focus on defining deficits and skill levels in social, language, communication, play, and reasoning, along with challenging behaviors. A practice parameter for the screening and diagnosis of children with autism and PDD has been published and provides excellent guidelines for practice.[9]

The clinical signs and symptoms of autism are the most severe in early childhood, but the course diverges dramatically thereafter, with a wide range of outcomes. Approximately one-half of autistic children make no developmental progress. The remainder makes small to large gains between 3 and 8 years of age. Thus, the manifestations of autism change substantially with age and the natural history is one of substantial improvement by school age in many children. With the increase in prevalence, a much higher percentage of children with PDD are now nonretarded at diagnosis, likely changing the natural history and developmental trajectories of autism and the PDDs in ways that are difficult to assess with the nearly universal intensive intervention.

Onset

In the majority of children, symptoms emerge in the form of developmental delays in the second year of life, though first-birthday videotapes have demonstrated impairments earlier. Early symptoms involve delayed language development, diminished or odd social contact, odd play with toys or preference for objects over people, and irritability related to change. Children with Asperger's disorder will not have the language abnormalities and in fact will often read early but will have the social oddities, the odd intense interests, and the unusual memory for facts. The social impairment in these high-functioning children may not be apparent until preschool, when they are first exposed to group social situations and it becomes apparent that they do not have group social etiquette and do not relate to other children. These children may be considered affectionate in terms of accepting or giving hugs,[9] and this should not preclude consideration of a diagnosis of PDD.

About 25 percent of children with PDD present with regression and loss of acquired language, social, and play skills, with the emergence of autistic behavior between 12 and 24 months. This usually takes place over a few months at most.

Social

The essential quality of the social deficit involves the lack of coordination or reciprocity. Social reciprocity requires the capacity to accurately judge and predict the reactions of others, to clearly grasp social situations and understand social cause and effect, and to subtly influence social interaction patterns. All of the components comprising social reciprocity are seriously impaired in autism. In its most severe form, it is expressed as a complete lack of comprehension of the social behavior of others and a profound incapacity for social responses. In moderate forms, the individual has a very rudimentary comprehension of common social situations and one- or two-step ways of interacting, such as repeating a few rote or canned phrases upon encountering and leaving people. In its least severe form, social exchanges are more extensive, involving conversation, but are actually no better coordinated. These children typically make off-topic comments, deliver monologues on their obsession, and make odd comments reflecting the disturbance in abstract reasoning. Their understanding of social situations is partial; as a result, they are extremely naïve, prone to being socially "exploited" and, at the same time, liable unwittingly to violate social conventions and infringe on the social rights of others. They are typically characterized as strange, odd, or weird. Persistent difficulties are present in peer relationships. They lack a best friend and do not establish close interpersonal connections based on a history of shared emotions and experiences. The level of social emotional function is often severely overestimated in these individuals and can range in adults from 18 months of age to 10 or 12 years. The developmental social-emotional level should be carefully assessed in every high-functioning individual with PDD.[10,11]

One of the key contributions to the understanding of the cognitive basis of the social deficit in autism was the discovery of the *theory of mind* deficit. This is the capacity for knowing that others have different thoughts from one's own and for automatically making inferences about what those thoughts are. This capacity is the basis for social reciprocity, empathy, understanding the motives and intentions of others, manipulation, and lying, none of which are within the repertoire of autistic individuals, although the most able individuals may develop some elementary capacity for empathy.

Verbal Language

The verbal language deficit in ASD is characterized by wide-ranging differences in the acquisition of spoken language and at times loss of language through regression, failure to compensate for verbal language deficits with nonverbal language, deviant language development, abnormalities in the use of all forms of language for social communication, and substantial residual deficits despite developmental progress. Parallel deficits are also present in language comprehension. Individuals with Asperger's disorder often have precocious language abilities, talking and reading early.

In its most severe form, neither expressive or receptive language abilities develop in autistic children, nor can they repeat. Unlike children with expressive and receptive language disorders, however, autistic children fail to compensate with alternate forms of communication, such as gesture, facial expression, eye contact, and body language. With some developmental progress, autistic children develop the capacity to repeat without the capacity to comprehend or speak using original language, resulting in echolalia, which can follow immediately after hearing the source or be delayed. With additional developmental progress, the child is able to associate the echolalia with an outcome and the echolalia is used to attain needs and thus is called functional. With further developmental progress, sufficient language comprehension is attained and correct grammar emerges. In the cases with the best outcome, grammatically correct complex sentence language is achieved between 5 and 6 years of age. Comprehension, though, remains below expressive language level, in that metaphoric and idiomatic language does not emerge automatically but must be taught. Use of language for communication is also abnormal in that at each level these individuals may have language but do not use it to ask for needs or to be social. Early on they do not know the basic elements of conversational etiquette or the mechanics of conversation, such as how to initiate, sustain, or appropriately terminate a conversation. It is also remarkable how even very long and sophisticated segments of talk can be scripted word for word.

Nonverbal Language

Impaired nonverbal communication is another defining characteristic of the ASDs. Abnormalities of prosodic language (see Chap. 21), both during development and at outcome, parallel those of left-hemisphere language. Speaking individuals with ASD may sound robotic, flat, and pedantic or "professor-like." Volume may be inappropriately loud or quiet.

Abnormalities in the quantity of eye contact are well known, but qualitative abnormalities have recently been emphasized, given the increase in high-functioning children who develop eye contact and the amount of training that is directed at achieving eye contact in ASD children. This impairment is seen earliest in the lack of eye contact to coordinate and share attention (joint attention, social referencing) with others, a skill evident around age 9 months among typically developing children. Later, qualitative abnormalities vary from eye gaze that is intrusive and persistent to atypical timing. A recent pilot study found that adults with ASD failed to use gaze to demonstrate a "listening response" while a social partner spoke with them. In either case, eye gaze is not used in a fluid, natural manner to demonstrate attentiveness to and social relatedness with others.

Expression and comprehension of facial affect are also abnormal. These individuals are often sober-faced. Alternatively, they have one expression, typically smiling, regardless of the situation. Facial expression has a parkinsonian character in that there is little or no affect or animation during social communication; if emotion originates internally though, the individual's face becomes animated. Comprehension of facial affect may be nonexistent throughout life, or comprehension of basic expressions, if dramatic, may develop. Interestingly, these deficits in comprehension are apparent in the way that individuals with ASD visually examine faces, focusing on details of faces and processing them as if they were objects.[12,13] In addi-

tion, they focus on the mouth region of the face rather than the eyes to ascertain emotion.[14] Using only photographs of the eyes, participants with high-functioning autism and Asperger's disorder, compared with normal adults, were impaired at recognizing complex mental states.[15]

Normally developing children use many gestures as part of coordinating focus and attention with others, including pointing and nods during conversation to indicate agreement or interest. Individuals with ASD often do not "check in" with a communicative partner to acknowledge understanding, as with the nod of the head or the shrug of the shoulders. Hand gestures during conversation may be nonexistent, clumsy, or awkward. In the first year of life, the absence of pointing to indicate needs and later interests are among the early signs of autism.

Imaginative Play

Interest in and appropriate use of toys for play is another area of delay and disturbance in ASD. In its most severe manifestation, there is no interest in toys, or the interest is in the taste, smell, or texture of the toys or in one piece of the toy. A slightly higher level of function involves lining up of the toys or hoarding or collecting them. With developmental progress, isolated appropriate actions emerge at first, and, later, sequences of actions, but play remains repetitive and does not have the imaginative quality seen in normal children. At a less impaired level of functioning, PDD children play with toys by emulating cartoons or videos verbatim.

The ability to pretend that one object is, in fact, a certain other object, known as meta-representation, is notably diminished among individuals with ASD. Beginning at around age $2\frac{1}{2}$ years, typically developing children begin to engage in pretend play. A block becomes a telephone, two sticks become an airplane, and a toy action figure can speak. Pretend play requires the ability to hold in mind two representations, what it is and, at the same time, what one is pretending it to be. Despite an interest in toys, moderately impaired children with autism show notable deficits in pretend play. Higher-functioning children with autism can be taught play sequences, but when asked to make up something new, they lack the ability to see things in any way other than the way they are from one's current perspective.

The typical developmental sequence of play with peers is also disturbed among children with ASD. Severely impaired children with ASD often do not interact with or even maintain proximity to peers during play. Parallel play can be observed among moderately to mildly impaired children with autism. At a mild degree of autistic impairment, greater degrees of cooperative interaction can be expected. The child with high-functioning autism will often help build the sand castle but then fail to reference his peers when he decides it is time to "knock it down." In other words, he attempts to interact and join in the cooperative play, but then lacks the ability to monitor his behavior and the reactions of others to keep the play truly cooperative. Another occurrence is for the child with Asperger's disorder to become a "social dictator." Hence, even at the highest level of functioning, children with Asperger's disorder tend to become stuck in the process of cooperative play, failing to achieve true cooperation.

Restricted Range of Interests and Activities

The final symptom category includes a number of diverse behaviors, but the common theme is a focus on details and a failure to understand the whole. These behavioral abnormalities include preoccupation with the sensory aspects of objects or the pieces of an object rather than the whole object, resistance to change or rituals for coping with change, and a narrow range of interests (collections or topics) with a focus on details. In all cases, there is a common focus on details and failure to appreciate the whole. Recent research suggests that the major cognitive determinants of this behavior are the abstraction deficit[16] and resulting dependence on piecemeal processing. One important study has demonstrated a dissociation between concept formation and concept identification abilities in nonretarded individuals with autism. Essentially, these individuals do not develop strategy or novel problem-solving abilities, nor do they form prototypes; consequently they are rule-bound and detail-oriented. These individuals rely on slow verbally mediated reasoning and classification; they lack the rapid automatic processing that includes concept-, prototype-, and strategy-formation abilities. For these individuals, rituals and sameness become a way of coping with change that is unpredictable because of the lack of concepts that normally provide the capacity to cope with variability in details while preserving an appreciation that the overall outcome remains the same. Less able individuals do not even develop rules or categories and are preoccupied with the elementary properties of objects. The most impaired individuals are oblivious to any meaning.

Associated Features

Some signs and symptoms are common in autism but are not considered diagnostic features of the disorder. These include hyperactivity with or without attention deficit disorder, alterations in sensory sensitivity (hyper- or hyposensitivity), delayed motor development, and apraxia.

Neurologic Examination

The neurologic examination is generally unremarkable except for subtle hypotonia and hyperreflexia. Head circumference is increased in autism. In pooled samples, the mean is shifted up to the 60 or 70th percentile, with the majority of autistic individuals having head circumferences above the 50th percentile and about 20 percent having macrocephaly (>97th percentile).[17-19] Macrocephaly is also present at increased rates among relatives.[20]

Complications in Individuals with PDD and in Family Members

Seizure disorder and affective disorder are two well-known complications of the PDDs. Both should be considered in the differential diagnosis of a sustained deterioration of function. The onset of seizure disorders is cumulative across the life span but has a peak in early childhood and a smaller peak at puberty. New onset of seizures can occur at any age, however. In the absence of tuberous sclerosis, seizures are usually secondarily generalized or partial complex in type, with the latter being especially difficult to detect because of the aberrant social behavior and attentional focus of individuals with autism. The tricyclic antidepressants and the traditional neuroleptics all lower the seizure threshold and can exacerbate or precipitate seizures in individuals with PDD. Even the newer neuroleptics are not without risk of precipitating seizures. The occurrence of depression has been thought to be more a complication of high-functioning individuals, reflecting the stress of being required to function in settings that exceed their social and emotional capability. Frequently high-functioning and especially nonretarded children and adolescents with PDD excel academically but have social and emotional capabilities that may be as low as those of a 2- or 3-year-old and rarely higher than those of a 7- to 10-year-old. Their inability to cope socially and emotionally leads to maladaptive behavior and depression, sometimes to the point of suicidal ideation and attempted suicide, while persistent efforts are made to continue them in this setting because of their academic success. Mania may also occur in autism but is far less common. Anxiety is a nearly universal accompaniment of PDD in individuals who are sufficiently aware of their environment to experience change or teasing by peers or to be cognizant of expectations and their inability to fulfill them. The relief of anxiety is thought to be the basis for the success of the selective serotonin reuptake inhibitors in improving function in individuals with PDD. Attention deficit disorder with or without hyperactivity may also co-occur with autism and may respond to traditional pharmacologic management.

Family members of individuals with PDD have an increased incidence of affective disorder, anxiety disorder, obsessive-compulsive disorder, and the broader autism phenotype or traits of autism. These conditions often go unrecognized and untreated, so that, although effective pharmacologic intervention is readily available, they interfere with the treatment of the child and the functioning of the family.

NEUROPSYCHOLOGY

This section is not intended to provide comprehensive coverage of the neuropsychology of autism but to highlight areas of most relevance or new findings. In the past, 75 percent of autistic individuals were mentally retarded with IQ scores below 70 and 25 percent were not mentally retarded. Recent prevalence studies have reported that as many as 40 to 50 percent are not mentally retarded, and a growing proportion of preschoolers have IQ scores in the normal range at the time of di-

agnosis. The introduction of the Asperger's Syndrome diagnosis in ICD-10 and DSM-IV has contributed to improved recognition of verbal school-age children and to a lesser extent adults with autism spectrum disorder.

Mental Retardation

Mental retardation in autism is part and parcel of autism and not the result of the chance co-occurrence of two rare disorders, which could not, in any case, explain the high frequency of this association. The mental retardation in autism is the more severe expression of the pattern of cognitive deficits and intact abilities seen in individuals with autism who are not mentally retarded. As a result, the mental retardation retains the peculiarities typical of cognition in autism, which distinguish it from mental retardation resulting from other conditions. In essence the distinguishing features are the marked dissociation between IQ scores and adaptive behavior scores, reflecting the disproportionate loss in social, language, and abstract reasoning skills with declining IQ, and the peculiarities of behavior. These higher-order skills are the basis of adaptive and flexible behavior in society and are not accurately assessed by IQ tests. IQ tests assess simpler abilities, and predictions about real-life function based on IQ scores depend on the degree to which simpler skills predict these higher-order abilities and thus on normal brain development. Behaviorally, mentally retarded individuals with autism can be distinguished from nonautistic mentally retarded individuals with comparable IQ scores by their much poorer social, verbal, and nonverbal language and reasoning abilities, the inability to use the skills they do have in these areas in a functional manner, and their greater facility with trivial details. In essence, mentally retarded autistic individuals are functionally much more retarded than their nonautistic mentally retarded peers. This distinction between autistic and nonautistic individuals with comparable IQ scores holds true across the IQ spectrum.

IQ Score Profiles

At Full Scale and Verbal IQ scores below 70, Verbal IQ is often significantly below Performance IQ. When Full Scale and Verbal IQ scores are above 80, this "prototypic" pattern is not present and most do not have a significant disparity; when present, it can be in either direction.[21] Essentially, the IQ test ceases to be a sensitive indicator of the language deficit in nonretarded individuals with autism. In terms of subtests, Comprehension is typically the lowest and Block Design the highest subtest scores. The Comprehension subtest assesses social, not language comprehension, and Block Design assesses visuospatial ability. In higher-ability individuals, the deviations are often not marked. The above "prototypes" are based on group analyses, but individual scores vary widely and none of these patterns can be used for diagnosis. In addition, many factors besides PDD can affect these scores.

Profile of Neuropsychological Functioning

The profile of neuropsychological functioning in autism has been examined to identify a shared feature of the deficits to determine why they might be occurring together as a syndrome. The most comprehensive of the few studies done to date involved 33 individually matched pairs of adults and community volunteers and found intact attention, sensory perception, elementary motor movements, memory for simple information, formal language (spelling, reading decoding, fluency), the rule-learning aspects of abstract reasoning, and visuospatial processing.[22] Deficits were present in motor praxis, memory for complex information (organizational strategies that support memory), the interpretative aspects of language, and concept formation. The implications of this profile were several, the most obvious of which was that information acquisition and visuospatial processing were intact. Deficits involved information processing abilities and, within those domains, the abilities that made the highest demands on complex information processing. The deficits respected domains, and thus complexity was determined within domain rather than across domains. This profile, therefore, suggested that autism was a disorder of information processing that disproportionately impacted complex information processing. In applying this construct across the autism spectrum, the severity of autism is equivalent to the overall information processing capacity, while the autistic quality of the symptoms is preserved by the disproportionate impact on complex information processing at all levels of severity. The

involvement of the motor domain, an area of relatively minor symptom involvement in today's society, suggests that the neuropathology involves a general architectural feature of the brain. This profile has now been replicated in a separate sample of adults and in a study of nonretarded children with autism. A similar neuropsychological profile has been observed in mildly mentally retarded autistic children.[23] Often, difficulties in function can be understood in terms of information processing demands, and reduction of these demands is effective in improving compliance and reducing behavior problems.

Part-Whole Processing

Another issue related to information processing that has been emphasized in autism is the performance advantage these individuals exhibit when piecemeal or local processing imparts an advantage. Thus, they are resistant to illusions and outperform controls on an embedded figures test.[24–26] However, for the same reason, they also have difficulty with face recognition and facial affect recognition, which require holistic processing. These issues are fascinating areas of research which involve the reciprocal cognitive and neural relationship between piecemeal or local processing and strategy or prototype formation. The failure of the latter cognitive abilities and neural substrate to develop leaves autistic individuals reliant on more elementary abilities and circuitry to perform tasks.[27]

Attention

Individuals with ASD may have attention deficit disorder, but it is not causative of their autistic symptoms. Purported deficits in shifting attention have been demonstrated to be deficits in executive function.[28,29]

Sensory Perception

Individuals with autism frequently complain of hypo- or hypersensitivity to sound, touch, and light, and nonverbal children have been reported to calm with sensory pressure or other input. These symptoms can be quite disabling, and yet there are no objective data regarding their neurologic basis. Evoked potential studies have demonstrated normal latencies and, in non-retarded individuals, normal perception of stimuli, so there is essentially no insight into the physiologic basis of this symptom. The only objective finding to date is that fingertip number writing is abnormal in a substantial percentage of nonretarded individuals with autism. These sensory perceptual distortions could be related to abnormal cortical integration or to abnormalities in thalamic gating.

Motor Function

A motor impairment is now widely accepted to be an integral part of the ASDs. The best-documented deficit involves motor praxis. Early in life, it may be apparent in the suboptimal formation of sign language. In higher-ability children, it is seen in their difficulty with scissors, crayons, tying shoes, handwriting, and motor coordination during walking and running. Gait is often visibly abnormal. A parkinsonian facies has also been described for decades, though its neurologic significance has been underappreciated.

Memory and Learning

Despite an early false analogy to amnesia, many studies have since demonstrated that basic memory processes are intact in autism. However, there is an inefficiency of memory and learning related to the failure to efficiently use organizational strategies to support memory. Thus, memory for simple material is intact but memory for larger amounts of material or material whose structure is inherently complex is deficient.[30] The particular test and material that will elicit deficits will depend on the general level of ability of the individual, as complexity or simplicity is relative to ability level. The implications of this deficit are that memory and learning can be improved by reducing the amount of material, preprocessing it, giving the bottom line, and increasing the processing time.

The impact of the memory deficit (which is actually a deficit in concept formation) on adaptive function has been demonstrated by Boucher[31] in a study of memory for a recently experienced event; she found that autistic children remembered less about a play activity than language-matched peers. Boucher proposed that autistic individuals would have difficulty with social situations because of the complexity of the infor-

mation and the demands this would place on memory. In a recent study, Williams and colleagues[32] examined the memory of autistic individuals for common social scenes and found they remembered less about common daily activities than matched controls. The ability of normal individuals to rapidly process and make sense of information enables them to cope with voluminous amounts of information. Having to deal with information without such organizing and processing capacities results in loss of information and considerable reduction in function.

Language

Enormous amounts have been written about the language impairment in autism.[33] Perhaps the most important clinical issue to emphasize is that these individuals are hyperlexic regardless of language level. Their comprehension is always below their expressive level. This means that what they mean by what they say is always different from what normal individuals mean if they say the same thing. It also means that they may do what the rule says they should *not* do while they are saying the rule. Thus, it is critical to constantly monitor what their function demonstrates their comprehension to be. In addition, they do not understand the idioms, metaphors, irony, and satire that adults learning English as a second language typically do not understand. Finally, their acquisition of information is reduced across all language modalities and nonverbal input deficits are often underestimated in terms of their contribution to communication.

TREATMENT

Though not well appreciated, the first line of intervention in autism should be management of the environment: the physical environment, the people, and the events. Because of their deficits, individuals with autism are unable or slow to process information and are easily overwhelmed by the environment. They function best when the environment is highly structured and supervised, which means that the world is simplified, interactions are limited and superficial, known rules govern actions, events and people are predictable, and they are protected from scapegoating. This type of environment has the equivalent therapeutic effect to neuroleptics in schizophrenia. No medication will accomplish in autism what this type of environment will.

Behavioral intervention should be approached with a full understanding of the autistic quality of these people's deficits and behaviors, as approaches used in other disabilities are not suitable for autism. Early childhood intervention programs are a current major focus in autism. A number of programs have reported improvement in outcome in children participating in preschool programs that involve 15 to 40 h of school-based intervention. These programs report substantial gains in IQ by school age, with 50 percent participating in mainstream education classes; this does not, however, mean that the children did not have significant deficits at outcome.[34] Also, the only true replication study to date has failed to demonstrate improvement in outcome with early intensive intervention.[35] Most such programs have had selection criteria that identify those children with evidence of communicative intent at entry to the program, the absence of dysmorphic features, and the absence of high rates of stereotypic behavior. Some programs also exclude children who fail to make progress after a few months. These selection criteria capitalize on early signs of less severe autism. It is not clear whether such programs would be equally effective in lower ability autistic children, nor is it clear how many hours of intervention are needed to achieve an optimal response. The National Research Council has published a comprehensive report entitled *Educating Children with Autism,*[36] which is essential reading for all involved in making or implementing treatment recommendations. Dawson's chapter reviews a number of programs reporting success in autism. Each of the programs has a different approach, but all focus on training five basic skills.[37] The first is the ability to attend to people and to cooperate with teaching exercises. The second is the ability to imitate others, both verbal imitation and motor imitation. The third is the ability to comprehend and use language. Most teaching strategies provide immediate positive reward to the child's smallest attempt to communicate, such as a glance or slightest body movement. The fourth domain is the ability to play appropriately with toys, and the fifth is the ability to interact socially with others.

All of these programs involve Applied Behavior Analysis (ABA), a method in common parlance and essential knowledge to all dealing with autistic children. The principles of ABA involve manipulating the environment to effectively reduce maladaptive behaviors, such as self-injury and aggression, as well as to teach functional skills including speech, academic skills, ability to sustain attention, fine and gross motor skills, language comprehension, and daily living skills. Reinforcement, extinction, chaining, and shaping are four basic techniques of ABA frequently used as part of intervention programs for individuals with autism. When tasks are broken down into their component parts and skills are taught through massed rote trials, individuals with ASD eventually develop some of the abilities that typically developing individuals gain through incidental learning.

Behavior modification has provided empirically demonstrated treatment gains to individuals with autism through functional analysis and treatment of self-injurious and self-stimulatory behavior, teaching appropriate skills, and building language.[34,36] A number of programs have reported substantial improvement in outcome in children participating in preschool programs that involve 15 to 40 h of school-based intervention.[37] Methods of ABA have been used to teach functional communication skills through the Picture Exchange Communication System (PECS)[38]; functional speech, daily living, and play skills through video modeling[39]; and language, imitation, and academic skills through discrete trial procedures.[34] Visual strategies, such as photographic activity schedules, are helpful to enhance independent functioning through the sequencing of tasks into component parts.[40] Further, treatments are beginning to be developed that focus primarily on the social deficits of persons with ASD. For example, the Relationship Development Intervention[10,11] provides an intervention approach to teach joint attention and experience sharing by breaking down the skills needed for successful interpersonal relatedness into component parts, which are then reinforced primarily through enjoyable social encounters.

NEUROPATHOLOGY

Relatively few neuropathologic studies, involving approximately 24 whole-brain specimens, have been performed in autism.[41-43] The initial study of 19 cases reported several major findings. The first was an increase in brain weight in children and average brain weight in adults. The second was a substantial increase in neuronal cell-packing density in the hippocampus, areas of the amygdala, entorhinal cortex, septum, mammillary body, and anterior cingulate gyrus. The increase in cell-packing density was the result of a 60 to 90 percent increase in neuronal number, a reduction in neuronal size, and decreased number and length of dendritic branches—signs of developmental immaturity. A third finding involved a 50 to 60 percent reduction in Purkinje cells in the posteroinferior regions of the cerebellar hemispheres. This was accompanied by abnormalities in the emboliform, globose, fastigial, and dentate nuclei; in children, the neurons were enlarged and numerous, whereas in adults, they were reduced in size and number. The olivary nuclei likewise displayed small pale neurons in adults and enlarged plentiful neurons in children. The preservation of the olivary neurons in the face of marked reduction in the Purkinje cells was indicative of an onset of these disturbances in circuitry prior to 28 to 30 weeks of gestation. A more recent study reported additional findings of megalencephaly in four of six adult brains and a variety of developmental abnormalities of the cerebral cortex.[41] Most recently, Casanova and colleagues[43] have reported bilateral increase in the minicolumns or vertical columnar units of cerebral cortex in autism. In order for the increased number of minicolumns to maintain local and distant cortical connections, it would require an increase in connections that would result in an increase in white matter.[43]

NEUROIMAGING

Structural Imaging

The most common clinical neuroimaging finding in autism is that of normal neuroanatomy when cases of autism secondary to other disorders such as tuberous sclerosis, fetal rubella, or fetal cytomegalovirus are excluded. Mild to moderate enlargement of the lateral ventricles is occasionally seen but is not related to hydrocephalus or to the severity of autism; thus its significance is unknown. Because gross anatomic abnormalities are not an integral part of this syndrome, routine scanning is not recommended in children with autism spectrum disorders in the absence of other neurologic indicators of a need for further investigation.[9]

Reports of imaging abnormalities in autism are based on research protocols and quantitative measurements rather than clinically apparent imaging abnormalities. These abnormalities are not diagnostic and are based on group differences, not individual differences. The most significant neuroradiologic abnormality to be reported in the past 5 years has been an increase in total supratentorial brain volume in children with autism, which has been a consistent finding of several studies.[44–46] The increase in total brain volume appears to be present by 3 years of age, the youngest age for which imaging data are available, and appears to normalize at puberty as a result of brain growth in the normal population and a slight reduction in brain size in the autistic population.[44–46] Both gray and white matter volumes are increased. In the posterior fossa, the cerebellar hemispheres are also increased in volume.[44,45] The significance of this increase in white matter volume appears to be related to the abnormality in cerebral cortical minicolumns and the accompanying developmental abnormalities in neural connectivity. The early overgrowth concludes with the onset of symptoms in the second year of life, disrupting the development of the intricate circuitry that underlies the emergence of social language, and reasoning abilities.

Several studies have reported a reduction in the area of the corpus callosum, though the region involved has varied from anterior to posterior.[47–49] Such abnormalities suggest fewer myelinated fibers and reduced interhemispheric connectivity.

Functional Magnetic Resonance Imaging

Because of the invasiveness of methods used before the development of magnetic resonance imaging (MRI), there are limited functional imaging data with such methods. Two early studies are of interest because they presage fMRI findings that will appear in the literature in the next 2 to 3 years. A positron emission tomography study with 2,3 DPG[50] reported a reduction in the intra- and interhemispheric connectivity of frontal and parietal cortices with both cortical and subcortical regions. A second study[51] reported delayed maturation of the frontal lobes in 3- to 5-year-old autistic children using single photon emission computed tomography (SPECT) to study blood flow.

Only a few fMRI studies have been published so far, but many such studies are in progress and in various stages of the publication process. Functional MRI studies of individuals with high-functioning autism and Asperger's disorder demonstrated that they did not activate the amygdala when trying to discern emotional expression from eyes and faces.[52,53] Studies using theory-of-mind tasks have in one case shown failure to activate the left medial prefrontal gyrus[54] and in another the amygdala.[52]

Studies of face recognition have reported that autistic subjects did not activate fusiform gyrus but instead activated inferior temporal gyrus, a region that normal subjects activate when viewing objects.[13] Within the field of visual cognition, there is active debate as to whether the fusiform area is specialized for faces or is an area of expertise used for all difficult distinctions. Studies have shown that architects activate the fusiform or "face area" when making refined distinctions in their areas of expertise. In autism, the significant implication is that clinically they have difficulty processing complex information, in this case faces, and their neural circuitry lacks the specialization to process this information.

Two PET studies of serotonin receptors have been completed, but sample sizes have been small and results therefore preliminary. The most significant reported that the autistic children had a gradual increase in serotonin levels between 2 and 15 years of age, in contrast to the high levels of synthesis until 5 years of age in normal children, which decline thereafter.[55]

PATHOPHYSIOLOGY

Ideas about the pathophysiology of autism have continued to evolve with research findings. Up until a few years ago, autism was thought to be the result of a single primary cognitive deficit and an anatomic abnormality in a single brain structure. Autism is now generally thought to be a disorder of multiple primary deficits resulting from underdevelopment of selected neural systems.

The major cognitive deficits proposed in recent years to underlie autism involve executive function, shifting attention, theory of mind, central coherence, and complex information processing. The executive dysfunction model subsequently ceased to be a viable hypothesis because of the emergence of studies demonstrating this deficit was not universally present in autism.[56] The deficit in shifting attention also proposed to underlie much of the symptomatology in autism has been shown by several studies to be a deficit in executive function, not in attention.[28,58] The theory of mind deficit, though a major contribution to the neurobehavior of autism, was not sufficient to accommodate the nonsocial deficits in autism such as abstraction, nonverbal language, and motor abilities. The central coherence theory or lack of drive to make sense of the environment was derived from the same constellation of deficits in higher-order abilities that gave rise to the complex information processing theory, and the terms are essentially synonymous. However, the term *central coherence* is unknown outside the field of autism and substitutes a new term for traditional terms used to describe well-known neuropsychological deficits. The disadvantage of central coherence theory is that it does not readily accommodate deficits in motor skills or nonverbal language or expressive language. *Complex information processing* is a general term that is used in most disciplines and is broad enough to accommodate both cognitive and noncognitive deficits as well as expressive and receptive deficits. It also makes it relatively easy to relate these deficits to neurophysiologic abnormalities in autism and to classes of neural circuitry that might be relevant.

Autism is now generally viewed as a neural systems disorder rather than a disorder of one or more brain regions. These systems involve neocortex, limbic structures, and cerebellum, but the relative contributions of these structures to the function of the affected neural systems is debated.[41,42,57,58] Other brain structures are also likely to be involved. Abnormalities in face recognition suggest that specialization of regional circuitry may also be affected, in addition to distributed neural networks. The next decade promises to bring exciting revelations about the neurobiology of autism and this entire category of disorders.

REFERENCES

1. American Psychiatric Association: *Diagnostic and Statistic Manual of Mental Disorders,* 4th ed, Text Revision (DSM-IV-TR). Washington, DC: American Psychiatric Association, 2000.
2. Baird G, Charman T, Baron-Cohen S, et al: A screening instrument for autism at 18 months of age: a 6-year follow-up study. *J Am Acad Child Adolesc Psychiatry* 39(6):694–702, 2000.
3. Bertrand J, Mars A, Boyle C, et al: Prevalence of autism in a United States Population: The Brick Township, New Jersey Investigation. *Pediatrics* 108(5):1155–1161, 2001.
4. Chakrabarti S, Fombonne E: Pervasive developmental disorders in preschool children. *JAMA* 285:3093–3099, 2001.
5. Perisco AM, Agruma LD, Maiorano N, et al: Reelin gene alleles and haplotypes as a factor predisposing to autistic disorder. *Mol Psychiatry* 6:150–159, 2001.
6. Cook EH Jr, Courchesne RY, Cox NJ, et al: Linkage-disequilibrium mapping of autistic disorder with 15q11-13 markers. *Am J Hum Genet* 62:1077–1083, 1998.
7. Gillberg C: Chromosomal disorders and autism. *J Autism Dev Disord* 28:415–425, 1998.
8. International Molecular Genetic Study of Autism Consortium (IMGSAC): A genomewide screen for autism: Strong evidence for linkage to chromosomes 2q, 7q, and 16p. *Am J Hum Genet* 69:570–581, 2001.
9. Filipek PA, Accardo PJ, Baranek GT: The screening and diagnosis of autistic spectrum disorders. *J Autism Dev Disord* 29(6):439–484, 1999.
10. Mundy P, Sigman M: Specifying the nature of the social impairment in autism, in Dawson G (ed): *Autism: Nature, Diagnosis, and Treatment.* New York: Guilford Press, 1989.
11. Gutstein SE: *Autism and Asperger's: Solving the Relationship Puzzle.* Arlington, TX: Future Horizons, 2000.
12. Hobson RP, Ouston, J, Lee A: What's in a face? The case of autism. *Br J Psychol* 79:441–453, 1988.
13. Schultz RT, Gauthier I, Klin A, et al: Abnormal ventral temporal cortical activity among individuals with autism and Asperger syndrome during face discrimination. *Arch Gen Psychiatry* 57:331–340, 2000.
14. Klin A, Jones W, Schultz R, et al: Defining and quantifying the social phenotype in autism. *Am J Psychiatry* 159(6):895–908.
15. Baron-Cohen S, Wheelwright S, Jolliffe T: Is there a "language of the eyes"? Evidence from normal adults, adults with autism or Asperger syndrome. *Vis Cogn* 4(3):311–331, 1997.
16. Minshew NJ, Meyer J, Goldstein G: Abstract reasoning in autism: a dissociation between concept formation and concept identification. *Neuropsychology* 16(3):327–334.
17. Fombonne E, Roge B, Claverie J, et al: Microcephaly and macrocephaly in autism. *J Autism Dev Disord* 29(2):113–119, 1999.
18. Lainhart JE, Piven J, Wrozek M, et al: Macrocephaly in children and adults with autism. *J Am Acad Child Adolesc Psychiatry* 36:282–290, 1997.
19. Fidler DJ, Bailey JN, Smalley SL: Macrocephaly in autism and other pervasive developmental disorders. *Dev Med Child Neurol* 42(11):737–740, 2000.
20. Miles JH, Hadden LL, Takahashi TN, et al: Head circumference is an independent clinical finding associated with autism. *Am J Med Genet* 95(4):339–350, 2000.
21. Siegel DJ, Minshew NJ, Goldstein G: Wechsler IQ profiles in diagnosis of high functioning autism. *J Autism Dev Disord* 26(4):389–406, 1996.
22. Minshew NJ, Goldstein G, Siegel DJ: Neuropsychological functioning in autism: Profile of a complex information processing disorder. *J Int Neuropsychol Soc* 3:303–316, 1997.
23. Fein D, Dunn M, Allen DA, et al: Language and neuropsychological findings, in Rapin I (ed): *Preschool Children with Inadequate Communication: Developmental Language Disorder, Autism, Low IQ: Clinics in Development Medicine.* Cambridge, UK: Cambridge University Press, 1996, vol 139, pp 123–154.
24. Happe FG: Studying weak central coherence at low levels: children with autism do not succumb to visual illusions. A research note. *J Child Psychol Psychiatry Allied Disc* 37(7):873–877, 1996.
25. Jolliffe T, Baron-Cohen S: Are people with autism and Asperger syndrome faster than normal on the Embedded Figures Test? *J Child Psychol Psychiatry Allied Disc* 38(5):527–534, 1997.
26. Shah A, Frith U: Why do autistic individuals show superior performance on the block design task? *J Child Psychol Psychiatry* 34:1351–1363, 1993.
27. Luna B, Minshew NJ, Garver KE, et al: Neocortical system abnormalities in autism: an fMRI study of spatial working memory. *Neurology* 59(6):834–840.
28. Goldstein G, Johnson CR, Minshew NJ: Attentional processes in autism. *J Autism Dev Disord* 31(4):433–440.
29. Pascualvaca DM, Fantie BO, Papageorgiou, et al: Attentional capacities in children with autism: Is there a

general deficit in shifting focus? *J Autism Dev Disord* 28:467–478.

30. Minshew NJ, Goldstein G: The pattern of intact and impaired memory functions in autism. *J Child Psychiatry* 42(8):1095–1101, 2001.

31. Boucher J: Memory for recent events in autistic children. *J Autism Dev Disord* 11(3):293–301, 1981.

32. Williams DL, Minshew NJ, Goldstein G: Impaired memory for faces and social scenes in autism: clinical implications of the memory disorder. *Arch Clin Neuropsychol.* In press.

33. Tager-Flusberg H: Understand the language and communicative impairments in autism. *Int Rev Res Ment Retard* 23:185–205, 2001.

34. Lovaas OI, Schreibman L, Koegel RL: A behavior modification approach to the treatment of autistic children. *J Autism Child Schizophr* 4(2):111–129, 1974.

35. Smith T, Eikeseth S, Klevstrand M, et al: Intensive behavioral treatment for preschoolers with severe mental retardation and pervasive developmental disorder. *Am J Ment Retard* 102(3):238–249, 1997.

36. Committee on Education Interventions for Children with Autism, Division of Behavioral and Social Sciences and Education, and National Research Council: *Educating Children with Autism.* Washington, DC: National Academy Press, 2001.

37. Dawson G, Osterling J: Early intervention in autism, in Guralnick MJ (ed): *The Effectiveness of Early Intervention.* Baltimore, MD: Brookes, 1997, pp 307–325.

38. Bondy AS, Frost LA: The picture exchange communication system. *Semin Speech Lang* 19(4):373–388, 1998.

39. Charlop-Christy MH, Le L, Freeman KA: A comparison of video modeling with in vivo modeling for teaching children with autism. *J Autism Dev Disord* 30(6):537–552, 2000.

40. MacDuff GS, Krantz PJ, McClannahan LE: Teaching children with autism to use photographic activity schedules: maintenance and generalization of complex response chains. *J Appl Behav Anal* 26(1):89–97, 1993.

41. Bailey A, Luthert P, Dean A, et al: A clinicopathological study of autism. *Brain* 121(Pt 5):889–905, 1998.

42. Bauman ML, Kemper TL: Is autism a progressive process? *Neurology* 48:A285, 1997.

43. Casanova MF, Buxhoereden DP, Switala AE, et al: Minicolumnor pathology in autism. *Neurology* 58:428–432, 2002.

44. Courchesne E, Karns CM, Davis HR, et al: Unusual brain growth patterns in early life in patients with autistic disorder: an MRI study. *Neurology* 57(2):245–254, 2001.

45. Sparks BF, Friedman SD, Shaw DW, et al: Brain structural abnormalities in young children with autism spectrum disorder. *Neurology* 59(2):184–192.

46. Aylward EH, Minshew NJ, Field K, et al: Effects of age on brain volume and head circumference in autism. *Neurology* 59(2):175–183.

47. Egaas B, Courchesne E, Saitoh O: Reduced size of corpus callosum in autism. *Arch Neurol* 52(8):794–801, 1995.

48. Hardan AY, Minshew NJ, Keshavan MS: Corpus callosum size in autism. *Neurology* 55(7):1033–1036, 2000.

49. Piven J, Bailey J, Ranson BJ, et al: An MRI study of the corpus callosum in autism. *Am J Psychiatry* 154(8):1051–1056, 1997.

50. Horwitz B, Rapoport SI: Partial correlation coefficients approximate the real intrasubject correlation pattern in the analysis of interregional relations of cerebral metabolic activity. *J Nucl Med* 29:392–399, 1988.

51. Zilbovicius M, Garreau B, Samson Y, et al: Delayed maturation of the frontal cortex in childhood autism. *Am J Psychiatry* 152(2):248–252, 1995.

52. Baron-Cohen S, Ring HA, Wheelwright S, et al: Social intelligence in the normal and autistic brain: an fMRI study. *Eur J Neurosci* 11:1891–1898, 1999.

53. Critchley HD, Daly EM, Bullmore ET, et al: The functional neuroanatomy of social behavior: changes in cerebral blood flow when people with autistic disorder process facial expressions. *Brain* 123:2203–2212, 2000.

54. Happé F, Ehlers S, Fletcher P, et al: "Theory of mind" in the brain. Evidence from a PET scan study of Asperger syndrome. *Neuroreport* 8:197–201, 1996.

55. Chugani DC, Muzik O, Behen M, et al: Developmental changes in brain serotonin synthesis capacity in autistic and non-autistic children. *Ann Neurol* 45(3):287–295, 1999.

56. Minshew NJ, Goldstein G, Muenz LR, et al: Neuropsychological functioning in nonmentally retarded autistic individuals. *J Clin Exp Neuropsych* 14:749–761.

57. Carper RA, Courchesne E: Inverse correlation between frontal lobe and cerebellum sizes in children with autism. *Brain* 123(Pt 4):836–844, 2000.

58. Minshew NJ, Luna B, Sweeney JA: Oculomotor evidence for neocortical systems but not cerebellar dysfunction in autism. *Neurology* 52(5):917–922, 1999.

Chapter 37

DEVELOPMENTAL READING DISORDERS*

Maureen W. Lovett
Roderick W. Barron

HISTORICAL BACKGROUND

For more than a century, it has been recognized that a sizable minority of otherwise intelligent, healthy children unexpectedly fail to learn to read. In 1895, Hinshelwood[1,2] described these specific reading acquisition failures as *visual word blindness* and Morgan[3] suggested a parallel between cases of acquired (alexia) and developmental reading disorders (dyslexia). The most influential early student of reading disability was Samuel Orton,[4,5] who described a condition he labeled *strephosymbolia,* proposing that it was caused by developmental delay in specialization of the left hemisphere for language. Orton's work formed the basis for a number of early educational therapies for the disorders,[6,7] some of which continue to be popular.[8]

In 1968, the World Federation of Neurology defined specific developmental dyslexia by exclusionary criteria as "a disorder manifested by difficulty in learning to read despite conventional instruction, adequate intelligence, and sociocultural opportunity." The disorder was attributed to "fundamental cognitive disabilities which are frequently of constitutional origin."[9] In 1979, Denckla offered a more specific definition that connected developmental dyslexia to speech and language disorders; she described it as the "index symptom of a developmental language disorder too subtle to lead to referral of the child in preschool life",[10] a view reiterated by other investigators since that time.[11-15]

Exclusionary definitions of dyslexia fostered diagnostic approaches based on a discrepancy between reading achievement and intellectual potential as measured by standardized psychometric tests. The working assumption was that higher-IQ disabled readers have a more specific form of dyslexia characterized by a uniquely deviant pattern of development in reading-related cognitive processes, while lower-IQ disabled readers were handicapped by developmental lags in many reading-related and reading-unrelated cognitive processes.[16] Some authors considered the IQ-discrepant group more purely dyslexic, with different etiology, than the IQ-consistent group of *"garden-variety"* poor readers.[17] Discrepancy-based definitions have dominated clinical practice and research for decades and have been legislated into eligibility requirements for special education services in many parts of the United States and Canada.[18,19]

CURRENT DEFINITIONS

Recent research, however, has demonstrated that disabled readers with and without discrepancies between aptitude (IQ) and reading achievement have similar profiles on the phonologically based information processing subskills that underlie word identification[20,21];

* **ACKNOWLEDGMENTS:** Preparation of this chapter was supported by a National Institute of Child Health and Human Development Grant (HD30970–01A1) to Georgia State University, Tufts University, and The Hospital For Sick Children/University of Toronto. The remediation research reported here was supported, in addition, by operating grants to the authors from the Ontario Mental Health Foundation, the Velleman Foundation, and the Social Sciences and Humanities Research Council of Canada. We gratefully acknowledge the conceptual contributions of our collaborators and colleagues over the years, particularly those of Robin Morris and Maryanne Wolf. We also gratefully acknowledge the intellectual contributions of senior members of the Learning Disabilities Research Program at The Hospital for Sick Children— Nancy J. Benson, Karen A. Steinbach, Maria De Palma, Jan C. Frijters, Léa Lacerenza, and the whole LDRP staff who have contributed so much to past and current intervention studies.

there is no support for greater specificity of cognitive deficits in relation to IQ-based discrepancies.[22,23] The current view is that reading disability is dimensional, like hypertension or obesity, and on the lower end of a normal distribution that includes both reading-disabled individuals and those with normal reading ability. An assessment of intellectual potential, while useful in practice, is not essential to the definition of developmental reading disorders; instead, the defining features of these disorders are found in the domain of language, particularly in impairments associated with phonological processing.[24]

The prevalence of developmental reading disorders is dictated by how they are defined. Some 4 to 10 percent of school-aged children in the United States are regarded as reading-disabled when an IQ-achievement discrepancy definition is used and 17 to 20 percent when the definition involves just low achievement.[25,26] These differences in prevalence have implications for educational practice, funding, and access to special education services. Research is required to determine reliable cutoffs for access to treatment that involve precise measurement of achievement in reading and reading-related skills.[23] Developmental reading disability is a chronic disorder that persists into adulthood,[27] and girls are as likely as boys to be identified when classroom-wide objective screening measures rather than teacher referrals are employed.[25]

The prevalence of developmental reading disorders varies across countries, with 1 percent reported in China and Japan to over 30 percent in Venezuela.[28] Although cultural values, educational practices, and opportunities for literacy experiences influence these differences, there is also evidence that the relationship between orthography and phonology in a language plays a significant role. In alphabetic languages such as Italian, Spanish, and German, the mapping between spelling and sound is relatively consistent and orthography tends to represent phonology almost directly. These phonologically shallow orthographies contrast with phonologically deep orthographies such as English, Danish, and French, where the consistency is much lower because the mapping between sequences of letters and phonemes is complex and permissible sequences are constrained by etymology and morphology as well as phonology.[29] As a result, the reported prevalence of developmental reading disorders in countries with shallow orthographies tends to be lower than that of countries with deep orthographies. Nevertheless, there is increasing agreement that deficiencies in phonological processes constitute the underlying basis of the disorders across different orthographies.[30]

WORD RECOGNITION AND PHONOLOGICAL PROCESSES

The most reliable indicator of developmental reading disorders is difficulty in acquiring rapid, context-free word-reading skill.[24,31–33] Many of the inconsistent results in this area of research can be traced to studies in which reading-disabled individuals were defined by criteria other than their ability to read aloud individual words that have been isolated from the context of a phrase or sentence.[12] Decoding nonwords, such as *nersh,* is a very sensitive measure for identifying problems in word reading.[34] Although disabled readers experience problems with comprehension when reading connected text, the correlation between nonword decoding and comprehension is high ($r = 0.79$), indicating that a substantial portion of the variability in comprehension performance can be attributed to print-to-sound decoding skill.[35]

Developmental reading disorders are accompanied by associated deficits in speech and language processing. Evidence accumulated over the past three decades indicates that deficient phonological awareness is a core linguistic deficit characterizing developmental reading disorders[12,20,21,24,36–38]; this deficit persists into adulthood even among individuals with childhood diagnoses of dyslexia who have attained reasonable standards of literacy as adults.[39]

The phonemes making up a syllable are coarticulated, resulting in a representation with considerable overlap in the acoustic and articulatory information for individual phonemes. Phonemes are not physically discrete units; they are embedded in syllables. Children have difficulty accessing phonemes as separate mental objects that can be associated with letters in the course of learning grapheme-phoneme correspondences.[40] The word *steep,* for example, consists of four phonemes: /s/,/t/,/i/,/p/.

Phonological awareness is demonstrated in oral language tasks in which the individual phonemes are matched, deleted, categorized, counted, *blended,* and reordered. Phonological awareness task performance is a unique and independent predictor of word reading in grades 1 through 5 even when the influence of the autocorrelated variable of word reading skill in previous grades is controlled statistically.[41] Phonological awareness tasks are memory-demanding, and verbal working memory is related to reading skill[42]; however, phonological awareness accounts for variability in reading skill when verbal working memory is controlled statistically. Results from longitudinal studies indicate that verbal working memory is not a unique predictor of reading skill in comparison to phonological awareness.[41]

Speed in naming sequences of familiar letters, numbers, objects, and colors is also a strong predictor of word reading skill.[43–45] Performance on these rapid serial naming tasks (also referred to as *rapid automatized naming tasks,* or RAN[46]) is a unique predictor of word reading skill, particularly early in the course of reading acquisition.[41] Naming speed is more strongly associated with measures of comprehension, fluency, and orthographic processing than phonological awareness performance.[47,48]

Phonological awareness and rapid serial naming, along with verbal working memory and oral vocabulary, have been conceptualized as a core set of processing skills which involve accessing, maintaining, and using precise phonological representations of verbal information.[21,24,38,49,50] Word reading and nonword decoding utilize core phonological processing skills extensively.[51] Deficiencies in these skills are the primary neurocognitive signature for the phenotype of developmental reading disorders[12,20,21,52] in studies of underlying brain and genetic bases of reading skill.[29,30,53–56] These deficiencies also are the focus of efforts to improve reading skill through early intervention and remediation.[57–68]

SUBTYPES

Developmental reading disorders have long been regarded as heterogeneous and subtypes have been reported to exist within the phenotype; hence the use of the term *disorders* rather than *disorder.*[69] In an influential study involving over 200 children, Morris and

colleagues[70] assessed core phonological processing measures (phonemic awareness, verbal working memory, serial naming tasks) as well as language (vocabulary and speech production tasks) and nonverbal skill measures identified as being associated with reading disorders (visuospatial, visual attention, and nonverbal memory tasks). Nine subtypes were identified: two subgroups were not disabled and two conformed to the profile of lower-IQ garden-variety poor readers.[16] Four of the remaining subtypes were deficient in phonological awareness, with different patterns of strength and weakness in verbal working memory and rapid serial naming as well as language and nonverbal processing. The ninth subtype was characterized by weakness in verbal and nonverbal rate of processing measures and relative strength on language measures. Consistent with a model of deficits in core phonological processes,[16,21] the most central finding was that of a pervasive deficit in phonological awareness across the four specific reading disability subtypes and the two garden-variety subtypes.

Two of the specific reading-disabled subtypes had deficiencies in phonemic awareness and rapid serial naming, whereas the other two were characterized by just one deficiency: phonemic awareness or rapid serial naming. This profile of results is consistent with Wolf and Bowers' double deficit hypothesis, in which it is proposed that children can be deficient in rapid serial naming or phonological awareness or they can also have a more serious double deficit that involves impairments in both.[44,45,71,72]

The dual-route model of word recognition as well as research on acquired dyslexia, both discussed in Chap. 20, provide the framework for another theoretically motivated subtyping scheme. Children were identified who fit the pattern of surface dyslexics because they were more impaired in exception (e.g., *have*) than nonword reading (e.g., *nersh*). *Have* is an exception word because it is pronounced differently from most _ave words. Other children fit the pattern of phonological dyslexics because they were more impaired in nonword than exception word reading.[73] Subsequent research, however, indicated that children in the surface dyslexia subtype could not be distinguished from younger normal readers who had less reading experience and therefore less opportunity to acquire the unique orthographic patterns characterizing exception words.[74,75] Consistent with evidence that nonword decoding is a primary impairment associated with developmental reading disorder,[12,34] the phonological dyslexics emerged as a robust subtype—a finding that is consistent with a deficit rather than a developmental delay pattern over time.[76]

Children classified as phonological dyslexics have a pattern of impairment in core phonological processing skills similar to that reported by Morris and colleagues for most of their subtypes.[70,74,75] The S-shaped function characteristic of categorical speech perception was markedly deviant for some of these children, even though their phonological awareness performance was very similar to other phonological dyslexics with normal categorical speech functions.[77] Furthermore, children who were impaired in both phonological awareness and speech perception were also impaired in morphological processing, a measure of language processing,[78] indicating that some children with developmental reading disorders may have comorbid language disorders that may warrant different approaches to treatment.[79]

VISUAL AND AUDITORY TEMPORAL PROCESSES

Developmental reading disorders involve deficits in phonological processing—a fundamental component of the language system. These phonological deficits cannot be further decomposed and understood as more basic deficits in sensory processing.[13,14,80] Despite this well-established theoretical perspective, there remains continuing interest in the visual and auditory foundations of developmental reading disorders.[81,82] Word recognition is initially visual, and basic neural mechanisms of vision are engaged during the act of reading[83,84] as well as eye movement control systems.[85] Visually based deficits tend to persist in the clinical profiles of disabled readers[86] and are associated with their word-reading performance.[87]

Compared to normal readers, dyslexic readers have been reported to have impaired contrast sensitivity in discriminating low-spatial-frequency grating patterns and in detecting flicker at high temporal frequencies; they are also characterized as having longer visible persistence for low-spatial-frequency

patterns.[88–90] Dyslexic children performed worse than normal reading controls on motion-detection tasks, with motion-detection measures related to word and nonword reading performance.[87,91–94] Dyslexic adults had lower levels of activation on functional magnetic resonance imaging (fMRI) in the extrastriate visual area V5/MT on motion-detection tasks than normal reading controls, but the two groups did not differ in activation in areas V1/V2 when processing stationary patterns.[95]

The distinction between the magnocellular and parvocellular pathways in vision has been used to interpret these findings.[81,82,96] Magno cells have relatively large cell bodies as well as dendrites that are dense and heavily myelinated; they are associated with fast conduction times and short response latencies. Magno cells ultimately project to the posterior parietal cortex and provide information about movement and coarse-grained information about form. Parvo cells are smaller, more numerous, and densely packed, with slower conduction times and longer latencies. Parvo cells ultimately project to the inferotemporal cortex and provide information about color and fine-grained information about form. Unlike magno cells, parvo cells give optimal responses to high luminance, spatial frequency, and contrast stimuli as well as to stimuli that are stationary (low-temporal-frequency) and chromatic.

The magnocellular system is involved in reading through eye-movement control; it inhibits the parvocellular system during a saccade and prevents visible persistence from the previous fixation from degrading a new fixation. The inhibitory capabilities of the magnocellular system are hypothesized to be deficient for dyslexic readers, resulting in less efficient reading. Evidence consistent with this hypothesis is mixed,[81,82,97–100] however, and it does not address the fact that reading words in isolation rather than in connected text is the primary area of difficulty for dyslexic readers.[101]

Two preliminary hypotheses have been proposed about how a deficient magnocellular system might influence individual word recognition. One is that the magnocellular system is involved in attentional allocation and it does not effectively inhibit the parvocellular system during the letter-to-letter shifts in attention that are involved in serial nonword decoding.[94] The other is that the magnocellular system prevents effective compensation for retinal slips (unintended eye movements) when fixating small targets such as letters in a word.[102,103] The retinal slip problem is increased with binocular perception. Stein and colleagues have reported that occluding the left eye tends to stabilize the binocular control of dyslexic children and increase their word-reading performance compared to a control (no occlusion) or those who were unable to achieve binocular stability.[104] These findings should be interpreted with considerable caution, however, because visual rather than reading problems may have been the primary basis for inclusion in this study, and direct comparisons were not made with phonologically based procedures for improving reading skill.

Specific language-impaired (SLI) children are reported to have an auditory temporal processing deficit for stimuli that is brief in duration, has a brief interstimulus interval, or is changing rapidly.[105] Tallal and Merzenich have shown that intensive training can improve the linguistic and nonlinguistic temporal processing deficits of these children,[106] and that their speech discrimination and language comprehension skills can be improved when the intensity and duration of critical speech cues (e.g., consonant format transitions) is increased online using computer speech algorithms.[107]

This interpretation of specific language impairment continues to be controversial, with evidence that is both consistent[108,109] and inconsistent.[110–113] Evidence for a connection between auditory temporal processing and developmental reading disorders is also very controversial, with positive results being reported for temporal order and same-different judgment tasks and for psychophysical tasks that involve thresholds for frequency and amplitude modulation.[94,114–116] Negative results have centered on failures to replicate and reports that reading-disabled children who differ in categorical speech perception do not differ when the stimuli are nonspeech analogues.[117,118] Although many of these studies indicate that auditory temporal processing measures are related to literacy and phonological processing, they do not address whether these sensory measures contribute uniquely to variance in word reading once the variance contributed by core linguistic processes, such as phonological awareness and rapid serial naming, have been controlled statistically.

Magno cells in the auditory relay nucleus of the thalamus (medial geniculate nucleus) are responsive to changes in frequency and amplitude, and postmortem evidence indicates that these cells, particularly on the side projecting to the left hemisphere, may be disordered in the brains of some dyslexic individuals.[119,120] Stein has hypothesized that visual and auditory magno cells may be similar and therefore both susceptible to influences that might alter their characteristics during the course of early brain development.[81,82] Recently, investigators have reported that measures of visual and auditory sensory processes index different aspects of developmental reading disorder; specifically, visual motion detection was correlated with orthographic processing and auditory temporal processing was correlated with phonological processing in the same individuals.[93,115,116]

These neuroanatomic and behavioral findings are consistent with the hypothesis of a more general temporal processing deficit.[55,81,82] Such a general deficit may also involve impaired motor development, which co-occurs with developmental dyslexia,[121] as well as functions of the cerebellum, which is the recipient of substantial magnocelluar input.[122] Although these speculations have the potential to push research on developmental reading disorders further into the mainstream of neuroscience research, the evidence for a nonlinguistic sensorimotor basis for developmental reading disorders continues to be preliminary and highly controversial. Even regarding visual, auditory, and motor deficits as different subtypes is inconsistent with current evidence indicating that virtually all subtypes associated with developmental reading disorders are characterized by deficits in linguistically based core phonological processes.[70]

GENETICS

Reading disabilities run in families, and family history is a critical risk factor for developmental reading disorders. Some 40 percent of boys and 18 percent of girls with an affected parent have been estimated to exhibit reading disability profiles.[123] Approximately 31 percent of the children in whom one or two of the parents were dyslexic were identified by their school as having difficulty learning to read by the end of second grade, and this prevalence doubled when their reading was assessed by psychometric tests.[29,124,125]

Comparison of monozygotic (MZ or identical) and dizygotic (DZ or fraternal) twins provides another methodology for exploring genetic contributions to reading orders. Using the Colorado Twin Study database, the unbiased concordance rate of reading disorder for MZ twins has been estimated at 68 percent and at 38 percent for DZ twins, providing evidence that reading disorder has significant genetic etiology.[126] In a subsequent study, reading performance was reported to be highly heritable for both disabled (0.82) and normal reader (0.66) groups while shared environmental influences were low (0.01 and 0.18, respectively). Both phonological and orthographic reading–related measures also appear highly heritable.[127,128]

Linkage analysis is currently used to assess "whether heritable variations at two loci (genetic positions on chromosomes) are transmitted together in relatives at a rate that is greater than would be expected by chance" (see Ref. 129, p. 513). A significant linkage to chromosome 15 was reported in a subset of nine multigenerational families in the first report of a genetic linkage to reading disorder.[130] This finding was not initially replicated with other families,[131–133] but recent evidence is consistent with a linkage to chromosome 15 involving reading[134] and spelling disability.[135]

Siblings can share several alleles or no alleles for a particular DNA marker. If those siblings who share more alleles also happen to have similar scores on a quantitative measure of a trait such as word reading (e.g., both scores are low), then it is possible to infer that a quantitative trait locus (QTL) linkage exits. This technique is more powerful when one of the siblings is selected because he or she has a very low score on the quantitative trait under investigation. Cardon and colleagues used interval mapping of genetic data from two independent samples of sibling pairs (fraternal twins and siblings) and identified a quantitative trait locus (QTL) for reading disability on chromosome 6 within the same area as the human leukocyte antigen (HLA) region.[132] This part of chromosome 6 had attracted interest because of a hypothesis about an association between autoimmune disorders and reading.[136] Although this hypothesis has not been supported,[137] the association of the HLA region on the short arm of chromosome 6 with reading disability has been a productive area of research.[53,138,139]

Grigorenko and colleagues reported loci for different components of reading disorder on chromosomes 6 and 15.[53] A phenotype related to single word-reading difficulties was linked to a marker on chromosome 15, and a correlated phenotype related to phonological awareness difficulties was linked to markers on the short arm of chromosome 6. The linkage findings implicating chromosome 6 and chromosome 15 in reading disability have been replicated, particularly the results for chromosome 6.[138,139] The distinction between the phonological awareness and word-reading phenotypes has not been replicated, however, possibly because the measures that identify them are highly correlated.

Initially, Grigorenko's results were interpreted as indicating that different components of reading skill might be linked to different genes. Pennington pointed out, however, that QTLs which appear to be localized to regions on chromosomes 6 and 15 should not be regarded as evidence that there are specific genes for reading ability or reading disability.[140] Instead, these and other genes may disrupt brain development in a way that eventually alters the developmental process of reading acquisition. Similarly, Plomin has argued that molecular biological techniques may not be productive when applied to the study of cognition and behavior if it is assumed that one or two major genes are responsible for genetic variation in complex behavioral traits and disorders. A more productive strategy would involve identifying multiple genes, each accounting for a relatively small amount of variance. Both genetic and environmental influences may be equally important in accounting for variation in the pheneotype according to this perspective.[141,142]

Fisher and colleagues[143] have recently published a complete genome scan for reading disorders that involved two reading-disabled families with a previously established genetic linkage to chromosome 6p. The most significant single point finding was for markers on chromosome 18p, with evidence of linkage at this locus for measures of single-word identification as well as orthographic and phonological processing skill. It is possible that a number of reading-related processes may be associated with this locus, and it may represent a more general risk factor for reading disability because it may influence several reading-related skills.[144]

Additional loci for reading disability have been reported, including a region on chromosome 2.[145,146]

While these linkage findings are encouraging, current evidence suggests that at least six different genes potentially influence reading disability,[147] and it is likely that more will be identified. Other developmental learning disorders that are frequently comorbid with developmental reading disorders may overlap genetically—such as attention deficit hyperactivity disorder (ADHD),[148,149] specific language impairment,[150] and mathematical learning disorders[151]—although the evidence to date is very preliminary. Recognition of the heterogeneity of both genetic and environmental contributions to the development of reading disorders has provided a more realistic and sophisticated perspective on the complexities involved in understanding these disorders.

NEUROBIOLOGICAL FOUNDATIONS

The neurobiological bases of reading disorder have been a topic of scientific interest since the first reports of visual word blindness over a century ago. Interest has been increasing and has been particularly strong in the past two decades.[29,55,152,153] Galaburda has provided unique neuroanatomic evidence for reading disorder in a series of postmortem investigations of individuals with a childhood history of dyslexia.[154,155] He reported that the planum temporale, which is located in the posterior aspect of the superior temporal lobe and is involved in language, was symmetrical in all seven of the dyslexic brains investigated.[156-158] In contrast, asymmetry is typical of normal readers, with the left side being larger in approximately 65 percent of the cases, and it may be a structural prerequisite for normal phonological development. Galaburda's finding reflects an unexpected increase in the size of the right planum in dyslexic individuals rather than a smaller left planum, a pattern interpreted as arising from reduced cell death during fetal brain development.[154,155]

Cortical malformations (ectopias, dysplasia, vascular micromalformations) in the frontal and language areas were also reported,[156-158] and Galaburda speculated that genetic factors may influence neuronal migration and contribute to establishing abnormal neuronal circuits in brain areas typically devoted to language functions. The result is that the dyslexic brain may have too many neurons in the posterior language areas, particularly in the right hemisphere, rather than too few.[154,155]

These autopsy investigations have been criticized, however, for the small sample of brains studied, the heterogeneity of the dyslexic symptoms, and comorbidity with other disorders. It is possible that symmetrical plana temporale may reflect a different pattern of early brain development common to several neurolinguistic disorders rather than just developmental reading disorder.[12,159] In addition, there is considerable variability in the planum temporale within the general population, and measurement problems prevent accurate comparisons across studies.[152,160,161]

Large samples of dyslexic and control twins have been investigated with quantitative MRI analyses in Colorado studies on the genetics of size variations in brain structure in dyslexia.[162] Individuals with reading disorders had the largest operculum, temporal, and posterior parietal/occipital regions and smaller bilateral insula and frontal cortex; there were no differences in subcortical structure volumes (e.g., basal ganglia, thalamus). Filipek[152] suggests that these findings provide evidence for developmental structural anomalies among individuals with developmental reading disorder in areas of the brain involved in receptive language. Despite progress in this area, there is relatively little evidence of substantial differences in anatomic brain structure between dyslexic and nondyslexic individuals but small sample sizes, measurement, and phenotype definition issues contribute to the conflicting evidence.[12,29,56] Nevertheless, this research is valuable because it encourages the hypothesis that developmental reading disorders are the result of anomalies in neural development arising from an event or sequence of events that occur in utero and may produce different patterns of brain development.[29,81,82]

Recent advances in functional brain imaging methods such as positron emission tomography (PET), functional MRI (fMRI), and magnetic source imaging (MSI) allow examination of the underlying neural systems involved in performing reading and reading-related tasks.[83,84] Using a subtraction paradigm common to fMRI studies (see Chap. 3), S. E. Shaywitz,

B.A. Shaywitz, and colleagues at Yale University[54] administered five tasks that varied the level of phonological/linguistic coding required: (1) visuospatial processing (do (\\\/) and (\\\/) match?), (2) orthographic processing (do *bbBb* and *bbBb* match?), (3) simple phonological analysis (do *T* and *V* rhyme?), (4) phonological assembly (do *leat* and *jete* rhyme?), and (5) lexical-semantic processing (are *corn* and *rice* in the same category?). As the phonological demands of print-to-sound mapping increased, adult disabled readers failed to increase activation within a large posterior cortical system that included the posterior superior temporal gyrus (Wernicke's area), the angular gyrus, and the striate cortex. Instead, these readers demonstrated overactivation in anterior areas, including the inferior frontal gyrus (Broca's area), on phonological tasks.

These data suggest disruption of a posterior cortical system that involves both visual and language processing areas as well as part of the association cortex. The association cortex includes the angular gyrus, which is thought to be recruited in the cross-modal processing involved in print-to-sound mapping during reading. S.E. Shaywitz, B.A. Shaywitz, and colleagues regard a pattern of relative *under*activation of posterior areas combined with relative *over*activation of anterior areas as "a neural signature for the phonologic difficulties characterizing dyslexia" (see Ref. 54, p. 2640).

Subsequent research by the Yale group[163] indicated that when task performance did not require phonological assembly (tasks 1 to 3), functional connectivity correlations between the angular gyrus and related posterior cortical areas relevant to reading were similar for dyslexic and nondyslexic readers. In contrast, functional connectivity correlations for the left hemisphere were weak on the word and nonword reading tasks (tasks 4 to 5) for the dyslexic readers because they require phonological assembly. When left hemisphere functional connectivity correlations were low for dyslexic readers on phonological assembly tasks, strong correlations were obtained at the corresponding right hemisphere homologues, suggesting that reading disabled individuals may be overly reliant on right hemisphere systems in performing phonologically demanding tasks.

Dorsal (temporoparietal circuit) and ventral (occipitotemporal circuit) left hemisphere systems are hypothesized to be associated with different functions in the normally developing reader's brain and in different phases of reading acquisition.[153] These two left hemisphere posterior systems and their functional connectivity are deviant in the brains of dyslexic readers. Individuals with reading disorders are characterized by increased reliance on the inferior frontal gyrus (Broca's area) during reading, possibly because it supports control and sequencing of articulatory recoding that may be recruited in response to phonological processing demands. These readers also show increased activation in the right hemisphere homologues of the impaired left hemisphere posterior systems. This right hemisphere shift may support word identification learning through nonphonological, visual-semantic pattern recognition processes.

The dorsal system includes the angular gyrus, the supramarginal gyrus in the inferior parietal lobule, and the posterior aspect of the superior temporal gyrus (Wernicke's area), and it is hypothesized to be dominant early in development. This system involves mapping visual units of print (graphemes) onto phonological units of language (phonemes) as well as analytic processing of the morphological and lexical semantic components of printed words. The ventral system predominates later in development and includes the lateral extrastriate areas and the left inferior occipitotemporal area. It involves rapid word identification, which is associated with the automatic, fluent word identification abilities of mature, skilled readers.[153]

Development of the ventral (occipitotemporal) system within the left hemisphere posterior reading system depends upon tight integration of the neural representations of the orthographic, phonological, and lexical-semantic information about words. Achieving this level of integration crucially depends upon first having an intact and functioning dorsal (temporoparietal) system. Deficits within the dorsal system, which supports the initial acquisition of word reading skill, preclude the subsequent development of the rapid ventral word-identification system.

Impaired temporoparietal circuitry, with its signature phonological processing deficits, disrupts the developmental trajectory of reading acquisition for children with developmental reading disorder by preventing them from developing a fast, ventral-occipital word-identification system. Activation of the inferior frontal gyrus and a shift to right hemisphere posterior processing by these readers is regarded as a response to the demands of word recognition and results in relatively inaccurate and nonfluent reading. This model of the course of reading development provides an initial characterization of both reading skill and reading disorder within the context of developmental cognitive neuroscience and provides a framework for understanding both the phonological decoding failures of struggling readers (impaired temporoparietal circuit) and their subsequent difficulty in attaining fluent and automatic word identification (impaired ventral-occipital circuit).[153]

The cross-linguistic nature of developmental reading disorders was examined by comparing cognitive and neuroimaging data on dyslexic and nonimpaired adult readers from three countries with alphabetic writing systems that varied in the depth of their orthographies.[30] Dyslexic Italian readers, who have a shallow orthography, were relatively better performers on literacy and phonological processing tasks than dyslexic French and English readers, whose orthographies are regarded as more complex (deep). PET brain scans taken during explicit and implicit reading activities revealed a common profile of reduced activation in the left middle, inferior, and superior temporal cortex and in the middle occipital gyrus for the dyslexic adult readers from all three countries. The nonimpaired control readers from each country showed a significantly greater activation in this large region of left cortex.

These results are consistent with the view that dyslexia is characterized by a universal neurocognitive profile in the brain that occurs regardless of whether the orthography is deep or shallow and is associated with characteristic phonological processing deficits. The depth of an orthography influences the extent to which the phonological deficits will impair the acquisition of reading skill and limit reading performance, but associated brain activation profiles during reading are similar across alphabetic languages regardless of their orthographic depth.

TREATMENT

Evidence indicates that reading ability improves with age and intervention for most reading-disordered children when adolescent and adult outcome data are examined. Core phonological deficits persist into adulthood, however, particularly among individuals who are severely impaired. Even in cases where the literacy outcome is good and educational success is achieved, phonological processing problems persist, as well as problems with spelling accuracy, word-recognition speed, and reading rate, particularly in the reading of technical expository text.[27,39,164,165] Dyslexic individuals who had pursued college education had the highest word-recognition achievement among a sample of adult dyslexics, but they were only at the 32nd percentile on a standardized word identification test. Standardized reading comprehension scores were higher, providing further evidence that aspects of word identification are the major area of difficulty for these individuals.[27,39]

Based on data from the Connecticut Longitudinal Study, children identified as reading-disabled in grades 2 through 6 continued to exhibit deficits in phonological coding in adolescence and to demonstrate continuing problems in reading, spelling, and reading rate compared to normally developing children with average and superior reading skills in the same grades. Children with persistent reading problems remained inferior readers relative to other students in high school despite having access to special education services during their schooling.[164] These findings are generally consistent with a deficit rather than a developmental lag model of reading disorder.[76]

There were no differences between good and poor readers in reports of legal problems, or use of alcohol or tobacco, or in the prevalence of conduct or attention problems in the Connecticut Longitudinal data.[164] Although there are differences in the composition of the different study samples, these results from the Connecticut Longitudinal Study appear inconsistent with other reports that adolescents with learning disorders have a threefold increase in their risk for substance abuse and elevated risk for adverse outcomes, including lower family socioeconomic status, IQ scores, and educational and occupational achievement.[166,167]

Many approaches to treating reading disorders have been advocated and attempted, but reports of reliable evidence from well-controlled studies on the efficacy of different interventions have emerged only since the mid- to late-1980s.[168] The absence of scientific evidence over so many decades led to inevitable questions about whether it is possible to treat these disorders successfully.[65,67,169] Within the last several years, a number of controlled and comparative research studies have been reported that have assessed the efficacy of different instructional approaches to remediating problems in reading acquisition in the early elementary grades.[57,64,170,171] Controlled intervention studies that focus on the core phonological and word-identification deficits of reading-disabled children in later grades have also been reported with positive results.[60–62,172–174]

These studies indicate that significant improvement can be achieved on speech-based and phonological reading measures for both young children at risk for reading disability and older children who are reading-disabled.[57,61,63,64,175,176] Furthermore, even with the most severely impaired readers drawn from a clinical sample, evidence from controlled intervention studies indicates that focused and systematic intervention, concentrated on remediating core deficits, results in measurable progress in learning phonological reading skills throughout the elementary school years.[59,72,172]

Remedial gains do not reliably generalize to other aspects of reading acquisition when children improve in phonologically based word attack and decoding skills. Although reading-disabled children could, after intervention, "sound out" new words or nonwords, they were not always improved in word recognition, text reading, or reading comprehension skills relative to a comparison group.[177] Generalization of remedial gains has been a substantial problem for many intervention methods evaluated in the literature[61,176] and for methods assessed in initial remediation studies we have conducted at The Hospital for Sick Children in Toronto.[178–180]

Generalization problems in these treatment studies may reflect the severity and complexity of the processing impairments exhibited by some disabled readers and the fact that the core processing deficits of many disabled readers extend beyond the realm of phonological awareness. Deficits in both phonological awareness and naming speed constitute a risk factor far more severe than either deficit alone.[45,72] There is also evidence that disabled readers have difficulty in specific aspects of executive functioning and strategy learning that are independent of their phonological processing impairments.[181–183] Many of the generalization fail-

ures may be due to difficulty in acquiring effective, flexible word-identification strategies and monitoring the effectiveness of strategy implementation.[60] It should be noted, however, that generalization and transfer-of-learning difficulties for disabled readers are specific to printed language learning; transfer occurs readily in learning tasks that have similar cognitive demands but do not require phonological processing.[184,185]

Difficulties children have in generalizing the gains they make following remedial instruction have motivated some of our most recent research with severely reading-disabled children referred to our laboratory classrooms at The Hospital for Sick Children in Toronto. Children with severe reading disorders were assigned randomly to one of two remedial reading programs or to a control treatment that dealt with classroom survival skills and consisted of instruction on study, organizational, and problem-solving skills.[59,72,172] Each reading program targeted generalization of treatment gains in word-identification learning but involved different instructional approaches and different levels of print-to-sound segmentation during training.

The PHAB/DI (Phonological Analysis and Blending/Direct Instruction) Program involves lessons from the direct instructional programs developed by Engelmann and colleagues; it trains phonological analysis, phonological blending, and letter-sound association skills in the context of word recognition and decoding instruction (see Reading Mastery I/II Fast Cycle, and Corrective Reading Programs).[186–188] The WIST (Word Identification Strategy Training) Program has a strong metacognitive focus in which children are taught how to use and monitor the application of four metacognitive decoding strategies. WIST was developed in our laboratory classrooms at The Hospital for Sick Children and is partially based on the original Benchmark School Word Identification/Vocabulary Development Program.[189] The dialogue structure for strategy instruction, the keywords, and the compare/contrast strategy (a strategy of word identification by analogy) were adapted from the Benchmark Program. WIST also includes, however, a direct training focus on the subskills necessary for strategy implementation, a metacognitive "Game Plan" for training flexibility in strategy choice and evaluating the success of those choices, and three additional word-identification strategies (Peeling Off,

Vowel Variations, and Spy). In summary, PHAB/DI focuses on grapheme-phoneme spelling-to-sound units while WIST trains recognition of larger subsyllabic units, particularly the rime. PHAB/DI promotes generalization of word-identification learning by intensive systematic remediation of basic sound analysis and sound blending deficits, while WIST involves teaching a set of flexible word-identification strategies as well as the specific skills and content required to implement them.

PHAB/DI and WIST proved much more effective than our previous interventions in achieving generalization of remedial gains.[178–180] PHAB/DI- and WIST-trained children were significantly improved on several standardized and experimental reading measures and showed evidence of generalization on a set of word-reading measures including words that varied in their spelling-to-sound similarity (distance) to the target words instructed in the PHAB/DI and WIST lessons. While both approaches were associated with large positive effects compared to the alternative treatment control condition (Classroom Survival Skills), different patterns of transfer were observed. PHAB/DI, with its emphasis on grapheme-phoneme analysis and blending, yielded broader-based and deeper generalization on speech- and print-based measures of phonological skill. WIST, with its strategy training focus, produced broader-based generalization for exceptions as well as regular words. These results indicated that children who were severely reading-disabled could learn phonological skills and letter-sound correspondences after extensive training, and they could generalize their word-identification skills to a range of uninstructed words. Furthermore, these effects could be obtained with relatively late intervention in grades 5 and 6.

The phonological processing and reading deficits of these children were not ameliorated after 35 h of intervention, but their speech- and print-based phonological skills were improved significantly and moved closer to age-appropriate levels; they showed substantially improved letter-sound knowledge, decoding abilities, and word-identification skills. These severely disabled readers were incorrectly identifying one-syllable words like *way, left,* and *put* before remedial intervention. Following PHAB/DI or WIST lessons, however, many were able to decode accurately, though often slowly, multisyllable words like *unintelligible, mistakenly,* and *disengaged.*

In a recent sequential crossover design involving 70 h of instruction, PHAB/DI and WIST were combined and compared to longer-term intervention, with each approach separately as well as with an alternative treatment control group (Classroom Survival Skills to Mathematics).[60] Generalized treatment effects were obtained on standardized measures of word identification, nonword reading, and passage comprehension, confirming the effectiveness of PHAB/DI and WIST on multiple indices of reading skill. The most important results, however, were the superior outcomes and steeper learning curves for children who had the sequential combination of PHAB/DI and WIST (PHAB/DI to WIST; WIST to PHAB/DI) compared to either intervention alone (PHAB/DI × 2; WIST × 2) on a variety of measures of word reading skill including nonword reading, letter-sound knowledge, keywords, near and far transfer words, and multisyllabic challenge words.

These results are important because they indicate that phonologically based approaches alone are not sufficient for achieving optimal remedial outcomes with reading disabled children. Phonologically based interventions appear necessary to achieve remedial gains, but generalization of those gains is more likely with a broader-based approach that combines direct and dialogue-based instructional methods, with children being taught different levels of subsyllabic segmentation and effective use of multiple decoding strategies. These results highlight the critical importance of strategy instruction and the promotion of a flexible approach to word-identification and text reading contexts.

Recent findings from a meta-analysis of the treatment outcome literature on learning disabilities are consistent with this conclusion. The optimal approach in instructing children with learning disabilities, according to a review of 180 intervention studies, is a combination of direct and strategy instruction methods. This combined approach appeared particularly effective in remedial reading interventions when the outcome measures required reading comprehension and text reading.[190]

We have begun to integrate these approaches into a single intervention program called the PHAST Track Reading Program (PHAST for Phonological and Strategy Training). It begins with PHAB/DI's program of phonological remediation and uses it as a foundation for introducing and scaffolding each of the four WIST strategies.[191] PHAST attempts to build context-free word identification skills and strategies to facilitate achieving the goal of reading connected text for meaning and is intended to be situated in a linguistically enriched and literature-based balanced literacy program. The dialogue structure of the PHAST Program and its metacognitive instructional focus are compatible with dialogue-based approaches to text comprehension and writing training. It could be implemented in the classroom as part of an integrated approach to reading, spelling, and writing instruction to allow intense instruction in spelling-to-sound and sound-to-spelling analysis at the subsyllabic, lexical, and connected text levels.

In a recent study, Torgesen and colleagues found significant improvements in generalized reading skills that were sustained over 2 years following intensive, phonologically based remediation programs (67.5 h).[62] These programs had little impact, however, on the disabled readers' impairment in reading speed. On average, children scored within the age-appropriate range on measures of word identification and passage comprehension 2 years after intervention, but they were two standard deviations below age norms on measures of reading rate despite increasing the number of words they could read per minute. There has been growing recognition that different models of remedial intervention will be required if disabled readers are to make gains in phonological processing skills, word identification and text reading accuracy, as well as in word-identification speed and text reading fluency.

RAVE-O is an experimental reading intervention program developed by Wolf that is designed to facilitate the acquisition of fluency.[192] It is to be taught in combination with a systematic phonologically based intervention program that provides instruction in letter-sound knowledge, decoding, and word-identification skills with the goal of improving speech-based phonological deficits in disabled readers. RAVE-O (Retrieval, Automaticity, Vocabulary Elaboration, Engagement with language, and Orthography) is designed to facilitate accuracy and automaticity in reading subskills and component processes and to develop fluency in word identification, word attack, and text reading and comprehension processes. RAVE-O

encourages children to learn to play with their language and it employs animated computer games[193] as well as minute-mystery stories, word webs, and word-retrieval strategies during instruction.

The PHAST Track Reading Program described above[191] and the RAVE-O Program[192] in conjunction with the previously described PHAB/DI Program[59,186–188] are being evaluated against both an alternative treatment control program (Classroom Survival Skills + Math)[60] and a phonological treatment control program (PHAB/DI + Classroom Survival Skills) in a large multisite intervention study funded by the National Institute of Child Health and Human Development.

Substantial increases in evidence-based treatment approaches to developmental reading disorder now allow more refined research questions to be posed about the combination of treatment components that are most effective, the characteristics of optimal treatment delivery, and mediators and moderators of long-term treatment outcome. New questions have also emerged about potential neurobiological correlates of the gains in performance that accompany effective intervention. Do the neurobiological substrates for reading behavior change with behavioral evidence of improvements in reading skill? And, if that is the case, what are the characteristics and limitations to the functional circuitry that underlie these newly acquired literacy skills?

Recent findings using magnetic source imaging (MSI) address some of these issues.[194] Eight dyslexic children (range 7 to 17 years of age, with a mean age of 11.4 years) received 80 h of intense, individualized, phonologically based remediation. They were given an MSI scan before and after the intervention while they performed a visual nonword rhyme-detection task (e.g., do *yoat* and *wote* rhyme?) which requires grapheme-phoneme decoding of each nonword. Eight normal readers were also scanned while they performed the rhyming task on two separate occasions 2 months apart, and no significant changes were observed in their activation profiles. Before the intervention, the dyslexic readers had limited activation in the left superior temporal gyrus as well as strong activation in the corresponding right hemisphere areas. After the intervention, the investigators reported that the brain activation profiles of the children were normalized, with an increase in the activation in the left superior temporal gyrus and a decrease in the right superior temporal gyrus.[194] These changes in activation were accompanied by behavioral evidence that the postintervention reading scores of the disabled readers had moved into the normal range. For the majority of dyslexic subjects, the postintervention brain activation profiles were indistinguishable from those of the age-matched normal readers, suggesting that the intervention had the effect of normalizing brain function rather than creating a compensatory reorganization. These findings, which require replication with larger samples and other measures, provide evidence that intense, phonologically based reading intervention procedures can alter the functional organization of the brains of developmentally reading-disordered children, even in adolescence.

REFERENCES

1. Hinshelwood J: Word blindness and visual memories. *Lancet* 2:1566–1570, 1895.
2. Hinshelwood J: *Congenital Word Blindness*. London: Lewis, 1917.
3. Morgan WP: A case of congenital word-blindness. *Bri Med J* 2:1378, 1896.
4. Orton ST: "Word-blindness" in school children. *Arch Neurol Psychiatry* 14:581–615, 1925.
5. Orton ST: Specific reading disability—Strephosymbolia. *JAMA* 90:1095–1099, 1928.
6. Gillingham A, Stillman BW: *Remedial Training for Children with Specific Disability in Reading, Spelling, and Penmanship*. Cambridge, MA: Educators Publishing Service, 1960.
7. Orton ST: *Reading, Writing, and Speech in Children*. New York: Norton, 1937.
8. Ansara A: The Orton-Gillingham approach to remediation, in Malatesha RN, Aaron PG (eds): *Reading Disorders: Varieties and Treatment*. New York: Academic Press, 1982, pp 409–433.
9. Critchley M: *The Dyslexic Child*. Springfield, IL: Charles C Thomas, 1970.
10. Denckla MB: Childhood learning disabilities, in Heilman KM, Valenstein E (eds): *Clinical Neuropsychology*. New York: Oxford University Press, 1979, p 550.
11. Bishop DVM, Adams C: A prospective study of the relationship between specific language impairment, phonological disorders and reading retardation. *J Child Psychol Psychiatry* 31:1027–1050, 1990.

12. Fletcher JM: Foorman BR, Shaywitz SE, et al: Conceptual and methodological issues in dyslexia research: A lesson for developmental disorders, in Tager-Flusberg, H (ed): *Neurodevelopmental Disorders*. Cambridge, MA: MIT Press, 1999, pp 271–305.
13. Liberman A: How theories of speech affect research on reading and writing, in Blachman, B (ed): *Foundations of Reading Acquisition and Dyslexia*. Mahwah, NJ: Erlbaum, 1997, pp 3–19.
14. Mann, V: Language problems: The key to early reading problems, in Wong B (ed): *Learning About Learning Disabilities*. San Diego, CA: Academic Press, 1998, pp 163–201.
15. Scarborough, HS: Early identification of children at risk for reading disabilities, in Shapiro BK, Acardo PJ, Capute AJ (eds): *Specific Reading Disability: A View of the Spectrum*. Timonium, MD: York Press, 1998, pp 75–119.
16. Stanovich, KE: Explaining the differences between dyslexic and garden-variety poor reader: The phonological core variable difference model. *J Learn Disabil* 21:590–604, 1988.
17. Gough PB, Tunmer WE: Decoding, reading, and reading disability. *Remed Spec Educ* 7:6–10, 1986.
18. Frankenberger W, Fronzaglio K: A review of state's criteria and procedures for identifying children with learning disabilities. *J Learn Disabil* 24:495–500, 1991.
19. Mercer CD, Jordan L, Allsop DH, et al: Learning disabilities definition and criteria used by state education departments. *Learn Disabil Q* 19:217–232, 1996.
20. Fletcher JM, Shaywitz SE, Shankweiler DP, et al: Cognitive profiles of reading disability: Comparisons of discrepancy and low achievement definitions. *J Educ Psychol* 86:6–23, 1994.
21. Stanovich KE, Siegel LS: Phenotypic performance profile of children with reading disabilities: A regression-based test of the phonological-core variable-difference model. *J Educ Psychol* 86:24–53, 1994.
22. Hoskyn M, Swanson HL: Cognitive processing of low achievers and children with reading disabilities: A selective meta-analytic review of the published literature. *School Psychol Rev* 29:102–119, 2000.
23. Stuebing KK, Fletcher JM, LeDoux JM, et al: Validity of IQ-discrepancy classifications of reading disabilities: A meta-analysis. *Am Educ Res J.* 39:469–518, 2002.
24. Share DL, Stanovich KE. Cognitive processes in early reading development: Accommodating individual differences into a model of acquisition. *Issues Educ Contrib Educ Psychol* 1:1–57, 1995.

25. Shaywitz SE, Shaywitz BA, Fletcher JM, et al: Prevalence of reading disability in boys and girls: Results of the Connecticut Longitudinal Study. *JAMA* 264:998–1002, 1990.

26. Shaywitz SE, Fletcher JM, Shaywitz BA: A conceptual model and definition of dyslexia: Findings emerging from the Connecticut Longitudinal Study, in Beitchman JH, Cohen NJ, Konstantareas MM, et al (eds): *Language, Learning, and Behavior Disorder*. New York: Cambridge University Press, 1996.

27. Bruck M: Outcomes of adults with childhood histories of dyslexia, in Hulme C, Joshi RM (eds), *Reading and Spelling: Development and Disorders*. Mahwah, NJ: Erlbaum, 1998, pp 179–200.

28. Tarnapol L, Tarapol M: *Comparative Reading Difficulties*. Lexington, KY: Lexington Books, 1981.

29. Grigorenko E: Developmental dyslexia: An update on genes, brains, and environments. *J Child Psychol Psychiatry* 42:91–125, 2001.

30. Paulesu E, Demonet JF, Fazio F, et al: Dyslexia: Cultural diversity and biological unity. *Science* 291:2165–2167, 2001.

31. Stanovich KE: Toward an interactive-compensatory model of individual differences in the development of reading fluency. *Read Res Q* 16:32–71, 1980.

32. Stanovich KE: Matthew effects in reading: Some consequences of individual differences in the acquisition of literacy. *Read Res Q* 21:360–407, 1986.

33. Perfetti CA: *Reading Ability*. New York: Oxford University Press, 1985.

34. Rack JP, Snowling M, Olson RK: The nonword reading deficit in developmental dyslexia: A review. *Read Res Q* 27:28–53, 1992.

35. Shankweiler D, Lundquist E, Katz L, et al: Comprehension and decoding: Patterns of association in children with reading difficulties. *Sci Stud Read* 3:69–94, 1999.

36. Bradley L, Bryant PE: Categorizing sounds and learning to read—a causal connection. *Nature* 301:419–421, 1983.

37. Wagner RK, Torgesen JK: The nature of phonological processing and its causal role in the acquisition of reading skills. *Psychol Bull* 101:192–212, 1987.

38. Wagner RK, Torgesen JK, Rashotte CA: Development of reading-related phonological processing abilities: New evidence of bidirectional causality from a latent variable longitudinal study. *Dev Psychol* 30:73–87, 1994.

39. Bruck M: Persistence of dyslexics' phonological awareness deficits. *Dev Psychol* 28:874–886, 1992.

40. Bryne B: *Foundations of Literacy: The Child's Acquisition of the Alphabetic Principle*. Hove, East Sussex, UK: Psychology Press, 1998.

41. Wagner RK, Torgesen JK, Rashotte CA, et al: Changing relations between phonological processing abilities and word-level reading as children develop from beginning to skilled readers: A five year longitudinal study. *Dev Psychol* 33:468–479, 1997.

42. Brady SA: The role of working memory in reading disability, in Brady SA, Shankweiler D (eds): *Phonological Processes in Literacy: A Tribute to Isabelle Y. Liberman*. Hillsdale, NJ: Erlbaum, 1991, pp 128–152.

43. Wolf M, Bally H, Morris R: Automaticity, retrieval processes, and reading: A longitudinal study in average and impaired readers. *Child Dev* 57:988–1000, 1986.

44. Wolf M, Bowers PG: The double-deficit hypothesis for the developmental dyslexias. *J Educ Psychol* 91:415–438, 1999.

45. Wolf M, Bowers, PG, Biddle K: Naming-speed processes, timing, and reading: A conceptual review. *J Learn Disabil* 33:387–407, 2000.

46. Denckla MB, Rudel RG: Rapid 'automatized' naming (RAN): Dyslexia differentiated from other learning disabilities. *Neuropsychologia* 14:471–479, 1976.

47. Bowers PG, Sunseth K, Golden J: The route between rapid naming and reading progress. *Sci Stud Read* 3:31–53, 1999.

48. Manis FR, Seidenberg MS, Doi L: See Dick RAN: Rapid naming and the longitudinal prediction of reading subskills in first and second graders. *Sci Stud Read* 3:129–157, 1999.

49. Goswami U, Bryant PE: *Phonological Skills and Learning to Read*. Hove, East Sussex: Erlbaum, 1990.

50. Stanovich KE: Early acquisition and the causes of reading difficulty: The contributions to research on phonological processing, in Stanovich KE (ed): *Progress in Understanding Reading: Scientific Foundations and New Frontiers*. New York: Guilford Press, 2000, pp 57–79.

51. Share DL: Phonological recoding and self-teaching. Sine qua non of reading acquisition. *Cognition* 55:151–218, 1995.

52. Bradley L, Bryant PE: Difficulties in auditory organization as a possible cause of reading backwardness. *Nature* 271:746–747, 1978.

53. Grigorenko EL, Wood FB, Meyer MS et al.: Susceptibility loci for distinct components of developmental dyslexia on chromosomes 6 and 15. *Am J Hum Genet* 60:27–39, 1997.

54. Shaywitz SE, Shaywitz BA, Pugh KR: Functional disruption in the organization of the brain for reading in dyslexia. *Proc Natl Acad Sci U S A* 95:2636–2641, 1998.

55. Habib M: The neurological basis of developmental dyslexia: An overview and working hypothesis. *Brain* 123:2373–2399, 2000.

56. Pennington BF: Dyslexia as a neurodevelopmental disorder, in Tager-Flusberg H (ed): *Neurodevelopmental Disorders*. Cambridge, MA: MIT Press, 1999, pp 307–330.

57. Foorman BR, Francis DJ, Fletcher, JM, et al: The role of instruction in learning to read: Preventing reading failure in at-risk children. *J Educ Psychol* 90:37–55, 1998.

58. Hatcher PJ, Hulme C, Ellis AW: Ameliorating early reading failure by integrating the teaching of reading and phonological skills: The phonological linkage hypothesis. *Child Dev* 65:41–57, 1994.

59. Lovett MW, Borden SL, DeLuca T, et al: Treating the core deficits of developmental dyslexia: Evidence of transfer-of-learning following phonologically- and strategy-based reading training programs. *Dev Psychol* 30:805–822, 1994.

60. Lovett MW, Lacerenza L, Borden SL, et al: Components of effective remediation for developmental reading disabilities: Combining phonological and strategy-based instruction to improve outcomes. *J Educ Psychol* 92:263–283, 2000.

61. Olson RK, Wise B, Ring J, et al: Computer-based remedial training in phoneme awareness and phonological decoding: Effects on the posttraining development of word recognition. *Sci Stud Read* 1:235–254, 1997.

62. Torgesen JK, Alexander AW, Wagner RK, et al: Intensive remedial instruction for children with severe reading disabilities: Immediate and long-term outcomes from two instructional approaches. *J Learn Disabil* 34: 33–58, 2001.

63. Torgesen, JK, Wagner RK, Rashotte CA et al: Preventing reading failure in young children with phonological processing disabilities: Group and individual responses to instruction. *J Educ Psychol* 91:579–593, 1999.

64. Vellutino FR, Scanlon DM, Sipay ER, et al: Cognitive profiles of difficult-to-remediate and readily remediated poor readers: Early intervention as a vehicle for distinguishing between cognitive and experiential deficits as basic causes of specific reading disability. *J Educ Psychol* 88:601–638, 1996.

65. Lovett MW, Barron RW: The search for individual and subtype differences in reading disabled children's response to remediation, in Molfese DL, Molfese VJ (eds): *Developmental Variations in Learning: Applications to Social, Executive Function, Language, and Reading Skills*. Mahwah, NJ: Erlbaum, 2002, pp 309–337.

66. Lovett MW, Barron RW: Neuropsychological perspectives on reading development and reading disorders, in Segalowitz SJ, Rapin I (eds): *Handbook of Neuropsychology:* Child Neuropsychology, 2d ed., New York: Elsevier, 2003, vol. 8, part II, pp 255–300.

67. Lovett MW, Barron RW, Benson NJ: Effective remediation of word identification and decoding difficulties in school-age children with reading disabilities, in Swanson HL, Harris K, Graham S (eds): *Handbook of Learning Disabilities*. New York: Guilford. In press.

68. Swanson HL, Hoskyn M: Experimental intervention research on students with learning disabilities: A meta-analysis of treatment outcomes. *Rev Educ Res* 68: 277–321, 1998.

69. Fletcher JM, Morris RD: Classification of disabled learners: Beyond exclusionary definitions. in Ceci S (ed): *Handbook of Cognitive, Social, and Neuropsychological Aspects of Learning Disabilities*. Hillsdale, NJ: Erlbaum,1986, pp 55–80.

70. Morris RD, Stuebing KK, Fletcher JM et al: Subtypes of reading disability: Variability around a phonological core. *J Educ Psychol* 90:1–27, 1998.

71. Wolf M, Goldberg A, Gidney C, et al: The second deficit: An investigation of the independence of phonological and naming-speed deficits in developmental dyslexia. *Read Writing Interdiscip J* 15:43–72, 2002.

72. Lovett MW Steinbach KA, Frijters JC: Remediating the core deficits of developmental reading disability: A double deficit perspective. *J Learn Disabil* 33:334–358, 2000.

73. Castles A, Coltheart M: Varieties of developmental dyslexia. *Cognition* 47:149–180, 1993.

74. Manis FR, Seidenberg, MS, Doi LM, et al: On the basis of two subtypes of developmental dyslexia. *Cognition* 58:157–195, 1996.

75. Stanovich KE, Siegel LS, Gottardo A: Converging evidence for phonological and surface subtypes of reading disability. *J Educ Psychol* 89:114–127, 1997.

76. Francis DJ, Shaywitz SE, Stuebing KK, et al: Developmental lag versus deficit models of reading disability: A longitudinal, individual growth curves analysis. *J Educ Psychol* 88:3–17, 1996.

77. Manis FR, McBride-Chang C, Seidenberg MS, et al: Are speech perception deficits associated with developmental dyslexia? *J Exp Child Psychol* 66:211–235, 1997.

78. Joanisse MF, Manis FR, Keating P, et al: Language deficits in dyslexic children: Speech perception, phonology, and morphology. *J Exp Child Psychol* 77:30–60, 2000.

79. Bishop DVM, Adams C: A prospective study of the relationship between specific language impairment, phonological disorders and reading retardation. *J Child Psychol Psychiatry* 31:1027–1050, 1990.

80. Studdert-Kennedy M, Mody M: Auditory temporal deficits in the reading impaired: A critical review of the evidence. *Psychonom Bulletin Rev* 2:508–514, 1995.

81. Stein JF: The neurobiology of reading difficulties, in Wolf M (ed): *Dyslexia, Fluency, and the Brain.* Baltimore, MD: York Press, 2001, pp 3–21.

82. Stein JF: The sensory basis of reading problems. *Dev Neuropsychol* 20:509–534, 2001.

83. Joseph J, Noble K, Eden G: The neurobiological basis of reading. *J Learn Disabil* 34:566–579, 2001.

84. Demb JB, Poldrack RA, Gabrieli JDE: Functional neuroimaging of word processing in normal and dyslexic readers, in Klein RM, McMullen PM (eds): *Converging Method for Understanding Reading and Dyslexia.* Cambridge, MA: MIT Press, 1999, pp 245–304.

85. Rayner K: Eye movements in reading and information processing: 20 years of research. *Psychol Bull* 124:372–422, 1998.

86. Willows DM, Terepocki M: The relation of reversal errors to reading disabilities, in Willows DM, Kruk RS, Corcos E (eds): *Visual Processes in Reading and Reading Disabilities.* Hillsdale, NJ: Erlbaum, 1993, pp 31–56.

87. Cornelissen PL, Hansen PC, Hutton JL et al: Magnocellular visual function and children's single word reading. *Vis Res* 38:471–482, 1998.

88. Lovegrove WJ, Bowling A, Badcock D, et al: Specific reading disability: Differences in contrast sensitivity as a function of spatial frequency. *Science* 210:439–440, 1980.

89. Lovegrove WJ, Garzia RP, Nicholson SB: Experimental evidence for a transient system deficit in specific reading disability. *J Am Optom Assoc* 61:137–146, 1990.

90. Lovegrove WJ, Martin F, Slaghuis W: A theoretical and experimental case for a visual deficit in specific reading disability. *Cogn Neuropsychol* 3:225–267, 1986.

91. Cornelissen PL, Richardson AJ, Mason AJ, et al: Contrast sensitivity and coherent motion detection measured at photopic luminance levels in dyslexics and controls. *Vis Res* 35:1483–1494, 1995.

92. Cornelissen PL, Hansen PC, Gilchrist I, et al: Coherent motion detection and letter position encoding. *Vis Res* 38:2181–2191, 1998.

93. Witton C, Talcott JB, Hansen PC, et al: Sensitivity to dynamic auditory and visual stimuli predicts nonword reading ability in both dyslexic and normal readers. *Curr Biol* 8:791–797, 1998.

94. Cestnick L, Coltheart M: The relationship between language-processing and visual-processing deficits in developmental dyslexia. *Cognition* 71:231–255, 1999.

95. Eden GF, VanMeter JW, Rumsey JM, et al: Abnormal processing of visual motion in dyslexia revealed by functional brain imaging. *Nature* 382:66–69, 1996.

96. Stein JF, Walsh V: To see but not to read: The magnocellular theory of dyslexia. *Trends Neurosci* 20:147–152, 1997.

97. Hayduk S, Bruck M, Cavanagh P: Low-level visual processing skills of adults and children with dyslexia. *Cogn Neuropsychol* 13:975–1016, 1996.

98. O'Brien BA, Mansfield JS, Legge GE: The effect of contrast on reading speed in dyslexia. *Vis Res* 40:1921–1935, 2000.

99. Skottun BC, Parke LA: The possible relationship between visual defects and dyslexia: Examination of a critical assumption. *J Learn Disabil* 32:2–5, 1999.

100. Skottun BC: The magnocellular deficit theory of dyslexia: The evidence from contrast sensitivity. *Vis Res* 40:111–127, 2000.

101. Hulme C: The implausibilty of low-level visual deficits as a cause of children's reading difficulties. *Cogn Neuropsychol* 5:369–374, 1986.

102. Stein JF, Fowler S: Visual dyslexia. *Trends Neurosci* 4:77–80, 1981.

103. Eden GF, Stein JF, Wood HM: Differences in eye movements and reading problems in dyslexic and normal children. *Vis Res* 34:1345–1358, 1995.

104. Stein JF, Richardson AJ, Fowler MS: Monocular occlusion can improve binocular control and reading in dyslexics. *Brain* 123:164–170, 2000.

105. Tallal P: An experimental investigation of the role of auditory temporal processing in normal and disordered language development, in Caramazza A, Zurif EB (eds): *Language Acquisition and Language Breakdown.* Baltimore, MD: Johns Hopkins University Press, 1978, pp 25–61.

106. Merzenich MM, Jenkins WM, Johnston P, et al: Temporal processing deficits of language-learning impaired children ameliorated by training. *Science* 271:77–81, 1996.

107. Tallal P, Miller SL, Bedi G, et al: Language comprehension in language-learning impaired children improved with acoustically modified speech. *Science* 271:81–84, 1996.

108. Habib M, Espesser R, Ray V, et al: Training dyslexics with acoustically modified speech: Evidence of improved phonological performance. *Brain Cogn* 40:143–146, 1999.

109. Wright BA, Lombardino LJ, King WM, et al: Defcits in auditory temporal and spectral resolution in language-impaired children. *Nature* 387:176–178, 1997.

110. Bishop DVM, Bishop SJ, Bright P, et al: Different origin of auditory and phonological processing problems in children with language impairment: Evidence from a twin study. *J Speech Lang Hear Res* 42:155–168, 1999.

111. Bishop DVM, Carlyon RP, Deeks JM, et al: Auditory temporal processing impairment: Neither necessary nor sufficient for causing language impairment in children. *J Speech Lang Hear Res* 42:1295–1310, 1999.

112. Bradlow AR, Kraus N, Nicol T, et al: Effects of lengthened format transitions duration on discrimination and neural representation of synthetic CV syllables by normal and learning disabled children. *J Acoust Soc Am* 106:2086–2096, 1999.

113. Nittrouer S: Do temporal processing deficits cause phonological processing problems? *J Speech Lang Hear Res* 42:925–942, 1999.

114. Tallal P: Auditory temporal perception, phonics and reading disabilities in children. *Brain Lang* 9:182–198, 1980.

115. Booth JR, Perfetti CA, MacWhinney B, et al: The association of rapid temporal perception with orthographic and phonological processing in children and adults with reading impairment. *Sci Stud Reading* 4:101–132, 2000.

116. Talcott JB, Witton C, McLean MF, et al: Dynamic sensory sensitivity and children's word decoding skills. *Proc Natl Acad Sci USA* 97:2952–2957, 2000.

117. Mody M, Studdert-Kennedy M, Brady S: Speech perception deficits in poor readers: Auditory processing or phonological coding? *J Exp Child Psychol* 64:199–231, 1997.

118. Studdert-Kennedy M: Deficits in phoneme awareness do not arise from failures in rapid auditory processing. *Read Writing* 15:5–14, 2002.

119. Galaburda AM, Livingstone M: Evidence for a magnocellular defect in developmental dyslexia. *Ann NY Acad Sci* 68:70–82, 1993.

120. Galaburda AM, Menard MT, Rosen GD: Evidence for aberrant auditory anatomy in developmental dyslexia. *Proc Natl Acad Sci U S A* 91:8010–8013, 1994.

121. Nicholson RI, Fawcett AJ, Berry EL, et al: Motor learning difficulties and abnormal cerebellar activation in dyslexic children. *Lancet* 353:43–47, 1999.

122. Irvy RB, Justus TC, Middleton C: The cerebellum, timing, and language, in Wolf M (ed): *Dyslexia, Fluency, and the Brain*. Timonium, MD: York Press, 2001 pp 189–211.

123. Pennington BF, Smith SD: Genetic influences on learning disabilities: An update. *J Consult Clin Psychol* 56:817–823, 1988.

124. Finucci JM, Gottfredson L, Childs B: A follow-up study of dyslexic boys. *Ann Dyslexia* 35:117–136, 1985.

125. Wood FB, Grigorenko EL: Emerging issues in the genetics of dyslexia: A methodological review. *J Learn Disabil* 34:503–511, 2001.

126. DeFries JC, Alarcón M: Genetics of specific reading disability. *Ment Retard Dev Disabil Res Rev* 2:39–47, 1996.

127. Hohnen B, Stevenson J: Genetic effects in orthographic ability: A second look. *Behav Genet* 25:271, 1995.

128. Gayán J, Olson RK: Reading disability: Evidence for a genetic etiology. *Eur Child Adolesc Psychiatry* 8: 52–55, 1999.

129. Smith SD, Kelley PM, Askew JW, et al: Reading disability and chromosome 6p21.3: Evaluation of MOG as a candidate gene. *J Learn Disabil* 34:512–519, 2001.

130. Smith SD, Kimberling WJ, Pennington BF, et al: Specific reading disability: Identification of an inherited form through linkage analysis. *Science* 219:1345–1347, 1983.

131. Bisgaard ML, Eiberg H, Moller N, et al: Dyslexia and chomosome 15 heteromorphism: negative lod score in a Danish material. *Clin Gene* 32:118–119, 1987.

132. Cardon LR, Smith SD, Fulker FW, et al: Quantitative trait locus for reading disability on chromosome 6. *Science* 266: 276–279, 1994.

133. Lubs HA, Duara R, Levin B, et al: Dyslexia subtypes: Genetics, behavior, and brain imaging, in Duane DD, Gray DB (eds), *The Reading Brain: The Biological Basis of Dyslexia*. Parkton, MD: York Press, 1991, pp 89–118.

134. Morris DW, Robinson L, Turic D, et al: Family-based association mapping provides evidence for reading disability on chromosome 15q. *Hum Mol Genet* 9:843–848, 2000.

135. Schulte-Körne G, Brimm T, Nöthen MM, et al: Evidence for linkage of spelling disability to chromosome 15. *Am J Med Genet Neuropsychol Genet* 74:661, 1997.

136. Geshwind N, Behan PO: Laterality, hormones, and immunity, in Geshwind N, Galaburda A (eds): *Cerebral Dominance*. New York: MIT Press, pp 211–224.

137. Gilger JW, Pennington BF, Harbeck RJ, et al: A twin and family study of the association between immune system dysfunction and dyslexia using blood serum immunoassay and survey data. *Brain Cogn* 26:310–333, 1998.

138. Fisher SE, Marlow AJ, Lamb J, et al: A quantitative-trait locus on chromosome 6p influences different aspects of developmental dyslexia. *Am J Hum Genet* 64: 146–156, 1999.

139. Gayán J, Smith SD, Cherny SS, et al: Quantitative-trait locus for specific language and reading deficits on chromosome 6p. *Am J Hum Genet* 64: 157–164, 1999.

140. Pennington BF: Using genetics to dissect cognition. *Am J Hum Genet* 60: 13–16, 1997.

141. Plomin R, Crabbe J: DNA. *Psychol Bull* 126:806–828, 2000.

142. Plomin R, Rutter M: Child development, molecular genetics, and what to do with genes once they are found. *Child Dev* 69:1221–1240.

143. Fisher SE, Francks C, Marlow AJ, et al: Independent genome-wide scans identify a chromosome 18 quantitative-trait locus influencing dyslexia. *Nat Genet* 30: 86–91, 2002.

144. Barr CL, Wigg K, Feng Y, et al: Linkage study of reading disabilities and attention-deficit hyperactivity disorder in the chromosome 6p region. American Society of Human Genetics 51st Annual Meeting, San Diego, CA. *Am J Human Genet* 69: 544, 2001.

145. Fagerheim T, Raeymaekers P, Tonnessen FE, et al: A new gene (DYX3) for dyslexia is located on chromosome 2. *J Med Genet* 36:664–669, 1999.

146. Petryshen, TL, Kaplan BJ, Hughes ML, et al: Supportive evidence for the DYX3 dyslexia susceptibility gene in Canadian families. *J Med Genet* 39(2):125–126, 2000.

147. Barr CL: Personal communication.

148. Willcutt EG, Pennington BF: Comorbidity of reading disability and attention-deficit / hyperactivity disorder: Differences by gender and subtype. *J Learn Disabil* 33: 179–191, 2000.

149. Willcutt EG, Pennington BF, DeFries JC: Etiology of inattention and hyperactivity/impulsivity in a community sample of twins with learning difficulties. *J Abnorm Child Psychol* 28:149–159, 2000.

150. SLI Consortium: A genomewide scan identifies two novel loci involved in specific language impairment. *Am J Hum Genet* 70:384–398, 2001.

151. Light JG, DeFries JC: Comorbidity of reading and mathematics disabilities: Genetic and environmental etiologies. *J Learn Disabil* 28:96–106, 1995.

152. Filipek PA: Neuroimaging in the developmental disorders: The state of the science. *J Child Psychol Psychiatry* 40:113–128, 1999.

153. Pugh KR, Mencl WE, Jenner AJ, et al: Functional neuroimaging studies of reading and reading disability (developmental dyslexia). *Ment Retard Dev Disabil Rev* 6:207–213, 2000.

154. Galaburda AM: Neurology of developmental dyslexia. *Curr Opin in Neurobiology* 3:237–242, 1993.

155. Galaburda AM: Developmental dyslexia and animal studies: At the interface between cognition and neurology. *Cognition* 50:133–149, 1994.

156. Galaburda, AM Kemper, TL: Cytoarchitectonic abnormalities in dyslexia: A case study. *Ann Neurol* 6: 94–100, 1979.

157. Galaburda AM, Sherman GF, Rosen GD, et al: Developmental dyslexia: Four consecutive patients with cortical anomalies. *Ann Neurol* 18:222–233, 1985.

158. Humphreys P, Kaufman WE, Galaburda AM: Developmental dyslexia in women: Neuropathological finding in three patients. *Ann Neurol* 28:727–738, 1990.

159. Morgan AE, Hynd GW: Dyslexia, neurolinguistic ability, and anatomical variation of the planum temporale. *Neuropsychol Rev* 8:79–93, 1998.

160. Filipek PA: Neurobiological correlates of developmental dyslexia: What do we know of how dyslexics' brains differ from those of normal readers? *J Child Neurol* 10: 62–69, 1995.

161. Westbury CF, Zatorre RJ, Evans AC: Quantifying variability in the palnum temporale: A probability map. *Cereb Cortex* 9:382–405, 1999.

162. Pennington BF., Filipek PA, Churchwell J, et al: Brain morphometry in reading-disabled twins. *Neurology* 53: 723–729, 1999.

163. Pugh KR, Mencl WE, Shaywitz BA, et al: The angular gyrus in developmental dyslexia: Task-specific differences in functional connectivity within posterior cortex. *Psychol Sci* 11:51–59, 2000.

164. Shaywitz SE, Fletcher JM, Holahan JM, et al: Persistence of dyslexia: The Connecticut Longitudinal Study at adolescence. *Pediatrics* 104:1351, 1999.

165. Scarborough HS: Continuity between childhood dyslexia and adult reading. *Br J Psychol* 75:329–348, 1984.

166. Beitchman JH, Wilson B, Douglas L, et al.: Substance use disorders in young adults with and without LD: Predictive and concurrent relationships. *J Learn Disabil* 34:317–332, 2001.

167. Beitchman JH, Wilson B, Johnson CJ, et al: Fourteen-year follow-up of speech/language-impaired and control children: Psychiatric outcome. *J Am Acad Child Adolesc Psychiatry* 40:75–82, 2001.

168. Lovett MW: Developmental dyslexia, in Rapin I, Segalowitz SJ (eds): *Handbook of Neuropsychology: Child Neuropsychology*. Amsterdam: Elsevier 1992, vol 7, pp 163–185.

169. Lovett MW: Defining and remediating the core deficits of developmental dyslexia: Lessons from remedial outcome research with reading disabled children, in Klein R, McMullen P (eds): *Converging Methods for Understanding Reading and Dyslexia*. Cambridge, MA: MIT Press, 1999, pp 111–132.

170. Foorman BR, Francis DJ, Winikates D, et al: Early interventions for children with reading disabilities. *Sci Stud Reading* 1:255–276, 1997.

171. Scanlon DM, Vellutino FR: A comparison of the instructional backgrounds and cognitive profiles of poor, average, and good readers who were initially identified as at risk for reading failure. *Sci Stud Reading* 1:191–216, 1997.

172. Lovett MW, Steinbach KA: The effectiveness of remedial programs for reading disabled children of different ages: Is there decreased benefit for older children? *Learn Disabil Q* 20:189–210, 1997.

173. Wise BW, Olson RK: Computer-based phonological awareness and reading instruction. *Ann Dyslexia* 45:99–122, 1995.

174. Wise BW, Ring J, Olson RK: Training phonological awareness with and without explicit attention to articulation. *J Exp Child Psychol* 72:271–304, 1999.

175. Wise BW, Ring J, Sessions L, et al: Phonological awareness with and without articulation: A preliminary study. *Learn Disabil Q* 20:211–225, 1997.

176. Torgesen JK, Wagner RK, Rashotte CA: Approaches to the prevention and remediation of phonologically-based reading disabilities, in Blachman BA (ed), *Foundations of Reading Acquisition and Dyslexia: Implications for Early Intervention*. Mahwah, NJ: Erlbaum, 1997, pp. 287–304.

177. Moats LC, Foorman BR: Components of effective reading instruction. *Sci Stud Reading* 1:187–189, 1997.

178. Lovett MW, Ransby MJ, Barron RW: Treatment, subtype, and word type effects in dyslexic children's response to remediation. *Brain Lang* 34:328–349, 1988.

179. Lovett MW, Ransby MJ, Hardwick N, et al: Can dyslexia be treated? Treatment-specific and generalized treatment effects in dyslexic children's response to remediation. *Brain Lang* 37:90–121, 1989.

180. Lovett MW, Warren-Chaplin PM, Ransby MJ, et al: Training the word recognition skills of reading disabled children: Treatment and transfer effects. *J Educ Psychol* 82:769–780, 1990.

181. Levin BE: Organizational deficits in dyslexia: Possible frontal lobe dysfunction. *Dev Neuropsychol* 6:95–110, 1990.

182. Swanson HL: Reading comprehension and working memory in learning-disabled readers: Is the phonological loop more important than the exdecutive system? *J Exp Child Psychol* 72:1–31, 1999.

183. Swanson HL, Alexander JE: Cognitive processes as predictors of word recognition and reading comprehension in learning-disabled and skilled readers: Revisiting the specificity hypothesis. *J Educ Psychol* 89:128–158, 1997.

184. Benson NJ: Analysis of specific deficits: Evidence of transfer in disabled and normal readers following oral-motor awareness training. *J Educ Psychol* 92:646–658, 2000.

185. Benson NJ, Lovett MW, Kroeber CL: Training and transfer-of-learning effects in disabled and normal readers: Evidence of specific deficits. *J Exp Child Psychol* 64:343–366, 1997.

186. Engelmann S, Bruner EC: *Reading Mastery I/II Fast Cycle: Teacher's Guide*. Chicago: Science Research Associates, 1988.

187. Engelmann S, Carnine L, Johnson G: *Corrective Reading: Word Attack Basics, Decoding A*. Chicago: Science Research Associates, 1988.

188. Engelmann S, Johnson G, Carnine L, et al: *Corrective Reading: Decoding Strategies, Decoding B1*. Chicago: Science Research Associates, 1988.

189. Gaskins IW, Downer MA, Gaskins RW: *Introduction to the Benchmark School Word Identification/Vocabulary Development Program*. Media, PA: Benchmark School, 1986.

190. Swanson HL, Hoskyn M: Experimental intervention research on students with learning disabilities: A meta-analysis of treatment outcomes. *Rev Educ Res* 68:277–321, 1998.

191. Lovett MW, Lacerenza L, Borden SL: Putting struggling readers on the PHAST track: A program to integrate phonological and strategy-based remedial reading instruction and maximize outcomes. *J Learn Disabil* 33:458–476, 2000.

192. Wolf M, Miller L, Donnelly K: Retrieval, automaticity, vocabulary elaboration, orthography (RAVE-O): A comprehensive, fluency-based reading intervention program. *J Learn Disabil* 33:375–386, 2000.

193. Wolf M, Goodman G: Speed wizards [computerized reading program]. Tufts University Boston, and Rochester Institute of Technology, Rochester, NY, 1996.

194. Simos PG, Fletcher JM, Bergman E, et al: Dyslexia-specific brain activation profile becomes normal following successful remedial training. *Neurology*. In press.

Chapter 38

MOLECULAR GENETICS OF COGNITIVE DEVELOPMENTAL DISORDERS

James Swanson
John Fossella
Deborah Grady
Robert Moyzis
Pam Flodman
Anne Spence
Michael Posner

Three disorders of childhood with important cognitive developmental components are addressed in this chapter: attention deficit hyperactivity disorder (ADHD), reading disorder (RD), and autistic spectrum disorder (ASD). The phenotypes (behavioral manifestations of these disorders) are discussed in Chaps. 35, 37, and 36, respectively. The cognitive neuroscience approach to understanding both phenotype and genotype (variations in DNA) to these disorders is discussed in a recent report by Posner et al.[1]

A first step in molecular genetic studies of ADHD, RD, and ASD is to find variations in DNA (genotypes) that may be associated with and linked to behavior of individuals with these psychopathologies (phenotypes). Two approaches are generally used to accomplish this: the genome scan approach and the candidate gene approach. The candidate gene approach starts with a hypothesis about a specific gene at a known chromosomal location, perhaps suggested by theories of the biological basis of etiology or treatment of the condition under investigation, and then tests whether a specific genotype is statistically associated with the disorder. The genome scan does not make such an assumption but instead starts with genetic markers spread across the entire genome and attempts to locate chromosomal regions by statistical methods (e.g., by finding markers that are shared at a greater-than-chance rate by affected relatives and thus are likely to be in chromosome regions harboring genes associated with and linked to the disorder). In general, the genome scan ap-

proach is most useful if the underlying genes are few, and their effect on predisposing risk is large. On the other hand, the candidate gene approach is more sensitive if the number of predisposing genes is large, and/or their individual effect on risk is small.

In this chapter, we present sections on some typical methods that are used to specify phenotypes of ADHD, RD, and ASD and some example methods used to specify genotypes used to investigate these disorders. Next we provide a brief review of quantitative statistical genetic methods that have been used to suggest a strong genetic basis for these three disorders. Then we will present a selective review of the literature of molecular genetic studies of ADHD, RD, and ASD, which fortunately provides excellent examples of candidate gene and genome scan approaches used to investigate genotype-phenotype relationships. Finally, we discuss the recent findings in each area that may point to important directions for future investigation of the genetics of cognitive developmental disorders.

PHENOTYPES OF ADHD, RD, AND ASD

One way in which phenotypes of ADHD, RD, and ASD have been specified is through clinical diagnosis of a psychiatric disorder. The criteria for clinical diagnoses are provided in the fourth edition of the American Psychiatric Association's *Diagnostic and Statistical Manual* (DSM-IV).[2] DSM-IV uses a categorical classification system that separates "mental" disorders into types based on consensus criteria (defining features) that are hierarchically organized. ADHD, RD, and ASD are classified as "Disorders Usually First Diagnosed in Infancy, Childhood, or Adolescence," which imposes a broad and overarching early age-of-onset criterion. This section of DSM-IV distinguishes 10 classes, each with multiple disorders having some common qualifying features: Mental Retardation, Learning Disorders (where RD is placed), Motor Skills Disorders, Communication Disorders, Pervasive Developmental Disorders (where ASD is placed), Attention-Deficit and Disruptive Behavior Disorders (where ADHD is placed), Feeding and Eating Disorders, Tic Disorders, Elimination Disorders, and Other Disorders. The DSM-IV criteria for ADHD, RD, and ASD are shown in Table 38-1.

The DSM-IV approach has an emphasis on phenomenology, not etiologies (which for psychiatric disorders are still treated as unknowns), and on reliability, not validity of diagnoses. DSM-IV is a categorical system, with diagnosis (classification) based on the presence of abnormal patterns of behavior assumed to be qualitatively different from the pattern of normal behavior in the population. This is appropriate

Table 38-1

DSM-IV criteria for three cognitive developmental disorders

ADHD (DSM-IV, pp. 78–85):
    (a) age-inappropriate levels of inattention and/or impulsivity/hyperactivity (at least 6 of 9 symptoms present in one or both domains)
    (b) onset by the age of 7 years
    (c) impairment in two or more settings
    (d) interference with appropriate functioning
    (e) not better accounted for by other psychiatric disorders

RD (DSM-IV, pp. 48–50):
    (a) a discrepancy between ability and achievement
    (b) significant impairment in activities that require reading
    (c) difficulties not solely due to a sensory deficit

ASD (DSM-IV, pp. 66–71):
    (a) impaired social interaction
    (b) impaired language used in social communication
    (c) restricted patterns of behavior

when the boundaries between classes are clear, when the classes are mutually exclusive, and when within-class homogeneity is high. For ADHD, RD, and ASD, these conditions may not hold, so the use of the categorical system of DSM-IV and the qualitative psychiatric diagnoses that it generates may not be optimal for specifying phenotypes to be used in genetic investigations. Dimensional descriptions of phenotypes of these cognitive developmental disorders have been used, based on quantification of attributes that are distributed continuously and do not have clear boundaries to define separate categories of psychopathology.

A typical way to provide a quantitative description of a disorder is to use rating scales to obtain a subjective impression of the degree of behavior that defines or underlies the disorder. For example, in the assessment of ADHD, two rating scales are freely available on the Internet: the Swanson, Nolan, and Pelham (SNAP) scale of Swanson et al.[3] and the Strengths and Difficulties Questionnaire (SDQ) of Goodman et al.[4] The SNAP (*www.ADHD.net*) asks for ratings of the degree of psychopathology defined by the 18 DSM-IV symptoms of ADHD, using a scale of 0 to 3 (e.g., not at all = 0, just a little = 1, pretty much = 2, and very much = 3). The SDQ (*www.sdqinfo.com*) asks for ratings of the presence of 30 common behavioral and emotional difficulties of childhood, 5 of which are designated as ADHD items, using a scale of 0 to 2 (not present = 0, present = 1, or very much present = 2). For both the SNAP and SDQ, the sum of the ADHD items or the average rating per item assigns a severity score that can be used as a quantitative phenotype of ADHD. There are many commercial versions of ADHD rating scales available. Tharpar et al.[5] provide a recent review of the quantitative phenotype of ADHD.

For the assessment of ASD, the Autism Screening Questionnaire (ASQ), also known as the Social Communication Questionnaire (SCQ), is a 40-item screening instrument based on DSM-IV criteria and the Autism Diagnostic Interview-Revised.[6,7] The SCQ is not available on the Internet. The Checklist for Autism in Toddlers (CHAT) also provides a quantitative description of ASD for screening at 18 months of age,[6] based on five items about simple pretend play and joint attention that are assessed by parental report and direct testing. Baird et al.[7] provide a review of a variety of instruments that have been used to define the quantitative phenotypes of ASD.

In the assessment of RD, scores on psychometric tests (e.g., the discrepancy between IQ and achievement test scores) are part of the criteria for RD and provide a quantitative description of the disorder. In fact, IQ-achievement discrepancy cutoffs are specified in psychiatric manuals[2,8] and educational laws and regulations.[9] The current view is that the distribution of IQ-reading achievement discrepancies is smooth and normal, suggesting a quantitative, not qualitative, phenotype that places an individual on a continuum not in a category (see Ref. 10). However, the use of an IQ-achievement discrepancy has been questioned and the use of low achievement alone has been suggested as an alternative.[11] In some molecular genetic studies of RD, composite reading scores rather than discrepancy scores have been used.[12] Furthermore, multidimensional phenotypes of RD have been proposed that are not directly related to the DSM or IDEA criteria for diagnoses, based on auditory (phonologic awareness) and visual (orthographic decoding) processes, and these phenotypes have been used in molecular genetic studies of RD (e.g., Ref. 13). Schulte-Korne[14] provides a recent review that includes discussion of methods to define quantitative phenotypes of RD.

BEHAVIORAL (QUANTITATIVE) GENETICS

Family and twin studies of ADHD, ASD, and RD have been conducted and provide evidence of genetic bases of these disorders. These studies capitalize on the statistical properties of relatives, which can be used to evaluate whether individuals who are exposed to similar genetic factors have similar phenotypes. For example, the coefficient of relationship (R) shows the proportion of alleles shared identical-by-descent from one relative to another (or from a common ancestor). For monozygotic twins, R = 1 and for dizygotic twins R = $\frac{1}{2}$. For first-degree relatives (parent-offspring, full siblings), R = $\frac{1}{2}$; for second-degree relatives (uncles, aunts), R = $\frac{1}{4}$; for third-degree relatives (first grandparents, cousins), R = 1/8 and so on (fourth degree, R = 1/16; fifth degree, R = 1/32; etc.). Thus, relatives of an individual with a disorder (e.g., ADHD, RD, or

ASD) can be chosen who share genotypes to a different degree (100 percent, 50 percent, 25 percent, 12.5 percent, etc.). Two important statistical terms are used to describe the results of family and twin studies of the genetics of ADHD, RD, and ASD: relative or recurrence risk (RR) and heritability (h^2).

To estimate RR, the population prevalence of the disorder and the prevalence of the disorder in different classes of relatives of the affected individual are obtained. Then, RR ratios (lambdas) are used to estimate the risks to relatives with different degrees of genetic relationship. Heritability (h^2) is defined as the ratio of genetic variance to phenotypic variance, but in a twin study it can be estimated from the observed correlation of phenotype and genotype in two types of twins (identical or monozygotic and fraternal or dizygotic). In a twin study, the genotypic correlation for monozygotic twins (1.0) and dizygotic twins (0.5) is known, and the correlations of phenotype across sets of the two types of twin pairs can be estimated. The difference in the correlations of the groups composed of monozygotic or dizygotic is used to estimate heritability: $h^2 = 2(r_{mz} - r_{dz})$. Even though heritabilty may change in different settings or for different measures of the phenotype, it is used as a way to estimate the percentage of total variation in the phenotype that may be due to genetic factors (whatever they might be).

Many family, twin, and adoption studies have been conducted to investigate the behavioral genetics of ADHD, RD, and ASD. For all three of these cognitive developmental disorders, estimates of lambda and h^2 are high and suggest that genetic factors play a large role in the etiologies of these disorders. Reviews of these studies are provides by Stevenson[15] and Faraone et al.[16] for ADHD, Pennington[17] and Schulte-Korne[14] for RD, and Smalley et al.[18] and Bailey et al.[19] for ASD.

These studies firmly establish that genetic factors play an important role in determining phenotype, but specific genetic factors are not uncovered by behavioral or quantitative genetic methods. Molecular genetic methods have this purpose, and some background on molecular genetics is provided in the next section.

Candidate gene studies are evaluated by simple statistical methods. For a population-based design, DNA is obtained from a group of affected probands and an unaffected (or randomly selected) control group. The prevalence of alleles (or a genotype) of the candidate gene are compared for the two groups, and a simple chi-square test is used to determine if the difference is statistically significant. In a family-based design, DNA is obtained from parents of the group of affected probands as well as from the affected probands. An initial step is to determine which two alleles (or genotype) were transmitted and which two were not transmitted to the child. For example, for four parental alleles (two for each parent), one allele from each parent (two of the four) are transmitted to the proband. The Transmission Disequilibrium Test (TDT) is used to determine whether the risk allele is "transmitted" more frequently than expected by chance in the group of affected probands. The alleles not transmitted represent a theoretical control group. A chi-square statistic is used to estimate if the candidate allele (or genotype) is prepresented at a greater-than-chance prevalence in the sample of affected probands. It is assumed that the actual transmission rate at meiosis is .5, but that the condition probability of having the disorder and being in the clinical group of affected probands is increased if the candidate allele increases risk for the disorder (or is close to a gene that does, and thus is in "linkage disequilibrium" with a risk allele).

Genome scan studies evaluate the marker alleles spread across the human genome. In an affected sibling design, families are recruited that have two children with the same disorder. DNA from the affected sib pair is used to determine the alleles present in markers spread across the genome. If the marker and the as-yet-unknown risk gene are far apart, then it is likely that recombination events over time would have separated them, but if they are close together, then recombination would be unlikely. The likehood of the observed data given linkage and nonlinkage are calculated, and the ratio is calculated. The logarithm of this ratio, labeled the "LOD" score, reflects the probability of linkage. A LOD score of 3.0 is typically required to confirm linkage. This represents 1000 to 1 odds of a chance occurrence, and it protects against false positive findings associated with the large number of markers and tests performed.

While genome scans are a useful tool for identifying DNA regions containing a major predisposing gene (for example the Huntington gene), they are less useful for complex genetic disorders, especially using reasonable sample sizes. In general, regions meet-ing the minimum acceptance for statistical significance (> LOD 3) have been difficult to find in studies of ADHD, ASD, and RD (Risch et al., 2000; Fisher et al., 2002).

MOLECULAR BIOLOGY

The starting point for the molecular genetic studies is the analysis of DNA, which is coiled up in long strings in the 46 chromosomes (23 pairs) in the nuclei of most cells. The basic building blocks of DNA are the four bases: adenine (A) and guanine (G) and cytosine (C) and thymine (T). When attached to a deoxyribose (sugar) and phosphate group, these bases form a nucleotide. Nucleotides have chemical properties that result in specific pairing of a "long" (A or G) and a "short" (C or T) base to a "base-pair" (bp). A long double string of bp forms Watson and Crick's famous double-helix structure. The length of a DNA string is measured in thousands of bp, or kilobases (kb). The 23 pairs of chromosomes are numbered based on length, from chromosome 1 (about 250,000 kp) to chromosome 22 (about 50,000 bp), plus the sex chromosomes X (about 100,000 kb) and Y (about 50,000 kb).

A gene is a segment of DNA that provides the code for a protein. A series of events occurs to build a protein from a gene. First, the double-stranded DNA unravels and the paired nucleotides separate into two complementary single strands. These single strands are translated into RNA. The specific order of the sequence in the single-stranded RNA provides a code for amino acids (the building block for proteins). Three nucleotides (triplets) are required to specify an amino acid. However, the four nucleotides taken three at a time can code for 64 different triplets, but there are only 20 amino acids incorporated into proteins. So, this is a redundant code, with 64 different triplets coding for one of 20 amino acids. The amino acids specified by the sequence of nucleotides are themselves chained together to form proteins.

Most of the 3 million kb of DNA in the human genome is "noncoding." The coding segments (genes) are spread out across each chromosome. Finding and counting genes was one of the primary purpose of the Human Genome Project (HGP), which identified far fewer (about 30,000 genes) than expected.[20,21] Even in a gene, not all of the DNA is used. The entire stretch is segregated into exons (which are used) and introns (which are not used). In the process of making a protein, the introns are cut out and the exons are joined to specify the final DNA sequence that provides the nucleotide code for a protein.

Although individuals have the same nucleotide sequence for 99 percent or more of the human genome, there are individual differences (polymorphisms) at many points in human DNA. Polymorphisms occur in the DNA segments comprising genes that build proteins (coding regions) as well as in the DNA segments that do not (noncoding regions). The polymorphisms in the noncoding regions of the human genome are used as markers in the genome scan studies (described below). The polymorphisms in the coding regions are used to specify genetic bases for structural differences in proteins of the body, and these are preferred (although not exclusively used) for specifying genotypes in candidate gene studies (also described below).

For particular locations on the human genome, DNA differences are called alleles. Some background is provided here about three methods for determining differences in DNA at a particular locus: SNPs, RFLPs, and VNTRs. At some loci, DNA varies across individuals at single points (nucleotides), and these differences are called single nucleotide polymorphisms (SNPs). Often, these single points can be detected by restriction enzymes that recognize and "cut" the DNA sequence into short or long fragments. These differences across individuals are called restriction fragment length polymorphisms (RFLPs). In some regions of chromosomes, a specific nucleotide sequence repeats, and the number of repeats varies across individuals. The length of the repeat sequence can be used to specify the number of repeats of the sequence in the variable number of tandem repeats (VNTRs).

MOLECULAR GENETICS OF ADHD, RD, AND ASD

ADHD and Candidate Gene Studies

The family and twin studies of ADHD (see above) stimulated molecular genetic studies to search for allelic variations of specific genes that are associated with this disorder. The initial investigations used the candidate gene approach (described above), and the following brief review of molecular genetic studies of ADHD provides excellent examples of the successful use of this approach. The candidate gene approach was based on two theories of ADHD: (1) the dopamine deficit theory of ADHD,[22,23] which suggests why the stimulant medications that are considered to be DA agonists (methylphenidate and amphetamine) are so effective for the treatment of this disorder, and (2) the neuroanatomic network theory of attention,[24] which suggests how DA is involved in the component processes of attention (alerting, orienting, and executive control). The candidate gene studies of ADHD have focused on two dopamine genes whose locations were known: the dopamine transporter (DAT) gene on chromosome 5 (5p15.3) and the dopamine receptor type 4 (DRD4) gene on chromosome 11 (11p15.5).

The DAT1 gene has a polymorphism (a 40-bp VNTR) in the 3′ noncoding region of the gene. In the human population, the primary allelic variants are defined by 3 repeats (in about 0.01 of alleles), 9 repeats (in about 0.25 of an alleles), or 10 repeats (in about 0.76 of alleles) repeats. Since a primary mechanism of action of methylphenidate is the inhibition of reuptake of DA,[25,26] an overactive DA transporter has been hypothesized as a factor in ADHD, and this suggests a plausible candidate gene based on the site of action of the primary treatment of this disorder.

In a family-based control association study, Cook et al.[27] investigated parent-to-child transmission rates of the DAT1 alleles. They reported an increased transmission of the most prevalent allele (10 repeat) in their ADHD sample. Subsequently, others have replicated this finding,[28,29] but some have not.[30–32] Nonreplication is expected for conditions with observed relative risk <1.5 when small sample sizes (<100) are used. Cook[33] performed a metanalysis that supported the statistical significance of this association.

The DRD4 gene has a polymorphism (a 48-bp VNTR) in a coding region (exon III). The polymorphism (from 2 to 11 repeats) produces differences across individuals in the size of an important region of the receptor (the third intracellular loop, which couples to G proteins and mediates postsynaptic effects). In humans, the allele frequencies of DRD4 vary across ethnic groups, but allele frequencies are well established within ethnic groups. For example, in a sample of 150 unrelated Caucasians (see Ref. 34), the allele frequencies were 0.10 (2R), 0.04 (3R), 0.67 (4R), 0.01 (5R), 0.02 (6R), 0.12 (7R), and 0.04 (8R).

We have described in detail elsewhere[35] why we chose the DRD4 as a candidate gene in our investigations of ADHD. Some contributing factors were that (1) the VNTR is in a coding region of the gene[36]; (2) the neuroanatomic foci of the gene product, D4 receptors, is in cortical areas including the anterior cingulate gyrus, a brain region that plays an important role in normal attention and motivation[24,37]; (3) the relatively less common 7R allele may code for a receptor that is subsensitive to DA,[38] although this is not just due to length[39]; and (4) the DRD4 7R allele is associated with higher-than-normal scores on the personality characteristic of novelty seeking (see Refs. 40 to 42).

Our initial candidate gene study,[43] using a case-control approach, reported that the percentage of DRD4 7R alleles was higher in a sample of ADHD subjects (29 percent) than in an ethnically matched control group (12 percent) (see Fig. 38-1, left). We noted that the percentage of subjects with at least one 7R allele (the 7-present genotype) in the ADHD sample was about 50 percent, which was greater than in the control group (about 20 percent), but that the presence of a 7R allele was not a necessary condition (since about 50 percent of the ADHD cases did not have this allele) or a sufficient condition (since about 20 percent of the non-ADHD cases did). Initial population-based candidate gene studies are always suspect, because for small sample sizes many positive findings turn out to be "false positives."[44] In a subsequent family-based association study of parent-child trios, we[45] replicated the percentage of 7R alleles in the probands (28 percent) and also reported that the transmission rate of the DRD4 7R allele from heterozygous parents to affected children was higher (64 percent) than expected (50 percent). This family-based design discounted the contention that the initial effect was a spurious association due to population stratification. Subsequently, many investigators replicated this finding,[46–49] but as expected for replications using a small sample size, some have not,[50–53] and others have only partially replicated the finding.[54,55]

Since there are so many genes expressed in the brain, it is typically assumed that an initial report of an association with any one gene will be a false positive.[44] However, when multiple replications of the same association are reported with family-based association methods, the assumption of a false-positive association is discounted. This is the case for the associations of the DRD4 and DAT1 genes and ADHD: at last count, over a dozen reports have confirmed these

Figure 38-1
Candidate gene studies of the DRD4 gene and ADHD.

Allele Frequency in ADHD & Control Groups

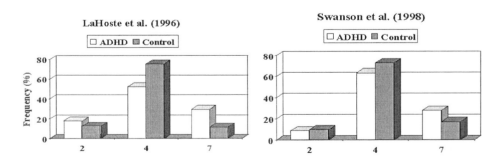

Allele (number of repeats)

associations (see Refs. 33 and 56). In the literature, multiple replications of a candidate gene association for a psychiatric disorder is unusual if not unprecedented.[44] Thus, these initial molecular genetic studies of ADHD provide excellent examples of the successful use of the candidate gene approach.

RD and Quantitative Trait Linkage Studies

The biological descriptions of RD have also capitalized on advances in molecular biology. After twin and family studies documented a genetic influence on RD, several molecular genetic studies converged to identify a chromosome location of specific genes involved. These studies have used a variety of approaches, differing in the ways the study population was ascertained, how the phenotype was defined, and the type of statistical analysis.

Almost 20 years ago, Smith et al.[57] reported linkage to a site on chromosome 15. Others have confirmed and extended this linkage[13,58] based on a variety of phenotypes for RD.

Smith et al.[57] reported linkage to sites on chromosome 6 and Cardon et al.[12] confirmed this using quantitative trait analysis. Others have used somewhat different phenotypes of RD and have failed to document linkage to chromosome 6.[59-61] Nevertheless, others have confirmed and extended linkage to chromosome 6 for a variety of phenotypes of RD.[13,62,63] Thus, three research groups studying five independent populations have found evidence for linkage of reading disability to markers on 6p21.3.

Cardon et al.[12] used reading achievement to define a quantitative trait and selected a candidate region (the HLA region of chromosome 6) to investigate with a set of DNA. markers based on an autoimmune hypothesis of RD.[64] Strong evidence for linkage was reported. Grigorenko et. al.[13] investigating subtypes of RD found linkage in chromosome 6 just for phonological deficits. Gayan et al.[63] claim that 8 DNA markers on chromosome 6 are linked to word recognition, orthographic coding, phonological decoding, and phoneme awareness. Recently, analysis of multiple genome scans has identified another marker for RD on chromosome X.[65]

As reviewed by McGuffin and Martin[66] and by Schulte-Korne,[14] this degree of replication in the investigation of complex disorders is rare, so these studies provides a successful use of linkage analysis to narrow the search for genes involved in RD. The next steps will be to look in the regions on chromosome 6 and 15 to find the genes that may be involved. One approach is to look for candidate genes in these regions that may be related to biological pathways related to visual (orthographic) and auditory (phonologic) processes that are involved in reading.

ASD and Genome Scan Studies

There has been considerable investigation of the molecular genetics of ASD, but instead of the candidate gene approach, most of these studies have used the genome scan approach. Rutter[67] describes the background for molecular genetic studies of ASD and outlines why an affected-sib genome scan approach was favored (i.e., high heritability of ASD, relative small set of genes hypothesized, and reliable and standardized diagnostic methods were available). The widespread interest in ASD led to a multisite international study as well as multiple individual genome scan studies. Two of these are review here: IMGSAC[68] and Risch et al.[69]

The IMGSAC study used an affected sib-pair design with a broad phenotype of ASD. The genotypes used were based on markers spread across the chromosome about every 10 cM. This study[68] showed weak linkage of a marker in chromosome 7 as well as possible sites on five other chromosomes. Risch et al.[69] used affected sib pairs and discordant sib pairs and over 500 anonymous markers in a genome scan and showed only a slight increase in allele sharing in the affected sib pairs (51.6 percent) than discordant sib pairs (50.8 percent). However, only one marker was even moderate in size, and it was on chromosome 1, which was different than the finding of the Consortium study, which identified linkage in a broad region of chromosome 7. This is not unexpected for a condition (such as the broad phenotype of ASD) that may be associated with many genes.

The genetic bases of ASD continue to be the subject of intensive investigations. The lack of vertical transmission initially discounted the genetic basis of ASD, but family, twin, and adoption studies[18,70] revealed a high relative risk to siblings (60 to 100) and high heritability (about 0.9). The broad phenotype was more heritable than the narrow phenotype, suggesting that a categorical disorder of autism was not inherited but rather a range of social and cognitive anomalies. However, the application of the genome scan approach has not produced a clear direction for the next studies. Risch et al.[69] concluded that the next step in the genome scan approach (positional cloning of susceptibility loci) would be a formidable task because no specific region of the human genome was implicated by the genome scans.

NEXT STEPS IN MOLECULAR GENETICS OF ADHD, RD, AND AS

Some very recent studies have set the stage for the next round of molecular genetic studies of cognitive developmental disorders. Two of these are genome scan studies[71] and two are follow-up studies of the DRD4 candidate gene.[72,73]

First, Fisher et al.[71] reported the results of a genome scan for RD that combined prior samples from the United Kingdom[62] and the United States.[12,63] Based on the larger sample and refined statistical methods, this study identified a new region on chromosome 18 that was linked to RD phenotypes based on phonologic and orthographic processing. Second, Fisher et al.[71] reported the results for the first genome scan for ADHD. Based on a quantitative ADHD phenotype (number of ADHD symptoms on a structured psychiatric interview), no chromosome region was identified that exceeded the established significance thresholds, but four regions were identified with less rigorous criteria for linkage on chromosome 5 (5p12), chromosome 10 (10q26), chromosome 12 (12q23), and chromosome 16 (16p13). None of these regions contained the DAT or DRD4 genes that have been shown to be associated with ADHD in the candidate gene studies.

While the Fisher et al. (2002) study could not detect a gene with a lambda < 2–3, what magnitude of risk could one expect for disorders such as ADHD? The DRD4 7R/ADHD association can be used to answer this question, since it is one of the most reproduced in complex behavioral disorders (Swanson et al.[32,35]; Faraone et al.[56]). The approximately twofold risk associated with the DRD4 7R allele and ADHD has been described as "small" (Faraone et al.[56]; Fisher et al.[71]). While a twofold risk may be considered small in some contexts, this risk needs to be put in the perspective of observed DRD4 allele frequencies (Ding et al.[73]) and the predictions of the Common Variant-Common Disorder (CVCD) hypothesis (Zwick et al.[76]). In the CVCD hypothesis, disease-related alleles that are "common," usually defined as a frequency greater than 0.01 (Zwick et al., 2000) are proposed to be predisposing to common disorders, such as ADHD. Indeed, it is hypothesized that the reason these disorders are common is that their predisposing alleles are common (Zwick et al.[76]). The frequency of the DRD4 7R allele varies in different populations (Chang et al., 1996; Ding et al., 2002). In the populations of predominantly European origin used in most investigations of the DRD4/ADHD association (Swanson et al.[32,35]; Faraone et al.[56]), the allele frequency of DRD4 7R is approximately 12–15 percent (Ding et al.[73]). Therefore, even if the presence of a DRD4 7R allele was a necessary predisposing condition for ADHD (i.e., 100 percent of ADHD probands had at least one copy of this allele), and assuming Hardy-Weinberg equilibrium, the increase in observed frequency would be only 3.6-fold, barely detectable using current genome scan approaches. While more extensive genome scans are in the planning stages, involving many more individuals and orders of magnitude more markers (Risch and Merikangas[77]), it is unclear at present when the resources will be available (in terms of families, technologies, and money) to conduct such searches successfully.

Swanson et al.[72] evaluated a small sample of individuals with ADHD who had been genotyped for DRD4 and separated these subjects into subgroups defined by the presence (7R-present) and absence (7R-absent) of the presumed risk allele. The prior association studies were based on allele probabilities, either by contrasting the allele probabilities of the ADHD and control groups or by testing for distortion of the expected parent to proband allele transmission probability of 0.5, but these probabilities do not provide information about possible functional significance of the alleles (or of some linked alleles of other genes responsible for functional differences). Swanson et al.[72] followed up the positive associations with a test for functional differences between candidate genotypes. For the measures of function, a neuropsychological battery of reaction time tests (the Stroop color-word task, the Posner cue-detection task, and the Logan stop-change task) was used; for the candidate DRD4 genotype, subgroups based on the presence or absence of the hypothesized "high risk" 7R allele (7-present versus 7-absent) were used. Thus, genotype was used as an independent variable to evaluate the functional significance of the 7R allele on the quantitative traits of response speed (RT) and variability (SD). It was predicted that the 7-present subgroup (i.e., consisting of those ADHD subjects with at least one 7R allele) would have the greatest impairment, based on the simple hypothesis that the 7R form of the receptor when stimulated by DA would be less likely than other forms to transmit signals and activate brain areas important for attention and motivation.[74,75] However, the performance of 7-present subgroup was not different from that of the control group. Instead, only the 7-absent subgroup showed abnormal performance (longer RT and higher SD). This suggested that the hypothesized "risk" allele may not be associated with a cognitive impairment, even though it is associated with abnormal behavior documented by subjective impressions of symptoms of ADHD.

Finally, Ding et al.[73] showed by DNA resequencing/haplotyping of 600 DRD4 alleles, representing a worldwide population sample, that the origin of 2R through 6R alleles can be explained by simple one-step recombination/mutation events. In contrast, the 7R allele is not simply related to the other common alleles, differing by greater than 6 recombinations/mutations. Strong linkage disequilibrium (LD) was found between the 7R allele and surrounding DRD4 polymorphisms, suggesting this allele is at least 5–10-fold "younger" than the common 4R allele. Based on an observed bias towards nonsynonymous amino acid changes, the unusual DNA sequence organization, and the strong LD surrounding the DRD4 7R allele, Ding et al.[73] proposed that this allele originated as a rare mutational event, that nevertheless increased to high frequency in human populations by positive selection. Ding et al.[73] asked why an allele that appears to have undergone strong positive selection in human populations never-

theless is now disproportionately represented in individuals diagnosed with ADHD? The CVCD hypothesis, discussed above (Zwick et al., 2000) proposes that common genetic variation may be related to common disease, either because the disease is a product of a new environment (so that genotypes associated with the disorder were not eliminated in the past) or the disorder has a small effect on fitness (because it is late onset). For early onset disorders (such as ADHD) Ding et al.[73] suggested the possibility that predisposing alleles are in fact under positive selection, and only result in deleterious effects when combined with other environmental/genetic factors. Thus, it is possible that the very traits that may be selected for individuals possessing a DRD4 7R allele may predispose behaviors that are deemed inappropriate in a classroom setting in certain cultures today, and hence lead to diagnosis of ADHD.

SUMMARY

It is unlikely that RD, ASD, or ADHD are simple Mendelian conditions in which a single gene is the cause of a disorder in individual cases. Instead, it is likely that they are complex conditions for which a set of genes alters the probability of a disorder and individual genes are insufficient to cause a disorder outright.[76] When statistical methods for genome scans that were designed for the investigations of Mendelian diseases (e.g., affected sib-pair designs for detection of linkage) are applied to the study of complex diseases such as ADHD, RD, and ASD (which have low values of relative risk <2.0 and high population prevalence of the putative risk allele >10 percent), very large sample sizes (5000 to 65,000) are required for adequate statistical power.[77] This calls for different designs for molecular genetic investigations of complex disorders, such as candidate gene studies of association that are intended to detect linkage disequilibria. However, even these designs will require much larger sample sizes than usual nongenetic studies of these disorders (e.g., 250 to 1000).

Most alleles associated with complex genetic disorders will be neither necessary nor sufficient to predispose to the disease (as clearly observed for the DRD4 7R allele/ADHD association), since other alleles at an unknown number of genes will be involved as well. Further, we can only guess, based on heritability studies, what fraction of cases have a genetic origin, versus other environmental causes. Therefore, if the CVCD hypothesis is correct, one will never observe anything other than a small increase in risk for a single gene/allele. Indeed, the observed twofold increase in DRD4 7R allele frequency in ADHD probands is approximately 50 percent of the maximum possible (if all ADHD is genetic). It is simple to demonstrate that this allele, in combination with as few as one or two other alleles of a yet unidentified gene (at a comparable frequency), could account for the majority of ADHD cases. Yet neither of these hypothetical genes would be detected in current genome scans, because of their small individual effect on risk. In summary, common alleles associated with a particular disorder are expected to have only modest increase in allele frequency (λ) in affected individuals. This suggests that for the immediate future, candidate gene approaches may be the most sensitive way to identify alleles likely associated with cognitive developmental disorders.

The current plans for the identification of a large number of genetic markers (e.g., 100,000 SNPs— see Ref. 77) for use in molecular genetic studies do not take into consideration why statistical procedures for Mendelian genetics may not be applicable to the study of complex disorders. The power of an anonymous genome scan relying on linkage (i.e., an affected sib-pair study) or linkage disequilibrium (a TDT association study) relies on the ability of the observed phenotype to predict the underlying risk genotypes.[78] Since there are many genotypes that can produce the same phenotype (a many-to-one relationship), the conditional probability of genotype given phenotype would still be low, so mapping approaches may not work or at best have very low power. Instead, Weiss and Terwilliger[79] assert that if association studies use markers that are not causative, then they must be done with several preselected markers per gene that effectively represent the variation in chromosome regions of interest. An understanding of these problems and the use of statistical designs specifically tailored for studies of complex disorders seems essential in molecular genetics of developmental psychopathologies.[80]

REFERENCES

1. Posner MI, Rothbart MK, Farah M, Bruer J: Special issue: The developing human brain. *Develop Sci* 4:253–387, 2001.
2. American Psychiatric Association: *Diagnostic and Statistical Manual of Mental Disorders,* 4th ed (DSM-IV). Washington, DC: APA, 1994.
3. Swanson J: *School-Based Assessments and Interventions for ADD Students.* Irvine, CA: KC Publishing, 1994.
4. Goodman R, Ford T, Simons H, et al: Using the strengths and difficulties questionnaire (SDQ) to screen for child psychiatric disorders in a community sample. *Br J Psychiatry* 177:534–539, 2000.
   Goodman R, Ford T, Simons H, et al: Strengths and difficulties questionnaire (SDQ) (1995). (www.sdqinfo.com)
5. Tharpar A, Harrington R, Ross K, McGuffin P: *J Am Acad Child Adolesc Psychiatry* 39(12):1528–1536, 2000.
6. Robins DL, Fein D, Barton ML, Green JA: The modified checklist for autism in toddlers: An initial study investigating early detection of autism and pervasive developmental disorders. *J Autism Dev Disord* 31(2):131–144, 2001.
7. Baird G, Charman T, Cox A, et al: Screening and surveillance for autism and pervasive developmental disorders. *Arch Dis Child* 84:468–474, 2001.
8. World Health Organization: *International Classification of Diseases.* Geneva: WHO, 1993.
9. IDEA: *Seventeenth Annual Report to Congress on the Implementation of the Individuals with Disabilities Education Act.* Washington, DC: Office of Special Education Program, U.S. Department of Education, 1995.
10. Shaywitz SE, Escobar MD, Shawitz BA, et al: Evidence that dyslexia may represent the lower tail of a normal distribution of reading ability. *N Engl J Med* 326:145–150, 1992.
11. Fletcher JM, Shaywitz SE, Shaywitz BA: Comorbidity of learning and attention disorders: Separate but equal. *Pediatr Clin North Am* 46(5):885–897, 1999.
12. Cardon LR, Smith SD, Fulker DW, et al: Quantitative trait locus for reading disability on chromosome 6. *Science* 266:276–279, 1994.
13. Grigorenko EL, Wood FB, Meyer MS, et al: Susceptibility loci for distinct components of developmental dyslexia on chromosome 6 and 15. *Am J Hum Genet* 60:27–39, 1997.
14. Schulte-Korne G: Annotation: Genetics of reading and spelling disorder. *J Child Psychol Psychiatry* 42:985–997, 2001.

15. Stevenson J: Evidence for a genetic etiology in hyperactivity in children. *Behav Genet* 22:337–344, 1992.

16. Faraone SV, Doyle AE: The nature of heritability of attention-deficit hyperactivity disorder. *Child Adolesc Psychiatr Clin N Am* 10(2):299–316, 2001.

17. Pennington BF, Van Orden GC, Smith SD, et al: Phonological processing skills and deficits in adult dyslexics. *Child Dev* 61:1753–1778, 1990.

18. Smalley SL, Asarnow RF, Spence MA: Autism and genetics: A decade of research. *Arch Gen Psychiatry* 45:953–961, 1988.

19. Bailey A, Phillips W, Rutter M: Autism: Towards an integration of clinical, genetic, neuropsychological, and neurobiological perspectives. *J Child Psychol Psychiatry* 37:89–126, 1996.

20. Venter JC, Adams MD, Myers EW: The sequences of the attention genome. *Science* 291:1304–1351, 2001.

21. International Human Genome Sequencing Consortium. *Nature* 409:860–921, 2001.

22. Wender P: *Minimal Brain Dysfunction in Children.* New York: Wiley Liss, 1971.

23. Levy F: The dopamine theory of attention deficit hyperactivity disorder (ADHD). *Aust NZ J Psychiatry* 25:277–283, 1991.

24. Posner MI, Raichle ME: *Images of Mind.* New York: Scientific American Library, 1994.

25. Volkow ND, Ding YS, Fowler JS, et al: Is methylphenidate like cocaine? Studies on their pharmacokinetics and distribution in the human brain. *Arch Gen Psychiatry* 52:456–463, 1995.

26. Volkow ND, Wang G-J, Fowler JS, et al: Relationship between blockade of dopamine transporters by oral methylphenidate and increases in extracellular dopamine: Therapeutic implications. *Synapse* 43:181–187, 2002.

27. Cook EH, Stein MA, Krasowski MD, et al: Association of attention-deficit disorder and the dopamine transporter gene. *Am J Hum Genet* 56:993–998, 1995.

28. Gill M, Daly G, Heron S, et al: Confirmation of association between attention deficit hyperactivity disorder and a dopamine transporter polymorphism. *Mol Psychiatry* 2:311–313, 1997.

29. Waldman ID, Rowe DC, Abramowitz A, et al: Association and linkage of the dopamine transporter gene and attention-deficit hyperactivity disorder in children: Heterogeneity owing to diagnostic subtype and severity. *Am J Hum Genet* 63(6):1767–1776, 1998.

30. Sunohara G, Swanson JM, Larosa G: Association of dopamine receptor genes in attention deficit hyperactivity disorder. *Am J Hum Genet* 54(Suppl):A4–38, 1996.

31. Castellanos FX, Lau E, Tayebi N, et al: Lack of an association between a dopamine-4 receptor polymorphism and attention-deficit/hyperactivity disorder: Genetic and brain morphometric analysis. *Mol Psychiatry* 3:431–434, 1998.

32. Swanson J, Flodman P, Kennedy J, et al: Dopamine genes and ADHD. *Neurosci Biobehav Rev* 24:21–25, 2000.

33. Cook E: Website, University of Chicago, 2000.

34. Petronis A, Vantol HH, Lichter JB, et al. The D4 dopamine receptor gene maps on 11-p proximal to HRAS. *Genomics* 18(1):161–163, 1993.

35. Swanson JM, Posner M, Fosella J, et al: Genes and ADHD. *Curr Psychiatry Rep* 3:92–100, 2001.

36. Lichter JB, Barr DL, Kennedy JL, et al: A hypervariable segment in the human dopamine receptor D-4 gene. *Hum Mol Genet* 2(6):767–773, 1993.

37. Seeman P: Dopamine receptors and psychosis. *Sci Am Sci Med* 2(5):28–37, 1995.

38. Asghari V, Sanyal S, Buchwaldt S, et al: Modulation of intracellular cyclic AMP levels by different human dopamine D4 receptor variants. *J Neurochem* 65(3):1157–1165, 1995.

39. Jovanic V, Guan HC, Van Tol HH, et al: Comparative pharmacological and functional analysis of the human dopamine D4.2 and D4.10 receptor variants. *Pharmacogenetics* 9:561–568, 1999.

40. Benjamin J, Li L, Patterson C, et al: Population and familial association between the DRD4 gene and measures of novelty seeking. *Nat Genet* 12:81–84, 1996.

41. Ebstein RP, Novick O, et al: Dopamine D4 receptor (D4DR) exon III polymorphism associated with the human personality trait of novelty seeking. *Nat Genet* 12:78–80, 1996.

42. Cloninger CR, Adolfsson R, Svrakic NM: Mapping genes for human personality [news]. *Nat Genet* 12:3–4, 1996.

43. La Hoste GJ, Swanson JM, Wigal SB, et al: Dopamine D4 receptor gene polymorphism is associated with attention deficit hyperactivity disorder. *Mol Psychiatry* 1:121–124, 1996.

44. Crowe RR: Candidate genes in psychiatry: Epidemiological perspective. *Am J Med Genet* 48:74–77, 1993.

45. Swanson JM, Sunohara GA, Kennedy JL, et al: Association of the dopamine receptor D4 (DRD4) gene with a refined phenotype of attention deficit hyperactivity disorder (ADHD): A family-based approach. *Mol Psychiatry* 3:38–41, 1998.

46. Smalley SL, Bailey JN, Palmer CG, et al: Evidence that the dopamine D4 receptor is a susceptibility gene in attention deficit hyperactivity disorder. *Mol Psychiatry* 3:427–430, 1998.

47. Rowe DC, Stever C, Giedinghagen LN, et al: Dopamine DRD4 receptor polymorphism and attention deficit hyperactivity disorder. *Mol Psychiatry* 3:419–426, 1998.

48. Faraone SV, Biederman J, Weiffenbach B, et al: Dopamine D4 gene 7-repeat allele and attention deficit hyperactivity disorder. *Am J Psychiatry* 156:768–770, 1999.

49. Sunohara G, Roberts W, Malone M, et al: Linkage of the dopamine D4 receptor gene and ADHD. *J Am Acad Child Adolesc Psychiatry* 12:1537–1542, 2000.

50. Hawi Z, McCarron M, Kirley A, et al: No association of the dopamine DRD4 receptor (DRD4) gene polymorphism with attention deficit hyperactivity disorder (ADHD) in the Irish population. *Am J Med Genet (Neuropsychiatr Genet)* 96:268–272, 2000.

51. Eisenberg J, Zohar A, Mei-Tal G, et al: A haplotype relative risk study of the dopamine D4 receptor (DRD4) exon III repeat polymorphism and attention deficit hperactivity disorder (ADHD). *Am J Med Genet (Neuropsychiatr Genet)* 96:258–261, 2000.

52. Kotler M, Manor I, Sever Y, et al: Failure to replicate an excess of the long dopamine D4 exon III repeat polymorphism in ADHD in a family-based study. *Am J Med Genet (Neuropsychiatr Genet)* 96:278–281, 2000.

53. Todd RD, Neuman RJ, Lobos EA, et al: Lack of association of dopamine D4 receptor gene polymorphisms with ADHD subtypes in a population of twins. *Am J Med Genet (Neuropsychiatr Genet)* 105:432–438, 2001.

54. Holmes J, Payton A, Barrett J, et al: A family-based case-association study of the dopamine D4 receptor gene and dopamine transporter gene in attention deficit hyperactivity disorder. *Mol Psychiatry* 5:523–530, 2000.

55. Mills J, Curran S, Kent L, et al: ADHD and the DRD4 gene: Evidence of association but no linkage in a UK sample. *Mol Psychiatry* 6:440–444, 2001.

56. Faraone S, Doyle A, Mick E, Biederman J: Meta-analysis of the association between the dopamine D4 gene 7-repeate allele and ADHD. *Am J Psychiatry* 158:1052–1057, 2001.

57. Smith SD, Kimberling WJ, Pennington BF, Lubs HA: Specific reading disability: Identification of an inherited form through linkage analysis. *Science* 219:1345–1347, 1983.

58. Morris DW, Robinson L, Turic D, et al: Family-based association mapping provides evidence for a gene for reading disability on chromosome 15q. *Hum Mol Genet* 22:843–848, 2000.

59. Schulte-Korne G, Nothen MM, Muller-Myhsok B, et al: Evidence of linkage of spelling disability to chromosome 15. *Am J Hum Genet* 63:279–282, 1998.

60. Field LL, Kaplan BJ: Absence of linkage of phonological coding dyslexia to chromosome 6p23-p21.3 in a large family data set. *Am J Hum Genet* 63:1448–1456, 1998.

61. Petryshen TL, Kaplan BJ, Liu MF, Field LL: Absence of significant linkage between phonological coding dyslexia and chromosome 6p23-21.3, as determined by use of quantitative-trait methods: Confirmation of qualitative analyses. *Am J Hum Genet* 66:708–714, 2000.

62. Fisher SE, Marlow AJ, Lamb J, et al: A genome-wide search strategy for identifying quantitative trait loci involved in reading and spelling disability (developmental dyslexia). *Am J Hum Genet* 64:146–156, 1999.

63. Gayan J, Smith SD, Cherny SS, et al: Quantitative-trait locus for specific language and reading deficits on chromosome 6p. *Am J Hum Genet* 64:157–184, 1999.

64. Gilger JW, Pennington BF, DeFries JC: A twin study of the etiology of comorbidity: Attention deficit hyperactivity disorder and dyslexia. *J Am Acad Child Adolesc Psychiatry* 31:343–348, 1992.

65. Fisher SE, Francks C, Marlow AJ, et al: Independent genome scans identify a chromosome 18 quantitative locus influencing dyslexia. *Nat Genet* 30:86–91, 2002.

66. McGuffin P, Martin NS: Science, medicine and the future: Behaviour and genes. *Br Med J* 319:37–40, 1999.

67. Rutter M: Genetic studies of autism: From the 1970s into the millennium. *J Abnorm Child Psychol* 28:3–14, 2000.

68. International Molecular Genetic Study of Autism Consortium (IMGSAC): A full genome scan for autism with evidence for linkage on chromosome 7q. *Hum Mol Genet* 7:571–578, 1998.

69. Risch N, Spiker D, Lotspeich L, et al: A genome screen of autism: Evidence for a multilocus etiology. *Am J Hum Genet* 65:493–507, 1999.

70. Fostein S, Rutter M: Infantile autism: A genetic study of 21 twin pairs. *J Child Psychol Psychiatry* 18:297–321, 1977.

71. Fisher SE, Francks C, McCracken JT, et al: A genomewide scan for loci involved in ADHD. *Am J Hum Genet* 70:000-000, 2002.

72. Swanson J, Oosterlaan J, Murias M, et al: Attention deficit/hyperactivity disorder children with a 7-repeat allele of the dopamine receptor D4 gene have extreme behavior but normal performance on critical neurpsychological tests of attention. *Proc Natl Acad Sci U S A* 97:4754–4759, 2000.

73. Ding YC, Chi HC, Grady DL, et al: Evidence of positive selection acting at the human dopamine receptor D4 gene locus. *Proc Natl Acad Sci USA* 99(1):309–324, 2002.

74. Swanson JM, Sergeant JA, Taylor E, et al. *Lancet* 351: 429–433, 1998.

75. Swanson JM, Deutsch C, Cantwell D, et al: Genes and ADHD. *Clin Neurosci Res* 1:207–216, 2001.

76. Zwick M, Cutler DJ, Chakravarti A: *Annu Rev Genomics Hum Genet* 1:387–407, 2000.

77. Risch N, Merikangas K: The future of genetic studies of complex human diseases [see comments]. *Science* 273:1516–1517, 1996.

78. Terwilliger JD, Weiss KM: Linkage disequilibrium mapping of complex disease: Fantasy or reality? *Curr Opin Biotechnol* 9:578–594, 1998.

79. Weiss KM, Terwilliger JD. Commentary: How many diseases do you have to study to map one gene with SNPs? *Nat Genet* 26(2):151–157, 2000.

80. Terwilliger JD, Goring HH: Gene mapping in the 20th and 21st centuries: Statistical methods, data analysis, and experimental design. *Hum Biol* 72:63–132.

GLOSSARY OF LINGUISTIC TERMS*

Affix A MORPHEME that must be attached to another morpheme. Also known as a bound morpheme. Prefixes attach to the beginning of a morpheme (e.g., *re-* in *redefine*), and suffixes attach to the end of a morpheme (e.g., *-er* in *worker*).

Case A set of affixes or word forms that are used to distinguish the roles of nouns. For example, in English, *I, me,* and *my* have different cases.

Categorical perception The phenomenon whereby a continuous change in a physical characteristic of a speech signal is perceived discontinuously. For example, "ba" and "pa" differ in voice onset time (VOT). If one starts with a "ba" and gradually increases VOT, English speakers find it difficult to detect any change until a categorical boundary is reached. When the categorical boundary is crossed, subjects' perception of the sound suddenly switches from voiced (ba) to unvoiced (pa).

Closed class word See FUNCTION WORD.

Content word A word that has lexical meaning (SEMANTIC content). Examples include nouns, verbs, adjectives, and adverbs. Because new lexical words such as *modem* or *fax* can freely be invented (i.e., the number of possible lexical words is infinite), lexical words are sometimes referred to as OPEN CLASS WORDS.

Discourse The organization of continuous stretches of language larger than a sentence in a conversation or text.

Function word or functor A word or bound morpheme whose role is strictly or mostly to signal grammatical relationships. Examples include

INFLECTIONS, conjunctions, articles, auxiliary verbs, and pronouns. A given language has a limited and finite number of functors and, hence, function words are sometimes referred to as CLOSED CLASS WORDS or closed class morphemes.

Inflection Refers to affixes that signal grammatical relationships such as plural, past tense, progressive tense, and possession (in English, *-s, -ed, -ing,* and *'s,* respectively).

Lexical access The process of looking words up in one's lexicon (mental dictionary).

Lexical decision In psycholinguistic experiments, subjects are sometimes asked to decide whether a string or letters (or sounds) is a word in their language. For example, subjects might be presented English words such as "table" and nonwords such as "bivel." Because the only way to determine that "table" is a word and "bivel" is not a word is to determine whether they are in one's lexicon, lexical decision tasks are used to study LEXICAL ACCESS.

Morpheme The minimal distinctive unit of meaning that can be combined to form words. Morphemes can be bound (see AFFIX) or free (able to appear by themselves).

Morphology The branch of linguistics that investigates the form or structure of words and the processes and rules that govern the ways in which MORPHEMES are combined.

Open class word See CONTENT WORD.

Orthography The writing system of a language.

Phoneme The minimal unit of the sound system of a language that can be used to signal a potential

* Prepared by Karin Stromswold.

difference in meaning. For example, /b/ and /p/ are phonemes in English because there are minimal pairs of words such as /bat/ and /pat/ and /cab/ and /cap/ that differ only in whether a /b/ or a /p/ is present.

Phonemic awareness The awareness that words and morphemes are composed of PHONEMES. Specifically, phonemic awareness refers to the ability to break words into their component phonemes (e.g., /bat/ → /b/ + /a/ + /t/), report the number of syllables in a word, report whether a particular phoneme appears in a word, etc.

Phonology The branch of linguistics that studies the sound systems of languages, including the sounds that are used in a language and the way these sounds may be combined.

Pragmatics The branch of linguistics that investigates phenomena associated with the use of the language by individuals. Of particular interest is the constraints that people encounter when they use language in social settings and the effect their language has on the people with whom they are talking.

Prosody The overall sound pattern or contour of a word or sentence, including pitch, loudness, tempo, and rhythm.

Semantics The branch of linguistics that studies meaning in language.

Syntax The branch of linguistics that studies the grammar of language, particularly the rules that govern the way words combine to form sentences.

Thematic role A term used for semantic roles such as agent, patient, location, source, or goal. For example, in the sentence *John eats spaghetti, John* is the agent and *spaghetti* is the patient. In Government Binding Theory, every argument is given a particular thematic role by its predicate. Thematic roles are drawn from a universal set of thematic relations.

CONTRIBUTORS

Geoffrey Karl Aguirre, M.D., Ph.D.
University of Pennsylvania
Center for Cognitive Neuroscience
Philadelphia, Pennsylvania

Michael P. Alexander, M.D.
Departments of Neurology
Beth Israel Deaconess Medical Center
    and Harvard Medical School
Boston, Massachusetts
Stroke Rehabilitation, Youville Lifecare Hospital
Cambridge, Massachusetts
Memory Disorders Research Center
Boston University School of Medicine
Rotman Research Institute
Baycrest Geriatric Centre
Toronto, Canada

Roderick W. Barron, Ph.D.
Professor, Department of Psychology
University of Guelph
Guelph, Ontario, Canada

Russell M. Bauer, Ph.D.
Professor, Associate Chair for Academic Affairs
Department of Clinical and Health Psychology
University of Florida
Gainesville, Florida

Kathleen Baynes, Ph.D.
Associate Professor of Neurology
University of California at Davis
Davis, California

D. Frank Benson, M.D.[*]
Augustus S. Rose Professor Emeritus of Neurology
University of California at Los Angeles
Los Angeles, California

Matthias Brand, Ph.D.
University of Bielefeld
Department of Physiological Psychology
Bielefeld, Germany

Anjan Chatterjee, M.D.
Department of Neurology
    and the Center for Cognitive Neuroscience
University of Pennsylvania
Philadelphia, Pennsylvania

Nomita Chhabildas
Department of Psychology
University of Denver
Denver, Colorado

H. Branch Coslett, M.D.
Department of Neurology
    and the Center for Cognitive Neuroscience
University of Pennsylvania
Philadelphia, Pennsylvania

Antonio R. Damasio, M.D.
M.W. Van Allen Professor and Head of Neurology
University of Iowa Hospitals and Clinics
Iowa City, Iowa

[*]Deceased

Hanna Damasio, M.D.
Professor of Neurology
University of Iowa Hospitals and Clinics
Iowa City, Iowa

Stanislas Dehaene, Ph.D.
Director, Cognitive Neuroimaging Unit
INSERM (The French Institute of Health and Medical Research)
Service Hospitalier Frédéric Joliot
Orsay, France

Maureen Dennis, Ph.D.
Institute of Medical Science, Department of Psychology
University of Toronto
Hospital for Sick Children
Toronto, Ontario, Canada

Leon Y. Deouell, M.D., Ph.D.
Helen Willis Neuroscience Institute
University of California, Berkeley
Berkeley, California

Martha J. Farah, Ph.D.
Professor of Psychology
   and Director, Center for Cognitive Neuroscience
University of Pennsylvania
Philadelphia, Pennsylvania

Todd E. Feinberg, M.D.
Chief
Betty and Morton Yarmon Division of
   Neurobehavior and Alzheimer's Disease
Associate Attending, Psychiatry and Neurology
Beth Israel Medical Center
New York, New York
Associate Professor, Neurology and Psychiatry
Albert Einstein College of Medicine
Bronx, New York

Ruth B. Fink, M.A.
Moss Rehabilitation Research Institute
Philadelphia, Pennsylvania

Pam Flodman, M.S., M.Sc.
Department of Human Genetics and Birth Defects
University of California, Irvine
Irvine, California

John Fossella, Ph.D.
Sackler Institute for Developmental Psychobiology
Department of Psychiatry
Weill Medical College of Cornell University
New York, New York

Karl J. Friston, M.D.
Head, Functional Imaging Laboratory
Institute of Neurology
University College London
London, England

Albert M. Galaburda, M.D.
Emily Fisher Landau Professor of Neurology and Neuroscience
Harvard Medical School
Chief, Division of Behavioral Neurology
Beth Israel-Deaconess Medical Center
Boston, Massachusetts

Michael S. Gazzaniga, Ph.D.
Director, Center for Cognitive Neuroscience
Dartmouth College
Hanover, New Hampshire

Joseph T. Giacino, Ph.D.
Associate Director, Neuropsychology
JFK Medical Center
Edison, New Jersey
Assistant Professor
Seton Hall University
Department of Neuroscience
South Orange, New Jersey
Clinical Assistant Professor
Department of Physical Medicine and Rehabilitation
University of Medicine and Dentistry of New Jersey
Robert Wood Johnson Medical School
New Brunswick, New Jersey

Georg Goldenberg, M.D.
Neuropsychologische Abteilung
Krankenhaus Munchen-Bogenhausen
Munich, Germany

Deborah Grady, Ph.D.
Department of Biological Chemistry
University of California, Irvine
Irvine, California

Murray Grossman, M.D.
Associate Professor
Department of Neurology
Hospital of the University of Pennsylvania
Philadelphia, Pennsylvania

Kenneth M. Heilman, M.D.
The James D. Rooks Jr. Distinguished Professor of Neurology
  and Health Psychology
University of Florida
Program Director and Chief, NF/SG VAMC
Gainesville, Florida

Richard B. Ivry, Ph.D.
Department of Psychology
University of California, Berkeley
Berkeley, California

Diane M. Jacobs, Ph.D.
Assistant Professor of Clinical Neuropsychology
Department of Neurology
Columbia University College of Physicians and Surgeons
New York, New York

Julene K. Johnson, Ph.D.
Institute for Brain Aging and Dementia
University of California at Irvine
Irvine, California

Margaret M. Keane, Ph.D.
Associate Professor
Department of Psychology
Wellesley College
Wellesley, Massachusetts

Robert T. Knight, M.D.
Department of Psychology
  and the Helen Willis Neuroscience Institute
University of California, Berkeley
Berkeley, California

Gilberto Levy, M.D.
Associate Research Scientist
Gertrude H. Sergievsky Center
Columbia University
New York, New York

Maureen W. Lovett, Ph.D.
Senior Scientist, Brain and Behavior Program
Director, Learning Disabilities Research Program
Hospital for Sick Children
Professor of Pediatrics and Psychology
University of Toronto
Toronto, Ontario, Canada

Karen Marder, M.D., M.P.H.
Associate Professor of Neurology
Gertrude H. Sergievsky Center
Columbia University College of Physicians and Surgeons
New York, New York

Hans J. Markowitsch, Ph.D.
Department of Physiological Psychology
University of Bielefeld
Bielefeld, Germany

Carrie R. McDonald, Ph.D.
University of Florida
Gainesville, Florida

Regina McGlinchey-Berroth, Ph.D.
Department of Veterans Affairs Medical Center
West Roxbury, Massachusetts

Mario F. Mendez, M.D., Ph.D.
Professor of Neurology and Psychiatry
  and Biobehavioral Sciences
UCLA School of Medicine
Los Angeles, California

Jessica A. Meyer
University of Miami
Miami, Florida

William Milberg, Ph.D.
Department of Veterans Affairs Medical Center
West Roxbury, Massachusetts

Bruce L. Miller, M.D.
A.W. & Mary Margaret Clausen Distinguished Chair
Professor of Neurology
Clinical Director, Memory and Aging Center
University of California at San Francisco
San Francisco, California

Nancy J. Minshew, M.D.
Associate Professor
Department of Psychiatry and Neurology
University of Pittsburgh School of Medicine
Pittsburgh, Pennsylvania

Robert Moyzis, Ph.D.
Professor
Department of Biological Chemistry
University of California, Irvine
Irvine, California

Alvaro Pascual-Leone, M.D., Ph.D.
Associate Professor of Neurology
Harvard Medical School
Director of Research at the Behavioral Neurology Unit
Beth Israel Deaconess Medical Center
Boston, Massachusetts

Bruce F. Pennington, Ph.D.
Department of Psychology
University of Denver
Denver, Colorado

Michael Posner, Ph.D.
Professor, Department of Psychology
Institute of Cognitive and Decision Sciences
University of Oregon Institute of Neuroscience
Eugene, Oregon

Cathy J. Price
Wellcome Department of Imaging Neuroscience
Institute of Neurology
University College London
London, England

Elliott D. Ross, M.D.
VA Medical Center
Oklahoma City, Oklahoma

Leslie J. Gonzalez Rothi, Ph.D.
Professor, Departments of Neurology, Clinical and Health
Psychology and Communicative Processes and Disorders
Program Director, VA Brain Rehabilitation Research Center
University of Florida
Gainesville, Florida

Eleanor M. Saffran, Ph.D.*
Department of Communication Sciences
Weiss Hall
Temple University
Philadelphia, Pennsylvania

Myrna F. Schwartz, Ph.D.
Moss Rehabilitation Research Institute
Philadelphia, Pennsylvania

Anne Spence, Ph.D.
Department of Human Genetics and Birth Defects
University of California, Irvine
Irvine, California

James Swanson, Ph.D.
Professor of Pediatrics
Executive Director, Child Development Center
University of California, Irvine
Irvine, California

Edward Valenstein, M.D.
Chair, Department of Neurology
The William L. and Janice M. Neely
    Professor of Neurology and Clinical and Health Psychology
University of Florida
Gainesville, Florida

Mieke Verfaellie, Ph.D.
Associate Professor
Department of Psychiatry and Psychology
Boston University School of Medicine
Boston, Massachusetts

Kytja K.S. Voeller, M.D.
Research Neurologist
Greenwood Genetics Center
JC Self Research Center
Center for Molecular Studies
Greenwood, South Carolina

Robert T. Watson, M.D.
Jules B. Chapman Professor in Clinical Care and Humaneness
Professor of Neurology and Clinical and Health Psychology
Senior Associate Dean for Educational Affairs
Vice-Chair, Department of Neurology
University of Florida
Gainesville, Florida

*Deceased

INDEX